EMERGENCY NURSING

PRINCIPLES AND PRACTICE

EMERGENCY NURSING

PRINCIPLES AND PRACTICE

SUSAN A. BUDASSI, RN, MSN, MICN, CEN

Clinical Specialist, Department of Emergency Medicine,
Brotman Medical Center, Culver City, California;
Assistant Professor of Clinical Nursing,
University of California, Los Angeles, California

JANET M. BARBER, RN, MS

Captain, USAF, Wilford Hall, USAF Medical Center (AFSC),
Lackland Air Force Base, Texas

with **418** illustrations

The C. V. Mosby Company

ST. LOUIS • TORONTO • LONDON   1981

The opinions or assertions in this book are the views of the
authors and are not to be construed as official or as
reflecting the views of the Department of the Air Force
or the Department of Defense.

The C. V. Mosby Company
11830 Westline Industrial Drive, St. Louis, Missouri 63141

Library of Congress Cataloging in Publication Data

Budassi, Susan A   1948-
   Emergency nursing.

   Bibliography: p.
   Includes index.
   1.   Emergency nursing.   I.   Barber, Janet Miller,
joint author.   II.   Title.
RT120.E4B82   610.73′6   80-21629
ISBN 0-8016-0451-6

GW/VH/VH 9 8 7 6 5 4 3 2 1   03/A/347

Contributors

SUSAN C. AUGUST, RN, BS, CEN

Head Nurse, Emergency Department, Brotman
Medical Center, Culver City, California

PETER A. DILLMAN, REMT-P, MS

Director of Education and Medical Quality
Assurance, Wishard Memorial Hospital,
Ambulance Service, Indianapolis, Indiana

REBECCA HATHAWAY, RN, MS

Assistant Director, Nursing, Critical Care
Division, UCLA Center for the Health Sciences,
and Assistant Clinical Professor of Nursing,
UCLA School of Nursing, Los Angeles, California

BARBARA WELDON KING, RN

Assistant Director, Department of Emergency
Medicine, Brotman Medical Center, Culver City,
California; Director of Clinical Support Staff,
Janzen, Johnston, and Rockwell, a Medical
Corporation, Santa Monica, California

ROBERT KOTLER, MD

Private Practice, Otorhinolaryngology,
Los Angeles, California

PEGGY McCALL, RN, BSN

Director of Emergency Center and Life Flight
Nursing, Hermann Hospital, Houston, Texas

CHARLES R. McELROY, MD

Director, Emergency Medicine Center, UCLA
Center for the Health Sciences, and Associate
Professor of Medicine, UCLA School of Medicine,
Los Angeles, California

MARGARET MILLER, RN, MSEd

Associate Professor, School of Nursing,
Creighton University, Omaha, Nebraska

GAIL PISARCIK, RN, MSN

Clinical Specialist, Psychiatric Nursing,
Emergency Department, Massachusetts General
Hospital, Boston, Massachusetts

MICHAEL L. RAINS, JD

Private Practice, Santa Monica, California

**JOAN KELLEY SIMONEAU, RN,
MICN, CCRN**

Director of Education, Prime Care Corporation,
Marina del Rey, California

NANCY SMITH

Assistant to Robert Kotler, MD,
Los Angeles, California

PEGGY STOKER, RN, MICN

Director of Education, Los Angeles County
Paramedic Training Institute,
Torrance, California

PATRICIA VARVEL, RN, BSN

Nursing Supervisor, Obstetrics and Gynecology,
St. Luke's Episcopal Hospital and Texas
Children's Hospital, Houston, Texas

Preface

Emergency care is at last a defined nursing specialty deserving its own comprehensive textbook. *Emergency Nursing: Principles and Practice* was specifically planned and written to meet this need.

The content has been selected and organized to provide a logical presentation of subjects germane to the emergency nurse. Initially, the reader is introduced to the role of the nurse within the contemporary emergency medical services (EMS) arena. Concepts and procedural aspects of basic triage, physical assessment, and life support are addressed, followed by in-depth chapters devoted to emergency considerations according to major problems and/or body systems. Emphasis has been placed on initial recognition of life-threatening circumstances and related intervention skills. A generous amount of psychosocial and behavioral content has been integrated throughout the book, and specific chapters have been provided to address psychiatric emergencies and crisis intervention strategies. Emergency department management, legal implications of emergency care, and prehospital care are thoroughly considered, too. Illustrations have been supplied in abundance to amplify important technical details of emergency department procedures.

Emergency Nursing: Principles and Practice may be used as a reference book, a comprehensive textbook, and a source book on emergency nursing. This book meets the basic and advanced needs of the emergency nurse by providing a single comprehensive source in which to find information. It can be used by nursing students wishing to increase their understanding of emergency nursing and by practicing nurses wishing to gain new information or validate information. This book was written primarily by nurses for nurses. It is our hope that it will be a valuable tool for our emergency nursing colleagues.

Susan A. Budassi
Janet M. Barber

Acknowledgments

Many thanks are extended to Cindy Allen for her assistance in obtaining the x-ray films for Chapter 19, Limb Trauma, and to Rick Lazar for the very creative photos found throughout the book.

Special thoughts and thanks are extended to the entire Brotman Medical Center Emergency Department staff for all their caring, enthusiasm, and desire to learn—especially to Barbara King, my dear friend and colleague, for all her special efforts on my behalf. Thanks also to the Los Angeles County Paramedics, who have made my career as challenging and exciting as it could possibly be.

Last, but not least, my thanks to Karen Hoxeng, Susan August, Gail Pisarcik, Gar and Nina LaSalle, Tom Hamilton, Joe Steglein, Al Downing, and Don Nowaski for listening, sharing, caring, and being my best friends, and to TK for teaching me "how to climb mountains."

SAB

As I recount the months I spent in researching and writing this book, I am painfully reminded that my contribution was essentially a solitary effort. My family, loved ones, and associates tolerated my endeavor, however, and understood—at least in part—my commitment to completing the project. I would be remiss, though, if I did not express appreciation to my students and the practicing emergency nurses, who have favorably responded to my teaching and my writing. It is this return that continues to motivate me.

I do want to thank Mary Woods for typing the manuscript, and for managing my book-related mail and phone calls. In addition to being a superior administrative secretary, Mary is a beautiful human being, who deserves a far greater accolade than this mere acknowledgment.

JMB

Contents

PART ONE

Principles of emergency nursing

Unit I □ Introduction to emergency nursing

1   An overview of emergency nursing, 3

2   Prehospital care, 11
Peggy Stoker

3   Communication in crisis, 21
Susan C. August

4   Legal considerations in the emergency department, 35
Michael L. Rains

5   Emergency department management, 51
Barbara Weldon King

Unit II □ Basic concepts of emergency nursing

6   Triage, 90

7   Patient assessment, 96
Joan Kelley Simoneau

8   Basic and advanced life support, 132

9   Laboratory specimens and intravenous fluid therapy, 196

10   Patient teaching in the emergency department, 214
Margaret Miller

11   Wound management, 228

12   Shock management, 237
Rebecca Hathaway and Janet M. Barber

PART TWO

Practice of emergency nursing

Unit III □ Medical and surgical emergencies

13   Multiple trauma, 263

14   Neurological emergencies, 270

15   Eye, ear, nose, throat, maxillofacial, and dental emergencies, 318
Susan A. Budassi, Robert Kotler, and Nancy Smith

16   Chest trauma, 349

17   Chest pain and respiratory emergencies, 365

18   Abdominal emergencies, 399

19   Limb trauma, 419

20   Genitourinary emergencies, 463

21   Obstetrical and gynecological emergencies, 473
Peggy McCall and Patricia Varvel

22   Pediatric emergencies, 494

23   Psychiatric emergencies, 516
Gail Pisarcik

24   Metabolic emergencies, 550

Unit IV □ Environmental emergencies

25   Outdoor emergencies, 567
Peter A. Dillman and Janet M. Barber

26   Burns, 599

27   Poisons and toxicology, 617

28 Disaster aspects in emergency
nursing, 641
Joan Kelley Simoneau

Appendices

A Joint Commission on Accreditation of
Hospitals requirements for emergency
services, 683

B Normal laboratory values, 692

C Conversions and equivalencies, 705

D Aftercare suggestions, 706

E Incubation periods, 711

F Major drug categories, 713

G Sample performance review, 739

PART ONE

PRINCIPLES OF EMERGENCY NURSING

Unit I ☐ **Introduction to emergency nursing**

Unit II ☐ **Basic concepts of emergency nursing**

CHAPTER 1

An overview of emergency nursing

THE NATURE OF EMERGENCY NURSING

Emergency nurses have a unique opportunity to combine their interests in every subspecialty of nursing into one, because the emergency care arena encompasses medicine, surgery, maternal-child nursing, psychiatry, and community health. Knowledge and skills, however, are well beyond those required of a generalist, who has a somewhat superficial base in each. The emergency nurse must be technically competent to perform physical assessments, hemodynamic monitoring, and cardiopulmonary resuscitation, and must possess the knowledge base to perform triage, collect meaningful data in a history, provide discharge or referral instructions, and anticipate the course of care for given medical and traumatic cases. Other day-to-day responsibilities relate to dealing with the emotionally disturbed, the grieving, the bewildered, and the unconscious. Task-oriented duties such as initiating an IV infusion, drawing arterial blood gases, recording a 12-lead ECG, assisting the physician with chest tube placement or peritoneal lavage, answering a Poison Control phone call, and directing field paramedics on a radio are among the other things emergency nurses do daily. They have, by nature of the setting and their role, the task of relating regularly to the general public and thus must always be cognizant of their human relations skills and the legal concerns of practice.

Emergency nurses interact with individuals of all ages, socioeconomic circumstances, cul-

tures, and religions. They must be sensitive to the special needs of individuals and their lifestyles, because such factors are often significant in health care problem solving.

Management skills and leadership functions are also inherent in the role of the emergency nurse, whether managing one shock room trauma team or an entire department. The unplanned, the unscheduled, and the unpredictable are everyday concerns for nurses in this setting.

Emergency nursing is a specialty, that has essentially been developed over the past two decades as part of a nationwide system of emergency medical service (EMS). Although one commonly associates this nurse with practice in an emergency department of a hospital, the settings may realistically include schools, clinics, industry, mobile intensive care units, and public gatherings. Emergency nursing is characterized by brevity of patient interaction, the stressful climate created by lack of control over the numbers of individuals seeking care, and the limited time frame in which to evaluate the effectiveness of intervention.

The American Nurses' Association's Division on Medical-Surgical Nursing Practice and the Emergency Department Nurses Association (EDNA) have developed standards of emergency nursing practice, which define the practice area and outline the scope of nursing activities.

Emergency nursing includes the care of individuals of all ages with perceived physical

3

or emotional alterations that are undiagnosed and may require prompt intervention. The care is unscheduled, and thus is episodic, primary, and acute.

The scope of practice of the emergency nurse encompasses activities that are directed toward health problems of various levels of complexity. Rapidly changing physiological or psychological status may be life-threatening, and it requires assessment, intervention, ongoing reassessment, and supportive care to significant others. Life support, health education, and referral are among the several roles and responsibilities.

Few nurses graduating from undergraduate programs are specifically prepared with the necessary content and skills, since today's typical curricula do not address emergency care. The education and training of this clinician are therefore relegated to on-the-job training. This is of concern when one considers that they will promptly be confronted with undiagnosed physical and emotional crises that demand prompt, skillful intervention.

Graduates of nursing education programs who choose to practice in small urban or rural areas are likely to find themselves in situations that demand a considerable degree of competency and specific preparation to function independently. Often they are called upon to provide initial life-support care, to clinically stabilize a patient before a long journey to another hospital, and to care for and monitor individuals who are critically ill while awaiting the arrival of an "on-call" physician. A well-educated emergency nurse who can deliver expert emergency care can help prevent the type of tragic circumstances that otherwise lead to increased morbidity and mortality.

There is a systematic effort by the EDNA and other special interest groups to enhance the practice of emergency care through educational endeavors of several sorts, including teaching institutes, seminars, standard curricula, self-study guides, the *Journal of Emergency Nursing,* and interdisciplinary involvement in EMS. A competency-based certification examination recognizing excellence in the practice of emergency nursing is now under development by the EDNA in close cooperation with the American Nurses' Association's other credentialling endeavors.

EMERGENCY NURSE PRACTITIONER

The federal and private foundation grants supporting nurse practitioner programs have created and sustained nearly 150 expanded role programs that offer certificates or advanced degrees. Certificate programs last from 16 to 68 weeks, whereas master's degree programs last from 44 to 72 weeks. These programs are designed to prepare the advanced nurse practitioner. Only six are designated for the "emergency nurse practitioner," however. The curriculum provides a balance of content on examining and treating the nonacute patient and caring for the critically ill or traumatized patient.

Emergency personnel of all types (physicians, nurses, paramedics, emergency medical technicians [EMTs]) must have a strong base in critical care theory and practice in order to effectively deal with the dynamic changes in field and in-hospital management of medical emergencies and trauma.

An inherent characteristic of EMS is the integrated nature of the emergency team. The quality of prehospital care of field paramedics depends on the physician or nurse direction from the base hospital's emergency department. In-hospital care is greatly influenced by the field team's efforts during initial stabilization and transfer and their ongoing communications.

The body of knowledge related to emergency and trauma is by nature multidisciplinary because of prehospital and hospital components. The combined efforts of field personnel and nurses and physicians are crucial to ensure optimum care for the ill and injured. These practitioners must work harmoniously, complementing and supplementing each other's roles, in order to accomplish the efficient, effective delivery of emergency services.

HISTORY OF THE EMS MOVEMENT

In the last decade or two, emergency care has come into its own. In the 1950s and 1960s it was common practice for funeral homes to provide ambulance service and for emergency rooms of the local hospital to be sparsely equipped and poorly staffed. Police, fire departments, and first-aiders provided the only prehospital care.

As emergency care needs became more apparent, agencies and organizations on several levels stepped in to engineer a plan to prevent prehospital death from illness and injury. The first efforts related to the establishment of the mobile intensive coronary care unit to prevent death from sudden-onset cardiac problems. The expansion and further diversity of these units' functioning formed the basis for today's exceedingly popular paramedic ambulances, which are equipped for the management of trauma and major medical emergencies. The 1966 National Highway Safety Act authorized the Department of Transportation (DOT) to establish EMS guidelines; under this law, funds were allocated for the purchase of ambulances, the installation of communications networks, and the development of EMT training programs as a part of statewide EMS plans. The proliferating 81-hour EMT training program soon became the minimum standard for prehospital caregivers. Other training programs, an advanced EMT II and an EMT-paramedic, were further efforts to upgrade the sophistication of prehospital care.

In June 1970, a National Registry of Emergency Medical Technicians was organized to unify educational requirements, examinations, and certification requirements of EMTs on a national level. Both EMTs and paramedics have specific requirements for continuing education in most states in order to ensure competency for recertification. The National Association of Emergency Medical Technicians (NAEMT) has been organized to meet the special needs of EMTs.

The Emergency Medical Services Systems Act of 1973 was designed to stimulate self-help regionalization of EMS programs in integrating the following 15 elements into a system.

1. Manpower
2. Training
3. Communications
4. Transportaiton
5. Facilities/categorization
6. Critical care units
7. Public safety agencies
8. Consumer participation
9. Accessibility to care
10. Transfer of patients
11. Standardized patient record keeping
12. Public information and education
13. Independent review and evaluation
14. Disaster linkages
15. Mutual aid agreements

The Division of Emergency Medical Services in the U.S. Department of Health, Education, and Welfare (HEW) has divided the country into approximately 300 EMS regions. States are rapidly demonstrating their own interest in maintaining and improving their system through funding, personnel licensing and certification, and facilities planning.

The 911 emergency telephone number is the result of concerted efforts to improve access to EMS by the consumer. Most emergency services—fire, police, and medical—are served by this universal service operating in hundreds of areas throughout the United States.

Concurrent with the growth of EMS has been a steady increase in the numbers of physicians, nurses, and other specialists whose prime concern is delivery of emergency care.

EMS MANPOWER

The manpower needs in the EMS system must include a cadre of first responders in the community who can establish contact with the system and meanwhile provide basic life support. Policemen, firemen, and citizens may fall within this group. The 911 emergency number or some other community-accepted number is then relayed by trained EMS dispatchers and communicators who triage the call, dispatch personnel and equipment, and provide instruction to first responders about what they should do until help arrives (Fig. 1-1). Those responding may be EMTs, EMT-paramedics, and even nurses, respiratory therapists, or physicians, depending on the type of call and the community-accepted protocol. For example, aboard specialized units, such as helicopters or neonatal mobile intensive care units, it is typical that respiratory therapists, transport nurses, and physicians accompany the victim, particularly if the distance from the scene to the target treatment facility is significant. In certain rural areas of the United States where terrain and

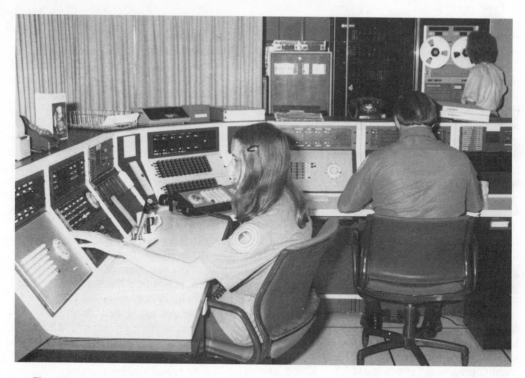

Fig. 1-1. Modern communications center. (Photo courtesy of Wishard Memorial Hospital's Ambulance Service, Indianapolis, Ind.)

weather conditions may present unusual problems, other rescue workers may join the medical team to ensure safety and efficiency in the transport. The MAST program (Military Assistance to Safety and Traffic), which links the Department of Defense and the other federal units (HEW and DOT), provides helicopters, fixed-wing aircraft, and military paramedical personnel to aid civilians in coping with on-the-scene and transport endeavors. Unfortunately this program serves only 20 to 30 sites throughout the United States at the present time.

EMERGENCY MEDICINE RESIDENCY TRAINING

The first postgraduate program in emergency medicine began in July 1970 at the University of Cincinnati Medical Center. During the ensuing years, 43 programs have been initiated

to train specialists in emergency medicine. The American College of Emergency Physicians has been working diligently for formal recognition of emergency medicine as a specialty, and in late 1979 was finally approved for this status by the American Board of Medical Specialists.

THE HOSPITAL EMERGENCY DEPARTMENT

Emergency departments provide care to 50 million people in the United States each year. Emergency departments serve as a trauma center, a convenience clinic on a 24-hour basis, and a physician's office, especially for the urban poor.

Emergency department visits totaled 85 million in 1979, a rapid acceleration of activity throughout the past decade. The use of the

Table 1-1. Classification of emergency facilities*

	Primary or comprehensive (PEF)	Auxiliary	First aid	No facilities (referral only)
MD				
In ER 24 hours	✔			
On call for ER 24 hours		✔		
None on call			✔	✔
RN				
In ER 24 hours	✔	✔		
On call for ER 24 hours			✔	✔
Specialty panel				
Yes	✔			
No		✔	✔	✔
Hospital radio net				
Yes	✔	✔		
No			✔	✔
Minimum 4-bed ER				
Yes	✔			
No		✔	✔	✔
CPR supplies defibrillator and monitor in ER				
Yes	✔	✔		
No			✔	✔
Laboratory technician 24 hours				
Yes	✔	✔		
No			✔	✔
Blood bank				
Yes	✔	✔		
No			✔	✔
X-ray technician available in 15 minutes				
Yes	✔	✔		
No			✔	✔
OR available 24 hours				
Yes	✔	✔		
No			✔	✔
Anesthesia available in 30 minutes				
Yes	✔			
No		✔	✔	✔
Intensive care unit				
Yes	✔			
No		✔	✔	✔
Disaster plan				
Yes	✔	✔	✔	✔
No				
Medical audit				
Yes	✔	✔	✔	✔
No				
JCAH accreditation ER under hospital's utilization committee of staff				
Yes	✔	✔	✔	
No				

*From Warner, C. G.: Emergency care: assessment and intervention, ed. 2, St. Louis, 1978, The C. V. Mosby Co.

emergency department has been growing steadily because of a lack (or inaccessibility) of primary care. Individuals who have low income or do not have a family physician must use the emergency department as their source of care in episodic illness. Few primary care physicians have office hours in the evenings or on the weekends, which forces their patients into another arena for care. One additional factor of importance relates to health insurance plans that favor paying emergency department charges over those of a regular office visit to a physician. It is also convenient for some individuals who prefer an unplanned or unscheduled approach to their health care delivery. (No appointments or reservations are ever required!) Some writers on the subject claim that emergency departments should not be labeled "emergency" departments but unscheduled or "unpredictable" medicine clinics.

The fact that emergency departments are available at all times to the public for health care has created an expectation of an open system of service.

Today's hospital emergency department is considerably more sophisticated in its management of medical and trauma cases than the emergency "rooms" of three or four decades ago. Statewide programs of facility categorization have ensured that the services available in any emergency department represent the highest quality for the intentions of the unit and that the health care industry make good use of the various types of unique capabilities. Criteria for categorization reference physical facilities, specialized equipment, medical subspecialists, types of services (for example, dialysis and computerized axial tomography), number and types of personnel, including their training in emergency care. The availability of key personnel according to full-time, part-time, and on-call status is also noted.

The outcome of categorization is a clear indication of the capabilities of facilities, so that all involved in the EMS will be able to more effectively utilize the services for limited emergencies, major emergencies, specialized trauma, and so on. States have each adopted unique schemes for grouping hospital emergency facilities into three to six categories (Table 1-1).

REGIONALIZATION

A systems approach to EMS is crucial in order to provide a high quality service with some consistency of the availability of services to persons, regardless of their place of residence. Furthermore, regionalization should help eliminate the costly duplication of critical clinical services such as centers for the high-risk neonate, and patients with severe burns, multiple traumas, or spinal cord injuries.

To utilize these facilities appropriately requires that candidates be identified using distinct criteria and that transfer to the specialized center be accomplished at the right time after stabilization of the victim.

Elaborate systems of ambulance and air transport have been developed that reflect special concern for the geographical location, terrain, and weather conditions inherent in the area. Communications, including telemetry, have become increasingly important in providing field direction for the prehospital team. Poison control networks have also proliferated in an effort to improve the early care of toxicological crises (Fig. 1-2). The interface of these innovations of physical resources with a sophisticated group of new specialists in emergency centers has brought credibility at last to the delivery of emergency care.

In some states there is a highly complex system of "base station" hospitals that are located strategically and serve as resources for field personnel, such as paramedics. Base station personnel communicate with the prehospital team on the scene and en route to a treatment facility, providing medical orders and supervision as required. Base station hospitals must be acute care facilities that have radio and telemetry equipment and specially trained physicians or nurses to communicate with field paramedics. California has specifically designated and trained nurses certified to issue emergency instructions to paramedics. This mobile intensive care nurse (MICN) operates within protocols established for the hospital and involves the physician in calls that require more than routine management.

The amount and type of independence exercised by field paramedics are determined by state legislation and local guidelines.

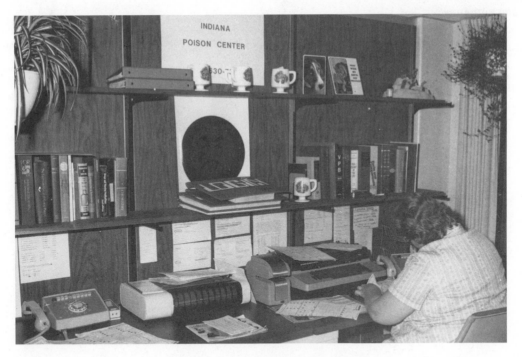

Fig. 1-2. Poison control center (Photo courtesy Wishard Memorial Hospital's Ambulance Service, Indianapolis, Ind.)

PHYSICAL FACILITIES IN THE EMERGENCY DEPARTMENT

The modern, well-equipped emergency department combines a clinic flow system with surgical suites and an intensive care area. Ordinarily, the design provides for an ambulance or vehicular entrance and a walk-in lobby.

A triage nurse functions at the intake point to make initial assessments regarding the individual's priority needs for care and directs them accordingly (see Chapter 6). Registration clerks and cashiers are usually available in the area to manage certain business functions and maintain records.

The treatment zones are usually subdivided into major shock rooms (often with full surgical as well as resuscitation capabilities), minor surgery rooms (wound cleanup, suturing, debridement), and medical examination and treatment rooms. Some larger emergency departments have an observation unit, isolation rooms, decontamination facilities, cast rooms, ophthalmological and ENT procedures room, obstetric and gynecological areas, and other specialized physical facilities. Small x-ray and laboratory units may also be a part of the overall department. Social services, pastoral counseling, and a quiet room for families of victims are available in some hospitals to meet psychological needs of the individuals served. Official city or county hospitals may have additional space to accommodate those who are being held by police for various reasons. Regardless of the design, the emergency department must be available 24 hours per day and staffed to deal with one or many victims of illness or injury who require resuscitation, stabilization, or routine management before transfer or discharge. (See Appendix A for JCAH Standards of Emergency Services.)

BIBLIOGRAPHY

American Nurses' Association: Standards of emergency nursing practice, Kansas City, Mo., 1975, ANA.

Cowley, R. A.: The resuscitation and stabilization of major multiple trauma patients in a trauma center environment, Clin. Med. **83:**14, 1976.

Geolot, D., Alongi, S., and Edlich, R. F.: Emergency nurse practitioner: an answer to an emergency care crisis in rural hospitals, J.A.C.E.P., **6**(8):355-357, 1977.

Gibson, C.: Emergency medical services: a facet of ambulatory care, Hospitals **47:**49, 1973.

Rockwood, C. A., Jr., and others: History of emergency medical services in the United States, J. Trauma **16**(4): 299-308, 1976.

CHAPTER 2

Prehospital care

Peggy Stoker

Paramedics have been dispatched to a private residence to a patient complaining of "chest pain." Within 4 minutes of the alarm, the paramedics arrive carrying a drug box, oxygen equipment, a portable radio, and a portable defibrillator. They find a 48-year-old male patient complaining of severe substernal chest pain that radiates to his jaw. One paramedic immediately applies oxygen, obtains vital signs, and applies ECG electrodes, while the second sets up radio communication with a nearby hospital and obtains a brief patient history. Before 2 minutes have elapsed, the "radio man" is prepared to communicate with the hospital.

A nurse in a busy emergency department is just completing her notes on a previous patient when a buzzer and flashing light over a door marked "Base Station" signal that paramedics need assistance with an emergency. Her response is immediate. Within 10 seconds, the radio console is prepared to receive voice communication and ECG transmission. The nurse is ready to provide the written documentation of the incident and to direct the care of the patient at the scene of the incident. The nurse's name tag identifies her as a "Mobile Intensive Care Nurse."

PARAMEDIC: Squad 1 to Metro Hospital. How do you copy?

MOBILE INTENSIVE CARE NURSE (MICN): Metro hospital to Squad 1. We copy loud and clear. Go ahead. Over.

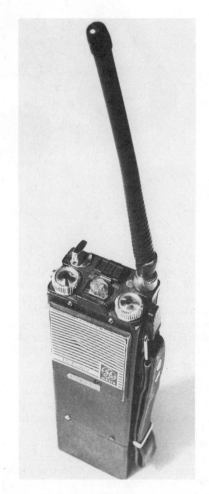

Fig. 2-1. Field radio. (Photo by Richard Lazar.)

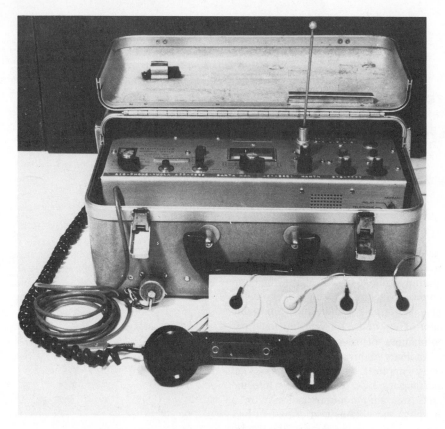

Fig. 2-2. Biocommunications radio. (Photo by Richard Lazar.)

PARAMEDIC: Squad 1 to Metro Hospital. We are at the home of an alert and oriented 48-year-old man complaining of severe crushing substernal chest pain radiating to the jaw of 1 hour duration. His skin is cool and diaphoretic. He has no history of cardiac or respiratory problems. He takes no medications. Vital signs are BP 120/70, P 88, R 18. Lungs are clear bilaterally.

MICN: Metro Hospital to Squad 1. 10-4. Start patient on O₂ at 6 L/minute per nasal cannula. Start an IV of D/5/W TKO. Administer morphine sulfate 4 mg/slow IV push and transmit a 5-second ECG rhythm strip. Over.

PARAMEDIC: Squad 1 to Metro Hospital. 10-4. Patient is on O₂ at 6 L/minute per nasal cannula. Orders are to start an IV of D/5/W TKO and administer 4 mg morphine sulfate slow IV push. ECG to follow. Over.

MICN: Metro Hospital to Squad 1. 10-4. Over.

The nurse flips the switch marked "ECG" on the communication equipment. The high-pitched whining sound of the telemetry coincides with the waves shown on the ECG strip. The nurse carefully studies the strip and recognizes that the patient is in a normal sinus rhythm with an occasional premature ventricular contraction.

MICN: Metro Hospital to Squad 1. We copy an NSR with occasional PVCs. Administer lidocaine 75 mg IV push, followed by a second bolus of 75 mg in 5 minutes. Over.

PARAMEDIC: Squad 1 to Metro Hospital. 10-4. The IV has been established and morphine sulfate administered. We will administer lidocaine 75 mg IV push followed by a second bolus of 75 mg in 5 minutes. Over.

MICN: Metro Hospital to Squad 1. 10-4. Give us an update on the patient status. Is he still having chest pain. Also, what is your destination and estimated time of arrival? Over.

PARAMEDIC: Squad 1 to Metro Hospital. 10-4. Patient states that his chest pain is almost gone. His BP is 120/70, P 80, R 16. His skin is cool and pale, but no longer diaphoretic. We are prepared to transport to Southside Hospital. Estimated time of arrival is approximately 5 minutes. Over.

MICN: Metro Hospital to Squad 1. 10-4. We will notify the Southside Hospital. Recontact enroute if there is any change in the patient's condition. Over.

PARAMEDIC: Squad 1 to Metro Hospital. 10-4. Over.

Over the last decade, the preceding scene has become commonplace in some rural as well as numerous metropolitan areas throughout the nation. And despite much initial controversy, the nurse's role in mobile intensive care (MIC) is now indisputable. The mobile intensive care nurse (MICN) is a vital member of the prehospital care team.

Who is this unique addition to the nursing community—the MICN? What special qualifications and what kind of training are required? More basic questions are: What is prehospital care? and What are the components of this emergency medical services system? These are a few of the basic prehospital care questions to be answered in the following pages. This chapter is designed primarily for the novice in this field as an introduction to prehospital care and the role of the MICN. In addition, prospective as well as functioning MICNs will find information contained in this section pertinent to their needs also. Prehospital care topics to be discussed include the history of prehospital care, system components and personnel, the role of the mobile intensive care nurse, and mobile intensive care assessment and treatment considerations.

HISTORY OF PREHOSPITAL CARE

Prehospital care is defined as the delivery of emergency care to the sick and injured at the scene of an emergency and during transport to an emergency facility.

The concept has grown rapidly over the last two decades and now is considered a true critical care specialty. MIC, as it is most often referred to, requires specially trained personnel, the MICN, the emergency department physician, and in particular, one of the newest additions to the health care team—the MIC paramedic. While at the scene of an emergency, the paramedic's major responsibility is to assess the patient, communicate the findings, and receive orders from an MIC nurse or physician at a remote hospital. As a result, the paramedic may be able to stabilize or to provide definitive emergency care for the patient before and during transport to the appropriate emergency facility. The paramedic functions as an extension of the acute care hospital's emergency department. He is the next best thing to having a physician at the scene of every emergency, whether it be at home, on the street, or at some remote location.

The prehospital care concept is not totally new. Prehospital care has roots, primarily in military medicine, that extend back decades. However, it was not until numerous outstanding developments in cardiac care, made primarily by Day in the early 1960s, that a definitive impetus to develop prehospital care systems capable of providing definitive therapy for specific cardiac disorders began. At that time (as today) coronary artery disease was the number one killer in the United States and in numerous other industrialized nations. Despite strides in patient monitoring technology and treatment modalities, two thirds of all patients dying from myocardial infraction were dying from potentially reversible ventricular fibrillation before reaching the hospital. The need for prehospital intervention was imperative. As a result of these statistics, it is not surprising that the individuals responsible for establishing most of the original prehospital care systems focused their attention primarily on the coronary care patient. In fact, these first prehospital care vehicles have generally been referred to as mobile coronary care ambulances or units. Pioneers in this area include Pantridge in Belfast, Ireland; Lorenz in Toulouse, France; and others in Moscow, Russia. In each of these systems, the mobile coronary unit was staffed by a physician and at least one assistant and was equipped similarly to an in-hospital coronary care unit.

In the mid 1960s, such individuals as Grace in New York, Warren in Ohio, and Nagel in Miami began experimenting with the prehospital care concept in the United States. However, the first real innovations in prehospital care did not take place until the late 1960s. In 1968, Nagel developed a system in Dade County, Florida, utilizing specially trained paramedical personnel under the direction of hospital-based physicians. The use of telemetry for prehospital care was born. For the first time it appeared that mobile coronary care could be provided for a vast population, at a relatively low cost, utilizing currently existing fire, police, ambulance, or other rescue personnel. The implications for the future development of prehospital care throughout the country were enormous.

Since 1968, the prehospital care system in the United States has grown at a phenomenal rate. Along with the growth, numerous changes and improvements have taken place. In fact, the concept of a prehospital care system designed primarily for the cardiac patient is a thing of the past. As more and more information becomes available, it is apparent that prehospital intervention can significantly reduce mortality and morbidity in a variety of noncardiac illnesses and injuries. For example, most trauma experts indicate that approximately 5% of the 150,000 persons who die from trauma each year in the United States could be saved with appropriate prehospital care. Mobile units are now utilized to provide prehospital care for all manner of illnesses and injuries. As a result, the units are no longer mobile coronary units, but instead are referred to as mobile intensive care units (MICU).

Today, in almost all prehospital care systems in the United States, paramedical personnel rather than physicians are used to staff the units. In most systems, the MIC paramedics receive direction by means of radio communications or telemetry with a hospital-based physician or the specially trained MICN.

Currently the largest and one of the oldest prehospital care systems in the United States is in Los Angeles. Developed by Criley and Lewis in 1969, the system currently serves approximately 7 million persons, covers approximately 4,083 square miles, and employs over 1,300 paramedics. Popularized on television, the Los Angeles system has served as the model for numerous systems throughout the United States. Although extremely complex, the components of the Los Angeles system are similar to those of almost all prehospital care systems in the country.

SYSTEM COMPONENTS AND PERSONNEL

Regardless of the size or complexity of a prehospital care system, there are several basic system components that are essential. These include:

1. The MICU vehicle, which is fully equipped to provide patient stabilization in the field.
2. The MIC paramedic, whose emergency medical care training prepares him to provide patient stabilization and, in a few specific instances, definitive patient care.
3. The base hospital and base hospital personnel, who direct prehospital emergency medical care by means of voice communications.
4. The biomedical communications system.

Mobile intensive care unit

The mobile intensive care unit (MICU) refers to the vehicle and personnel required to provide MIC. In almost all communities, the MICU designation is approved only for those units meeting strict criteria regarding vehicle standards, staffing, and equipment.

The MIC vehicle is most often an ambulance, capable of transporting at least two paramedics, two patients, and the driver. The type of ambulance is by no means standard, and may be either a specially equipped van, utility-type or carry-all vehicle, or station wagon.

Although most systems appear to favor ambulances, many other types of vehicles have functioned very successfully as MICUs. These units possess all MICU capabilities, but are not equipped to transport patients. Most often these are rescue trucks or fire engines. In systems utilizing these nontransport vehicles, patients are transported in the conventional ambulances with the MICU personnel in attendance.

Most prehospital care systems require that MICUs be staffed by at least two MIC paramedics 24 hours a day. Although a few systems do function with one MIC paramedic and one Emergency Medical Technician I (EMT-I), the difficulty of adequately handling the critically ill patient or patient in a full cardiopulmonary arrest without at least two MIC paramedics is apparent.

Readily available backup personnel are a necessity in all prehospital care systems. Most frequently, fire department or police personnel, usually with EMT-I–level training, provide this backup. Recognizing the frequent need for more than two persons at the scene of emergencies, many communities automatically dispatch backup personnel to all rescues.

MICU inventory must include the standard complement of EMT-I ambulance equipment: litter, extrication tools, portable suction unit, protable oxygen equipment, bandages, dressings, splints, and backboards. In addition, a variety of advanced life support equipment and medications are necessary.

1. Cardiac telemetry unit for transmitting patient's ECG to the base hospital.
2. Portable, battery-operated monitor/defibrillator.
3. Drug box containing the full complement of approved MIC medications and IV equipment.
4. Laryngoscope, endotracheal (ET) tubes, esophageal airway (EA), and other airway equipment.

Mobile intensive care paramedic

The MIC paramedic is trained to provide emergency medical care to the sick and injured at the scene of an emergency and during transport to a general acute care hospital. In California, as in most states, the training program must be approved by the county health officer or the state. The paramedics, upon successful completion of the training, must pass written and practical and/or oral examinations before becoming certified. In Los Angeles the MIC paramedic training program consists of approximately 960 hours.

The initial 2 months' (320 hours) didactic training consists primarily of lectures, workshops, laboratory sessions, and hospital rounds. The student is also given the opportunity to practice field techniques during weekly patient simulations. The didactic phase is followed by a 1-month (160 hours) inhospital clinical phase in which trainees practice patient assessment and other paramedic skills introduced previously. Following successful completion of the clinical phase, the student is assigned to an MICU with two certified paramedics for field practice and evaluation before certification.

Base hospital

The base hospital is a strategically located general acute care hospital having radio and biomedical communication equipment for the purpose of directing prehospital emergency medical care given by MIC paramedics. When at the scene of a medical emergency, the MIC paramedics contact the base hospital, transmit all vital information, and are given specific patient care orders by the hospital personnel. The base hospital is staffed 24 hours a day by registered nurses and physicians trained in emergency and prehospital care medicine and radio communication techniques.

In many systems, paramedics have base hospital contact before initiating even the most fundamental advanced life support techniques, such as starting an IV, inserting an EOA or ET tube, or administering sodium bicarbonate. Based on this fact, the MIC paramedic functions as an extension of the hospital's emergency department. As long as communication has been established, responsibility for prehospital care rests with the base hospital as well as the MICU personnel. Therefore, base hospitals in most areas of the country monitor the performance of not only their in-hospital professional staff, but the MIC paramedic as well.

In addition, base hospitals provide a formal program of continuing education, both didactic and clinical, for all MIC paramedics.

Biomedical communications system

A reliable communications system is an essential element of prehospital care. The development of such a system involves three aspects.

1. The initial dispatch of the rescue vehicle.
2. Communication with the base hospital for the supervision of patient therapy.
3. The direction of the rescue vehicle to a hospital having appropriate patient care facilities.

The initial dispatch in many systems is accomplished over already existing communications channels (for example, by the fire department dispatcher). A separate communications system then links the paramedic in the field with the MICN at the base hospital.

The essential elements of the paramedic-hospital communications network include the following.

1. The ability to transmit both voice and ECG.
2. The ability to transmit over radio or telephone. Since relatively few radio frequencies are available for this type of communication, it is not unusual for two or more MICUs to be communicating with a base hospital at the same time on the same frequency. The telephone is used whenever feasible in order to avoid this type of radio frequency overcrowding. The telephone is also useful when the radio cannot be used (for example, because of topographic obstacles, radio interference, or equipment failure).
3. In areas where there are multiple base hospitals utilizing different radio frequencies, each MICU should have the capability of selecting more than one channel. Hence, if radio communication cannot be established with the primary base hospital (for instance, because of a topographic obstacle such as a hill or tall building), a second hospital can be contacted.
4. It is essential that the base hospital be

able to interpret ECG transmission in order to direct appropriate therapy, so a "duplexed" system (that permits paramedics to both transmit and receive at the same time) is required.

The concept of "central emergency medical dispatch" is particularly pertinent to large metropolitan areas. It involves the direction of all requests for emergency response to a single center (by the use of the universal emergency telephone number, 911) and the dispatch of the rescue vehicle by that center. In addition, such a facility can maintain a current status report on all hospitals within its area (bed availability in the CCU, and so on). In this way, a critically ill or injured patient is taken to a hospital capable of treating him.

Communications equipment. Every base hospital must have equipment and personnel available to permit two-way voice communication with the MICU 24 hours a day. The two-way communication is accomplished through the base hospital communications console, which contains the ECG demodulator, cassette tape recorder, strip chart recorder, oscilloscope, radio control unit, and telephone. Voice communication can be maintained either by radio or telephone.

Base hospital voice and telemetric communications with the MICU are accomplished quite simply. The paramedics' portable communications unit utilizes a radio transceiver, which is capable of transmitting as well as receiving voice communications. The paramedics' communications unit also contains a modulator, which converts the patient's ECG to an FM tone. The voice and the ECG are transmitted on a predetermined radio frequency to the base hospital. The base hospital's console receives and, for medical-legal reasons, tape records on cassette the voice communication. The ECG transmission passes through the base console's ECG demodulator and is converted back to the ECG recording. The MICN can then use the strip chart recorder to make a permanent visual record of the ECG.

In the event that the radio signal is of poor quality, the ECG radio signal can also be "patched" to the telephone. The telephone "coupler mode" allows a paramedic team to use a common telephone circuit to transmit ECG telemetry and voice to the base hospital.

Communications techniques. In order to utilize any biomedical communication system effectively, MICNs must have a thorough knowledge of basic communication principles.

The extensive use of radio jargon in the prehospital care situation is unnecessary and in many instances can be detrimental to effective communication. However, there are several universally accepted and understood terms that facilitate communication and should be utilized. The most standard of these are listed below.

Term	Meaning
Affirmative	Yes
Clear	All communications are over, that is, "general hospital base clear"
Copy	Receive, for example, "We do not copy your transmission"
Go, go ahead	Proceed with your message
Negative	No
Over	Message completed
Roger	Yes
Say again	Repeat your communication
Stand by	Wait, there will be a delay in communications
10-4	Transmission received

In addition to using the appropriate radio terminology, the MICN should follow several specific communication rules (many mandated by the Federal Communications Commission) when on the radio.

1. Speak slowly and distinctly. Even under the best of conditions, voice communications are seldom received as clearly as one would like.
2. Be concise. Avoid unnecessary verbiage.
3. Ask paramedics to repeat doubtful messages. State, "Say again," or "We do not copy your transmission."
4. Request that paramedics repeat all base hospital orders, especially drug orders.
5. Avoid the use of radio jargon, except that which is approved for prehospital care communication in your area.
6. Identify yourself as well as the MICU

before every transmission. For example, state, "Rescue 51, this is General Hospital."

7. Because courtesy is implied, avoid the use of such terms as "please" and "thank you."
8. Avoid emotion in tone of voice as much as possible.
9. Avoid the use of abbreviations, except those standard abbreviations approved for prehospital communications in your area, such as ETA, ED, CPR, and IV.
10. As required by the Federal Communications Commission, close each call with the base hospital call letters assigned by the Federal Communications Commission.

ROLE OF THE MOBILE INTENSIVE CARE NURSE
Definition

The MICN is defined as a registered nurse who has been certified as qualified to provide emergency care and issue emergency instruction to MIC paramedics. The MICN, although certified by the state or the county, receives authority to provide prehospital care direction from the base hospital physician. Although the physician may not be physically present at the base hospital radio during every call, he must be readily accessible on the premises.

Responsibilities

The MICN's primary responsibility is to direct paramedics in the provision of optimal prehospital care. After evaluating the paramedic's initial patient assessment, the MICN must recognize when additional information is necessary and interpret the information appropriately. For patients for whom prehospital intervention is essential, the nurse must order the approved therapy, evaluate the results of this therapy and order appropriate patient transport. This enormous responsibility requires an extensive knowledge of critical and emergency care nursing, as well as thorough training in the principles of prehospital emergency medicine.

It is the MICN's responsibility to decide when, how, and to which hospital a patient will be transported. In many situations, primarily those dealing with critically ill patients who cannot be stabilized in the field, immediate transport is indicated. In contrast, it is not unusual for a patient in full cardiopulmonary arrest to remain in the field for up to 30 minutes.

How a patient is transported should also be a responsibility of the MICN. "Red lights and siren" (referred to as Code 3 or Code R in many regions) should be reserved only for those patients who cannot be stabilized in the field (for example, the full cardiopulmonary arrest or critical trauma patient). In most other situations, the benefit of arriving in the emergency department a minute or so sooner does not offset the increased possibility of vehicular accidents.

In most situations, the patient should be transported to the most accessible emergency facility equipped, staffed, and prepared to care for the patient. This generally will be the closest emergency facility. Although it is advantageous for the personnel providing emergency care for a patient to have also directed that patient's prehospital care, this alone is seldom justification for bypassing an appropriate emergency facility in favor of the base hospital.

There has been much controversy in recent years regarding the advisability of transporting patients having specific disorders, such as multiple trauma, to predetermined treatment centers. The decision to establish such a center would depend on regional topography, population density, and financial and medical resources.

Just before transport, the MICN should remind the paramedics to recontact the base hospital if the patient's status changes during transport. During transport, a patient's condition may deteriorate rapidly. It is the MICN's responsibility to ensure continued care during transport, which may include stopping the vehicle to stabilize the patient.

The provision of prehospital care is a team effort coordinated by the MICN and MIC physician. Therefore, it is necessary for the MICN to be leader and teacher, as well as prehospital care expert. It is the nurse's responsibility not only to monitor and direct MIC paramedic field activities, but to informally critique field care whenever possible with the paramedics. With this assessment, paramedics are able to improve their skills, and cooperation between base hospital and field personnel is enhanced.

Qualifications for mobile intensive care nurse certification

Although MICN certification requirements vary from region to region, there are several basic prerequisites which most systems agree upon. The candidate:

1. Must be a registered nurse licensed in the state in which MICN status is sought.
2. Must have demonstrated proficiency in extensive critical care and emergency department experience (as specifically outlined by her community).
3. Must be certified by the American Heart Association in the provision of Basic Cardiac Life Support (BCLS) and Advanced Cardiac Life Support (ACLS).
4. Must successfully complete an MICN course that includes training in the structure of the local prehospital care system, role of the MICN, communication techniques, and prehospital emergency care.
5. Must ride with an MICU and observe a minimum number of field responses in order to appreciate the adversity of prehospital patient care delivery and gain an understanding of the prehospital care system and the MIC paramedic's role.
6. Must successfully complete an MICN certification examination process, which should include a written as well as a performance examination.
7. Must successfully complete and internship, during which the candidate directs a minimum number of prehospital care calls under the supervision of an experienced MICN or MIC physician.

Following certification, the MICN must maintain and update her skills through participation in a formal program of continuing education. MICN continuing education should consist of attendance at a minimum number of hours of formal lecture pertaining specifically to prehospital emergency care. In addition, the MICN should be required to participate in formal critiques of numerous prehospital care field responses (usually referred to as tape reviews). The tape review is a vital component of the paramedic's as well as the MICN's continuing education and is an important tool in evaluating the effectiveness of MIC. These regularly scheduled reviews allow the prehospital care team members the opportunity to critique their own performance as well as the performance of others. In addition, the review allows paramedics, MICN's and MIC physicians the opportunity to exchange ideas and opinions on patient care management, thus improving rapport and promoting appropriate communication.

MICN continuing education should also include periodic field experience observing MIC paramedics in the delivery of prehospital care.

As is the case with MICN certification requirements, MICN recertification requirements vary considerably. However, regardless of the community, an MICN recertification program should have the following components. The candidate must:

1. Earn a minimum number of hours of continuing education credit in approved prehospital care lectures and tape reviews and observe a minimum number of prehospital emergency responses.
2. Function continuously as an MICN by directing prehospital care or coordinating related MICN and/or MIC paramedic training activities.
3. Successfully complete a comprehensive testing process that includes a written as well as a performance examination.

PREHOSPITAL CARE ASSESSMENT/ TREATMENT CONSIDERATIONS

The goal of an MIC system is to begin care of the acutely ill or injured patient as soon as possible in order to reduce morbidity and mortality. This philosophy does not include providing definitive care for all or even most patients. Because of a lack of equipment, diagnostic tools, personnel, and facilities, definitive care at the scene of most medical emergencies is impossible. In numerous instances, paramedics must assess and treat their patients under extremely adverse conditions. Patients may be found trapped inside or beneath a vehicle, unconscious in a crowded theater or restaurant, or clinging to the side of a cliff. Fortunately, definitive care in the prehospital setting is unnecessary for most prehospital care emergencies. The emphasis is on stabilization in cases in which definitive care is impossible. In situations in which even stabilization is impossible, rapid transport to the nearest emergency facility equipped to provide definitive therapy is necessary. In other situations, a delay in medical treatment presents no danger to the patient. Therefore, in prehospital care, there are three principles to be considered.

1. Patients who can be stabilized with or without definitive care in the prehospital care setting (such as the myocardial infarction patient) should be stabilized in the field.
2. Patients who cannot be stabilized without definitive in-hospital therapy (for example, the patient with a critical head injury) must be transported *as soon as possible* with attempts at stabilization made en route.
3. The stable patient who has a nonlife-threatening disorder for which treatment either cannot or need not be provided at the scene (for example, a woman in labor with her first pregnancy who shows no signs of imminent delivery) should be transported without attempts at definitive treatment.

With these principles in mind, the patient evaluation will now be addressed.

Patient evaluation

In the prehospital care system the paramedic is the eyes, ears, and hands of the physician. With appropriate training, the paramedic is capable of painting a concise and accurate clinical picture of the patient. But the paramedic's assessment in many situations could be viewed as tremendously incomplete when contrasted with in-hospital techniques. For this reason, it is essential that the MICN recognize the principles of prehospital patient assessment. Simply stated, this practical philosophy dictates: "If the imformation provided by a physical or historical finding will not have an impact on the patient's prehospital care, the information should not be requested." With this in mind, prehospital patient assessment becomes tremendously simplified.

Because of the unique environment, the paramedic's first priority at the scene of any emergency is to remove himself and the patient from any danger. This requires an immediate assessment of the situation and paramedic decision making regarding:

1. The removal of the patient (and the paramedic in some instances) from sources of physical danger, such as fire, falling debris, and electrical wires.
2. The initiation of specific crowd control maneuvers to ensure optimal working conditions.
3. A request for additional assistance, whether police, fire personnel, or additional paramedic units.

Although these initial decisions are usually made before base hospital contact, base hospital personnel may be informed of changes in the situation at the scene of the accident after contact has been made. In these situations, it becomes necessary for the base hospital to intervene and request the appropriate intervention to eliminate hazards at the scene.

After evaluating the environment, the paramedic makes an immediate assessment of the patient, utilizing the ABCs (airway, breathing, and circulation). Although in many instances the ABCs are accomplished at a glance (such as when the patient is alert and talking), base hospital personnel must always request this information if it is not provided initially.

For a more complete review of patient assessment, refer to Chapter 7 and to specific chapters dealing with the chief complaint.

BIBLIOGRAPHY

Baldwin, L., and Pierce, R.: Mobile intensive care: a problem-oriented approach, St. Louis, 1978, The C. V. Mosby Co.

Barber, J., and Budassi, S.: Mosby's manual of emergency care: practice and procedures, St. Louis, 1979, The C. V. Mosby Co.

Caroline, N.: Emergency care in the streets, Boston, 1979, Little, Brown and Co.

Cosgriff, J., and Anderson, D.: The practice of emergency nursing, Philadelphia, 1975, J. B. Lippincott, Co.

Gazzaniga, A., Iseri, L., Baren, M.: Emergency care: principles and practices for EMT paramedic, Reston, Va., 1979, Reston Publishing Co.

Stephenson, H.: Immediate care of the acutely ill and injured, ed. 2, St. Louis, 1978, The C. V. Mosby Co.

Stewart, R., and others: Los Angeles County Paramedic Training Manuals, all four volumes (unpublished), 1975, Los Angeles County Paramedic Training Institute.

Walraven, G., and others: Advanced pre-hospital Care, Bowes, Md., 1979, Brady Co.

Wasserberger, J., and Eubanks, D.: Advanced paramedic procedures, St. Louis, 1977, The C. V. Mosby Co.

CHAPTER 3

Communication in crisis

Susan C. August

The mind has a tremendous influence on the relative health and well-being of an individual. The emergency department staff is faced with a myriad of patient complaints and anxieties ranging from stitching a cut thumb to delivering a baby or performing lifesaving measures on a heart attack victim. All these patients require not only assessment of their physical needs and intervention, but also an evaluation of their psychological state. The impact that injury or illness has upon the psyche of each individual must be assessed so that appropriate intervention can be taken and thus promote a return to a high level of wellness. "Just as the body is affected by injury, so will the mind react to stress caused by the injury" (Riehl, 1970, p. 231).

If we are to give adequate total care to emergency department patients, then it becomes paramount that we develop assessment skills not only in physical assessment and diagnosis but also in psychological diagnosis. So many times we are intensely involved with management of the vital organs—watching monitors, checking blood pressures, and measuring intakes and outputs—and yet we fail to acknowledge or deal with the patient's psychological state, which is functioning concomitantly with the other vital functions. The patient's level of anxiety, understanding of the events, and coping mechanisms are just as critical to evaluate as all other vital signs, since all these factors influence the way in which a patient responds to treatment.

Specific treatment plans should be developed to meet the needs of each patient. Obviously, lifesaving measures are first priority; after the patient is stabilized, attention can be turned to identification of all other needs. The car accident victim will have not only physical injuries but also psychological trauma that may include questions of loss of function, hospitalization expense, concern over family members, or dismay over body image change. A sudden death in the emergency department may leave relatives stunned, requiring staff to offer emotional support or temporary guidance. Even the mother who brings in the child with chest congestion may have concerns over payment of bills, problems of child rearing, family squabbles, and so on. These not only increase her level of anxiety, but may also be reflected in the child at the time of evaluation.

Ideally, every emergency department should have a specialist skilled in the psychosocial aspects of emergency health care delivery. Since this is often impossible, it becomes the responsibility of the other health care professionals to develop skills in patient assessment and provide the benefits of adequate intervention.

MAINTAINING HOMEOSTASIS

Humans at all times seek to main equilibrium between the external and internal environments

(Schnaper, 1975, p. 94). This equilibrium is maintained by a series of homeostatic mechanisms operating on both an intrapsychic and an interpersonal level. These adaptive maneuvers allow us to function and fluctuate from day to day. Whenever stressful events occur in life situations that threaten homeostasis, certain biopsychosocial mechanisms adjust to return the organism to its previously balanced state, in the same way that, when there is an acute loss of a large blood volume, the body reacts with compensating mechanisms that cause vasoconstriction of peripheral vessels so that blood is shunted to the vital organs. Similarly, if one is faced with a stressful situation, as is often seen in the emergency department, each person's life-style places at his disposal a range of problem-solving techniques from which he may choose, according to his perception of the demands of the situation.

Along with these problem-solving techniques, each person has an array of psychological defenses that have been developed by the ego for the defense of self-esteem, self-worth, and self-preservation. In most situations, these often unconscious defenses are the psychological mainstays of homeostasis. If these habitual protective resources are stressed to the limit in any particular person, then both cognitive and behavioral breakdown occurs, leading to disorganization. This is identified as a state of crisis. Simply defined, crisis is an "upset in a steady state" (Bowlby, 1960, pp. 11-12).

PHASES OF REACTION

Social psychiatrist James Tyhurst identifies three predictable phases of an individual's reaction to a crisis at the time of major disasters. The phases are impact, recoil, and the posttraumatic period. Each of these phases has specific characteristics, including time, stress, and psychological phenomena.

Impact

Impact is the time that the acute illness or injury takes place. The time span of initial impact varies with the incident, normally lasting from seconds to hours. It may be as sudden as a gunshot wound or motorcycle accident, or as persistent as chest pain with angina or a nosebleed. The initial stress is maximal and continues until the stress is no longer operating on the individual. The individual's thinking is concerned with the immediate present, and response is usually automatic. The reactions or psychological patterns of people seen in the impact phase can be divided into three rather typical groups. The first group is "cool and collected" during the acute situation. These persons are aware of the situation and are able to evaluate, plan, and implement a course of action. The second group exhibits the most commonly seen reaction. They are stunned and bewildered, and their field of attention is restricted. They act on reflex rather than thinking things out. They lack an awareness of any subjective feelings or emotions, although they manifest "the physiological concomitants of fear" (Tyhurst, 1957, p. 756). The third and final group shows inappropriate responses and appears in a state of confusion and paralyzing anxiety.

Recoil

Again, the time span of this recoil phase varies according to individual differences. This is the phase most often observed in emergency department patients. The initial stress has ceased, and the patient is out of the immediate, life-threatening danger. Some stress may persist, but it is significantly decreased in nature, type, and severity. These stresses are often discounted psychologically by the patient, after the magnitude of his initial stress.

During this period, there is a gradual return of self-consciousness and awareness of the immediate past. While giving a history, he will be recalling his experience for the first time. The first overt emotional expression and subjective feeling of emotion will become apparent. He will achieve his first awareness of what he has just passed through. There is a need to talk, to get angry, or to express himself in some way. Tyhurst likens the need to talk to a childlike attitude of dependency, which is a major force in this phase. There is a need to talk and get support that may appear only at this time.

Once his defenses are mobilized, the patient may refuse to seek or accept help. This is why the initial interaction in the emergency department can be so critical.

Posttraumatic phase

The posttraumatic phase includes rehabilitation and, according to some theorists, continues for the remainder of one's lifetime. This is then the time when the person experiences his first full awareness of the true significance of his recent disaster. A change in body image, loss of a loved one, and continued medical care may now become major concerns. The posttraumatic phase is a period of readjustment. Temporary fatigue or anxiety, dreams about the incident, anorexia, and mood swings may be observed. This phase, although not frequently seen in the emergency department, is just as important as the first two in terms of patient recovery.

FACTORS PRODUCING CRISIS

Gerald Caplin, a major contributor to crisis theory, identifies three general factors that may produce a crisis state.
1. A precipitating event that poses a threat to an individual or family.
2. A threat to basic securities, which may be symbolically linked to earlier events that resulted in vulnerability or conflict or may be reminiscent of an earlier, inadequately resolved crisis.
3. An inability to respond with adequate coping mechanisms.

These three factors will now be discussed relative to emergency department patients.

Precipitating event

Almost any kind of event can pose a threat to homeostasis at any place or time. We are often confronted daily with threats to such basic securities as the need for love or affectional ties, the knowledge of body integrity, and the continuance of the organism. The individual may or may not have developed adequate coping mechanisms from past experiences that he is able to mobilize and integrate into a behavior to combat a previously unencountered threat. A crisis ensues when the person is unable to deal with precipitating events and thus succumbs to the threat.

There are three types of precipitating events. The most commonly seen in the emergency department is the sudden or unexpected event. This includes accidents, disaster, or illness. The second type is usually from chronic illness, such as diabetes, renal dialysis, hypertension, or other diseases, which may precipitate a crisis at any unforeseen time. The third type is seen as a series of cumulative minor stresses that add up to trigger a period of disequilibrium.

An unexpected event, often referred to as an emergency, is defined as an "unforeseen isolated incident, which, if unresponded to will result in life-threatening or psychological damage" (Resnick and Ruben, 1975, p. 5). Commonly encountered events that may precipitate crisis include: an auto accident with or without physical injury; death of a significant person; catastrophic environmental events, such as earthquakes, floods, or hurricanes; and catastrophies of our technological age, such as plane crashes, train derailment, or nuclear accidents. Sudden physical illness, such as heart attack or stroke, can precipitate fears related to loss of life, body function, and image, and social and sexual relationships.

The second type of precipitating event, prolonged stress, is often not a priority in the emergency department but still produces anxiety and therefore may lead to a potential crisis. A diabetic patient who has a sore on his foot may be distraught and coping poorly; the patient on dialysis whose shunt has clotted may act demanding; and finally, the hypertensive patient whose presenting complaint is a headache may be mainly concerned about the possibility of a stroke. All these represent prolonged stress situations with potential crisis possibilities.

The third type of precipitating event is identified as a series of minor incidents that accumulate to eventually cause a major disruption in the patient's equilibrium. The young woman who is despondent over the loss of her job, the breakdown of her car, and the recent death of her mother suddenly becomes unable to cope when her boyfriend decides to end their relationship. She decides to end it all with a bottle of pills—a common emergency department event.

Each of these three types of precipitating events may be seen in the emergency department. Defining the precipitating events gives the staff a better "handle" with which to approach patient management. This coupled with a further understanding of the significance or meaning of the event may lead to the development of adequate coping skills.

Meaning of the event

Individuals vary greatly in the way they react to a stressful situation. The meaning or significance of the event is the key that determines how the individual will respond. Each person's response is influenced by a variety of factors that together define the meaning of the event. These factors include the current situation relative to past events, the person's perception of the problem, and other influences such as personality and socioeconomic, religious, and cultural elements, which all play a factor in defining the meaning of the event.

Sometimes what may seem like a very insignificant event to the staff causes a major crisis for the patient. That present event may be linked to unresolved conflicts, which may in turn amplify or distort the patient's response to the present event. To illustrate, a 76-year-old woman is brought into the emergency department after tripping on the curb in front of her home. X-ray films show a fractured hip. When told she needs to be admitted, she becomes very upset and insists on being transferred to another hospital. After appropriate staff intervention, it is learned that her husband died at the same hospital 1 year previously. She is certain that her admission will also lead to her death. Overreaction such as this may be the first clue that a crisis is at hand.

Confusion at the time of the event or about the nature of the problem may also significantly contribute to the level of stress. Emergencies are characteristically accompanied by chaos and confusion. The elements of the sudden impact of a car collision—stunned passengers, injured persons, possible fire, blocked traffic, people screaming, and the wail of distant sirens—add up to pandemonium. By the time victims from such a scene arrive in the emergency department, they may be so distraught that the unfamiliar medical environment may be enough to trigger a crisis.

On rare occasions, a stressful situation may be seen as a challenge and may be approached with a positive attitude by a patient. Often, the success a person has had with past experiences may contribute to his positive attitude. For instance, if a carpenter who has been the victim of multiple injuries in previous years comes in with a severe laceration to his forearm from an electric saw, he may consider it no problem. He may see this as "just one more to add to my list of scars."

On the other hand, the person who sees the situation as problematic may find it a difficult and trying time in his life. For example, the aspiring high school fullback is brought to the emergency department during his first game of the season with a torn knee ligament. Upon learning that he will be out for the season, he becomes angry, tearful, and withdrawn.

Other factors that can possibly influence the meaning of a crisis situation are personality and socioeconomic and cultural elements. If a person has a tendency for a high anxiety level in his most routine times, then added stress will usually cause even higher levels of anxiety. Here it can be valuable to establish premorbid behavior patterns of the patient from the patient and family and associates. Cultural influences may often be seen in methods of expressions and both verbal and body language. Customs and ceremonies and manners and vocabulary are important aspects to remember when working with people of unfamiliar cultures.

The meaning of the event is obviously a multifactoral component in the development of a crisis. It is perhaps the key to assessment, because often the precipitating events may appear to the staff to be quite severe, yet the patient may not perceive the event as drastic, and will therefore not manifest a crisis. The staff interpretation must always be tempered with an evaluation of the patient's coping mechanisms.

Coping mechanisms

"Human beings placed in a stressful environment react in a variety of ways, but the response common to all is anxiety" (Holmes, 1978, p. 139). Anxiety is defined as "feelings of uncertainty in the face of danger" (Holmes, 1978, p. 231). Any threat to the security of an individual produces a certain degree of anxiety.

Anxiety affects people's physical, cognitive, and psychological well-being. In a stressful situation, anxiety triggers defense mechanisms, which may or may not alter behavior and physiological patterns. These defenses are activated in order to help us bear whatever misfortune has befallen us. They are the mind's protective devices, nature's way of allowing us to maintain homeostasis. These responses have been developed by the ego for the protection of one's self-esteem.

In addition to anxiety, certain behaviors are commonly seen at the time of injury or illness. A greater or lesser area of functioning may be interfered with, according to the significance of the problem and the intensity of the behavior. These behaviors include numbness, confusion, fear, discomfort, urgency, and helplessness.

Term	Meaning
Numbness	Typically described as "frozen" behavior; people appear to be in a dazed state
Confusion	A difficulty making any sense or order out of the situation
Fear	A feeling of alarm provoked by a sense of danger
Discomfort	An unpleasant sensation
Urgency	A need for immediate attention
Helplessness	A feeling of inability to care for oneself

All these components may be compounded by the presence of anxiety.

Depending on the level of anxiety, clinical presentation may or may not be greatly affected. A certain amount of anxiety can be a positive thing and "an effective stimulant to action. It . . . helps the individual to mobilize his resources in meeting the problem" (Aguilera and Messick, 1978, p. 63).

With an initial rise in anxiety, behaviors are mostly appropriate, although there is an increase in sensitivity so that the person is very alert and sees, hears, and grasps more. The person is in control of his emotions and is able to verbalize any fears. There is an associated physiological reaction that causes a rapid pulse, increased respiration, dilated pupils, and diaphoresis.

With further increase in tension, a person's perceptual field is narrowed. One sees, hears, and grasps less but can attend to more specific details if directed to do so. This is noted as "selective inattention," where one fails to notice what goes on in the environment peripheral to the immediate situation, but can shift his attention if instructed. A person attempts emergency problem-solving mechanisms, which may be seen in repeating of procedures, becoming task-oriented, or focusing upon one aspect of the problem and not involving the whole entity.

With unresolved stress, the level of anxiety will continue to escalate. The clinical picture will show definite signs of disorganization, primarily in the behavioral and cognitive components. There will be identifiable alterations in all major areas of functioning.

There will be an accentuated use of one or more behavioral patterns. The person feeling very uncomfortable may become demanding, indecisive, repetitive, or withdrawn. Behavior will be less organized and more regressive. Inappropriate emotional reactions, impaired attention span, an altered level of consciousness, and a loss of memory or concentration may be noted. In very severe cases, there may be a distortion of reality or "cognitive confusion" (Parad, 1965, p. 28) in which the individual does not know how to think about his problem, formulate, or evaluate a possible outcome.

CRISIS-PRONE PEOPLE

In his article, "Crisis Theory: a Formulation," Ralph Hirschowitz identifies characteristics of healthy and unhealthy crisis coping.

The person who reacts adaptively or healthily in a stressful situation has some of the following characteristics:

• Is able to deal with the tasks and exhibit appropriate affective dimensions in a stressful situation.
• Is able to use defenses to decrease anxiety in constructive ways.
• Is able to acknowledge needs for dependency and see, receive, and use assistance.
• Is able to deal with medical uncertainties without behaving impulsively.
• Is able to accept environmental challenges and recognize value in personal growth.

As opposed to the preceding adaptive reactions, some people with the following characteristics may go into crisis. They may:

• Exhibit excessive denial or withdrawal and utilize fantasy to replace or merge with reality.
• Exhibit impulsive behavior and use scapegoats such as hospital personnel or family on whom to ventilate rage.
• Deny or overcontrol emotions, thus suppressing feelings.
• Meet dependency needs by either clinging excessively or, at the other end of the spectrum, completely denying the need for assistance—actions interpreted by others as not wanting or needing help.
• Be unable to ask for help or use it when it is offered.
• Resort to hyperritualistic behavior, which serves little or no purpose.

CRISIS AND CRISIS INTERVENTION

When an event is perceived as threatening, and there is an imbalance between the difficulty of the problem and the resources immediately available to deal with it, then there is an increase in the anxiety level. The usual homeostatic, problem-solving methods are unsuccessful, and alternative emergency problem-solving techniques do not work. Disorganization follows, which leads to a state of crisis.

Gerald Caplan defines crisis as occurring "when a person faces an obstacle to important life goals that is, for a time, insurmountable through the utilization of customary methods of problem-solving. A period of disorganization ensues, a period of upset, during which

many abortive attempts at solutions are made" (1964, p. 38).

It is during this time that people are very vulnerable and have an opportunity either to fail or to grow. The outcome of disequilibrium depends on availability of appropriate help and the interaction that takes place with others and the self. W. I. Thomas, a social theorist, views crisis as a positive force, "a catalyst that disturbs old habits, evokes new responses and becomes a major factor in charting new developments" (Caplan, 1964, p. 23). The goal of crisis intervention in this instance is to return the individual to his previous state of homeostasis, but perhaps with new problem-solving techniques, enabling him to cope at a higher level.

When one works with people in crisis, it is helpful to know that a crisis does not continue idefinitely. Caplan noted that within 4 to 6 weeks, a resolution will be made either with or without help. However, the patient may return to the same level or even a lower level of equilibrium. With crisis intervention, it is possible to facilitate a return to a higher level with new insights and better coping skills.

Balancing factors

Attempts to regain equilibrium are influenced by three recognized balancing factors: perception of events, situational supports, and coping mechanisms. When one perceives threats from a stressful situation, the strengths or weaknesses in these factors can be a direct influence toward the onset of crisis or a return to equilibrium.

Perception of events. The way in which a person perceives an event affects his return to equilibrium. If the person perceives the situation realistically, identifying a relationship between the event and the onset of his feelings, then related problem-solving methods can be effective. If, on the other hand, the event is perceived unrealistically, with distortions or inaccurate information, then problem-solving efforts will most likely be unsuccessful.

Situational supports. People depend on others for support in times of stress. Different figures in a person's life may or may not be available when needed. The patient finds support most often from family or close friends. The most significant finding here is that the family or friend is a familiar and trusted source of support. Given the time and energy to develop a rapport with a patient, others (for example, emergency department personnel) can fill this role in times of stress.

Coping mechanisms. Through daily living we acquire methods of relieving anxiety, which over a period of time may become routine ways of reducing tension. We may or may not be consciously aware of the manner in which we react in certain situations. Our methods of handling problems are called our "coping mechanisms." These vary from person to person and, depending on previously attempted success or failure, these mechanisms become incorporated into one's life-style.

Focus of crisis intervention

The focus of crisis intervention in the emergency department is basically "psychological first aid" (Klinman, 1978, p. 11). It is designed to prevent further disorganization of one's emotional equilibrium. By providing immediate intervention at the time of the crisis, it avoids the development of more permanent or harmful psychosocial problems. Patients are especially receptive to professional interventions when they are in a crisis-induced, regressed emotional state. During periods of instability when forces are teetering in the balance, the patient is often more willing to accept guidance than during periods of stability.

Assessing patients in crisis

The impact a situation has on a person can have from little effect to an extremely severe influence on a person's life. Each person's reaction is different. Staff must assess each patient individually, in order to intervene appropriately.

Assessing the impact is done by observing the patient's behavior, emotions, and cognition during his stay in the emergency department. With no emotional impact, behaviors are appropriate, emotions are in control, and the person is able to think clearly. Behavior, emo-

tions, and cognition are only slightly affected with mild impact. There may be some anxiety, although the person is basically calm and thinking clearly. With moderate impact, the patient is noticeably affected, but the response is neither continuous nor highly intense, and he responds to help. With severe impact, the patient is clearly affected in one or more life areas. The patient is visibly upset yet responds to reassurance. The patient experiences difficulty conceptualizing strategies for future planning. When there is a very severe impact from the situation, the patient may be either crying or withdrawn throughout the examination, and there is a generalized feeling of fear or anger, or both. The patient is unable to comprehend the situation or develop problem-solving strategies. The patient who has an extremely severe impact is incapacitated by the situation and may need hospitalization. Extreme nervous disorders or psychotic reactions may be seen. The level of impact and its related behaviors, emotions, and cognition are summarized in Table 3-1.

Intervention techniques to maintain equilibrium

Situational support. In the emergency department, patients can be greatly influenced by those around them. Staff as well as family and friends can help the patient confront the stressful situation and identify ways of promoting a healthy return to equilibrium. Patients under stress are acutely aware of messages that we as staff may send, both verbal and nonverbal. These methods of support given by staff, family, and others will now be discussed in light of the emergency department patient, who can be extremely sensitive and susceptible to influence while under stress.

STAFF AS SUPPORT

NONVERBAL COMMUNICATION. The outward appearance of confidence is easily noticed by the patient. Ideally, one communicates confidence, openness, and warmth in a manner that supports the patient's reaction to the highly stressful situation. What realistically happens is that with certain patients on certain days and at certain times, one may not be as supportive

Table 3-1. Guidelines for assessing patients in crisis*

Impact	Behaviors	Emotions	Cognition	Examples
No emotional impact				
No observable effect of the situation on the person's behavior	Questions, responses, activities are appropriate for the situation May ask questions, request information, obtain knowledge correctly Not withdrawn or anxious	Expresses that he is "all right" Feels in control of emotions Expresses concerns and reactions clearly	Evidences clear thinking Able to make decisions Plans well Is reality-oriented	Reports that "I will be OK" Reports that he can "handle it"
Mild impact				
Behavior, emotions, and cognition are only slightly affected by the situation	Questions, responses, and activities are mostly appropriate May evidence some anxiety, fear, stress May be cooperative and responsive; displays few visible signs of upset	Seems in control of emotions and basically calm May report a little embarrassment Is able to talk about the situation	Clear, good to very good future plans	Reports some confidence that he will be OK Feels sure that with help "I"ll handle it"
Moderate impact				
Is noticeably affected by the situation but response is not continuous or highly intense Responds to help and reassurance Can conceptualize strategies for dealing with the future	May tear or cry a little during the examination, but visible affect or distress is minimal May display some silly or inappropriate behavior May be anxious, unable to absorb information easily, somewhat confused	May seem somewhat affected by the situation but will respond to reassurance from others Expresses worry, fear, some inability to concentrate Somewhat dependent	Asks for help and has good plans and strategies for coping with the problem	Asks for help and support Reports concern about the future impact; "Will I be OK?"
Severe impact				
Is clearly affected by the situation in one or more life areas Behavioral response occurs more than once and is somewhat intense Needs reassurance, and experiences difficulty conceptualizing strategies for future planning	Is visibly upset during part of the evaluation, yet responds to reassurance; the signs of distress can be pinpointed to certain factors (the questions about incident, the examination, the outcome and future problems)	Expresses feelings of guilt, self-blame, helplessness, either with strong emotion or he repeats this concern	Appears confused or disoriented Is visibly upset, yet has some plans for handling problems arising from the situation	Says he is very frightened "doesn't want to go out anymore," or states other unrealistic plans

*Developed by Dr. Susan Meyers Chandler, School of Social Work, and Dr. Libby O. Ruch, Sociology Department and Women's Studies Program, University of Hawaii, Honolulu, Hawaii.

Table 3-1. Guidelines for assessing patients in crisis—cont'd

Impact	Behaviors	Emotions	Cognition	Examples
Very severe impact				
Has a strong reaction in one or more areas Is not incapacitated but highly affected by the situation Behaviors are continuous and intense Seems only somewhat responsive to reassurance and is only somewhat able to conceptualize strategies for dealing with the future	Is visibly upset during most of the exam Crying, trembling, withdrawal evident throughout the exam Responses occurring almost continuously—*not* focused only on the situation —*generalized distress*	Verbalizes strong reactions; may repeat responses with intensity Generalized fear and/or anger	Very confused, disoriented, unable to comprehend situation May deny responses No plans for the future; evidences little ability to consider alternatives or develop strategies for the future	Reports that he will "never drive again," "never look the same," or "can't go home"
Extremely severe impact				
Is incapacitated by the situation; may be hospitalized for psychiatric observation or treatment Behaviors are multiple, continuous, and extremely intense Unaware of efforts to reassure	May be suicidal, catatonic, hysterical, or crying May have phobias or other psychological symptoms that indicate he is incapacitated in some way	Shows extreme nervous disorders, psychotic reactions	Is unable to deal with the situation or the future Is unable to make decisions for self	Has no awareness of what happened or where he is; out of touch with reality

as usual. It is important to realize that we are only human and each of us has an "off day." At these times we should communicate this to other staff so that they are aware and may intervene in our behalf. So many times, when an emergency occurs, the patient reflects the staff's mood. If staff members are anxious, this may be felt by the patient and will increase his level of anxiety. If staff members project a sense of calmness and control, then this can influence the patient toward a positive way of handling the situation. Nonverbal communication is also greatly influenced by physical closeness or contact. Where a person positions himself when communicating can influence a patient's perception of a message. The nurse who stands behind the desk reassuring a frightened mother may be able to make a more effective contact if she comes around and stands next to her. So often we give our patients instructions when they are lying flat, or take a history from a woman in stirrups set up for a pelvic exam, or yell across the room to the patient, explaining to him how to take medications. All these situations communicate a nonverbal as well as a verbal message. In fact, the nonverbal message may be so overpowering that the patient fails to assimilate the verbal message.

Other important forms of nonverbal communication are eye contact and facial expression. These are nonphysical ways of touching and can often be used to reassure the patient. Often, when physical touch is impossible or inappropriate (for example, with a burn patient or a quadraplegic patient), then eye contact may be the only way of reaching that person other than with words. Facial expression can often acknowledge feelings, both the patient's and our own. This is particularly important to remember when the staff is faced with a repugnant sight or smell. We must, for example, avoid showing dismay at disfigurement when uncovering the bandages. Often, the patient is unable to see the trauma and is watching for the reaction of the nurse to gauge the seriousness of the wound.

Perhaps the most important of the nonverbal entities of communication is physical touch. An arm around the shoulder, a firm handshake, or a reassuring pat on the knee is usually warmly received, especially by those who are apprehensive. Everyone has a need to be touched, and at distressing times a touch can be very comforting. Sometimes staff members may hold back with the fear that some people do not feel comfortable being touched, whereas others may use touch liberally. Perhaps it is best to say that each situation and each person is unique, necessitating assessment and evaluation of how each patient will respond. It is important to remember that there are many taboos about touching. It follows then that it is important to identify nonverbal cues and be aware of patients' reactions to touch.

VERBAL COMMUNICATION. Everyone knows how much a calm, reassuring voice can lower anxiety levels. Just the tone of the voice can often communicate much more than the words themselves. Anxiety can be picked up in the voice before other behavioral signs become apparent. In an emergency situation in which people are intensely working in life-threatening situations, their hands may be steady, and quick motions may go unnoticed, but shouting or rapid speech will be an obvious clue to the high level of tension.

In addition to the verbal input, there are other factors that serve to relay a message. Small courtesies, often neglected, can help make the emergency department a friendlier environment. With each patient and family, it is important for the staff to take time to introduce themselves and their roles. By identifying people, the patient is soon able to recognize familiar faces and names. This then becomes an identifiable resource in an unfamiliar environment. Often, however, people run in and out of the room, and the patient has no one to ask questions of or tell problems to.

Brief explanations are often more valuable than lengthy technical details. With an increased level of anxiety, a patient is unable to absorb complicated messages, so that communicating small amounts at frequent intervals is usually most effective.

The gift of verbal communication is one that we often take for granted, yet it is by far the most important of our senses for communication. For the care of the patient and the safety of the emergency department, it is important that messages be correctly transmitted and received.

FAMILY SUPPORT. The involved family can be as much an integral part of the patient's recovery as staff participation. Sometimes in critical care it is not always possible to have the family at the bedside, but as soon as feasible, all efforts should be made to reunite the family with the patient. The family reminds the patient of reality and of the outside world. It is often his only link. In addition, family members can be very useful in problem solving and in offering more effective means of coping for the patient.

We must also remember that families can be just as anxious as patients. They have been isolated from the patient and may be frightened, because they initially saw the patient when the injury occurred and have most likely not seen him since. Their concern and desire for care to be given for their loved one may be displayed as impatience or complaints, which mask a cry for help. They need to be kept informed, just as the patient does. Again, brief descriptions at frequent intervals are most easily understood.

OTHERS. Patients encounter many other persons in the emergency department besides health care personnel and family. These may include paraprofessionals, law enforcement officers, friends, volunteers, and ministers. When the patient does not have family members available, other possible relationships should be explored that could be supportive at the time of stress. Because the patient's thinking may become clouded, it may take several attempts for the patient to clearly recall names and numbers of friends.

If no support appears available, it is important to have ancillary personnel in the form of clergy and community volunteers. Even a call to a hot line may get the patient some needed support.

Perception of events. The emergency department is a strange and threatening environment to most people who come for treatment. Equipment may look and sound overwhelming even to the casual observer, but especially so to patients. Oftentimes we are unable to prevent patients from observing other patients with severe medical problems. It is frightening to see another patient convulse, bleed, or exhibit psychotic behavior. It is no wonder that very often a patient's level of anxiety is high, not only from his own injury but also from the unfamiliar environment as well. When a patient does not understand what is going on, he may often become confused or have an unrealistic perception of events about him.

If a person is able to have a clear understanding of what is happening or is about to happen, his ability to cooperate will significantly increase. Obtaining a history, explaining emergency department procedures, keeping the patient informed, and explaining medical findings are all ways of increasing patients' abilities to cope.

TAKING A HISTORY. It is essential to emergency department diagnosis and treatment that an accurate history of events, signs, and symptoms, and a past medical history be taken. As we have patients relate this information, we are facilitating an increase in their perception of events. By reviewing their story, we are helping them realize that there was a beginning and an end — bringing order into a chaotic situation. We can redirect the patients' congition and action to the most critical, or at least the most

malleable, elements of their illness. Recognition and realistic response to the precipitating stress is infinitely more productive than preoccupation with the symptoms. Skillfully guiding patients to see the relationship between high anxiety and events will encourage them to deal with their feelings.

EXPLAINING EMERGENCY DEPARTMENT PROCEDURES. By providing information that encourages a more accurate perception, we decrease feelings of apprehension felt by patients. Telling them what is going to happen and when and how it will feel is only fair. Giving them reasons for needed tests, possible side effects, and what the expected outcome will be prepares them so that they are more aware and in better control of the situation. Nothing is more frightening than to be totally helpless with no feeling of control.

Talking to the patients in language that they can understand is important. This first requires finding out if they have any medical background in order to relate at this level. It is just as frustrating to be talked down to as it is to be lost in a barrage of medical jargon. For example, the physician who told his patient, "John, you have a fractured femur," was surprised when the patient replied "Oh, really, is it broken?" Asking him to explain to you in his own words his understanding of what was said will assess if the patient really comprehends.

The routine emergency department procedures, such as registration, vital signs, disrobing, and the physician's examination should be explained. These procedures become routine for staff but are unfamiliar to patients, who should be asked if they have questions. These steps will help eliminate uncertainty, "the most fertile source of anxiety" (Kliman, 1978, p. 236).

If there is a significant time delay between your initial contact and when the physician will see the patient, he should be told that there will be a wait. There is nothing more frustrating than to sit in an empty examining room and wait, wondering if one has been forgotten. The patient should be told where his family will be, especially if the family is coming in or if others are injured. Other patients' conditions should not be discussed unless the patient asks or unless you have been instructed to do so. His silence or avoidance should be respected as an inability to cope with that particular information at that time.

Often patients will request medication before completion of the examination. If they cannot have medication, as is the case with patients with neurologic injuries, possible surgery candidates, or those with pain of unknown origin, it should be explained why medicine cannot be given. Patients should be reassured, however, that their needs will be dealt with as soon as the medical regimen allows it.

Ominous prognostic and extraneous medical discussion should be avoided. Care must be maintained at all times to avoid discussing unrelated cases in front of a patient. Overheard comments can often be misinterpreted or exaggerated. In the same manner, comments directed to the patient should be realistic and, as pointed out previously, not cluttered with jargon. False reassurance—such as, "Everything will be all right," or "You'll be well in no time"—should not be offered; rather an honest appraisal should be given, tempered with optimism.

The complexities of illness or injury can be overwhelming to the medically naive individual. A clear understanding of emergency department procedures is facilitated by an appropriate history, clear, concise explanations of procedures at the person's own level of understanding, skillful handling of medical questions, and, most important, an awareness of the needs of the patient.

Coping mechanisms. The third of the three forces that serve to maintain equilibrium is the promotion of adequate coping mechanisms. This can be a difficult and time-consuming task. Simple formulas cannot ease the distress caused by uncontrolled traumatic events. A high level of energy is necessary on the part of the staff to be able to observe behavior and identify ways of meeting patients' needs. Some of the ways to intervene include helping the patient confront the crisis, identify feelings and past problem-solving methods, and develop new

methods of coping. The goals are to decrease anxiety, gain control, increase confidence, and reinforce desired behavior.

CONFRONTING THE CRISIS. After establishing rapport, we must begin to help the patient acknowledge the crisis. Many times patients are still dazed by the event, and in these situations it takes time, but slowly they begin to realize the reality of their situation. Very often, people deal with a crisis only briefly at first, in comprehensible and manageable doses that do not produce overwhelming pain or fear. As a patient begins to confront the crisis, it may at times be necessary to "back off" and discuss other things less painful. It is essential to be patient and realize that repeated small doses of confrontation will eventually lead to healthy confrontation of the events.

As the patient begins to deal with the crisis, the staff will need to prevent further disorganization by providing impulse control and implementing limit setting. Efforts to relieve anxiety may mean that staff will have to direct patients' actions. Deep breathing exercises, concentrating on specific objects, or other methods of relaxation may help calm the patient. As anxiety decreases, the patient can then begin to take control in order to help counteract the feelings of helplessness so common at stressful times.

IDENTIFYING FEELINGS. Not all people are able to identify and verbalize their feelings. Some may need assistance to talk about how they perceived the events and what they were feeling at the time. As a patient tells a story, it is important to help the patient gain some understanding of the relationship between the events and the distress he is feeling now. He must realize that fear, anger, and tension are normal responses at stressful times. In this frightening time, what is needed most is understanding. The patient needs to talk about fears related to hospitals, doctors, or medical procedures. The patient is not expecting staff to take these fears away, but he does need to talk and be taken sincerely. Even a simple "I'd be upset, too" or "I don't blame you. Nobody likes a shot" will help the patient feel less frightened and better able to cope with the situation.

Cheerful and well-intended statements, such as "You're lucky to be alive" or "Everything will be okay," are more likely to increase anxiety rather than boost spirits. The patient may know from experience that everything may not be okay.

PROMOTING PROBLEM SOLVING. After the patient has adequately ventilated his feelings, the nurse can help the patient set up problem-solving tasks that can handle the previously overwhelming experience in a more systematic and effective manner. The nurse reflects to the patient past events and related feelings. It is important to point out strengths, to help the patient begin to develop a plan with an awareness of what has been effective in the past, and to identify any situations in which he had to find new ways of working things out and what worked. Now the patient should be helped to redefine the present situation in terms of old problem-solving techniques. What expectations does he have about the outcome? Is there any information that has been previously omitted?

The patient must begin to examine possible alternative solutions. It is essential not to give advice, but to listen to or propose alternative solutions and let the patient make the decision. It may take some prodding, but most often patients are able to come up with alternatives. Helping the patient identify the plan that seems most likely to work and then encouraging him to carry through with the decisions made effectively promote problem solving.

SUMMARY

The typical emergency department is a specialized area reflecting turmoil and crisis at all hours of the day and night. An individual seen in this setting may be thrown from complacency into a full-blown crisis. How the patient copes with this change in his homeostasis determines how to intervene with crisis management.

The three phases of a reaction must be identified: impact, recoil, and the posttraumatic period. Staff must note where the patient fits on this time line, and then must identify the factors that produced the particular crisis at hand, including the precipitating events, the meaning of the event, and a clarification of the available coping mechanisms that the patient has at hand. Once these mechanisms are brought to light, an evaluation of the individual's perception of the event and the available support structures can be carried out.

This particular structural approach to crisis intervention can lead to specific problem-solving techniques for those individuals bordering on homeostatic disequilibrium. Emergency department staff should:

- Create a calm environment that fosters trust, understanding, and a rational approach to problem solving.
- Make contact with the patient, realizing that important parts of communication take place verbally as well as nonverbally with eye contact, facial expressions, touch, and reassuring voice tones.
- Include the family with updates on the patient's condition, and allow them to provide needed support.
- Explain procedures in nontechnical language, giving reasons, side effects, and expected outcome, using familiar words, and encouraging questions.
- Help the patient confront the crisis when and as he is ready, and help him regain control of lost self-esteem.
- Help the patient identify and "get in touch with" his feelings.
- Finally, help the patient begin problem solving by identifying past similar events, previous coping mechanisms and techniques, and alternative solutions.

These interventions may appear to be mostly common sense, but it is surprising how often and how easily they are forgotten on a day-to-day basis. It is important to imagine ourselves in the patient's situation. The few minutes spent with a patient checking a blood pressure, giving a shot, or transporting him to the x-ray department can be so much more valuable if we are attuned to the needs of another human being. When we use the above techniques, we will find a new world of patient care that most people never take the time to discover.

BIBLIOGRAPHY

Aguilera, D., and Messick, J.: Crisis intervention: theory and methodology, ed. 3, St. Louis, 1978, The C. V. Mosby Co. p. 63.

Bowlby, J.: Grief and mourning in infancy and early childhood, Psychoanal. Study Child **15:**11-12, 1960.

Caplan, G.: Principle of preventative psychiatry, New York, 1964, Basic Books, Inc., pp. 23 and 38.

Hirschowitz, R.: Crisis theory; a formulation, Psychiatr. Ann. **3:**36-47, December 1973.

Holmes, J.: Stress and anxiety in the emergency department. In Barry, J., editor: Emergency nursing, New York, 1978, McGraw-Hill Book Co., pp. 149 and 231.

Klinman, A.: Crisis: psychological first aid for recovery and growth, New York, 1978, Holt, Rinehart and Winston, Inc., pp. 11 and 236.

Parad, H.: Crisis intervention: selected readings, New York, 1965, Family Services Association of America, p. 28.

Resnick, H. L. P., and Ruben, H.: Emergency psychiatric care, Bowie, Md., 1975, The Charles Press Publisher, Inc., p. 5.

Riehl, L.: Emergency nursing. Peoria, Ill., 1970, Chas. A. Bennett Co., Inc., p. 231.

Schnaper, N.: The psychological implications of severe trauma; emotional sequelae to unconsciousness, J. Trauma **15**(2):94, 1975.

Tyhurst, J. S.: The role of transition states — including disasters — in mental illness. In Proceedings of the Symposium on Preventative and Social Psychiatry, Washington, D.C., 1957, Walter Reed Army Institute of Research, p. 766.

ADDITIONAL READINGS

Barten, H. H.: Brief therapies, New York, 1971, Behavioral Publications, Inc.

Bartolucci, L., and Drayer, C.: Overview of crisis intervention in the emergency rooms of general hospitals, Am. J. Psychiatry **130:**953-959, September 1973.

Beland, I., and Passos, J.: Clinical nursing pathophysiology and psychosocial approaches, New York, 1975, Macmillan Publishing Co., Inc.

Brammer, L.: The helping relationship, Englewood Cliffs, N.J., 1979, Prentice-Hall, Inc.

Edwards, R. V.: Crisis intervention and how it works, Springfield, Ill., 1977, Charles C Thomas, Publisher.

Hatton, J.: Performance evaluation in relation to psychosocial needs, Superv. Nurs **8:**30-35, July 1977.

Jacobson, G., Strickler, M., and Morley, W.: Generic and individual approaches to crisis intervention, Am. J. Public Health **58**(2):338-343, 1968.

Johnston, D. H.: Crisis intervention training for emergency medical personnel, J.E.N. **3:**27-30, May-June 1977.

Lee, J.: Emotional reaction to trauma, Nurs. Clin. North Am. **5:**577-587, December 1970.

O'Connor, G.: Psychiatric changes in the acutely injured, Postgrad. Med. **48:**210-214, September 1970.

Rapoport, L.: The state of crisis: some theoretical considerations. In Parad, H. J.: Crisis intervention: selected readings, New York, 1965, Family Services Association of America.

CHAPTER 4

Legal considerations in the emergency department

Michael L. Rains

"Look at those jerks over there. When I first came to work here 26 years ago, we would have taken those bench bums for a ride into the mountains and administered some employment incentive through indiscriminate use of the police night stick." It was my first day as a police officer in October 1975, and I was being "treated" to the observations of a veteran police sergeant who, I believed, had wallowed in the filth of the vice detail too long before his latest reassignment to uniformed patrol. I was embracing a panorama of the Pacific Ocean from the coast highway, the beauty of the moment being filtered through my supervisor's caustic remarks and the Remington shotgun barrel that protruded over the dashboard of the car directly in front of where I sat.

"Things have really changed for cops—all for the worse. People don't respect us any more, but by the same token, they expect us to be a likeness of Jack Webb and triumph over crime, as well as perform the services of social workers, priests, doctors, lawyers, the Chamber of Commerce, and miracle faith healers. Of course, no one helps us when we try to accommodate their wishes. The nurses and doctors at the local emergency hospital are often obstacles when we have to interview victims there or take suspects there for treatment. Don't ever count on cooperation from them, and you'll never be disappointed. Of course, the way the law is today, we have to take arrestees to the hospital for treatment any time they cut their finger and want a Band-Aid, or we get sued. I can remember when all we used to have to worry about was catching crooks—without worrying about how we went about it—without considering any threat of civil liability—without being required to waste valuable coffee-break time sitting in the hospital while the nurses and doctors malingered—without worrying about gathering evidence or treating victims or arrestees before we talked to them."

Whether you as a nurse realize it or not, the comments made by this training sergeant are more than the rambling reflections of a cynical man. Rather, two distinctive themes emerge from his statements, which will reoccur virtually every day that you are working as a nurse in the emergency department. First, times have changed, and you can no longer perform your duties as a nurse with your *sole* consideration being the welfare of your patient. You must be alert to the ever present threat of *civil liability,* and your actions in the emergency department should be premised with an understanding of general concepts of liability, *as well as* the welfare of the patient. Second, there will be many times in which local law enforcement officers will bring crime victims into the emergency department for treatment, or will call upon your assistance to help gather evidence for criminal prosecutions. In both cases, the possibility of conflict between the emergency department staff and the officers is present. Hence, you must understand your obligations to assist law enforcement officers, and, equally important, understand those actions that you are *not* required to take even though ordered to by a law enforcement officer. Unfortunately, many of the conflicts between emergency department nurses and police officers have traditionally been the result of the misunderstanding on the part of the officers as to your role as nurses in performing certain services, and a similar misunderstanding or misinterpretation of the law upon which officers request your assistance.

This chapter attempts to explain a few of the various theories under which emergency room nurses have been sued civilly, to explore the different ways in which nurses can expect to interact professionally with police officers, and to provide general guidelines as to the law-imposed obligations in these instances. Finally, it will provide some thoughts on civil liability arising out of the interaction of emergency nurses with the local police. This material should be prefaced by the observation that the concepts of liability and guidelines provided herein are offered in a very *general* sense, with an understanding that various state laws and court decisions will differ. Although much of the material discussed will be applicable throughout the United States, specific inquiries concerning subjects discussed in this chapter should be made through your respective hospital legal counsel.

GENERAL LIABILITY CONCEPTS

As a general rule, an emergency department has an obligation toward all patients to exercise that degree of care, skill, and diligence generally used by hospitals in the community where the hospital is located, or that degree of care, skill and diligence that is used by hospitals in similar communities (*Foley v. Bishop Clarkson Hospital,* 1970). This rule has been criticized as tending to perpetuate different standards of care—the nurse in the "country" emergency department will be held to a lesser degree of care and skill than the "city" nurse. Because of this, some states have abandoned the "community standard" and have adopted a standard encompassing all hospitals wherever located (*Alden v. Providence Hospital,* 1967). In addition, once a hospital, whether public or private, has established an emergency department, that hospital has a duty to admit emer-

gency patients, since the maintenance of an emergency facility creates a reliance on the part of the public that medical care will be available whenever an emergency arises (*Manlove v. Wilmington General Hospital,* 1961).

As a nurse in the emergency department, you are expected to abide by professionally accepted standards of nursing practice, and before a person can sue you and/or your employer, that person must prove that your departure from this accepted standard has been the cause of his or her injury. If a patient believes that he or she has suffered an injury as a result of mistreatment in the emergency department or that his original injury was aggravated by such mistreatment, there are generally two theories upon which suit may be brought. These theories, or "causes of action," as they are often called, include *breach of contract* and *tort*.

In order for the injured patient to hold your employer/hospital liable for breach of contract, the patient has to show that there was an express agreement in the contract to achieve a particular cure or result with respect to the injury involved and that the hospital, through the actions of its doctors and nurses, has not complied with this agreement. Thus, in breach of contract causes, the injured patient cannot prevail merely by showing that his injury was the result of your departure as a nurse from professional standards, but must additionally show a contractual provision wherein the hospital agreed to protect him from the action(s) that allegedly resulted in his injury. It is because of this seemingly insurmountable burden imposed on the civil plaintiff (the party bringing suit against you and the hospital) that breach of contract actions are rare. Where such actions are brought against hospitals, however, the defendant/hospital may attempt to introduce provisions in the contract, or patient consent form, that attempt to negate any liability arising out of the treatment of the patient. Such *disclaimer clauses* are often held invalid as being violative of public policy (*Funkl v. Regents of the University of California,* 1963).

By far the greatest number of lawsuits being filed against emergency department personnel today are in the nature of *tort actions*. Generally, these civil actions allege that the plaintiff has been injured by the actions of the emergency department (who are called defendants in this context) and that such injuries were the result of the failure of the emergency department personnel to abide by the standards of the profession.

An injured patient suing to recover for his hospital-induced condition will often sue those who actually caused the injury, including the nurse(s) responsible for his care and treatment, as well as the *hospital itself,* under the theory of *respondeat superior,* which makes the hospital liable for the torts of its employees if committed within the scope of their employment. Although the hospital/employers in the past attempted to avoid such liability by claiming that the alleged negligent nurse was an "independent contractor," many jurisdictions have refused to recognize such defenses and have ordered the hospital to defend the employee, and if it is proved that the employee's conduct was not consistent with professional standards, to pay any monetary damages to the injured party on behalf of the employee (*Seneris v. Haas,* 1955).

The law may help a patient prove his case against the emergency department through providing him with a doctrine called *res ipsa loquitur.* This doctrine, which was used to impose liability on an entire surgical team (doctors and nurses) in a 1944 California case *(Ybarra v. Spangard),* is usually applicable where it appears that the patient's injury is of such a nature that it can be said, in the light of past experience, that it *probably* was the result of negligence (failure to abide by professional standards) by someone and that the defendant (hospital and employees) is probably the person/entity who is responsible (*Zentz v. Coca Cola Bottling Co.,* 1952). Thus, *res ipsa loquitur* can be used to establish care below acceptable professional standards where there is no other evidence consistent with the patient's injury or where the patient was unconscious at the time the alleged injury occurred in the emergency room. Although this doctrine was originally introduced to overcome the "conspiracy of silence" that was believed to exist

among medical professionals when a patient was injured, it still lingers on today, even though professional testimony is readily available to establish conduct falling below professional standards.

Nurses and physicians in emergency departments have been sued on theories as varied, numerous, and creative as Walt Disney characters. Some of these suits are listed below to give you an idea of the type of actions that could give rise to civil liability against you and your employer.

In *Johnson v. St. Paul Mercury Insurance Co.* (1969), the hospital was sued because a nurse's *aide* had taken the patient's history, instead of a registered nurse, as was customary. The court held that the aide was not responsible for the doctor's failure to diagnose the patient properly.

In *O'Neil v. Montefiore Hospital* (1960), the court held that the jury should be entitled to decide whether the nurse had been negligent in failing to obtain the services of doctors after the patient's wife informed the nurse that she believed her husband was having a heart attack. After failing to obtain the services of doctors associated with the husband's insurance plan, the nurse refused to have the husband examined or treated at the hospital, and the husband died shortly after arriving home.

Wilmington General Hospital v. Manlove (1961) indicates that liability of a hospital may be based on the *refusal* of services to a patient in case of an "unmistakable emergency." In this case, the nurse on duty in the emergency department informed the parents of a child that the hospital could not provide care because there was a danger of conflict between medicine given by the attending physician and what the hospital physician might prescribe. Although the infant had a temperature of 102° F, the nurse did not examine him, take his temperature, feel his forehead, or look down his throat. The court said that this may fall below the standards of the nursing profession generally.

Petry v. Nassau Hospital (1944) awarded a patient damages against a hospital where the nurse in charge of the emergency department left a patient on an examination table 2½ to 3 feet wide without side rails, and the patient fell from the table, injuring himself.

Quick v. Benedictine Sisters Hospital Association (1960) was a similar case, in which the patient/plaintiff had fallen out of bed while being treated for mental and nervous disorders. The court held that the failure of the nurses to prevent the patient from falling constituted conduct below the acceptable standards of nurses generally and could be *imputed* to the hospital/employer through the doctrine of *respondeat superior*. The court, in announcing the decision, noted:

We adopt the rule that a hospital is liable for the negligence of its nurses in performing mere administrative or clerical acts, which acts, though constituting a part of the patient's prescribed medical treatment, do not require the application of the specialized technique or understanding of a skilled physician or surgeon. This rule, in recognizing that the right of control remains with the hospital as the general employer, is consistent with the nature of such acts and is in accord with the custom which in everyday practice governs the relationship between the hospital staff and the attending physicians (*Quick v. Benedictine Sisters Hospital Association*, 1960, p. 46).

In *McDowell v. County of Alameda* (1979), members of a public hospital emergency department determined that a patient just admitted who was exhibiting bizarre behavior was entitled to medical services under the health plan of another local hospital. The staff requested the patient's private hospital to send an ambulance to transport him for observation, but the hospital refused. The public hospital then placed the subject in a taxi and instructed the driver to take the patient to the private hospital. The patient alighted from the cab soon afterward, never arriving at the private hospital. Two days later the same patient shot and killed another man, whose heirs sued the public hospital for failing to see that the patient safely arrived at his private hospital, thereby protecting the victim from the attack. The court dismissed the case, saying that a governmental immunity statute protected the hospital in its determination not to confine the patient there and that, since the patient had not communicated any threats toward his victim in the presence of the staff, they were not thereby obligated to take action to prevent an act of hostility that they had no way of foreseeing.

Austin v. Regents of the University of California (1979) involved a situation in which a husband was allowed admittance to the delivery room of the hospital where his wife was giving birth to a baby. The wife died during the delivery procedure, but the husband asked the attending physician to deliver the as yet unborn child; the doctor refused, and the husband sued the hospital and the delivery team, contending that after the death of his wife, he was able to feel life in the child, causing him emotional distress for which he sought damages. The California District Court indicated that damages were recoverable against the hospital under the circumstances, although a strong dissent was filed by a Justice that indicated that previous California decisions have allowed recovery in these situations *only* when the person suffering distress at the sight of the death of a loved one has witnessed the death *involuntarily*. In this case, the husband had requested to be admitted to the delivery room where he witnessed the death of the wife and child. Although policy decisions concerning whether or not to allow relatives of badly injured patients into the emergency department to converse with them or see any treatment performed should be dictated by hospital management and the legal staff, decisions such as this seem to give support to a nonadmission policy.

Finally, in *Ramsey v. Physicians Memorial Hospital* (1977), the court of Special Appeals of Maryland held that the failure of a nurse to notify the examining physician of the mother's removal of ticks from the bodies of her infant sons caused the death of one of her sons and the other's near fatal illness. It should be noted in this case that the failure to communicate this information to the physician was largely the fact that the nurse had not written down the mother's statement on the patient's charts when she received the information. Damages were awarded against the hospital for the nurse's negligent omission under the theory of *respondeat superior,* with the court indicating that such damages may encourage nurses to record such critical information on patient's treatment records.

Liability can also be premised on treatment without the patient's consent, which constitutes a technical assault (*Rogers v. Lumberman's Mutual Casualty Co.,* 1960). There are a limited number of situations in which patient consent may be dispensed with, such as in prisons where treatment may be required for the collective good of the inmates, or in emergency situations where actions are required to save a life. In the latter situation, treatment is justifiable on the grounds that a reasonable person would, if *able* to give consent to the treatment, give the required permission for the life-saving measures (*Cobbs v. Grant,* 1972). "Emergency" situations are those that render immediate treatment advisable because of an unexpected or sudden situation (*Moran v. Board of Medical Examiners,* 1947).

In nonemergency situations, as a general rule, even when dealing with a police officer who says that consent of the patient to a particular procedure or treatment is not required, it is advisable, for your own protection, to seek the patient's consent. In this context, the consent of the patient may be obtained orally, although a written consent is certainly preferable. Where such consent is sought, the consent in order to be valid must be "informed," meaning that it must be given by one who is legally and physically *capable* of understanding the nature of the treatment that is being undertaken, the expected result of the proposed treatment, any available alternatives, and most important, any risks associated with the treatment. In addition, consent, to be valid, must be given by a person *legally* competent to consent, meaning an adult of sound mind in most states. In many instances, if an adult is temporarily unable to give an informed consent because of unconsciousness resulting from trauma or sedation, consent may be obtained from another person, provided that person was authorized previously to give such consent by the patient undergoing treatment (Edwards, 1970).

In the case of minors, California courts have required that if the minor is younger than 14

years, consent must be obtained (in nonemergency situations) from either parent, if any, or legal guardian, or person *in loco parentis* (one standing in the place of a parent with a parent's rights, duties, and responsibilities) (*Cobbs v. Grant,* 1972). When minors who are 14 or older are involved, consent is required from the minor patient and either a parent or legal guardian or person standing *in loco parentis*. However, it is advisable that, if the minor does not appear to be capable of understanding and executing an informed consent, the rules for a minor under 14 years be followed. (D'Amico and Sherman, 1978).

In some instances, persons may be admitted to the emergency department who are not legally adults but are *emancipated*. Emancipation of a juvenile may be established by marriage, the earning of one's own living, the maintenance of a home separate from one's parents, or psychological maturity (*Bach v. Long Island Jewish Hospital,* 1966). In the case of an emancipated minor, it is generally permissible to provide treatment upon the minor's consent, without the additional consent of the parent(s).

Some state statutes or court decisions indicate that a finding of "mental illness," even by a judge or jury, does not raise a presumption that the patient is legally *incompetent* to give an informed consent to treatment (California Welfare and Institutions Code, Section 5368). However, any consent given by a patient who is either physically or emotionally traumatized is not likely, in retrospect, to be considered as "informed" by its very nature. Although emergency department personnel are encouraged to seek the consent of patients who have noticeable psychiatric problems, such consent may be ineffective in limiting the hospital's liability for any injuries suffered by that patient while undergoing treatment. Further discussion concerning your dealings as an emergency room nurse with psychiatric patients will be provided at a later point in this chapter.

Finally, in the area of "consent," you will probably hear in your career on one or more occasions the term "implied consent." This term may be used in the context of emergency situations requiring lifesaving measures, as noted above, but more often arises in the discussion of certain state statutes that make driving *privileges* conditional on a driver's "implied consent" to take a chemical test if suspected by a police officer of driving under the influence of alcohol. Under most of these laws, if the suspected drunken driver refuses to submit to a test, he may not generally be forced to do so, but his license may be revoked. As in the area of psychiatric patients, more discussion of the implied consent law and the responsibilities of emergency department personnel in extracting blood samples from suspected drunken drivers upon the request of a police officer is discussed in greater detail later in this chapter.

During this general discussion concerning liability that can arise through your employment in the hospital's emergency department, it has become apparent that your attentions and energies as a nurse should be premised on an ideal of avoiding liability, both for yourself and your employer. Recent attempts in California on the part of some emergency department personnel to defend themselves against alleged acts of negligence have proved largely unavailing, thus making it even more important to avoid the mere allegations in the first place. One such attempt to defend against alleged emergency department malpractice arose in the California case of *Colby v. Schwartz* (1978). In this case, a *physician* accused of negligence in handling a patient in the emergency department defended his conduct by alleging that he, as an emergency department employee, was entitled to be judged by a *less strict standard* than physicians in other parts of the hospital who did not have to undertake desperate emergency lifesaving measures without research and deliberation. Rather, the doctor argued that he should be entitled to the more relaxed standard of liability under California's "good samaritan" act (California Business and Professions Code, Sections 2144 and 2144.5). The court rejected the doctor's argument, holding that he (and presumably all other emergency department personnel) would be judged according to whether the conduct in question fell below that expected of other medical personnel *generally*.

Nevertheless, there have been some encouraging changes in California statutes that are responsive to the difficult situations that emergency department personnel are often confronted with. Thus, a law enacted in California in 1978 provides that when an allegation has been made against an emergency department *physician* that he or she has been negligent, it must be proved that his or her treatment fell below that exercised by reputable members of the physician's or surgeon's profession in the same or similar locality *in like cases and under similar emergency circumstances* (California Health and Safety Code, Section 1768) (emphasis supplied). Unfortunately, the California legislation in its present state is protective only of emergency department physicians and is not addressed to other staff.

DUTY TO REPORT CERTAIN CRIMES TO THE POLICE

Many states, such as California, have statutes that impose an obligation on hospital personnel to report certain crimes to the local law enforcement agency. In California, nurses are mandated to notify the police department when a person is admitted suffering from a wound or other injury inflicted by his own act or the act of another by means of a knife, gun, or other deadly weapon, or in cases in which injuries have been inflicted in violation of a criminal law of the state (California Penal Code, Section 11160). Although nurses faced with a statute such as this may be in doubt as to whether injuries inflicted on a patient by another person using a comb, or kicking the patient with his feet, would constitute injuries inflicted with "deadly weapons," a simple rule for nurses is to *always* contact the local police agency when in doubt as to whether a patient's injuries have been inflicted by a "deadly weapon" or in violation of a criminal law of the state.

One caution may be interjected at this point: In those states whose laws require emergency departments to report certain crimes to the police, it is possible that the law will indicate that any person admitted to the hospital suffering from a psychological or physical condition that has been brought about by an overdose of drugs is *not* an "injury" within the meaning of the law, and hence, there is *no duty on the part of the nurses to report such an overdose to the police* (California Penal Code, Section 11160). This exception to the general rule that self-inflicted injuries should be reported is a result of the California legislature's determination that those who have been plagued with emotional crises resulting in drug abuse should not be discouraged from seeking medical assistance. Certainly, requiring the emergency department nurses to report those seeking medical assistance for drug overdoses to the local police is counterproductive to public policy, which encourages those with problems to seek assistance without the fear of being arrested.

Again, using California law as a guide, you may be required to report another type of criminal violation to the police—that offense commonly called "battered child syndrome." California law requires that in any case in which a minor is brought to the emergency department for diagnosis, examination, or treatment, or when such minor is observed by a registered nurse in the employ of a public health agency, and it *appears* that the minor has been *sexually molested,* or that any other injury has been inflicted on the minor by *willful neglect,* the local police or the county welfare or county health department should be contacted and a report made by one of those agencies (California Penal Code, Section 11161.5). Normally, when a statute mandates such action on the part of nurses, it also provides that they will be *immune* from civil liability for reporting *suspected* battered child syndrome as long as they believed in good faith that the child's injuries were just as consistent with *intentional misconduct* of the parents as they were with a series of accidents or mishaps that normally accompany that child's age group (California Penal Code, Section 11161.5).

Although the California courts have declared that the crime of child abuse or child neglect applies only to children who are born, as opposed to fetuses (*Reyes v. Superior Court,* 1977), this does *not* mean that instances wherein a pregnant woman is beaten and the life of the fetus jeopardized should go unreported to the police. In the first place, the beating of anyone is a violation of the criminal law that

should be reported to the police. Thus, even if the fetus does not die from the beating of the mother, the assailant can still be charged with assault and battery, or aggravated assault against the mother. On the other hand, if the fetus has died as a result of the beating, the assailant may be charged with homicide in some states (California Penal Code, Section 187), if it can be shown that the fetus was viable, which normally occurs about 28 weeks after gestation, but may occur as early as 24 weeks (*Roe v. Wade,* 1973). If the dead fetus was not viable the assailant may still be charged with criminal abortion in some states when it can be proved that the beating of the mother was perpetrated with the intention of killing the fetus (California Penal Code, Section 274).

Although the failure to report crimes in general, or battered child syndrome in particular, is usually treated as a misdemeanor offense, punishable by a short-term jail sentence or a monetary fine, there are more serious potential civil liabilities for failing to carry out these statutory duties. The California Supreme Court, for instance, has indicated that the failure of the hospital staff to report battered child syndrome constitutes medical malpractice (*Landeros v. Flood,* 1976). In *Landeros v. Flood,* the child was initially admitted to the hospital suffering from a spiral fracture of the right tibia and fibula, which gave the appearance of having been caused by a twisting force. The child also had bruises over her entire back, and superficial abrasions on various parts of her body, along with a nondepressed linear fracture of the skull, which was in the process of healing. Despite these injuries, the physician who examined the child failed to notify the police and released the child to her parents, who repeated their acts of inhumanity at a later date.

The *Landeros* decision provided a guideline that can be used by emergency department physicians and nurses alike, although the language is decidedly directed more at the examining physicians. According to the court, the question that must be asked any time that it is alleged that there has been a failure to report battered child syndrome is "whether a reasonably prudent physician examining this [child] in the first place would have been led to suspect that she was a victim of battered child syndrome from the particular injuries and circumstances presented to him, would have confirmed that diagnosis by ordering x-rays of her entire skeleton, and would have promptly reported his findings to the appropriate authorities, to prevent a recurrence of the injuries.''

Two other examples have provided additional guidelines as to when it would be proper to report cases of suspected battered child syndrome and avoid criminal prosecution or imposition of civil liability, or both. According to *Fare v. Maria R.* (1976), the fact that the teenage mother jeopardized the life of her infant by giving her overdoses of aspirin was not sufficient to charge the mother with neglecting or endangering the child. Here, the mother was concededly ignorant of the effects of giving the child too much aspirin, and the court indicated that normally child endangering and child abuse require a *willful,* conscious attempt to bring about the injuries that the child suffered.

Further guidelines are provided by another case (*People v. Beaguez,* 1965), which held that a parent may be charged with child beating or child neglect ''if the parent intentionally places the child in a situation in which serious physical danger or health hazard to the child is reasonably foreseeable, and has knowledge, either actual or constructive, that the act tends to endanger the child's life.''

When you are unsure whether to contact the police because of a patient's suspiciously received injuries, when an infant is admitted for diagnosis or treatment and the injury might have been received by an *intentional* act of another, a good rule of thumb is to contact the police and allow them to determine whether to take a report.

COMMITMENT OF PSYCHIATRIC PATIENTS TO AN EVALUATION FACILITY

There are many instances in which persons with psychiatric problems—either drug-induced or congenital—wander voluntarily into emergency departments. In many cases, these individuals are seeking a sympathetic ear; in some

isolated cases, these individuals become predisposed to trying to attack and bite off that same sympathetic ear. In any event, the possibility of violence perpetrated by a person exhibiting abnormal behavioral characteristics should be guarded against by the presence of several persons in the immediate area of an employee interviewing the patient.

Often after a person who has apparent psychological problems is interviewed, it becomes obvious that the person will require longer-term therapy than he will likely receive from emergency department medical personnel. The question then becomes what to do with the patient. Most states have a law that provides that involuntary detention is permissible for a person who, as a result of a mental disorder, is a danger to himself or herself, to other persons, or is gravely disabled (California Welfare and Institutions Code, Section 5150). The term ''gravely disabled'' is defined in California to mean that the patient is in such a condition that he is ''unable to provide for basic personal needs for food, clothing, or shelter'' (California Welfare and Institutions Code, Section 5008 [h] [1]). When these criteria are apparent, the patient can be detained for up to 72 hours in a mental health facility for psychiatric evaluation and treatment, which can be extended in duration if required.

What happens if a psychiatric patient comes to the hospital, and communicates information to you that he is going to ''kill Barbara, the girl who lives down the street,'' but that other than this one indication of being violent, the patient appears to be lucid, calm, and rational? In *Tarasoff v. The Regents of the University of California* (1976), two psychotherapists employed by the university (who were empowered to sign an involuntary commitment) determined that a patient who had communicated threats toward another person still did not appear to meet the definitional parameters of ''gravely disabled, a danger to himself, or others.'' Hence, they released the patient, who carried out his threats and killed the victim soon afterward. The California Supreme Court indicated that the two psychotherapists were *immune from liability* for failing to confine the patient for 72-hour evaluation, under a governmental immunity statute (California Government Code, Section 856). However, liability was imposed, nevertheless, because the psychotherapists, according to the Court, *had a duty to warn the victim of the threats made by the patient*.

The Court imposed liability on the psychotherapists in *Tarasoff* out of the recognition that when they become aware of the possibility of violence being perpetrated against the victim, they were vested with a *duty* to act to protect the victim—not necessarily by confining the threatening party—but certainly by warning the possible (ultimate) victim. Citing the language of another California case (*Vistica v. Presbyterian Hospital,* 1967), the Supreme Court noted:

When a hospital has notice or knowledge of facts from which it might reasonably be concluded that a patient would likely harm himself or others unless preclusive measures were taken, then the hospital must use reasonable care in the circumstances to prevent such harm.

Thus, the language of *Tarasoff* provides some authority for the proposition that, if a member of the emergency department is informed by a possible psychotic patient of his or her intention to do harm to a *specifically named or identified* individual, such statement should be documented, and the information relayed to the person threatened if possible, or to the police department. Certainly, if the patient made general threats against the community at large, or unnamed individuals with whom he associates, it would seem highly unlikely that the law would impose a duty on the nurse or physician to whom the comments were made to locate and warn the spectrum of potential victims.

Since the *Tarasoff* decision, one case has indicated that a professional person who hears a patient threaten to *commit suicide* may not be held liable for failing to communicate that threat to relatives if the patient does in fact take his or her life at a later date. Thus, the court in *Bellah v. Greenson* (1978) refused to impose liability on a psychiatrist for failing to tell a young girl's parents that she had threatened

suicide. The girl later took an overdose of sleeping pills. The court based its ruling of nonliability on the fact that no duty exists to communicate threats to harm or kill *onself* (as opposed to another person). Nevertheless, it should be noted that this case involved a *professional relationship* between a psychiatrist and patient, where confidentiality of the client's secrets is of utmost importance.

HELPING POLICE OFFICERS GATHER EVIDENCE

There may be some instances in which you can be considered as an "agent" of the police, in addition to being an "agent" of the hospital. One such situation in which an agency relationship with the police may occur is in those instances where you find *contraband* (any items that are illegal to possess) in the clothing or on the person of a patient. This situation most often arises when a patient is admitted in an unconscious or semiconscious condition, and removal of the clothing is necessary to determine the nature and location of injuries. If during such a process an item is discovered that you believe is forbidden (such as a small handgun or restricted narcotics), it may be best to note when and where you discovered the item and contact the police. Although you should never go into the pockets of a patient affirmatively seeking out possible incriminating evidence, if such evidence is discovered *inadvertently,* there is case authority for using it in a subsequent criminal proceeding (*People v. Gonzales,* 1960).

Most of the time you will become an agent of the police at their *request*. The most frequent contact you can expect to have with the police in this context is when you are requested to take blood from a suspected drunken driver for blood alcohol analysis. Many states have what are commonly called "implied consent" laws, which require drivers detained by police officers to take one of several chemical tests (usually blood, breath, or urine) to determine the alcohol content of their blood (California Vehicle Code, Section 13353[a]). Refusal by the driver to take or complete one of the chemical tests will normally result in suspension of the driving privilege for a specified time period, usually 6 months to a year. Normally, when a police officer brings a suspected drunken driver into the hospital and requests a blood sample to be taken by the nursing staff, it is the result of the *driver's request* after being advised of the alternative tests available by the arresting officer. There are other occasions when a police officer may request a blood sample to be taken for an arrestee who is suspected of driving under the influence of drugs, or a combination of drugs and alcohol. It is common, for instance, for an officer to request a blood sample in instances when the driver is suspected of having ingested any form of *barbiturate* or sedative. Obviously, a breath sample would not help the officer determine the amount of drugs ingested, and analyses of barbiturates are, according to many crime laboratories, difficult to obtain from urine samples.

Most arrests involving drunk drivers, whether by drugs or alcohol, are *misdemeanors,* meaning they are less serious than felony crimes, and usually carry a possible monetary fine, and in some instances a short jail sentence. A driver will be charged with *felony* drunk driving in most states if he or she causes an accident and the *injury* of another person while driving in an inebriated condition (California Vehicle Code, Section 23101[a] [alcohol], and 23106 [a] [drugs]).

You are going to be faced with situations in the emergency department in which a police officer attempts to make you an "agent" for purposes of taking a blood sample from a drunk driving arrestee who *has not consented* to the taking of such blood. What do you do? First of all, although this is not a text on police procedures, I cannot envision any instances in which a police officer will request that a blood sample be taken forcibly from a suspected drunk driver charged with a mere *misdemeanor,* with the exception of driving under the influence of drugs, to which the implied consent law does not apply. This is because, if such a driver refuses to give a test voluntarily, the arresting officer should recommend the suspension of the driving privilege under the state's "implied consent" laws, and not force the driver to take any test. Courts who scrutinize blood tests taken forcibly in misdemeanor arrests may not believe that such a procedure is warranted in a relatively minor offense, especially when the drunk driver who has refused the test may lose his or her driving privilege altogether and still be prosecuted for drunk driving without the presence of a chemical test. The vast majority of instances in which you will be requested to withdraw blood forcibly from a drunk driver will be those situations in which the driver is charged with a *felony* offense (he has caused an accident and injured another person).

The forcible taking of blood is governed by guidelines established by the United States Supreme Court in *Schmerber v. California* (1966). *Schmerber* says that blood can be taken from a nonconsenting arrestee *"provided it is done in a reasonable, medically approved manner,* is incident to the person's arrest, and is based on the [officer's] reasonable belief that the person is intoxicated." Obviously, the requirement that the blood be taken in a reasonable, medically approved manner is critical to those in the emergency department. The significance of conforming to this standard for personnel taking the blood is twofold: First, if the blood is taken in an "unreasonable" manner, it cannot be used against the arrestee at his trial. Second, and more important to you, it *could* result in the arrestee suing you and the hospital for assault and battery.

One case involved the forcible taking of blood from a drunken driver that was determined to be unreasonable. The case, *People v. Kraft* (1970), involved two police officers wrestling the arrestee to the floor in the emergency department, with the arrestee screaming and kicking the entire time, and one of the officers placing a "scissor-lock" around the arrestee's body with his legs. The court trying the arrestee for misdemeanor drunk driving refused to allow the blood sample as evidence and chastised the officers (and nurses) in open court, saying, "strong arm behavior by police officers cannot be tolerated, even while we recognize the importance of prosecuting and convicting drunken drivers."

Another case (*People v. Fite,* 1968) provides further guidelines for the forcible taking of blood, holding, ''The implied consent law does not call for the exclusion of blood alcohol tests over the defendant's refusals to submit, when such taking is in *no way brutal or shocking to the conscience.''* Unfortunately, the court decisions to date make it incumbent upon *you* —the person taking the blood—to determine if the taking will be ''unreasonable'' or ''brutal or shocking to the conscience.'' It would seem to be a safe conclusion that if there is going to be a ''tug-of-war'' between the arresting officer(s) and the arrestee, which will involve flying night sticks, profanities, and leather restraints, there is a good possibility that the taking of blood in such a situation would come within the parameters of ''brutal and shocking to the conscience.'' On the other hand, if the arrestee merely verbally protests the taking of the blood, but does not physically resist, or only resists momentarily, the taking of blood would seem to be permissible by contemporary standards, especially in felony arrests, where the leeway given officers is generally greater in gathering evidence against the accused.

What if the suspected drunken driver is unconscious or incapable of consenting because of his or her degree of intoxication? Many states have provided that blood may be taken from such a person without his consent (California Vehicle Code, Section 13353[a]). Other important considerations to keep in mind when taking blood include remembering that arrestees for suspected drunken driving do not generally have the right to have their attorney present before or during the taking of blood (*Skinner v. Silas,* 1975), nor do they have the right to consult an attorney before determining which of the three chemical tests they take under the ''implied consent'' law (California Vehicle Code, Section 13363[a]). You should always inform the arresting officer of the sterilizing agent used on the arrestee's arm when drawing blood and take the actual sample in the *physical presence* of the officer, which will be important from the standpoint of ''chain of evidence.''

Here is a final, but very important reminder

with regard to the taking of blood at the request of officers. Most states provide that blood should be withdrawn after *written request* by the law enforcement officer and that, if such procedure is followed, the nurse/hospital will incur *no civil or criminal liability* (unless, of course, the sample was taken negligently and the needle was broken under the arrestee's skin, for instance) (California Vehicle Code, Section 13354). Moreover, where such general grant of immunity to the emergency department is given by statute, the statute may recognize that only the signature of the *arresting officer* is needed, and it is *not necessary* for the *arrestee* to sign the consent form in order to exempt the hospital from civil or criminal liability.

ADMINISTERING LAXATIVES AND EMETICS

It is a common practice among heroin dealers to package the powder in balloons that can easily be ''transported'' in the mouth (as many as ten balloons at a time). The balloons, which generally sell for a minimum of $25 apiece, can be readily swallowed by the dealer when approached by the police and will be later eliminated and retrieved through the excretory process. The United States Supreme Court has declared that an officer's act of choking a heroin dealer to prevent his swallowing the balloons is ''brutal and shocking conduct,'' and that officers should not resort to such measures to obtain the evidence (*Rochin v. California,* 1952). Because it may take hours or days after the balloons are swallowed before the arrestee defecates, and because it is necessary to keep him under constant observation during that period in order to seize the evidence before it is flushed, officers have understandably started seeking other, more expeditious means of obtaining the balloons.

One means of obtaining the evidence is to have the local emergency department nurse administer either a laxative or emetic to the arrestee and force him to eliminate the balloon(s) in either the excrement or vomitus. If this happens to you, there are several things that should be kept in mind. First of all, unlike the taking of blood samples, there is no peace officer request form that authorizes the hospital to administer a laxative or emetic and exempts the staff from civil and criminal liability for so doing. There should be an *express understanding* between the officer requesting and the nurse administering that the procedure is being undertaken upon the officer's request and authorization and that such indication will be reflected in the police report of the incident. Moreover, the *arrestee's consent* should be noted on the chart.

If the arrestee refuses to submit to the procedure *voluntarily,* there is case law that suggests that an officer should not request the forcible elimination of this evidence, unless it is done pursuant to a search warrant issued by a magistrate (yes, a search warrant can be issued for the contents of one's digestive system), which makes the procedure presumptively lawful (*United States v. Jeffers,* 1951). Two relatively recent cases (*People v. Bracamonte,* 1975; *People v. Rodriguez,* 1977) indicate that, without such a warrant or voluntary consent of the arrestee or a medical *emergency that is life threatening,* the intrusion into the body through the administration of a laxative or emetic to obtain evidence of this nature violates the patient's right to privacy. In these situations, the courts have instructed officers to allow the normal process of digestion and elimination to occur before retrieving the balloons (*People v. Rodriguez,* 1977). More important, since the procedure does not have the general approval of the courts (unless the arrestee consents, the officer has a search warrant, or one of the balloons has burst inside the body, creating a medical emergency), your participation in the gathering of evidence could lead to a lawsuit charging you with violation of the patient's constitutional rights to privacy (42 United States Code, Section 1983).

DEAD PATIENTS: INTERACTION WITH THE LOCAL CORONER'S OFFICE

Recently, a nurse told me of an incident in an emergency department of a hospital where a stabbing victim had been admitted in very critical condition and had died shortly thereafter.

The poor man had apparently not yet gasped his last breath before the local police detective was clamoring for the nurse to release clothing and other personal effects to him, which would be used as evidence in prosecuting the murderer. The detective was told—quite properly—to sit down and be patient until the local coroner's office representative arrived, who would release any property to the detective.

In deaths attributable to sudden, violent, or unusual circumstances, where the deceased has not been attended by a physician in a certain number of days before death; in deaths related to or following known or suspected self-induced or criminal abortion; in cases of known or suspected suicide, homicide, or accidental poisoning; in deaths attributable to accidents, drowning, fire, hanging, gunshot, stabbing, exposure, acute alcoholism, drug overdose, drug addiction, or any other death caused by criminal means; the involvement of the coroner's office is usually mandated by statute (California Government Code, Section 27491). California law requires the coroner's office to be notified upon the death of any patient in a hospital operated by the State Department of Health of any successor agency (California Government Code, Section 27491). These statutes usually require the coroner's office to inquire into the circumstances surrounding death and to sign the death certificate.

However, even though the coroner's office should be contacted by the emergency department in any of the situations described above, most states also require the police to be notified of deaths that appear to be the result of criminal conduct (California Government Code, Section 27491.1). Although the police should be aware of such situations *before* the patient is admitted, personnel in the emergency department should contact the police if it becomes apparent that they have not been apprised of the death. In addition, those police detectives who are eager to take property of the deceased before the arrival of the coroner's office should be made to comply with the laws of the majority of states, which indicate that it is unlawful for anyone—nurse, physician, or police officer—to remove "paper, money, or property'' from the deceased before the arrival of a representative of the coroner's office, or without permission of the coroner. (California Government Code, Section 27491.3). In those instances where an officer is allowed to take property of the deceased, it should only be with knowledge and consent of the coroner and only after a receipt is prepared listing the property, which is acknowledged by the police officer in writing (California Government Code, Section 27491.3).

OBTAINING PHYSICAL EVIDENCE IN RAPE INVESTIGATION

There has been an encouraging trend in the area of criminal procedure and evidence that has made the prosecution of a defendant charged with rape less traumatic and embarrassing to the victim, who, under earlier laws, was herself often on trial for promiscuity. Many new laws prohibit the use of evidence of a rape victim's past sexual conduct to prove a lack of chastity in the particular encounter (California Evidence Code, Sections 1103[2] and 782), thus encouraging women to report this crime without the fear and stigma associated with the courtroom ordeal. However, the burden is still on the prosecution (and the police) to gather sufficient evidence to convict the accused rapist, and if the prosecution fails to introduce sufficient evidence, the defendant must *necessarily* go free. Hence, you may again become an ''agent'' of the police in the collection of vital evidence for a rape investigation.

Rape, which is defined with minor variances by different states, normally requires three factors, all of which must be proved: (1) lack of consent, (2) penetration, however slight, and (3) unlawfulness. Medical evidence may be necessary to establish both penetration and lack of consent, but is generally of little value in determining unlawfulness, which depends on the applicable state law (Root, Ogden, and Scott, 1974). From the standpoint only of the police, the medical records of a rape victim should contain the following information (Fisher, 1975):

1. General physical appearance and demeanor of patient.

2. Presence or absence of marks on clothing, and condition of clothing.
3. Presence or absence of violence and tissue damage to the body and its character and location.
4. Secretions for microscopic examination, if requested.
5. Blood, hair, or any other specimen collected, and their disposition.

Keep in mind that, when you record any of the above information or any other information on the patient's chart, the rape victim is required to sign a consent to release any copies of the record to the law enforcement agency. Otherwise, these records should be obtained by the use of a *subpoena duces tecum* (a writ requiring documents in court) (Fisher, 1975).

Physical evidence normally requested in rape investigations can be expected to include vaginal, anal, and oral smears and swabs, vaginal or anal aspirate, suspected seminal stains on the skin of the victim, pubic hair from the victim, and saliva and blood samples.

If these evidentiary items are gathered at the behest of a law enforcement officer, they should normally be turned over to the officer, who will then place them in evidence and give them to the crime laboratory for examination. Perhaps the soundest word of advice with respect to examinations of suspected rape victims is that if the examination is to be performed on a female victim by a male physician, a female nurse should be present in the same room the entire time. Recently, a male physician examined a teenage woman who claimed she had been raped. The physician informed the woman that this examination indicated no trauma to the genital area. The woman made an allegation to the hospital administration that the physician had exceeded the boundaries of a permissible examination, and an investigation was launched, which was highly damaging to the integrity of the physician's reputation. Luckily for the physician, one of the officers who had brought the female to the hospital had placed his ear to the door of the examination room. He was able to refute the women's allegations and substantiate the testimony of the doctor. If there is a moral to this tale, it is that female nurses should insist on physical presence during the examination of suspected rape victims, for the welfare of both their patients and their co-workers.

TESTIFYING IN COURT PURSUANT TO SUBPOENAS

Some of the various ways in which you will be asked to become an "agent" of the police include instances in which you have heard a patient make an incriminating statement, in which you inadvertently find evidence, or in which you take blood or other evidence at the request of a police officer. In many cases where you have helped gather evidence (blood samples, for instance), special rubber stamps may be used to affix a standard format to the arrestee's hospital records (which will be subpoenaed), indicating the nature of your actions in the matter. Your verbal testimony in most of these instances will not be essential. Other methods may be used in some states to relieve the emergency room staff from having to personally testify in court. California, for instance, has just enacted a law that permits nurses who have taken blood samples from persons arrested for drunk driving to testify through the use of written affidavits, negating the requirement for physical presence in court (California Evidence Code, Section 712). This legislation is the result of a recognition that the interests of justice can be served without interfering with the personal and professional life of the emergency department staff. Nevertheless, there will be other instances in which you will be expected to make a physical appearance in a courtroom because of the seriousness of the case, the nature of your participation, or the desires of the defense attorney or prosecutor for your testimony.

The means by which the government will require your presence in court is a subpoena. A subpoena is normally defined as a documentary order signed by a magistrate, court clerk, district attorney or his investigator, or public defender or his investigator, compelling attendance before the court on the date and time noted (California Penal Code, 1326). Most states require that in order for service of a sub-

poena to be effective, the nurse must be personally served with the subpoena. Many conversations I have had with emergency department staff (nurses and physicians alike) have revealed that it is a rather common practice for the emergency department secretary to accept service of all subpoenas *on behalf* of the individuals subpoenaed. This process is administratively easier on the issuing authority, but is still technically invalid. Hence, the members of the emergency staff could conceivably demand that all subpoenas be served personally, or refuse to obey them entirely.

The language of this discussion has thus far focused on the technical aspects of the subpoena process. Although technically you should be served with subpoenas personally, there is no reason why—speaking now from the practical standpoint—you should object to the emergency department secretary accepting service on your behalf. If the hospital that employs you has an efficient procedure that relays copies of subpoenas to you as they are received without fail, you are probably well advised to continue utilizing it. If, on the other hand, copies of subpoenas are strewn about the emergency department in various places "in the hope" that the subpoenaed party will miraculously locate the subpoena, it is highly recommended that the procedure for accepting and relaying the subpoenas be changed, or that you demand to be served personally.

Upon receiving a subpoena, check to see if it requires your physical presence in a particular court on a given date and time, or if it places you "on call." If the subpoena indicates that you are on call, you will be expected to be someplace where you can be contacted by the emergency department (which is usually called by the court, if an on-call witness is needed) and from which you can arrive at the court in a short time, usually within an hour. If you are placed on call during a day off it is best to plan your activity in such a way that you can be near a telephone and to let the emergency department secretary know the number at which you can be contacted.

In the event that you have been "effectively" served with a subpoena, but you fail to appear as ordered or you cannot be located pursuant to an on-call subpoena, you may find yourself the participant in an exciting but unexpected trip—to the local courthouse—handcuffed in the rear of a sheriff's or marshall's car. Most state laws pertaining to subpoenas in criminal cases make failure to obey the subpoena punishable as contempt of court, which may result in your incarceration for a short period of time, or in the assessment of a monetary fine (California Penal Code, Section 1331). Although as a practical matter the contempt power of the court is not used in all cases wherein a party has failed to appear as ordered, it is an ever present "incentive" for prompting your attendance before the court. If you have failed for some reason to appear as ordered in the subpoena, it would greatly benefit your cause if you have a plausible explanation for your failure.

BIBLIOGRAPHY

Alden v. Providence Hospital, 382 F.2d 163 (D.C. Cir. 1967).
61 American Jurisprudence 2d., Physicians, Surgeons, and Other Healers.
Austin v. Regents of the University of California, 2 Civ. No. 53279 (Cal. Ct. App., 2d Dist., Feb. 9, 1979).
Bach v. Long Island Jewish Hospital, 48 Misc. 2d 207, 267 N.Y.S.2d 289 (Sup. Ct., 1966).
Bellah v. Greenson, 81 Cal. App. 3d 614, 146 Cal. Rptr. 535 (1978).
California Business and Professions Code, Sections 2144 and 2144.5.
California Evidence Code, Section 712 (Effective 1-1-79).
California Evidence Code, Section 1103(2) and 782.
California Government Code, Section 856.
California Government Code, Section 27491.
California Government Code, Section 27491.1.
California Government Code, Section 27491.3.
California Health and Safety Code, Section 1768.
California Penal Code, Section 187.
California Penal Code, Section 274.
California Penal Code, Section 1326.
California Penal Code, Section 1331.
California Penal Code, Section 11160.
California Penal Code, Section 11161.5.
California Vehicle Code, Section 13353.
California Vehicle Code, Section 13353(a).
California Vehicle Code, Section 13354.
California Vehicle Code, Section 13363(a).
California Vehicle Code, Section 23101(a) (alcohol), and 23106(a) (drugs).
California Welfare and Institutions Code, Section 5008(h) (1).
California Welfare and Institutions Code, Section 5150.
California Welfare and Institutions Code, Section 5157.
California Welfare and Institutions Code, Section 5368.
Cobbs v. Grant, 502 P.2d 1, 104 Cal. Rptr. 505 (1972).
Colby v. Schwartz, 78 Cal. App. 3d 885, 144 Cal. Rptr. 624 (1978).
D'Amico, S., and Sherman, S. L.: Legal considerations. In Warner, C. G., editor: Emergency care: assessment and intervention, ed. 2, St. Louis, 1978, The C. V. Mosby Co., p. 17.
Edwards, S. L.: Failure to inform is medical malpractice, 23 Vanderbilt L. Rev. 754 (1970).
Fare v. Maria R., 64 Cal. App. 3d 731, 135 Cal. Rptr. 2 (1976).
Fisher, B. A.: Physical Evidence Utilization in Rape Cases. In Physical Evidence Bulletin, Los Angeles County Sheriff's Department, March, 1975.
Foley v. Bishop Clarkson Hospital, 195 Neb.89, 173 N.W.2d 881 (1970). See also American Jurisprudence 2d, Hospitals & Asylums, Section 26, p. 869.
Johnson v. St. Paul Mercury Ins. Co. 219 So.2d 524 (La. App. 1969).
Landeros v. Flood, 17 Cal. 3d 399, 131 Cal.Rptr. 69, 551 P.2d 389 (1976).
Manlove v. Wilmington General Hospital, 53 Del. 338, 169 A.2d 18 (1961).
McDowell v. County of Alameda, 1 Civ. No. 43452 (Cal. Ct. App. 1st. Dist. Jan. 16, 1979).
Moran v. Board of Medical Examiners, 187 P.2d 878 (1947).
O'Neil v. Montefiore Hospital, 202 N.Y.S.2d 436 (1960).
People v. Beaguez, 232 Cal.App.2d 650, 43 Cal.Rptr 28 (1965).
People v. Bracamonte, 15 Cal.3d 394 (1975).
People v. Fite, 267 Cal.App.2d 685, 73 Cal.Rptr. 666 (1968).
People v. Gonzales, 183 Cal.App. 2d 276, 5 Cal.Rptr. 920 (1960). See also Coolidge v. New Hampshire, 403 U.S. 443, 91 S.Ct. 2022, 29 L.Ed 2d 564 (1971).
People v. Kraft, 3 Cal.App. 3d 890, 84 Cal.Rptr. 280 (1970).
People v. Rodriguez, 71 Cal.App. 3d 547, 139 Cal.Rptr. 509 (1977).
Petry v. Nassau Hospital, 48 N.Y.S.2d 277, 50 N.Y.S. 2d 436 (App. Div. 1944).
Quick v. Benedictine Sisters Hospital Association, 102 N.W.2d 36 (1960).
Ramsey v. Physicians Memorial Hospital, Inc. 373 A.2d 26 (1977).
Reyes v. Superior Court, 75 Cal.App.3d 214, 141 Cal. Rptr. 912 (1977).
Rochin v. California, 342 U.S. 165, 72 S.Ct. 205, 96 L.Ed. 183 (1952).
Roe v. Wade, 410 U.S. 113 (1973).
Rogers v. Lumbermen's Mutual Casualty Co., 119 So.2d 649 (La.App. 1960).
Root, I., Ogden, W., and Scott, W.: The Medical Investigation of Alleged Rape, West. J. Med. **120:**329, 1974.
Schmerber v. California, 384 U.S. 757, 86 S.Ct. 1826 (1966).
Seneris v. Haas, 45 Cal.2d 811, 291 P.2d 951 (1955).

Skinner v. Silas, 58 Cal.App. 3d 591, 130 Cal.Rptr. 91 (1975).

Tarasoff v. Regents of the University of California, 17 Cal.3d 425, 131 Cal.Rptr. 14 (1976).

Tunkl v. Regents of the University of California, 50 Cal.2d 92, 383 P.2d 441 (1963).

United States v. Jeffers, 342 U.S. 48, 72 S.Ct. 93, 96 L.Ed. 59 (1951).

42 United States Code Section 1983.

Vistica v. Presbyterian Hospital, 67 Cal.2d 465, 62 Cal. Rptr. 577, 432 P.2d 193 (1967).

Wilmington General Hospital v. Manlove, 54 Del. 15, 174 A.2d 135 (1961).

Ybarra v. Spangard, 25 Cal.2d 486, 154 P.2d 687 (1944).

Zentz v. Coca Cola Bottling Co., 39 Cal.2d 436, 247 P.2d 344 (1952).

CHAPTER 5

Emergency department management

Barbara Weldon King

Emergency department management is one of the most exciting, challenging fields in health care today. Emergency medicine is a relatively new, dynamic, and rapidly changing specialty. There are still many areas of controversy and many areas yet to be researched. Opening a chest in the emergency department was unheard of 10 years ago. Twenty years ago hardly anyone had heard of prehospital care.

The people who work in emergency departments are unique and challenging to manage. Most emergency people do not like routine; they enjoy bringing order out of chaos; they are motivated, aggressive, and not content in a static environment. Keeping up with an ever changing field and with people who are easily bored is not an easy task; but it certainly can be rewarding.

This chapter does not present new scientific studies in management. It does present some basic, practical, and easily understood ideas about people and systems. In a single chapter, it is not possible to explore in depth all the aspects of management. Entire books have been written about motivation, goal setting, performance reviews, and various other management topics.

As you read about management, it is important to remember that there are as many management styles as there are managers. Although it is hoped that the ideas presented here are sound and useful ideas, in management, unfortunately, there are no absolutes. What works in

one system or with one person may not be appropriate in every system or with every person. Part of the chapter will discuss the importance of common sense and perspective in the manager. If there were true absolutes in management, that need for common sense and perspective could be deleted.

The first section of this chapter addresses a few of the "systems" parts of management: goal setting, problem solving, and dealing with structure and change. The second section deals with the management of people. The emphasis in this chapter is more on the people part of management for two reasons. First, I tend to be more "people-oriented" (sometimes an asset, sometimes a liability) than "systems-oriented"; and second, people everywhere are pretty much the same (collectively speaking, that is), but systems vary widely.

Many of the sections here will overlap and repeat ideas from other sections. Management is an integrated process, and it is not possible to totally isolate one component from another—either in practice or on paper.

I would like the reader to take away from the discussions the ideas and concepts—not formulas. There are no magic formulas. Management is primarily an art, not a science.

MANAGEMENT OF THE SYSTEM

According to Webster, a system is "an established way of doing something." Having a collection of the most talented, motivated people in the world is nice, but if there are not systems for guiding their efforts, confusion and chaos result, and the overall output is significantly decreased. To illustrate, suppose you did not have a system for scheduling and simply called around every day looking for people to work. Most of the available administrative time would be spent on the phone. Imagine, also, a patient's chart that did not have specific areas labeled to indicate what should be recorded. Much time would be spent trying to locate the patient's name, address, and orders on the chart. The same principles apply to less obvious areas, including goal setting and problem solving.

The first portion of the chapter discusses a few of the systems areas of management: goal setting, problem solving, project management, and structure and change. The intent here is to convey that systems are essential to smooth operation. This section provides some examples of systems for managing certain areas, but the important thing is that the manager understand the *need* for a defined method of operating. It is certainly easy to understand the need in scheduling and in chart design, but it is also important to have a systematic process for setting goals and resolving performance problems. For example, a staff member comes to you and says that nobody is restocking the rooms anymore. If you do not understand the need for a defined method of approaching these problems, your response might be to simply *demand* at the next staff meeting that everyone stock his or her room. If you have a defined approach, the investigation might reveal that someone moved all the supplies and nobody can find anything to restock with.

Systems are essential. Develop your own, use somebody else's, or do both, but don't assume you can successfully manage without them.

Setting goals and objectives

If you don't know where you are going, you will end up somewhere else.

L. Peter

In emergency care, the only predictable thing is change, usually rapid and often dramatic.

Medical care changes, health care systems change, prehospital care changes—nothing seems to stabilize for more than a few days at a time. In the midst of all this, it is very easy to get caught up in daily "fire-fighting" and lose sight of long-term goals.

"Fire-fighting" (dealing with the 1,001 problems that crop up every day) can be a full-time job if you allow it to be. The only way to avoid this fire-fighting syndrome, (or "management by crisis" as it is sometimes called) is to be zealous in your commitment to goal setting and goal achievement.

Laurence Peter is accurate: "If you don't know where you are going, you will end up somewhere else." The importance of goal setting cannot be overemphasized. Conscious attention to where you are versus where you want to be is imperative if you expect to establish and maintain a progressive emergency service. Although no one goal-setting method is right for every environment, the following guidelines may be useful in establishing a goal-setting process.

Goal-setting activities should be a cooperative effort between nursing and physician administration. If goals are established independently, it is likely that too many projects will be activated simultaneously, resulting in staff frustration, stress, and confusion. It is also important that all members of the team understand the objectives, which is difficult to achieve if goals are not mutually agreed on ahead of time.

The medical director and nursing supervisor may be the only ones directly involved in the goal-setting process, or all the administrative staff may be involved. Representatives may be selected from the department staff to participate in the process, or written input may be solicited from all staff members.

The first step in this goal-setting process is to define the *strategic goals* for the department. There are two kinds of strategic goals: the first represents the overall philosophy of the department. Some examples of overall strategic goals are "provide optimal emergency care"; "meet the needs of all client groups" (that is, patients, physicians, community); "provide opportunities for professional advancement."

There should be few overall strategic goals —no more than five—and they do not change. These philosophical "goals" essentially represent the department's "reason for existence," and they provide the basis for all other goal setting. Outlining these philosophies is therefore a very important part of the goal-setting process.

The second kind of strategic goals are established annually. Every department should, formally and *in writing*, define the departmental goals for the year. Each of these annual goals should relate to one or more of the "philosophical" goals. For example, "Ensure appropriate initial patient screening" is an annual goal and relates directly to the overall goal of providing optimal medical care. "Minimize patient processing time" is a goal that relates to meeting the needs of the patient client group. Annual strategic goals represent *where you want to be*. Annual goals, therefore, require that you first know where you are.

Emergency department status survey. The emergency department status survey on p. 54 is an assessment tool developed by Dr. James K. Fulcher for use in the goal-setting process. This survey is an outline of those areas of emergency department operation that should be assessed annually to provide a clear picture of *where you are*. The outline lists several key areas of operation and subcategorizes each of these areas. Use of this assessment tool is invaluable when establishing annual goals.

The status survey must be done in writing. Each subcategory should be honestly reviewed. This tool is for *internal* use only. Keeping the status survey within the department will enable the reviewer(s) to be accurate and honest in their assessment. Hospital administration may receive the results of the survey—the annual goals—but need not see the survey. For instance, if your survey of the billing/collection system says "collections are at an all-time low," one of your annual goals may be "improve collection at time of service," but it is reasonable that your superiors see only the goal and not the survey statement. This is *not* to say that one should try and keep secrets, but it is easier to be truly honest if this survey is not widely circulated, particularly since it contains information about other departments that could be misunderstood.

Each category of the status survey should be assessed, even if it is a simple statement such as "no major problems." All categories should be assessed based on their relationship to what would be "perfection." Clearly, perfection in all areas, at all times, is not a realistic goal, but aiming for less than 100% will only lower the ultimate result.

Ideally, the status survey should be completed by two or three key administrative people independently and then compared. It is most interesting to look at different perceptions of the same areas. For even more diverse views, ask two or three of the staff members to complete the survey.

After the survey has been completed and compiled, the people responsible for annual goal setting should meet to review this assessment and set goals for the year. Annual goal setting requires three "Cs": commitment, compromise, and common sense.

The people involved in goal setting must have a *commitment* to the process and an understanding of its importance. They must also be mature enough to be committed to the achievement of the final goals even if some of the goals decided on are not the ones they would have chosen.

Goal setters must be willing to look at all perceptions and *compromise* when necessary. There should be a spirit of cooperation and mutual respect among the individuals involved.

Finally, goal setting calls for *common sense*. The worse shape the department is in, the easier it is to set goals; major deficiencies are then much more obvious. As a department becomes more finely tuned, the lines become much grayer, and deficiencies are not so glaring. Common sense is essential when priorities are established for departmental improvement. "Thorough knowledge of renal pathophysiology" is probably unrealistic if no one in the department is certified in basic CPR. An exaggerated example, for sure, but it is not unusual to see lofty goals set when the basics are not yet covered. So, assuming that all the goal setters have the three "Cs", you should be able to come up with annual goals without a great

Emergency department status survey*

I. Facility and equipment
   A. Size and design
   B. Emergency equipment
   C. Stocking and control procedures
   D. Equipment checking procedures

II. Charts and records
   A. Design
   B. Chart procedures
   C. Storage and retrieval
   D. Statistics

III. Administration/management
   A. Personnel
   B. Policy/procedure manual
   C. Communications
   D. Administrative procedures
   E. Budget

IV. Personnel
   A. Staffing
   B. Back-up procedures
   C. Morale
   D. Evaluation
   E. Orientation
   F. Recruitment standards

V. Logistics of patient care
   A. Triage
   B. Admission procedures
   C. Discharge procedures
   D. Hospital admission
   E. "Processing" paperwork
   F. Telephone communications
   G. Billing/collection

VI. Ancillary services
   A. Radiology
   B. Laboratory
   C. Pulmonary
   D. ECG
   E. Social services
   F. Other

VII. Attending staff relationships
   A. Private physicians
   B. Back-up physicians
   C. Emergency committee

VIII. Interhospital relationships
   A. Administration
   B. Medical staff office
   C. Business office
   D. Nursing administration

IX. Extrahospital relationships
   A. Police department(s)
   B. Fire department
   C. Others

X. Paramedic/ambulance services

XI. Quality monitoring
   A. Chart review
   B. Standards/protocols

XII. Education
   A. CPR training
   B. Continuing education
   C. Reference materials

*Developed by James K. Fulcher.

Examples of assessment following.

EXAMPLE 1: Section I, Part A.
   A. Size and design: The size of the emergency department is adequate for our current census and would probably remain adequate up to an increase of another 300 to 400 patients per month. The design of our cardiac/trauma room is, however, inefficient. During major cases, there appears to be much unnecessary running around for equipment and supplies. This problem warrants further study.

EXAMPLE 2: Section VI, Part F.
   F. Other (Medical Records): The current handling of the emergency department records by the medical records office is unsatisfactory. It often seems that the medical records department has difficulty locating our previous records in a timely fashion. We should work with the medical records director to attempt to resolve this problem. The emergency department handling of the patient record presents no major problem at this time.

EXAMPLE 3: Section VIII, Part D.
   D. Nursing administration: Our relationship with the critical care units is, overall, not a problem. It would, however, be helpful to develop a more regular system of communication and feedback with these units.

deal of difficulty. Before we move to objectives, there is one final goal-setting warning, especially to those who are new to the goal-setting process: *Be realistic*. Tackling lab and x-ray delays, the collection system, medical record problems, new emergency department charts, a facility redesign, and the care of multiple trauma patients all in one year will only result in frustration and discouragement at the end of the year. There should be only two or three major goals for a year. There may be some minor "clean-up" goals in addition, but attempting to resolve four or more major deficiencies in 12 months is unrealistic.

Tactical objectives. Once the annual goals have been decided on, each *goal* should be broken down into *tactical objectives*. Writing objectives helps determine the cause of the deficiency and work toward resolution. "Ensure thorough documentation of all cardiac arrests" is an excellent goal, but the statement itself is hardly a sufficient basis for action. Going to the emergency department staff and saying "improve your CPR documentation" will not be well received or productive. Tactical objectives for the above goal follow.

1. Establish criteria for CPR documentation.
2. Review 20 CPR charts and compare with criteria.
3. Assess cause of deficiency.
4. Implement staff education, charting format, and so on to correct deficiency.
5. Review results (re-audit).

There is one more step in the process, and that is the task outline. A *task outline* is a listing of specific activities necessary to meet each *objective*. Each *objective* should have a *task outline*, and that is discussed in the section on project management.

At this point, there are undoubtedly a number of readers who are wondering when one has the time to actually resolve deficiencies after spending all this time outlining the deficiency itself and the mechanisms for resolution. There are several responses to that query.

1. With practice, the time involved to do this becomes less and less
2. All these activities already go on in your head if you do any kind of goal setting.

3. Knowing the steps ahead of time helps diminish confusion and delay later on.
4. Although goal setting should be a formal activity with meetings and the involvement of all key people, the objectives and responsibility for achievement may be parceled out to individuals.
5. Task outlines (to be discussed later) need not be a formal-typed-submit-to-committee activity. Task outlines can be jotted down and kept for reference so that as one step is completed you can move rapidly on to the next.

Summary. Goal setting is essential. No one can keep up with changes, new regulations, and requirements and maintain systems that are already in progress unless there is an organized system for doing so. If you doubt this, check with managers who you know have a well-run, progressive department and find out how they have achieved that state. It is probably not run by "crisis management."

In summary, the goal-setting process is:
1. Establish *philosophical goals* (no more than five).
2. Complete *emergency department status survey* (annually).
3. Establish *annual* strategic *goals* (based on status survey; no more than four major goals).
4. Write *objectives* for each strategic goal.
5. Complete *task outline* for each objective.

Problem solving (goal barriers)

There is always an easy solution to every human problem—neat, plausible and wrong.
H. L. Mencken

This section is (knowingly) mistitled, and the two explanations for that are appropriate here.

First, although the title is problem solving, the discussion relates primarily to problem identification, because I believe that identification is more difficult than resolution. Once the real reasons for a deficiency have been determined, correcting that deficiency, although sometimes tedious and time-consuming, is usually the easier of the two tasks. If your car periodically stalls, the difficult part for the mechanic is finding out *why*. Fixing it may be expensive and take a long time, but once the reason is known, the biggest challenge has been met.

Second, this section is titled problem solving because that is a familiar term to most of us. The word "problem," however, carries some negative connotation and already sounds discouraging. I prefer the term "goal barrier" simply because it presents a different mental picture, and because all "problems" are really barriers to a goal. A semantics game? Yes, but at times it is psychologically helpful to choose those words that most accurately represent what we mean. "X-ray is really a problem!" sounds different from "there is a barrier to speedy processing of our patients."

Reading this section will likely not change established, familiar terminology, but attitude is important to resolving goal barriers, and the more positive the approach, the better. There is a familiar axiom that illustrates this concept: "There are no problems, only *opportunities*."

In emergency department management, there are many "opportunities." Goal barriers abound and proliferate. In fact, much of our effort is directed toward resolving goal barriers. Lack of a MAST suit is a barrier to temporary correction of hypovolemic shock; inadequately trained staff may be a barrier to appropriate patient triage; medicines in unlockable cabinets may be a barrier to JCAH accreditation; and personnel conflicts are barriers to teamwork. Each goal barrier represents an opportunity to utilize our skill and creativity.

Before a goal barrier can be resolved, it is important to identify the difference between *symptoms* and *diseases* and between *people* barriers and *system* barriers. For the purposes of clarity in this discussion, the differences between symptoms and diseases and the ones between people barriers and system barriers will be separated. Often, however, when one is differentiating goal barriers, the *symptoms* look like *people barriers* when the *disease* is the *system*.

Symptoms versus diseases. "We have a morale problem" is not an accurate statement. Low morale is a symptom of a disease and not the disease itself. High staff attrition rates are often symptoms of the job satisfaction disease (barrier); a decrease in thorough charting, in the presence of increased census, may be a symptom of inadequate staffing, and so on.

As one approaches goal barriers, it is very important that one deal with the "disease" and not the symptom. Weekly requests for "better charting" are not going to produce results if there are simply not enough people to care for the patients and thoroughly document that care at the same time.

For those who are new to resolving goal barriers, it is a good idea to practice identifying "diseases" every time a goal barrier (problem) is identified. Working on symptoms alone will not produce long-term results and is a waste of valuable time.

People barriers versus system barriers. A lot is blamed on people when the system is at fault. Saying that Mike doesn't care about doing proper chest compression is unfair if Mike has never had a CPR class or hasn't practiced for a couple of years. Criticizing staff members for not reporting deficiencies when they have never seen results of their reporting is also unfair. "Adequate" documentation can only be expected if "adequate" documentation has been concretely outlined. Many, many complaints about inadequate performance can be traced to inadequate education, poor feedback, or poorly designed systems, rather than to laziness or apathy.

Any time that there is a significant decrease in overall output, efficiency, or effectiveness in a department, it is unlikely that suddenly all the staff members quit caring. Even isolated, person-specific deficiencies are often the result of poor orientation or lack of positive feedback. If we assume that the manager has hired reasonably intelligent, well-intentioned people, then probably 90% of all barriers are system-related.

There is a simple mechanism for differentiating between symptom and disease and identifying people barriers and system barriers: all statements about goal barriers (problems) should be followed by *because*. For example:

The morale is low *because*. . .

Patients are leaving without a medical exam *because*. . .

Theresa was rude *because*. . .

Charting is inadequate *because.* . .

The use of "because" will start the thought process on the path to identifying the true barrier. The "because" technique should be taken to its conclusion. For instance, the morale is low *because* there hasn't been enough feedback *because* the head nurse hasn't had the time *because* there were too many simultaneous projects *because* of poor planning. Only when taken to its final stage can the real barrier be determined.

If you are seriously looking for real barriers, you will only rarely arrive at becauses that end with laziness, apathy, or bad attitude. And even when you do, there are usually personal problems (family, school, money) that have caused the behavior in a particular individual.

Once the barriers have been identified, you can proceed to resolution decisions. Goal barriers come in many sizes—and so do solutions. Solutions to barriers may range from 3-minute chats to 12-month projects—and some barriers warrant "waiting it out."

When resolving goal barriers, one must also be careful not to overtreat or undertreat the disease. When caring for patients, the same kind of decisions must be made. It is costly and time-consuming to order a CBC, tests for electrolytes, urinalysis, blood sugar, blood gases, a chest x-ray film, and lung scan on an emotionally upset patient with rapid respirations, numbness, and tingling that were relieved by paper-bag breathing. It is also overtreatment to call a 12-person conference for an isolated abrupt exchange between staff members.

Conversely, a young patient who has sudden onset of severe headache and no prior history of headaches should not be sent home without a neurological examination with instructions to take aspirin every 4 hours; just as an incident of a staff member truly going berserk in the middle of a cardiac arrest should not be written off as a "bad day."

Resolving deficiencies calls for common sense and good judgment—and no one is always right in that decision-making process. Keep in mind, however that the treatment should fit the disease.

In summary, the system for identifying goal barriers and the need for resolution is:

1. Is this a symptom or disease?
2. Is this a people barrier or a system barrier?
3. Have I taken the "because" to its conclusion?
4. What is the magnitude of the problem?
5. What will happen if I do nothing?
6. Does this barrier constitute a real hindrance to a goal, and if so, *what is the goal?*

When you have identified the goal and the barrier, you now have the basis for a project.

Project management

"Project" in this context will be used to mean any activity that is undertaken to resolve a barrier to a goal. Remember that nearly 100% of our work is directed toward achieving a goal that is important to the care of patients and the smooth operation of the department.

There are a variety of approaches and terminologies used in the goal-setting process. Many people, when setting goals will use opening words such as "improve," "increase," or "decrease." Some people will argue that "improve CPR documentation" is really an *objective* for the *goal* of "ensuring optimal care of the cardiac arrest patient." However, the *important* thing is to use terminology that is understood by all. It is also helpful to use the same language approach throughout a project outline. The project outline here uses a 'pure" goal-setting format, but if "improve" is more understandable to the reader than "ensure," use "improve." Whatever works is a good tool.

If you have a clear understanding of the goal-setting and goal-barrier concepts, outlining objectives, solutions, and tasks is not difficult. An example of goal setting through goal achievement in outline form follows. This outline is detailed to provide a clear picture of the process. It is not necessarily recommended that one go through this entire written outline for every barrier that arises. It *is* recommended that the objectives/task outline be used for annual goals, however. (For the reader's information the goal outline identifies the "philosophical" [strategic] goal to which the activ-

Project outline

Project chairperson: M. Smith
Project name: Triage
Philosophical (strategic) goal: Provide optimal emergency care*

PART I: Goal/Objectives
   A. Goal: Ensure appropriate patient triage
   B. Objectives
      1. Develop triage criteria/coding system
      2. Provide staff education regarding triage coding
      3. Audit coding system for accuracy
      4. Reinforce if indicated
      5. Re-audit

PART II: Task outline
   Objective 1: Develop triage criteria/coding system

Task	Assigned to	Deadline	Report to
1. Select three staff members to assist with task	M. Smith	1/15	D. Jones
2. Collect data from three area hospitals about triage systems	J. Rogers	2/1	M. Smith
3. Establish criteria for priority of patients	All	2/28	M. Smith
4. Develop coding system	All	3/15	D. Jones

   Objective 2: Provide staff education regarding triage coding

Task	Assigned to	Deadline	Report to
1. Prepare written guideline for coding system	J. Rogers	3/20	M. Smith
2. Schedule staff meetings	J. Rogers	3/30	M. Smith

   Objective 3: Audit coding system for accuracy

Task	Assigned to	Deadline	Report to
1. Select 30 patient records	S. Brown	6/1	J. Rogers
2. Audit for triage accuracy	J. Rogers	6/15	M. Smith
3. Report to staff	J. Rogers		M. Smith/ D. Jones

*For reader information only

ity relates. However, it is not usually necessary to include philosophical goals in the project outline.)

Ideally, each *task outline* should be on a separate page and should be given to the persons involved in completing the task.

As you can see, much of the material contained in these outlines represents the step-by-step process that usually goes on in one's mind. Sitting down in advance and outlining the necessary tasks, objectives, and responsible parties will help avoid delays and eliminate overlooking essential steps in the project.

Creativity in project management. Within each project lies the opportunity to creatively meet the challenge of management. Many management mistakes are made because of the tendency to see only what is known or has been experienced. When working toward a goal, do not confine yourself to tradition, and do not put up barriers that do not exist. During the initial brainstorming process, do not limit suggestions and ideas. In a true brainstorming session, the individuals "think out loud" without regard to feasibility of an idea. Each brainstormer states every idea that pops into his mind, and the other people are not permitted, at that point, to make judgments such as "that won't work," or "that's too expensive." Once all ideas have surfaced, the group then begins to eliminate those ideas that are truly not feasible, but the reasons for lack of feasibility must be stated before an idea is eliminated.

If you are unhappy with the hospital review format, do not assume that the personnel office wouldn't accept an "emergency department addendum" that is specific to your area. If you think a full-time collection person would be helpful, ask for a 3- or 6-month trial program. If the hospital is on a one-to-one restock system and that is inefficient for your area, request a trial program there also. Visiting other emergency departments is another good way to open up your "tunnel vision." After 2 or 3 years at one facility, we all tend to see it only as it is and not as it could be. If there are efficiency problems, see if some physical redesign would be helpful.

Projects are also a golden opportunity for staff involvement. Those people out there in the "trenches" have lots of good ideas that will surface if they are asked. Some of the best improvements come from the folks who have to face the inefficiency and frustration on a daily basis. For example, the emergency department in which I work has *separate* ambulance and walk-in entrances. Unfortunately, the *ambulance* entrance is the most visible as you approach the emergency department. The ambulance entrance doors are automatic and operated by press-plates on the walls—both inside and out. Many of our patients, upset and in a hurry, did not see the walk-in entrance. We put up more signs—no improvement. There were daily complaints about the problem, and it was a source of great frustration to all the staff to have patients and family members suddenly appear through the ambulance doors. This went on for 18 months until finally one of the clerks meekly said "is there any reason why we

couldn't take the outside handles off the ambulance doors?" It worked!

Administrative structure and change

Structure. Finding the administrative structure that meets the department's needs is one of the greatest challenges faced by the department manager. Administrative structure refers to the assignment of responsibilities for people and functions. Administrative structure is that entity on which organizational charts are based; a traditional administrative structure follows.

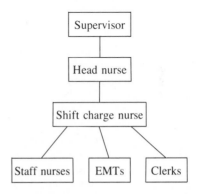

Each of these categories of staff member has some defined area(s) of responsibility. Unfortunately, no one structure works in every environment, and it may take several tries to find the best method of operation.

Because no one structure works in every department, it would not be reasonable here to recommend a particular structure for administrative activity, but there are three consistent guidelines to follow in the process of developing an appropriate *(workable)* method for operating a department.

1. Define your needs.
2. Be creative.
3. Match people and functions.

DEFINING NEEDS. Much defining of needs in administrative structure is instinctive. You have a "feeling" that certain activities are inefficient or not thorough or inadequate, or you feel pressured for time—indicating either poor time organization or the need for additional administrative help or the need to redistribute some duties.

If you are setting up a new department or have the above feelings about a department you are already managing, there are several approaches that can be taken when attempting to define the needs. Only one approach will be presented here. The important thing is that the problem be looked at in its entirety and not just as a "slice." In the approach below, there are several steps to follow to define the needs:

1. Make a list of all the functions that are not direct "hands-on" patient care or direct registration/discharge activity. The list should include all the usual administrative duties, such as interviewing, orientation, education, ordering, and restocking, and should also include those things that are related to patient care but may not be built into the current system, such as triage, expediting patient flow, social service, and checking equipment.

2. After the list is made, take each item on the list and categorize it as specialized or nonspecialized. A specialized function is one that requires special knowledge or training—nursing education, for instance, can not be done by the departmental secretary. Ordering medical supplies also requires some knowledge of emergency medicine. Recording departmental statistics, however, can be done by anyone with minimal training.

3. After categorization, you should also indicate those things on the list that are currently not being done and *why* they are not done, for example, inadequate time available, no system set up, inadequate monitoring, or no trained person available.

When you have completed these activities, you should have a clear picture of what needs to be done and by whom, and you should be ready to move on to *creativity*.

CREATIVITY. One of the most common errors made when developing a management system is the tendency to see what is and not what could be. Tradition says that there is an official charge nurse on each shift, that supervisors do the

ordering, that only social workers can do social service functions; and many managers are unable to clear out the "tradition cobwebs" and look at alternatives without preconceived ideas about the structure.

After you have listed your needs, categorized the activities, and compared what is done with what you feel is desirable, you can begin to develop alternatives for correction of the management deficiencies. This is the time to get the department's creative thinkers together and have a true brainstorming session, one that opens up the mind so new ideas and concepts are not automatically blocked out.

Many administrative activities can be distributed to people in the department who traditionally do not have the responsibilities. It is difficult to teach creativity on paper, but below are examples of some structural resolutions to management problems.

Problem	Solution
Students in the emergency department are getting fragmented education.	Staff nurse "preceptors" have been assigned (volunteered, actually); the students work that staff nurse's regular shift and work only with the *one* preceptor.
New staff members are not getting individual attention during orientation.	"Big brothers/sisters" have volunteered to help orient, answer questions, and encourage the new person for the first 4 weeks in the department (1 to 2 weeks past orientation)
Much staff shift rotation is making it difficult for shift charge nurses to do staff reviews.	Charge nurses assigned to specific shifts have been deleted. Reviews have been reassigned to supervisor and head nurse. Review input is obtained from co-workers who are selected *by the staff member being reviewed.*
Dual problem 1. No social worker is available.	A new position of patient representative has been created. Patient representatives do initial

Problem	Solution
2. Patients are not getting appropriate attention at time of registration; they are being greeted with pure "business" tone.	patient registration (the usual clerical work) and are also responsible for the social service aspects of the emergency department operation: they help with placement problems and do emergency department death/crisis counseling. Since "social service" kinds of people are recruited for the position, patients get more appropriate initial attention.
Another dual problem 1. Administrative time available is insufficient to do quality audits. 2. Staff involvement/concern with quality assurance is low.	Departmental audit committee has been created, chaired by and composed of emergency department staff.
And another 1. Morale is low among EMTs. 2. Increasing patient census is creating greater demands on RN time.	A new EMT grade has been created: the EMT II. EMT IIs are internally certified (based on classes, written tests, and performance tests) to give tetanus toxoids, do plaster splinting, and insert Foley catheters and NG tubes.
There is insufficient time for supervisor to order all items and supervise restocking/ordering activities.	"Chief EMT" position has been created. Chief EMT supervises all supply/stocking activity, does all departmental ordering, and hires and orients all EMTs.

This list could go on and on, but the general idea should be clear by now. And don't overlook your secretarial talent. Most secretaries are good organizers and do an excellent job of setting up systems.

Brainstorming to develop alternatives works well whether you are changing an entire structure or merely working on one particular area. After you have developed the ideas for new administrative structure, you should begin the process of matching people and responsibilities.

MATCHING PROCESS. Some controversy exists over whether one should define job responsibilities and look for someone who can fulfill those responsibilities or whether one should use available resources and match people to responsibilities. In the real world, probably a combination of both these approaches is appropriate.

Matching people and functions is a challenge that often results in an odd distribution of duties. The concept of matching is simple: each of us has areas of talent, and each of us has areas in which we do not excel. Compulsive, superorganizers are often not outstanding in interpersonal relationships—and vice versa. And there are people who are very good teachers but who cannot develop a budget. The goals of matching are to (1) combine the right people with the right job and (2) balance the talent areas in the department as a whole so that the department has people who excel in interpersonal relations and people with organizational ability.

There is one caution concerning the matching process. Although there is no law that says individuals have to supervise functions *and* supervise the people doing those functions, it is very difficult to monitor functions unless you also have responsibility for the people who do those tasks. To clarify: suppose you assign an EMT to oversee all restocking activity. If that EMT does not have "authority" over the people doing the restocking, it can be very frustrating. This is not to say that such a system cannot work, but it does require a special combination of people and it also requires that the person who supervises the function and the persons with responsibility for the people work very closely.

Change. Much has been written about change: people's response to it and how to cope with it. There are even "stress points" assigned for certain changes in one's life—for job change, for divorce, for moving, for vacation, and so on.

In relationship to emergency medicine and its people, there are some observations to be made. Emergency people are an interesting group.

They have the same responses to change as most people, but, in general, people attracted to a field as diverse and chaotic as emergency care are usually aggressive and motivated and do not tolerate *stagnation* any better than they tolerate change. So, although they may resist change, they also will find it difficult to work in an environment that maintains the "status quo" for long periods of time. And if the status quo goes on too long, they will often come with many ideas of their own for "improvements"—change.

Implementing changes in work procedures and policies in often difficult. The guidelines below may be helpful in avoiding some of the resistance.

1. *Don't* make more than one major change every 3 months—preferably no more often than every 6 months. Major changes in structure and ways of operating are very difficult to adjust to. Also, if you have an option, don't fire people at intervals any closer together than every 3 months; even if everyone understands why, they all tend to get nervous.
2. Get as much input as possible before making changes, large or small. If there has been preparation and discussion, the "change resistance quotient" is lowered. In addition, you will often receive input you hadn't thought of, which will avoid mistakes in system design.
3. When introducing a change, *be sure* that everyone understands that if it doesn't work, they will *not* be stuck with it forever. For internal changes in procedures, staff members should be assured that the goal is to find a *workable* method.
4. *Always* explain the reason for any change. Having a new procedure "dumped" on you without explanation is very frustrating, and it significantly elevates the "resistance quotient."

Summary. Structuring an emergency department and making changes in an emergency department can be very difficult. *Nobody* starts out with a perfect system, and even perfect systems eventually require some changes.

One last note about structure and change: something that worked well a year ago does not necessarily work well forever—needs change, people change, census increases, census decreases, health care changes. Always be on the lookout for methods of operating that are outdated. If you do, you will likely not fall into the "tradition" trap, and you will have a good chance at maintaining a progressive and dynamic department.

MANAGEMENT OF THE PEOPLE

The best systems developed by mankind are worthless if you don't know how to manage the people. People run the system. The right people run it better. Get the right people in a good system and manage them well, and you have the makings of an outstanding department.

People are complex. Much of what motivates them and causes them to respond so differently is not well understood. Being responsible for a group of people, therefore, is sometimes frustrating, an incredible challenge, and one of the most exciting parts of the management task.

This section has to do with people: how to find them, motivate them, schedule them, review them, select their leaders, resolve their conflicts, and promote teamwork among them.

The information presented in this section is primarily a philosophy of management, though some "how-tos" are included. If you are currently a manager or are thinking about becoming one, the first thing you should explore is your philosophy about people. The intent here is to convey *concepts*. People differ, leadership styles differ, and it is the manager's responsibility to develop his or her own specific techniques for dealing with other people. It is hoped that the pages that follow will be of help in developing a philosophical approach conducive to a well-run department and reasonably satisfied staff members.

Selection of staff members

Finding a person to fill a particular position can be difficult. Finding the *right* person can be very difficult. The selection process is one of the most important tasks that the manager faces. The responsibility for selecting permanent members of the team should not be taken lightly. Selection of staff is a four-step process.

1. Definition of needs
2. Recruiting
3. Interviewing
4. Making the decision

NOTE: This section is concerned primarily with selecting staff for nonadministrative positions. Selection of leadership staff is discussed later in the chapter.

Step 1: Defining needs. There are several selection needs that should be considered before you start the recruiting process: the basics, the need for experience, and the personality needs of the department.

BASIC NEEDS. Some needs are easily identifiable. If you are filling an RN position, you should only interview RNs. Are your nonlicensed personnel staff aides and orderlies, or do you require EMT certification? Do you need people with billing experience for admitting clerks? Most of these questions are easily answered.

EXPERIENCED OR INEXPERIENCED? Before you start recruiting, you must decide whether you need someone with experience, or decide that you are willing to train someone. This decision should be based on (1) the position and its requirements and (2) the emergency department census.

THE POSITION. If you are looking for a full-time triage nurse or one who will be the only RN on the 11 to 7 shift, you cannot take someone fresh out of State Board exams, give her 3 weeks of orientation, and put her in charge. The hazards to patients and to the individual are obvious. If you are looking for a clerical person to type charts, file, and answer phones, you can train a person without jeopardizing patient care. You must decide ahead of time what you need and not waste time on people who do not meet the criteria. Occasionally you will miss the one in 100 who could do the job without experience, but the alternative is to interview the 99 others.

THE CENSUS. If your monthly emergency department census is 800, you probably have the time, and an environment in which to train someone. If your monthly census is 3,000, you need somebody who knows the basics: which patients can wait and, more important, which ones cannot. There are many gradations between 800 and 3,000—and many other "busyness" factors: do you have resident staff or full-time emergency physicians? You must examine your department and come to a decision about what the needs are.

PERSONALITY. The third and final step in determining needs is to look at what "personality" would benefit the department. This area, unfortunately, is rarely considered when looking for a new staff member, probably because it is viewed as something of a luxury.

What is meant by "personality"? Most applicants can be divided into two categories: job seekers and career seekers. Before we define these terms, it should be made clear that the terminology is not intended to divide applicants into "desirable" and "undesirable"; they are merely different—not better or worse.

Job seekers are usually looking for a position that will provide them with an enjoyable means of support while they pursue other interests such as school, family, or even skiing. Some of them are undecided about their career, some about how much of their lives to commit to a career, and others about what specific area to pursue. They may do their work well, but usually do not have a high level of involvement.

Career seekers are those who are aggressive, highly committed, full of ideas, and willing to devote the time and energy required for growth and change.

On the surface, it would appear that, given a choice, you would want only career seekers. Look again. Do you really want 30 people with strong convictions about where the copying machine should be placed? Probably not. What you do want is a balance. If your department is full of job seekers, start looking for some career people. If you already have enough leaders, look for followers. Both are required to accomplish the goals.

Step 2: Recruiting. Recruiting is the next logical step, and probably the most difficult. The ability to recruit depends on many factors: the geographical location, time of year, and what you have to offer. Having a vacancy at

Christmas and knowing that you pay less than anyone in the city can easily cause panic.

Applicants are obtained primarily by means of three mechanisms: referral, drop-ins, and advertising.

REFERRALS. Of the three ways to obtain new staff, this is the most preferable. If someone whose judgment you trust has worked with or knows an applicant, you already have access to much valuable information that cannot be obtained any other way. The applicant's strengths, as well as potential problem areas, are already identified. The hazard in referral is that the person doing the referring may have poor judgment.

In any case, put the word out. Tell the department staff, and call professional friends and acquaintances. Out there, somewhere, is the right person looking for a new opportunity.

DROP-INS. These are the ones who call or stop by, not in response to an ad. They are usually:
1. New in the area, or
2. Aggressive and bright enough to know how to bypass the personnel office, or
3. Not bright enough to know there is a personnel office, or
4. Seventeen years old and looking for their first job.

The chances of finding a successful applicant are about the same as when you actively advertise.

ADVERTISING. Advertising is an art. There are people who do it for a living. Those who have had the pleasure of writing their first ad have all wished they had taken a journalism elective. It is very difficult, especially when paying by the word, to say everything you want to say about what you have to offer and what you're looking for. A few hints about advertising follow.
1. Don't write a narrative, "Hospital was founded in 1920 . . . "
2. Title it "EMERGENCY NURSES" in big letters.
3. Make the criteria known; it will avoid unnecessary telephone calls.
4. Include those things that will attract the kind of applicant you are looking for, for example, "excellent medical care,"

"full-time emergency physicians," "progressive educational program."
5. Have other people review the ad to tell you if it sounds attractive.

Now that the ad is written, you must decide where to place it. Professional journals are an obvious choice, but you need to know about the vacancy well in advance. It is usually 6 weeks before the ad appears. Try local and metropolitan newspapers. You can also place ads in out-of-town or out-of-state papers.

Other possibilities include the newsletter for your professional organization (usually needs less lead time than a journal), placement centers at colleges and universities, and your own hospital's placement bulletin—there may be hidden talent lurking in the hallways.

Recruiting "blind," that is, by means of advertisements and drop-ins, is always more risky than the referral method. You have to rely solely on references and your astute judgment, and that's why interviewing is so critical to the selection process.

Step 3: Interviewing

There is something that is much more scarce, something finer far, something rarer than ability. It is the ability to recognize ability.

E. Hubbard

If there were a fool-proof method for weeding out the undesirables during the interview process, we would not spend nearly so much time documenting so we could fire those people who impressed us so at the interview. In this section some common interview techniques, their advantages and disadvantages, and the responsibility of the interviewer are discussed.

INTERVIEW TECHNIQUES

THE PANEL METHOD. The panel method consists of bringing various representatives from the staff (the interview committee) together to conduct the interview. The representatives are usually people such as the supervisor, clinical instructor, a charge nurse, staff nurses, and the medical director. The structure is generally formal. The advantages are that there is more input, the burden for decision making is shared, the staff feels more involved, and group perspective may be better than an individual one. The disadvantages are that it is difficult to schedule all people, administrative cost is increased, the applicant tends to be uncomfortable, and a decision is sometimes difficult to reach.

ONE-TO-ONE METHOD. One person only does the interviewing, usually the supervisor. The interview tends to be informal. The advantages are that it is easy to schedule, administrative costs are decreased, decisions are less time-consuming, and the applicant is usually more comfortable. If the supervisor's judgment is poor (or variable), the disadvantages can be disastrous. The staff feels less involved, the burden on the interviewer is increased, and there is no input into the ''can't-decide-between-the-two-candidates'' situation.

ONE-TO-ONE SERIES METHOD. The applicant interviews on a one-to-one basis with several selected interviewers. This method is usually used when hiring leadership staff. The advantages are that it is easier to schedule than a panel, there is more input into decisions, and it is more comfortable for the applicant than the panel. There are two disadvantages. The applicant must make several appointments, which increases administrative costs. There is also an increase in the time involved to collect information from all the interviewers to make a decision.

ONE-TO-TWO METHOD. The applicant interviews with (usually) the supervisor and one other representative of the staff. The advantages are that it decreases the burden on one individual, it is easier to schedule than a panel or a series, there is more input than in the one-to-one method, and the staff is involved. The disadvantages are that it is slightly more difficult to schedule and there is a slight increase in administrative costs.

SUMMARY. Is any one method preferable to the other? With the exception of the panel method, probably not. Each of the other techniques may be favored in a given situation. My personal preference is a one-to-one series for leadership positions and one-to-one or (preferably) one-to-two for staff positions. The panel method is cumbersome, costly, rigid, and tends

to promote the asking of questions such as, ''What is your nursing philosophy?''

The important thing in deciding interview techniques is to allow flexibility. No one method is perfect for every situation, and the freedom to choose the most desirable will save the department much time and energy.

INTERVIEWER RESPONSIBILITIES. Selecting the right people is one of the keys to success in any program. Most of the deciding factors in selection come from the interview. Therefore, knowing how to conduct an interview and learning how to obtain the information you need are critical to the selection process. There are as many interview styles as there are interviewers. Each individual must develop a style that is personally comfortable. There are, however, responsibilities that should not be ignored.

BE SURE YOU KNOW THE BASIC NEEDS. Do not interview inexperienced people if you know that the job requires experience. Take a good look at the entire department, and decide whether you need job-seekers or career-seekers.

HAVE A CLEAR PICTURE OF YOUR ENVIRONMENT. Emergency department environments differ widely. Universities, private hospitals, and public hospitals all offer different challenges and require different kinds of people. A critical care nurse who really enjoys one-to-one or two-to-one patient care would probably not be happy as a full-time triage nurse. If your environment is flexible, calling for a lot of teamwork and mutual give and take, a person with a militaristic view of things might have difficulty adjusting. Be sure you understand what your environment calls for.

BE SURE YOU ARE UP FOR IT. I have, on occasion, postponed interviews purely because I was not up for them. Interviewing is exhausting, especially if you get a one-word reply to every question and are basically doing a monologue. You should be rested and fully enthusiastic about your department. Do not forget that the applicants may be interviewing elsewhere. Don't risk losing a good candidate because you're tired and cranky, and don't schedule more than two in a day. By the time you say, for the fifth time in a day, ''We have a wonderful educational program,'' you'll sound like a recording.

PUT THE APPLICANT AT EASE. It is difficult enough to find out what you need to know about the applicant. Don't complicate it by increasing his or her anxiety level. If applicants are relaxed, they are more likely to reveal who they really are. Offer a cup of coffee, chat about the energy shortage, ask if they had any trouble finding the hospital, talk about a patient you just had—anything. Don't just start out with "What are your career goals?"

ASK QUESTIONS THAT HAVE ANSWERS, AND BE DIRECT. Top on the list of ridiculous interview questions are "What is your nursing philosophy?" "How would you compare 2-, 3-, and 4-year graduates?" and "Where do you plan to be in 15 years?" You will find out more by asking if their favorite patients are medical or surgical than you will asking about their nursing philosophy. Often I directly ask such questions as "Are you fairly comfortable with arrhythmias?" and "What are your strengths in nursing care?" Most applicants will be honest when approached directly; there is very little future in bluffing.

ASK IF THEY HAVE ANY QUESTIONS—AND LISTEN. If the first question is "How long before I'm eligible for vacation?" or "How many MediCaid patients do you see?" beware. You will learn a lot about what is important to them by *listening* to their questions and answers.

REVIEW THE INTERVIEW. Initially, this should be done in writing. List the things you liked and your negative observations or any questionable areas. If you have interviewed with someone else, review your list with her. See if your impressions are the same. Ask yourself if this is someone you would want to work side by side with 40 hours a week, and pay attention to your instinct. If there is something you "just can't pinpoint," be cautious. Remember, the best resumes in the world are still only resumes.

CHECK REFERENCES. *Always* check references. Getting a thorough reference is becoming increasingly difficult. In most states, the only information that can be given is hire date, termination date, and eligibility for rehire. Some clues for checking references follow.

1. Get the name of the immediate supervisor, and call him or her directly. Do not call the personnel office.

2. If the supervisor hedges, be cautious. If the applicant was a "model employee," the tone of voice is usually different than if he or she was not.
3. If the applicant is not eligible for rehire, he or she is usually someone you would not want.
4. If you had negative observations or questionable areas in the interview, ask about those specific points.

Now that you have decided what you need, recruited, and interviewed, the only thing left is to make the decision.

Step 4: Making the decision. Do not panic. If all the applicants were washouts, *do not hire anyone,* no matter how your schedule looks. Keep looking. Hiring someone and firing her 3 months later only doubles your work. Remember number 3 of Murphy's laws: "It is easier to make a commitment or to get involved in something than to get out of it."

If you have interviewed with other people, review all the candidates when you are finished. (During a 2-year period in my career, I interviewed jointly with one other person. We hired only those applicants we were both enthusiastic about. If either of us had reservations about someone, he or she was disqualified. Our success rate was unusually high.)

Finally, if possible, take a mental break for a few days. Do not make a decision immediately. Put recruiting, interviews, and your tight schedules out of your mind for 2 or 3 days. You will find your perspective is different and your mind clearer to make the final decision.

Motivation

Motivation. Everybody talks about it. "How can I motivate so and so? He's bright and has so much to offer, but he's just not motivated." Much research has been done to enable us to better understand human behavior. Following is a brief review of some of the better-known theories of motivation.

Motivational theories

HIERARCHY OF NEEDS. Abraham Maslow was among the first to propose a motivational theory (Maslow, 1954). Even though it has been the source of considerable controversy since its

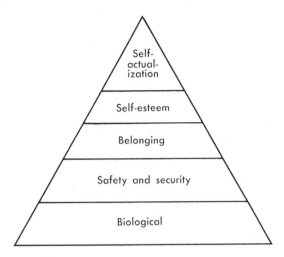

Fig. 5-1. Maslow's hierarchy of needs. (From Maslow, A.: Toward a psychology of being, New York, 1962, D. Van Nostrand Co.)

first appearance, a brief summary may still provide the manager with insight.

Maslow identified five needs that serve as motivators (Fig. 5-1). To understand the hierarchy, one must know the two basic assumptions: (1) A need emerges only when the lower level need has been met. (One would have little concern for self-actualization if one were having severe difficulty breathing.) (2) More than one need may be operating at once, but only one will dominate. Most managers today are concerned primarily with the top two or three needs in the hierarchy. Physiological and safety needs are generally adequate in the work environment, and so our attention must be directed toward the higher motivational levels.

N ACH THEORY. In his article, "That Urge to Achieve," David McClelland discusses what divides people in the world into two broad groups: "There is that minority which is challenged by opportunity and willing to work hard to achieve something and the majority which really does not care all that much" (McClelland, 1966). This minority, those with a high *n*eed for *ach*ievement (n Ach) are still a puzzle to psychological researchers. According to McClelland, the need for achievement is "a distinct human motive, distinguishable from others" (McClelland, 1966). People who score

high in n Ach testing have several characteristics in common.

1. They set moderately high, but not unachievable, goals for themselves.
2. They respond only if they can influence the outcome by doing the work themselves.
3. They show strong preferences for situations in which the results of their effort are readily visible.
4. They consistently look for ways to "do things better."

There are, as yet, no concrete answers about why certain people seem to have a higher level of n Ach than others, but "the evidence suggests it is not because they are born that way, but because of special training they get in the home from parents who set moderately high achievement goals, but who are warm, encouraging and nonauthoritarian in helping their children reach these goals" (McClelland, 1966). Can n Ach be increased in a given individual? McClelland's research suggests that it is, in fact, possible to change an individual's thinking process and increase his need for achievement.

EXPECTANCY THEORY. Developed by Victor Vroom, the expectancy theory states that a worker's motivation depends primarily on what he perceives as the result of a given behavior and the value he places on these results (Vroom, 1964). For instance, if a staff nurse highly values a promotion to charge nurse and believes that demonstrating commitment (that is, schedule flexibility and educational participation) will produce the desired promotion, she or he will probably be motivated to work extra shifts and attend lectures. A staff nurse who is content as a staff nurse and has no desire for promotion will probably have less motivation (or at least different motives) to put in additional time and energy. Vroom's theory suggests, therefore, that employees can be motivated by changing how they perceive the *value* of the outcome of their behavior.

MOTIVATION-HYGIENE THEORY. The motivation-hygiene theory, developed by Frederick Herzberg, divides worker motivation into two distinct categories: *satisfiers* (motivators) and *dissatisfiers* (hygiene or maintenance factors) (Herzberg, 1967). When hygiene factors (dissatisfiers) are inadequate or absent, the results are worker dissatisfaction. Dissatisfiers are factors such as working conditions (lighting, space, and so on), salaries, relationships with management and co-workers, and company policies. If these factors or conditions are inadequate, the employee will be dissatisfied. Adequacy in all hygiene factors does *not,* however, produce motivated employees. Even if the salary is adequate, co-worker and management relationships are good, working conditions acceptable, and company policies reasonable, the employee is not *necessarily* motivated to achieve or contribute.

Satisfiers (motivators) are such things as achievement, responsibility, recognition, the work itself, and promotion. If these factors are available in the environment, the results are employee satisfaction and motivation.

Motivation methods. Managers do not study motivation theory solely to understand why people *don't* produce. Clearly, the goal is to find motivation methods that encourage greater efficiency and productivity. Before you can start trying to motivate others, you must first address three questions.

1. How do you personally feel about people and what it takes to motivate them? Are you of the school that believes people are basically lazy and stupid, or do you believe that, given the opportunity, most people are eager to contribute something to their jobs and capable of doing so. This is an important question. If you *really* believe people are inherently lazy, you will probably find it difficult to interact in ways that will have a positive effect on others' productivity.

2. What is your usual way of interacting with other people? Do you tend to avoid confrontation? Would you rather "do it yourself" than teach, or even ask someone else to help? Do you give orders or request assistance? Do you ask what happened or accuse others of mistakes before you have all the facts? Take a good look at your usual behavior. It may surprise you.

3. Does your usual style of interacting correspond with your answer to question number 1? If not, you have a conflict that needs to be resolved. If you do believe people are willing to contribute, but you accuse, dictate, and "do it yourself," something is amiss.

Motivation is not a single interaction with another person. It is not a yearly performance review. It is not remembering once a week to pat somebody on the back. It *is* something that should be an integral part of your style as a manager. Motivation can be very difficult if you have to consciously remember to do it. If it is a natural outgrowth of how you feel about people, it is not nearly so taxing. The paragraphs that follow outline four components of motivation that are key in the motivational process.

Communication. People are, by nature, social creatures, and communication, both verbal and nonverbal, is an integral part of our daily lives. Communication is vital to motivation.

Later in the chapter, the section on leadership addresses the issue of personal communication styles. For the moment, the discussion will be limited to those areas of communications that should be routine in your motivational system.

EXPECTATIONS. If you want complete vital signs on every patient, but don't tell anyone that you do, you would then be ill-advised to criticize staff members for not doing them. A simplistic example, to be sure, but if you were to begin questioning the staff in your department, you will likely be amazed at how many gray areas exist. Do you expect all staff to cheerfully rotate shifts every 3 months or only occasionally? Does everyone in your department really understand his role in a disaster? Are your patient records supposed to be signed with the beginning of treatment or at the end? *Who* is supposed to call the blood bank for uncrossmatched blood for trauma patients? Are tennis shoes really okay? How *many* lectures a year are considered "educational enthusiasm"? People need to know what criteria are being used to make judgments about their performance. The art here is to be sure the expectations are clearly understood, *without* creating an atmosphere of dictatorship.

FEEDBACK. If you have ever made a suggestion to your supervisor for improving your department and not received a response, you may already understand the importance of feedback. Any question or suggestion deserves a prompt response, even if the response is that you will not be able to deal with the problem right away. When a staff member takes the time (and has the good sense) to question a procedure or recommend an improvement, it is essential that you reply as soon as possible. Write a note to yourself, put it on your calendar or "to-do" list, but don't forget it. Even the worst suggestions warrant discussion and an explanation of why they won't work.

Another feedback area is constructive criticism. When a staff member makes an error, do not write it down and present it at a performance review 6 months later. The best of us make mistakes, and timely discussion will have the most benefit. There are three rules for constructive criticism that should never be broken.

1. *Never* criticize or reprimand in the presence of others.
2. *Always* ask for the person's version of the story. Many times there is a very logical explanation for what you observed or heard fifth hand.
3. *Always* explain why it was an error. People remember if they understand the rationale.

RECOGNITION

A pat on the back is only a few vertebrae removed from a kick in the pants, but it is miles ahead in results.

V. Wilcox

The third communication practice that should be an integral part of your style is recognition. When was the last time you complimented someone on her handling of a difficult patient? When did you last express appreciation to a nurse, technician, or clerk who *always* does the assigned duties? We all need recognition for our accomplishments—large or small. It is much too easy to get so wrapped up in problems that you don't even see the good. *Take the time to notice and communicate.* Another cardinal sin, too frequently committed by supervisors, is not giving credit where credit is due. If someone makes a suggestion or an unusual contribution, be sure that you publicly recognize his effort. Taking someone's suggestion and presenting it as your own will ensure that the person involved will never make another suggestion.

GOALS. The last communication practice, often ignored, is the communication of goals. If you expect to get support from the staff, they must know what the goal is. Communicating goals includes *all* goals—from the overall departmental goals for the year to the reason for instituting a new procedure. Again, people cooperate if the rationale is clear. If you are talking about departmental goals, it is also beneficial to explain the mechanisms that will be used to accomplish the goal. For instance, if one of the goals for the year is to "improve clerical efficiency," it is essential to explain that you are planning to preprint the patient's number on the charts and add an addressograph, rather than making the clerks work harder.

Staff involvement. The second component of the motivational system is *staff involvement.* To effectively involve staff members in the growth and progress of the department, there are two things the manager should understand: why and how.

WHY SHOULD THE STAFF BE INVOLVED? There are two reasons. Herzberg's theory states that satisfiers (motivators) are recognition, responsibility, and the work itself. Most of use are more enthusiastic about a project into which we have had direct input. Involving the staff in goal setting and decision making also gives them some control over their work environment. Very few people respond positively to dictatorship.

The second reason that the staff should be involved is that managers are not all-knowing. Unfortunately, no magic answers go with a promotion. Experience (usually the trial-and-error variety) may have taught the manager how *not* to do things, but managers still have not cornered the market on good ideas. What good managers *really* do is find good people and figure out how best to utilize their talents.

HOW SHOULD THE STAFF BE INVOLVED? Every staff member is, at some level, *involved* in the progress of a department. One is either (1) a hindrance to progress or (2) a help to progress. The old adage "if you are not part of the solution, you are part of the problem" is true. Rarely is anyone a neutral force. Every time someone "complains," he or she is involved in identifying barriers to a goal. Although it may be true that the barrier is of one's own making, it is a barrier nonetheless. Allowing individuals to be an asset to progress requires some skill and patience, but the benefits far outweigh the disadvantages.

The use of the word "allowing" is not accidental. It is important to remember that managers do not *get* people involved. They allow the individual to express a natural inclination, and they establish the mechanisms that encourage the expression of that inclination.

There are really only two activities that any staff member, manager or otherwise, is involved in: goal setting and goal achievement. Here is a simple example: Objective*: "correct

volume depletion" (more commonly heard as "start an IV"); to achieve: take IV bottle from shelf, remove cap, and so on. *Everything* we do is directed toward achieving a goal. So the real questions, when we discuss staff involvement, are: (1) What are the goals of the staff member? (2) What are the department's goals? (3) Are they compatible?

What are the goals of the staff member? Before you read further, choose one member of your department's staff, and write down what you think he or she wants from the 8 hours a day spent at work. Now, having done this exercise, you have a list of the goals for that staff member. If you wrote things such as "get paid for 8 hours of doing nothing," or "make everyone's life miserable," you need to either do some extensive reading about human behavior or seriously assess your interviewing/hiring abilities. More likely, however, you have written goals related to learning, being recognized for achievement, or simply enjoying their workday experience.

What are the department's goals? Every member of the emergency department team should be able to list the department goals—both the ongoing, permanent goals and the specific objectives for the year. One of the keys to establishing a successful mechanism for staff involvement is ensuring that everyone knows what the goals are. When new staff members are oriented, they should be given a clear picture of the overall philosophy of the department; when specific yearly, monthly, or weekly objectives are established, those objectives should be shared with all members of the team.

Are the staff member's goals and departmental goals compatible? It is probably safe to say that nearly everyone who sought employment in your department had a reason for choosing that specific area. A critical care nurse may have wanted to broaden his or her base of experience, an EMT may have wanted a change from prehospital to hospital-based care, a clerk may have wanted exposure to health care to assist in future career decisions. Some of the staff may have been looking for an exciting way to support their ski habit. Everyone came for a specific reason.

The manager's responsibility is to combine:

---

*The words "goal" and "objective" are used interchangeably in this section. In the previous section, they were separately defined.

(1) those goals of the staff member that are specific to emergency care; (2) the personal goals of *all* individuals: recognition, achievement, and responsibility; and (3) the departmental goals, in such a way that all can be fulfilled—no easy task, to be sure, but not as difficult as it may sound. Meeting all these objectives simultaneously offers another golden opportunity for creativity.

There are many methods that can be established to promote the involvement of staff members. Involvement may take any form—from helping establish annual objectives to figuring out how to get the blood off the wall before the next trauma case. The opportunities for input and assistance are endless, and the mechanism will vary from department to department, from year to year, and from individual to individual. The manager is responsible for creating the methods best suited for the environment.

ANNUAL GOAL SETTING. Although it would probably be unwise to get all staff members to agree on annual goals, it is possible to select representatives to assist in the process, or to ask each category of personnel (nurses, EMTs, clerks) to establish one or two group goals, or to solicit input from staff, formally or informally, concerning their perception of the "improvement needed" areas.

PREESTABLISHED PROJECTS. After objectives have been established, ideally, they are achieved by one method or another. Solicit assistance. Tell everyone what you are trying to achieve and see who is interested. You may define the overall objective and let the team members break it down into tasks. You may define the tasks and ask for assistance in a specific area. There are long-term projects, short-term projects, ongoing tasks, one-shot projects. You may want the chairman of a group, a group member, or a single individual to complete a specific activity. Someone can chair the audit committee; another can take responsibility for all CPR education; someone else may want to take responsibility for follow-up phone contact of sexual assault patients. Everyone has some talent and an area of special interest.

PERSONNEL PROBLEMS. If you are having difficulty with a new staff member, ask one of his or her colleagues to be a big brother or sister for awhile. Working out performance problems with a peer is often less threatening and more successful than "supervisory counseling."

ORIENTATION. The folks who do the work every day know what their new colleague *really* needs to know, and many of them are good at sharing that knowledge: Utilize that talent.

COMPLAINTS. As stated before, complaints are the identification of a barrier to achieving a particular goal. If someone has identified a barrier, ask if he is interested in helping find a solution.

NEW IDEAS. Everyone who comes up with a new idea for improving patient care, efficiency, interpersonal relations, or anything should be encouraged and praised. Grab on to that interest, and channel it.

INTERVIEWING. Create a rotating interviewer position, or simply allow those who are interested to sit in on interviews.

RECRUITING. If you are looking for a new staff member, ask the staff to help recruit. Be sure to thank anyone who refers an applicant, *and* be sure to explain why you did not hire the applicant if you do not.

SCHEDULING. Anyone who expresses an interest in scheduling should certainly be encouraged to help with it.

HAZARDS IN STAFF INVOLVEMENT. Any system comes with a full complement of potential hazards. These hazards must be identified to be avoided.

If you are trying to improve your relationship with hospital administration and the least tactful nurse in your department volunteers to be the liaison, you may want to channel that enthusiasm into another area, or at least spend some time discussing the art of diplomacy. If the clerical staff unilaterally decides to increase collections by 200%, you should investigate what methods they intend to use.

Obviously, these are extreme examples, but occasionally we all tend to get carried away by our enthusiasm, and it is the manager's responsibility to be sure that projects and new ideas are carried out in a manner consistent with departmental philosophy.

Another potential hazard is allowing too

many projects to be going on at one time. Change is difficult for everyone, and a barrage of new procedures may create chaos and fatigue among the staff.

Along the same vein is the third warning: All good ideas do not warrant implementation solely because they are good ideas. Calling every emergency department patient 24 hours after treatment may be very good idea, but probably impractical. The institution of a new policy or procedure should be consistent with current departmental needs.

The last hazard warning has to do with priority setting. Advanced cardiac life support certification for emergency department staff is an excellent idea, but should follow a well-organized basic cardiac life support certification system. Offering a 12-week advanced arrhythmia course is also a good idea, but not if only one nurse is ready for advanced arrhythmias. Again, the available time, effort, and energy should be utilized to meet objectives that are consistent with needs.

It would be unwise to move on to the next section without addressing the questions that many readers are undoubtedly now asking:

1. Staff involvement may work fine for someone else, but what about a department like *mine* where everyone is apathetic?

> Lots of folks confuse bad management with destiny.
>
> *E. Hubbard*

This problem will be discussed directly when we discuss the third component of the motivational system: leadership and its effect on motivation. It will also be addressed indirectly in the portion of this chapter that deals with leadership as a single issue. For the time being, it is sufficient to summarize: If you have a department filled with apparently apathetic, unenthusiastic, unmotivated people, the problem is probably not with the staff members.

2. "What do I do about the people who aren't motivated?" Actually, dealing with this issue is a relatively simple, two-step process: (1) ascertain the reason(s) and (2) correct the barriers, *if possible*. People choose to be uninvolved for any number of reasons. They may

not have received enough recognition, and therefore feel they have "nothing to offer"; they may not understand that they can be involved without devoting 100% of their life energy to work; they may be insecure enough personally that they feel everyone else has better ideas; they may be temporarily hostile about the administration; they may not yet have seen a project they are interested in; or they may simply be one of those people who have chosen not to devote additional energy to their job.

In all but the last example, most of the barriers can be corrected, and your efforts should be directly toward dealing with the real problems and not the symptoms. In the last example, do nothing. As long as the individual is fulfilling his or her job responsibilities and not creating a negative atmosphere, don't waste valuable time trying to significantly alter someone's view of the world. Nobody gets 100% participation, and expending a lot of energy on the 1% or 2% who have chosen not to be involved only diminishes the energy available to the other 98%. And keep in mind, in the circumstances described above, there is nothing inherently wrong with someone who has actively decided to direct his extra efforts to activities outside of work. Remember, you don't *get* people involved, you allow them to express a natural inclination.

If these individuals are not fulfilling their responsibilities and are creating a negative atmosphere, then you aren't dealing with a motivation problem. You are dealing with either an isolated personnel problem or, in the Herzberg theory, an unresolved "dissatisfier" factor.

Leadership: its effect on motivation. The third and final component of any motivational system is its leadership. Whether they are titled managers, supervisors, administrators, directors, coordinators, or chiefs, the people we are talking about are those who have been given the responsibility of guiding the efforts of others to achieve a defined set of objectives.

Anyone who has ever worked under an incompetent manager knows well the effect that incompetence has on motivation. Eventually the best, most motivated people will give up trying to make changes, suggestions, or improvements. Managerial incompetence should probably be clarified here, although most people, sadly, probably already know firsthand what the characteristics are. Incompetent managers are those who are always right or cannot take criticism, or don't listen or appear unconcerned with people's problems, or dictate without explanation, or don't know what they're doing, or always take sides, or never delegate, or are power happy—and keep their job forever it seems.

Incompetence is, however, different from inexperience. Inexperienced managers, as distinguished from incompetent managers, learn from mistakes and make a genuine effort to correct their deficiencies. No one knows everything about how to lead, but good managers listen, try to learn, make changes if indicated, and enjoy their work.

Trying to maintain enthusiasm when you work for someone you do not respect as a professional or as a person is very difficult. Note the use of the word respect, as opposed to like. It is highly improbable that even the best of managers are liked by everyone. If the manager is respected as a reasonable, capable person, being liked is not essential.

Many "motivation" problems could be easily resolved by a change in leadership. This is not to say that any time there is a motivation slump, the supervisor should be fired, but if a majority of the team members exhibit chronic apathy and discontent, someone should at least take a look at the quality of leadership.

The flip side of the issue is the positive effects of good leadership. When the manager is respected and is enthusiastic about his or her work, that enthusiasm quite naturally filters to all staff members. Genuine enthusiasm is contagious. Think about the times you have worked on a project with someone who was really excited about it, and compare that with the projects you have worked on where the leader presented it all as drudgery. It makes a difference, doesn't it?

Summary. Motivation is complex and no one approach works in every environment. Each manager must tailor his or her motivational system to fit the milieu. In any system, how-

ever, the three components remain the same. Your motivational system should include:

1. *Communication:* Expectations, feedback, recognition, and goals.
2. *Staff involvement:* It must be *allowed,* and the mechanisms established to encourage it.
3. *Leadership:* Supervisors, directors, and charge nurses should be respected and enthusiastic.

Scheduling

Emergency care is stressful—mentally, physically, and emotionally; and it is a 24-hour-a-day operation. Scheduling for 24 hours a day, 365 days a year is not an easy task. When staff members are vacationing or ill, emergency departments don't have the luxury of working "short." When trying to fill every position every day, one has an understandable tendency to create a lot of rules and to become insensitive to individual needs and differences.

The nursing profession is currently experiencing great unrest, and since much of the unhappiness is directly related to scheduling, it seems appropriate to discuss scheduling as a single issue.

There are three objectives the manager attempts to meet when he or she sits down to do a schedule.

1. Provide staffing that is adequate to ensure that patient care is not jeopardized.
2. Meet individual needs and preferences.
3. Be fair.

These are difficult objectives particularly because they must be met simultaneously.

The most frequent complaints you will hear from disgruntled staff members have to do with their schedule. "'They' put me on night shift and didn't even tell me. I had plans for that evening." It is imperative when doing a schedule, to remember that you are scheduling people's *lives,* and indiscriminate use of that power can rapidly create a morale crisis, and subsequently, a high attrition rate.

There are no easy answers to the problems of scheduling, but the following guidelines are offered.

1. Have as *few* rules as possible. If a nurse

wants an extra weekend off, and he or she can find appropriate coverage, there is no logical reason to deny that request. Ditto if someone wants to trade a shift. Don't create rules dictating that people can never leave early, arrive late, or work only 1 day a week. Scheduling policies *are* necessary, but only when there is solid justification for them. Solid justification is *not* manager stress, "hospital policy" (hospital policies *can* be changed and exceptions granted), or abuse of the system by an isolated staff member.

2. Try to have extra help available. Call them "per diem," "casual," or "subject-to-call," but try to keep enough help available that you are able to ensure some flexibility. On the surface this sounds costly, but if you weigh the cost of per diem help against the cost of "quit-recruit-interview-orient," you will probably find that you come out ahead.

3. *Do not* make schedule commitments that you cannot keep, and once you have made them, do not renege. If you have hired someone for 4 days a week in the emergency department, give her 4 days a week *in the emergency department*. Don't ship her off to CCU. If you promised 3 to 11, don't schedule her for 11 to 7 without permission.

4. Have an employment agreement. Employment agreements should spell out, at the minimum:
   a. Category: full-time, part-time, per diem, exempt.
   b. Number of hours a week commitment.
   c. Wages.
   Employment agreements are "clarity" tools for both the employee and the staff member. Be sure to get a new agreement if an employee's status changes.

5. Communicate. If you need coverage for the 11 to 7 shift, and want to use someone who ordinarily doesn't work 11 to 7, ask her if she is willing. *Never* put someone into an unusual slot, or change her rotation without speaking with her first.

6. *Grant all schedule requests.* Obviously

this isn't always possible, but it should always be your goal. If you are absolutely unable to, explain why.

7. Deal directly with abuses. Making rules that affect everyone in the department solely to resolve one or two offenders is unwise. It is better to be rid of one or two offenders than everyone in the department.

In spite of the fact that the above may sound (1) unworkable and (2) like an administrative nightmare, it is usually well worth the effort. In general, if people are treated with consideration, you will find them willing to help out when you are in a bind, and your attrition rate will reflect that consideration.

Performance review systems

A performance review, if done appropriately, can be a positive, motivating experience for both the staff member and the reviewer. If not done appropriately, a review can be a frightening, negative experience for the staff member and an energy drain for the reviewer.

This section outlines the two types of performance reviews and the objectives of each, lists the responsibilities of the staff member and the reviewer, and briefly discusses review format.

Performance review—formal. When we combine Webster's definitions of "performance," "review," and "formal," we arrive at an understanding of this process.

Term	Meaning
Performance	The act of performing, . . . accomplishment, fulfillment, . . . operation or functioning, usually with regard to effectiveness
Review	A look at, . . . a general survey, report or account
Formal	Of external form or structure, . . . of or according to fixed customs, rules, . . . done or made in orderly, regular fashion . . .

A formal performance review is a structured method of looking at accomplishments and effective function. Probably the most common mistake made in interpreting this definition is assuming that the review process is a one-sided monologue. Good reviews are dialogues. Before a formal review is conducted or a review system is designed, there are some questions that should be answered.

- What are the objectives of the formal review?
- What are the responsibilities of the staff member?
- What are the responsibilities of the reviewer?

FORMAL PERFORMANCE REVIEW OBJECTIVES

1. To establish rapport, particularly with new staff members. Scheduling an uninterrupted hour or more to talk with a staff member provides a rare opportunity for the individuals involved to become better acquainted. This time should be used to open or reopen lines of communication.

2. To provide an opportunity to discuss staff member goals, methods of achievement, and deadlines. Many staff members, especially those who have not previously been involved in personal goal setting, may need to explore that process with a "guide." Outlining work-related goals does not come easily to everyone. Those staff members who list such things as "finish school" and "enroll in scuba diving class" as personal goals probably do not yet have a clear enough picture of goal setting in a work environment. Those who do understand goal setting may need education in methods of achievement. For instance, if someone lists "improve my attitude about nonemergent patients" as a goal and writes "try harder" as a method, she could probably benefit from suggestions to read about the health care system, or talk with her colleagues about nonemergent patients, or spend more time with these patients to ascertain why they came to the emergency department. Finally, many people set unrealistic deadlines for themselves. Any nurse who sets a 3-week deadline for "understanding 12-lead ECGs" is either unrealistic or a genius.

   When a review is conducted, the staff member and reviewer should look over the goals, methods, and deadlines from the previous review and ask:
   a. Was she able to meet her goals; and if not, why not?
   b. Did the methods work, or did they have to be altered?
   c. Were the deadlines realistic?

3. To provide an opportunity for feedback to the staff member regarding her performance. This is, traditionally, the primary focus of the review—and probably should not be. There are still supervisors who keep a little black book with all the "bad" things a staff member has done; and, at review time, this list is dutifully read to the offending party. Inappropriate behavior, in attitude or clinical performance, should be discussed at the time of the incident and not weeks or months later. Reviews should be a general survey of strengths and "improvement-needed" areas, and that survey should be conducted primarily by the staff member and only secondarily by the reviewer.

4. To provide an opportunity for education of the staff member. This refers not to clinical education but to education about the changing world of health care, the reasons for internal procedural changes, or the reason why the hospital or emergency department administration have selected certain goals for the year. The reviewer has a captive audience and an opportunity to answer questions about health care systems, prehospital care systems, hospital and emergency department methods of operating—even if the questions are not directly asked.

5. To provide an opportunity for feedback *to the reviewer* regarding departmental problems and administrative performance. *This* should probably be the primary focus of the review or, at the very least, should get equal time with No. 3. The people who take care of the patients, fill out the forms, answer the phone, and interact with other agencies, department heads, and patients' families every day know what the real problems are. They

also know who works and who does not. Don't pass up this chance to pick their brains and to find out what you, personally, are doing (or not doing) that makes their lives more difficult.

6. To document the above items. We live in a world of rules, regulations, and laws. Documentation serves two purposes: protection of the staff member and protection of the employer. Lengthy discussion of the importance of documentation is unnecessary, but one thing deserves attention: *nothing* should go into a staff member's personnel file unless he or she has signed it.* People have a right to know what could potentially be released to a future employer.

Performance review—informal. Adapting from the definition of formal review, we can define the informal performance review as a casual or unceremonious method of looking at effective function. More specifically, informal reviews are the discussion of single incidents or transient attitudes. In the formal review section we briefly talked about the supervisor who keeps a black book in preparation for formal review. Informal reviews have made these books obsolete and, more to the point, ridiculous. If there is a problem with an individual's clinical performance, attitude, or behavior, these problems should be discussed at the time they occur or very soon thereafter. Nobody will remember why he went to lunch early 6 months after the fact.

Informal reviews take on many forms. They may be in the form of anecdotal records or as casual as "I heard there was a problem with the lab last night—what happened?" Informal reviews are conducted on a daily basis, even though we may not have identified them as such. They are not restricted to discussing problems and negative behaviors. They should be

equally balanced with compliments and pats on the back.

INFORMAL REVIEW OBJECTIVES

1. To collect data. Frequently the story you heard initially is the end result of the gossip game and bears little or no resemblance to the actual incident. There is also the old saying, "There are three sides to every story—your side, my side, and the truth."

2. To correct misunderstandings. Maybe the lab didn't really hang up on the offended party; perhaps the switchboard disconnected the call at the most inopportune moment. Maybe the charge nurse was conducting two conversations, and when she said "yes" it was in answer to the person who asked if Mrs. Smith was still here and not in answer to the staff nurse who asked if she could go to lunch now.

3. To correct for the future. Some of the best teaching/learning experiences are "What would you do differently next time?" and "What can we do to ensure that this doesn't happen again?"

4. To maintain contact. Much of our daily contact with staff members is in the form of reviewing specific situations. If we keep black books instead of handling problems at the time they occur, we could easily and rapidly become isolated from those things that are important in the daily lives of the staff.

Performance review responsibilities. This segment applies primarily to the formal review process, although some of the principles are readily adaptable to the informal process as well.

There are usually two primary parties involved in the formal review. Each of those individuals has responsibilities in the review process. For clarity, we will call the person who is celebrating a 3-month, 6-month, or annual anniversary in the department the "staff member" and the person to whom he or she is directly responsible, the "reviewer."

STAFF MEMBER RESPONSIBILITIES. Opposite is an excerpt from a memo of mine that I give to

---

*If obtaining a signature would be inappropriate, the documentation should go into a confidential departmental file and *not* into the individual file. The confidential file should be flagged to indicate that the information is used only after consultation with the hospital attorney. Any documentation placed in the confidential file should be signed by at least two people.

emergency department staff members in preparation for review.

Do I have to do anything for the review?

Yes.
You will be notified when a review is near. You are then responsible for the following:
1. Contact the reviewer to set up a mutually convenient time for the review.

2. Prepare a staff performance objectives sheet *before* the review. If you have never set professional goals, talk with the reviewer ahead of time to discuss your questions.
3. Be prepared to discuss:
   a. Your strengths (what you think you're good at)
   b. Your "improvement-needed" areas (what you want to learn and attitudes you want to change)

Emergency department

Name: _____ Date: _____

Staff performance objectives

Please list below your goals for professional growth in the coming six months or year in the first column. The second column should outline your proposed methods for achieving those objectives. In the third column, please indicate your projected deadlines for achievement.

Performance objectives may be of an individual or group nature, personal or departmental, and may include such items as clinical expertise, attitude changes, departmental restructure, and so on. If your goals incorporate group or departmental objectives, please indicate what your personal contribution would be toward achieving this objective.

Goals	Methods	Deadline

c. What you like about the emergency department

d. Areas of deficiency or inefficiency in the emergency department

e. What you like about "the administration" (charge nurses, assistant director, medical director, and so on)

f. What you would like to see changed about "the administration."

4. If you are eligible for a merit increase and feel you should have one, write out and bring with you a list of the reasons why you feel an increase is warranted.

RESPONSIBILITIES OF REVIEWER. Some of the reviewer's responsibilities are concrete, obvious, and relatively simple to fulfill. Other responsibilities are intangible and sometimes difficult to achieve or measure.

1. Notify the staff member at least 1 week, and preferably 2 to 6 weeks, before her anniversary date that a review should be scheduled.

2. Provide the staff member with written information about the review process. The written material should include information concerning when reviews are done, why they are done, a list of the staff member's responsibilities, a goals sheet, the format to be used in the review, and an outline of procedure in the event of disagreement with the reviewer.

3. Provide adequate time for the review. Fifteen minutes is not enough. Usually the review will take an hour or more.

4. Provide uninterrupted time. Phone calls and drop-in visits should not be permitted during the alloted review time. It is rude and may break the train of thought of the staff member and the reviewer.

5. Prepare for the review. Write down the points you wish to cover, spend time thinking about the overall performance of the preceding months, talk with the staff member's direct co-workers, and review the previous goals list.

6. Be honest. That means you must be able to directly confront problem areas without beating around the bush.

7. Be fair. Make sure your information is accurate and reflects the opinion of more than one person.

8. Do not attack. Reviews should *not* be structured as criticism. They should be an honest appraisal of the strengths of the staff members as well as those areas (we all have them) where further growth and improvement are indicated.

9. Be receptive. If you are going to ask for sincere feedback, you must be prepared to look at your own performance and analyze its strengths and weaknesses. Staff members are a valuable source of input about how others perceive you, and if that input is met with immediate defense or attack, you will lose a potential source of information that may be helpful to your growth as a manager. This does not mean that you must accept all input as a 100% accurate reflection of your abilities, but do listen and ponder.

Learning to conduct true dialogue reviews takes time and practice. Nobody is so completely secure, fair, honest, and receptive that every review goes smoothly and results in enthusiastic, motivated, and happy staff members. If you feel the review isn't going well, discuss it before you go on, for example, "I feel some tension here. Did I say something that bothered you?" "I need to clarify something you just said that is bothering me." Do not expect to develop rapport and totally honest dialogue overnight, and remember that there will always be those few people who are not able to be open and direct in communicating no matter how they are approached.

REVIEW FORMATS. A review format is the written document on which the formal review is based. There are probably hundreds of different formats in use, and most hospitals have some sort of standardized, required format for their institution. Don't feel confined by that. If the hospital standard form does not meet your needs, request the use of an addendum specific to your area.

Formats run all the way from the ten-question, quality-of-work, quantity-of-work, job-knowledge review to a totally new, start-with-a-blank-page appraisal.

The start-with-a-blank-page appraisal, when based on a key responsibilities format is an excellent review tool (Smith and Brouwer, 1977). It works best, however, when you have no more than five people a year to review. It is time-consuming to write a review with no specific format, and that alone usually means long delays in producing the written document.

The ten-question quality/quantity, job knowledge format may meet the needs of the personnel office, but beyond that serves little useful function.

The best formats are those specifically designed to review those areas that you and the staff consider important in your environment. "Relates well with house staff" is appropriate in teaching institutions only. "Completes restocking assignments thoroughly" is appropriate unless there is a full-time restock person. Design a format that addresses the special needs and philosophies of your department. See Appendix G for sample of emergency department review format.

Leadership

In this context, the discussion of leadership is concerned with those people who have a title—supervisor, charge nurse, head nurse, manager, coordinator. They are the people who have been selected to assume a level of responsibility that is beyond what is expected of a regular staff member.

Essential qualities for leader selection. There is a long-standing tradition in many professions that leaders are selected on the basis of "years of service." It is a puzzling tradition that brings to mind a story.

According to legend, the Roman emperor Hadrian once found himself in an analogous position. One of his generals, the story goes, felt overdue for promotion. He took his case to the emperor and cited his long service as justification. "I am entitled to a more important command," he declared. "After all, I'm very experienced—I've been in ten battles."

Hadrian, a shrewd judge of men and their abilities, did not consider the man qualified for higher rank. He waved a casual hand at some army donkeys tethered nearby. "My dear general," Hadrian said dryly, "take a good look at those donkeys. Each of them has been in at least *twenty* battles—yet all of them are still donkeys (Gellerman, 1963).

An old quotation also comes to mind: "You can have either 20 years of experience or 1 year of experience 20 times."

The nursing profession does another very puzzling thing. The profession has somehow come to the conclusion that clinical excellence automatically equals management excellence. How all of this came to pass is a mystery. The effects of these traditions, however, are not very mysterious and have probably been experienced by all readers. The importance of having leaders who are respected and the results of incompetent leadership have been discussed. In this section the qualities that should be looked at when selecting a manager are outlined, not necessarily in order of priority.

"NATURAL" LEADERSHIP. If you put 15 people in a room and give them 10 minutes to resolve a problem, one or two will "naturally" lead the

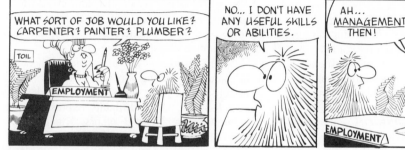

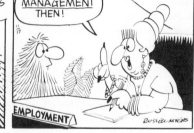

Fig. 5-2. Reprinted by permission of the Chicago Tribune—New York News Syndicate, Inc.

discussion. You know the type—title or no title, they are the people in your department to whom everyone automatically goes when a question arises. It does appear to be true that certain people are "born" leaders. Deciding whether or not they are actually *born* with this talent will be left to the heredity-versus-environment folks. The practical effect is the same. A percentage of the population seems to have an abstract quality that is different from the other percentage of the population.

The importance of this quality deserves an illustration. Picture that person in your department who is capable, does his work thoroughly, but is always quiet, rarely enters into discussion, and doesn't socialize much. Now picture that same person in charge of a project that represents a major change for the department, or picture him recruiting and interviewing. The value of natural leadership is readily apparent. It is essential to reiterate, however, that these qualities do not divide people into desirable or undesirable categories. They are simply different—*not* better or worse.

COMPETENCE. If you are asking someone to serve as a leader, he should have the skills to do so. Obviously, no one person excels in all areas, but he should be competent in his area of responsibility. For instance, a nurse who doesn't know a paramedic from a fireman should not be selected as paramedic liaison nurse; the weakest clinical nurse should not be asked to be responsible for the overall departmental in-service training, the least tactful person in the department should not be assigned all performance reviews, and a supply technician should know the difference between 4 × 4s and 2 × 2s.

Staff members will not respect or follow the guidance of someone who is incompetent in his area of responsibility. Leaders should be skilled in their area—whether it be interpersonal skills, organizational skills, educational skills, or clinical skills, a leader should be the most competent person you can find.

HIGH LEVEL OF COMMITMENT. Commitment is very difficult to quantify, but everyone knows who the committed people are. Their career development is important to them; they take the

time and effort to look for answers; they help resolve problems; they take the time to leave a note if something needs repair; they attend classes; and they demonstrate in word and deed that they do not take responsibility lightly.

They do *not* routinely goof off at work, call in sick when they are not, refuse to help out in scheduling, hang out in the lounge, leave their mess for the next shifts, or refuse to pitch in because it's "not my job."

ENTHUSIASM. Enthusiasm may look like commitment—and in fact you don't usually find enthusiasm without commitment, but in relationship to leadership, there are subtle but important differences. An emergency nurse, technician, or clerk may be highly committed to emergency care and the progress of his or her career, but may not have any enthusiasm for the responsibilities associated with management. Good leaders *genuinely* enjoy the kind of work they do. The good leaders are those who accepted the position because of *the work itself* and not because they wanted a title, or more money, or weekends off, or power.

This quality cannot be overemphasized. It is imperative that those people selected as leaders get true enjoyment out of the work itself. Taking a leadership position for *any* other reason will have disasterous effects. Besides which, if a leader doesn't enjoy the work, nothing else really makes it worth the hassle. A leader who does not like the job can destroy a department.

EGO STRENGTH. I recognize that no one is 100% secure. Everyone comes fully equipped with a full complement of assets and liabilities. Ego strength, in this context, means a variety of things, listed below.

SELF-CONFIDENCE. A good leader should have enough self-assurance that she is not afraid to voice opinions, make decisions, or speak with some degree of authority.

INTERPERSONAL SKILLS. Interacting with others in a genuinely caring way requires some degree of self-love. People whose personal esteem is very low often have difficulty expressing concern and appreciation to others. This difficulty may be demonstrated by abruptness with others, an inability to say "thank you," or a need to "put people down." Frequently, these people take sides and do not make an effort to help staff members support each other and "see the other side."

CONFRONTATION SKILLS. A good leader must be able to confront both people and problems. If one's opinion of oneself is regulated solely by external factors, other people's approval carries such impact that confrontation becomes very difficult. Good leaders confront without attack, never accuse, and interact in ways that promote trust in their objectivity and fairness.

Leaders must also confront problem areas and not be afraid to pursue resolutions. They should possess confidence in their ability to solve problems.

SELF-ASSESSMENT. People who are reasonably secure are not afraid to examine their own behaviors and motivations. They are not afraid to admit error. They are not defensive and hostile when criticized, and they don't always need to be right. They solicit feedback from colleagues and make sincere effort to improve their areas of deficiency.

Good managers know their strengths *and* their weaknesses and are not afraid to surround themselves with talented people. They are able to delegate, when appropriate, and are not concerned when other people have skills that they do not possess. They also know when stresses are interfering with their judgment and are willing to admit it.

REALNESS. People who like themselves are willing to be themselves. They can admit anger, fear, frustration, and "bad days." No one is "in control" all the time. This does not mean that good leaders routinely shout, throw things, or cry a lot. But occasionally everyone reaches a stress limit, and staff members will find the manager more believable as a person if she is not reluctant to express the feelings we all experience.

Recruiting: "inside" or "outside." The leadership selection topic would not be complete without addressing the age-old inside promotion versus outside recruitment issue. To begin, when a management position is available, the staff members in the department should have a realistic picture of what is required to fulfill the responsibilities. If previous

leaders have had the qualities described above, staff members probably already have a reasonable understanding of the effort and energy that is necessary to meet the needs of the department. If the leadership has previously been too low-key, then the people responsible for recruiting have an obligation to explain to all internal candidates that the former level of output was not sufficient and that greater commitment, time, and energy will be required. A clear picture of the job will, by itself, eliminate many applicants.

The next step is to open interviews to anyone in the department who is interested. Those who wait to be asked and do not show the initiative to actively seek the position can be eliminated from the running.

The third step is to evaluate all candidates by the criteria outlined previously. If the recruiters (there should be more than one) honestly feel that none of the candidates is capable, then it is necessary to look outside. It's that simple.

If you have made an honest assessment and decided to look outside and you are concerned about resentment from other staff members, then you might try asking those staff members who did not apply if there is anyone in the department who they feel is capable of doing the job. If your assessment is accurate, they will ponder a bit and concur that there is not. When employees are presented with the possibility of working under someone who is not right for the position, much of their resentment will rapidly fade away.

The applicants themselves should be directly, kindly, and honestly informed of the reasons why they were not selected. If the recruiters feel they could be developed, then their areas of deficiency should be identified and a program begun to develop them for future positions. If the applicants are mature and the denial is based on reasonable assessment, they will have some understandable adjusting to do, but it should be short-term.

When internal candidates are reviewed, another possible situation may arise. There may be a candidate who is questionable—perhaps good in some areas, but deficient in others. If there is such a person internally, and there is sufficient reason to consider her for the position, the opportunity should be extended. However, the areas in question should be discussed with the candidate and she must have a clear understanding of what is expected. If she is, in time, able to fulfill the responsibilities, great; if not, *do not leave her in the position*. The probationary period should not exceed 3 months. And there should be documentation that the requirements and concerns were understood. If possible, some measurable criteria should be established. There should not be weekly conferences to discuss performances and establish direction for the following week; self-assessments and initiative are the responsibilities of a leader. Her performance and abilities should stand (or fall) on their own merit. A conference at 6 weeks is probably indicated to avoid the "I didn't know I wasn't doing well" allegation, but constant counseling should not be necessary for people who are in a position to lead others.

The above paragraph is not intended to be interpreted as a harsh, insensitive approach to managing people. It is simply true that some people are not yet ready for leadership positions or are wrong for the environment or are not leadership material at all. The effects of leaving these people in management positions are devastating and serve to demoralize the nursing profession.

If such a situation occurs, the person involved should be given every consideration and be provided graceful, supportive alternatives. She should be commended for her willingness to try. It is occasionally even possible to keep her in the same department. Not working out in a "titled" position should not be viewed as a social disgrace. The individual should be reminded of her talents and encouraged to pursue areas where these talents can be utilized.

One of the great mistakes in nursing is that those who don't "move up" have somehow been looked upon as "failures" or "lacking in commitment." Patients have lost some of the best clinical care available because good nurses felt pressured into "moving up." Good clinical nursing should be recognized and encouraged and should never take a back seat to titles.

Responsibilities of a leader

ROLE MODELING. The leader described earlier is understandably expected to serve as a role model to other staff members in attitude and perspective. No one is a "model of perfection", but the departmental leaders should exemplify maturity and professionalism.

ENTHUSIASM. The leaders should be expected to serve as a positive motivating force in the department. If a member of the leadership staff is consistently cranky, depressed, short-tempered, and appears to hate coming to work, the effects are self-explanatory.

SUPPORT/PERSPECTIVE. The leadership staff should serve as a support system to the department. Support and perspective translate into many behaviors. Department leaders should have the most thorough knowledge of procedures and policies so that they can be looked to for answers. They should also have a level of understanding of departmental philosophies and objectives that enables them to support changes. They should serve as a sounding board for other staff members and should help resolve minor problems before they become major problems. They should be expected to handle their own complaints in a mature manner without creating morale crises by inappropriate "behind-the-back" complaining. They should have a mature perspective of the department and its relationship to other departments and to outside agencies. Ideally, they serve as public relations officers for the hospital and the department.

PROBLEM SOLVING. Good leaders should be able to reason through a problem, even when there is no "policy," and come to a logical resolution. They should be able to think clearly, weighing advantages and disadvantages, and not jump to hasty conclusions without knowledge of all the facts. They should also know when it is appropriate to refer a problem to the hospital administrator or the medical director. When situations arise that are unfamiliar, they should make it their business to find out how to deal with them the next time.

COMMUNICATION. Good leaders are skilled in communication. They know that you question—not accuse. They know that part of their responsibility is to teach perspective, understanding, and "lets'-look-at-it-from-their-side." They also know how to confront their colleagues when differences arise.

They know the importance of communicating to their superior when a problem has occurred. If the state governor was a patient on Friday night and not happy with the care received, a good leader knows it is wise to advise the department director and hospital administrator.

INITIATIVE. Leaders are expected to possess some initiative. It is not necessary to call the hospital administrator and tell him that the air conditioning is broken. Good leaders don't "dump" problems that they could easily resolve themselves. Good leaders also know what is going on in the department. If there is the sound of breaking glass coming from a treatment room, the charge nurse does not wait for someone to file a report before investigating whether or not the security guard should be called.

Effective leaders take initiative in helping resolve long-term problems too. If there seems to be a department-wide deficiency in documenting the care of chest pain patients, they help devise education, audit, new forms, or whatever it takes to resolve the problem.

DECISION MAKING. It has been said that good managers make decisions—if it's the right decision, so much the better. Although this may be a slight exaggeration, when leaders (particularly those with overall responsibility) are afraid to risk being wrong, they may immobilize the growth of the department. A weekend charge nurse who is afraid to call the copier repair people before Monday may risk an uprising if the staff has to run three flights of stairs to get copies made over the weekend.

CLINICAL TIME. The final behavior that should be expected—demanded—of nursing leaders is that they spend some portion of their time working in actual patient care. There are several advantages to adopting this practice.

1. The nurse leader is able to maintain some percentage of his or her clinical skill.
2. It maintains perspective about the real purpose of the job. It is too easy to drown in papers and rapidly forget that the reason for being a nurse is the care of patients.

3. It is good for mental health. Caring for patients is very rewarding, and the feedback is more immediate than the feedback in management. The nurse leader can, at least for 8 hours, forget about meetings, phone calls, and administrative hassles and do something with rapid visible results.
4. It diminishes Monday morning quarter-backing. If you were not there at 2:00 AM Saturday, it is easy to second-guess and say "This is what I would have done." You don't know what it's like unless you do patient care occasionally.

Leadership styles—or how to put together a management team. Teams are two or more people working together to achieve a goal (or goals). When putting a management team together, you should attempt to do the job with the minimum number of people with titles. Having 30% of the department staff in charge of something creates confusion and hassle.

No matter what the size of the team, there are three essential ingredients: people skill, clinical skill, and organizational skill.

People skill involves the ability to interact in a genuinely caring, nonthreatening manner, to confront, counsel, and see the good qualities. These are people who (1) remember to ask how your weekend was and (2) really do care if it was rotten.

Clinical skill includes clinical expertise, educational enthusiasm, and commitment to learning and teaching. These are nurses (1) whose eyes light up when a new, sophisticated procedure is introduced and (2) who actually understand how it works.

Organizational skill is the ability to define systems that improve efficiency, to identify inefficiencies, think logically, and organize projects. These are the ones who (1) cannot *stand it* when everything is out of place and jumbled up and (2) are in fact able to design a *workable* system for resolving the problem.

Ideally we would be able to find a leader with an equal balance of all these skills. Unfortunately, there are few people who possess *all* these skills.

The trick in putting together a management team is to assess what the current skills are and add to the deficient areas. It does not work out well if all the leaders are people-oriented but don't care that there aren't any 4 × 4s. Nor does it work well if there are lots of 4 × 4s and no pats on the back for getting them there.

The truth is that most leaders have some amount of each skill but are generally weighted more heavily in one area. If possible, you don't want people who have only one skill. If you have a real organizer who has no time for people, somebody has to soothe the ruffled feathers, and if you have a 100% people person, there won't be any 4 × 4s, and if you have a 100% clinician, everyone will know how to do the new procedure, but the right equipment will not always be available.

When filling (or creating) a position, assess the current leadership talents and the departmental deficiencies and write a summary of what kind of abilities are needed to resolve the problem areas. Many leaders make the mistake of choosing people who are like themselves because they may see eye-to-eye and be easier to get along with. But if you want a happy, well-organized, and clinically excellent department, that usually can't be done with people who are all cut from the same bolt of cloth. Always seeing eye-to-eye may make for a very peaceful working environment, but growth, change, and progress come only with new perspectives, some opinion differences, and varied ways of viewing the world.

Should you be a leader? This last portion of the leadership section speaks directly to those people who are already leaders and to those who may be considering it.

Management requires a different set of skills than patient care does. Anyone who has even organized a small project understands that fact. And management is not for everyone, just as emergency care, geriatric nursing, oncology nursing, and OR nursing are not for everyone.

Discovering that management is not for you should not be perceived as failure or disgrace. People do not criticize nurses who choose oncology over critical care; neither should they criticize nurses who choose direct patient care to management. Nurses try many areas before they find their niche, and management is only one of many possibilities.

Back to the original question. Should you be a leader? The answer to that is two-parted. Do you really enjoy it? Are you good at it? Usually those go hand-in-hand, but there are sadly still those people who enjoy the title and prestige and do not have the skills.

A self-quiz designed to help you arrive at the answer to the two questions above follows.

Do you enjoy the work?

1. What has been the happiest, most rewarding period in your career? If your answer is "when I was a staff nurse," perhaps you should reevaluate your career.
2. Do you look forward (at least 90% of the time) to going to work? If not, why not?
3. Do you find yourself longing to take care of patients and avoid the management hassles?
4. What is your assessment of your mental health? Do you smile often and go home feeling as if you have accomplished something, or do you find yourself grumpy, withdrawn, and always tired and depressed?
5. Do you look forward to new changes and problem-solving challenges with enthusiasm? Or do you find yourself procrastinating and avoiding new projects?
6. How do you feel about your colleagues? Do you think that they are basically a good group with whom you feel comfortable, or do you find you are consistently angry with them, routinely cranky and critical of their behavior? Colleagues include all department staff—physicians, nurses, technicians, and clerks, as well as nursing and hospital administration.
7. Are you physically healthy most of the time? If your sick days have dramatically increased, that may be an indication of stress.
8. How do your loved ones feel about your job? If your family and friends have expressed concern about your job's effect on your outlook, you may need to look carefully at your career choices.
9. What was your original reason for accepting the position?
10. Do you often feel that it is not worth the hassle?

Are you good at it?

1. What is the status of the overall morale in your department?
2. What is the attrition rate?

3. Have you noticed an increase in sick calls?
4. Do staff members come and talk with you regularly in a relaxed and comfortable way?
5. Have you accomplished the goals you set out to accomplish?
6. Do your colleagues feel free to offer advice, input, and suggestions for improvement?
7. Are people in the department actively involved in helping to make changes and improvements in the department?
8. Are there many people in the department whose talents exceed yours in certain areas?
9. Are you ever complimented by your superiors or the staff for the kind of job you are doing?
10. Is there chronic tension and friction between nurses, doctors, technicians, and clerks? Are they consistently critical of one another?
11. Do you regularly have to intervene in resolving petty personnel conflicts?
12. Do the people in the department enjoy coming to work, and do they treat patients with empathy and respect?

This self-assessment should give you a fairly accurate picture of whether this is the right career choice for you.

If you are really unsure and are willing to risk the outcome, go to your immediate supervisor and tell her that you are questioning whether you are effective in management. If she says "You're doing an excellent job," you probably are. If you get a reply such as "Not everyone is cut out for management" or "Do you have other options in mind?" you may want to consider a change.

Making a change is simply that. It is deciding that there are other options that would provide you with a happier, more rewarding career. It is not failure. Your colleagues will respect and appreciate your willingness to assess yourself and admit that you are not happy in that position. And your superiors will probably do everything possible to help you find a position that will meet your needs. Chronic frustration and unhappiness are not healthy for you or for the department.

Teamwork/personnel conflicts

No member of a crew is praised for the individuality of his rowing.

Ralph Waldo Emerson

Emergency care offers unique opportunities and challenges in the area of teamwork. It is the only area in health care where physicians, nurses, technicians, and clerks work side-by-side on a 24-hour basis. It is also a stressful area, and emergency personnel have a relatively short period of time in which to meet a variety of goals. First and foremost, the patient's medical needs must be met; in addition, his emotional needs and those of his family must be met. There are forms, requisitions, reporting laws, and legal problems to be reckoned with. All this must be done, and done right, and emergency department staff members have anywhere from 30 minutes to a few hours to accomplish these varied objectives.

To expect, in such an environment, that staff members will always interact in a calm, quiet, and reasonable manner and never ruffle each other's feathers is unrealistic. However, if an atmosphere of professionalism and mutual respect is established throughout the department, peer conflicts and related problems can be minimized.

Establishing and maintaining this atmosphere present a genuine challenge. People who are attracted to emergency care are generally not low-keyed. They have definite ideas and opinions and usually are not at all reluctant to share their perceptions of things. This individualism is, overall, an asset: dealing with immediate threats of life and limb require some assertiveness, and it is much easier to tone down assertiveness than it is to gear up apathy. However, these qualities can also create many injured egos and, if not properly handled, some boulders on the road to teamwork.

Providing an atmosphere of professionalism and respect is a two-part task. The atmosphere must first be established, and then it must be maintained.

Establishing the atmosphere. Establishing a teamwork milieu is primarily the responsibility of the leadership staff.

MEDICAL DIRECTOR/NURSING SUPERVISOR RELATIONSHIP. If the top leadership people in a department are not able to interact in a mutually supportive manner, the groundwork is already laid for trouble. The physician director and the nursing director should be the role model for teamwork. The planning for a department's growth and progress should be a joint effort between physician and nursing leadership in order to ensure that goals are agreed on, understood, and supported by both parties. When the top leadership is pulling together, departmental teamwork is a natural result.

Obviously, leaders are going to disagree on occasion, but these disagreements should not be the topic of general discussion throughout the department. The leadership staff should be mature enough that they do not find it necessary to grouse about the department, slandering the others and soliciting allegiance, directly or indirectly, for their "side." The goal should always be to arrive at a mutually agreeable method of operating. If these two people are absolutely unable to work together, one of them should go—perhaps both.

SELECTION OF STAFF. Earlier in the chapter the selection of staff members was discussed. Selecting staff members who are mature and professional in their outlook will prevent personnel conflicts. Staff members whose entire life is focused on work, whose friends are all work friends, tend to get a skewed perspective of the work environment. There is also the "chronic complainer," whose investment is solidly in keeping problems going and not in resolving them. These are the people who say *nothing* directly, whose complaints are always heard third hand and who never actively work toward resolution of a problem. Do not let one of them get transferred to your department.

LAYING THE GROUNDWORK. When new staff members are hired, they should, as part of their orientation, be given a clear picture of how complaints and problems are to be handled. It must be communicated from the outset that the goal is problem resolution, not problem continuance and magnification. New staff members should understand that there are only one of two people to whom they should go when problems arise: the person they have the conflict with or the immediate supervisor. Magnifying problems by grumbling to many people should not be tolerated. If the message is delivered early in the game, it may help avoid serious morale problems in the future.

ROLES/TEAMWORK. If the leadership staff makes it known that no one job category is more important than another—that it takes the cooperative effort of all to meet the goals—the hierarchy problems can be minimized. Although it may be true that good physicians are harder to acquire than good clerks, an emergency department cannot function adequately without good clerks—or nurses or technicians. No one category can effectively operate without cooperation and expertise in the other categories. It should be understood that all personnel will be treated with respect. Another factor that ensures a smoothly running department is teamwork. Nurses should not be sitting in groups of two and three while technicians clean suture sets. Clerks should not be sitting while nurses are up to their eyebrows in requisitions. The "whose job is it?" problem can be difficult. For efficiency's sake, there must be defined sets of responsibilities, but 5 minutes after duties lists are distributed, someone will invariably say "That's not my job." Getting over the hurdle takes time and patience. People are naturally inclined to heave a sigh of relief when their duties list is completed and are apt to ignore the fact that there are five other people who have been working diligently without break for the past 8 hours.

During orientation, it should be communicated that, although there are defined responsibilities, it is also *expected* that each person will help out if his colleagues are overloaded.

SEMANTICS. Our primary method of communication is words, and the words we use should be carefully chosen. Part of laying the groundwork for genuine teamwork is being selective in our terminology. For instance, "the 3 to 11 charge nurse hates the new doctor" has a different sound from "the 3 to 11 charge nurse came to talk to me about the new doctor." "She's really stupid when it comes to arrhythmias" sounds different from "I think she needs some arrhythmia education."

The word "employee" immediately says that there is an "employer" or "boss." When it comes right down to it, *everyone* is really a *staff member,* and there should be *personnel* manuals, not *employee* manuals.

Finally, do not call the people in the department ''my'' nurses or technicians or clerks. Staff members do not belong to anyone. They are the nurses in the emergency department, or the department secretary—but not ''my'' anything or anybody—and it is ''our'' department not ''my'' department.

It may be difficult to change years of terminology habits, but try listening to yourself, and assessing the psychological impact of your word choices. Whenever possible, use words that are not ''loaded.''

Maintaining cooperation. The responsibility for maintaining a cooperative atmosphere lies primarily with the leadership staff and secondarily with all members of the team. A mutually supportive, understanding environment requires empathy, the recognition of conflict and differences, and conflict resolution.

EMPATHY. Encouraging empathy among staff members is one very good way to promote teamwork. When a new physician works her first shift and seems slow and uncertain, staff members should be reminded that they all had a ''first day.'' ''Slowness'' complaints seem to be related to physician more often than any other job category. Somehow, people expect that a physician should be able to drop into any environment, not knowing the procedures and ways of working, and function at top speed.

One of the ways to promote empathy is to arrange some role switching. Unfortunately, this cannot be done with all personnel. An emergency department technician cannot be ''physician of the day,'' but nurses can be technicians, and clerks can help out with nursing duties, and physicians can be nurses. From a cost standpoint, routine role changing is not often feasible, but if the opportunity presents itself, it should not be passed up.

Complaints about other staff members should be met with some dialogue about the possible reasons for the behavior. These dialogues should also reflect some of the good points about that person. ''Yes, I know he can be a little short-tempered occasionally, but there isn't a better nurse in the department, and he really is concerned that the patient gets the best care available.''

Department personnel should also be reminded that everyone has idiosyncrasies: some people can't get to work on time, others hate checking the equipment, some are occasionally grumpy, others are slow, still others are too compulsive. Each person has something that is not 100% perfect. And each person has some redeeming qualities.

This is not to say that all personnel conflicts should be handled by playing the ''glad game,'' but investigating reasons for the behavior and looking at overall patterns of performance may take some of the steam out of the complaint.

CONFLICT RECOGNITION. Recognizing conflicts is an important part of maintaining a teamwork environment. Differentiating minor transient problems from conflicts that will interfere with good working relationships is sometimes difficult. Although personal conflicts should not be ignored, they should also not receive more time and attention than they warrant. Calling an eight-person group therapy conference every time there is an impolite exchange only adds to the problem. Most adults realize that life is full of annoyances, many of which are not worth a lot of emotional energy. Overemphasizing minor situational problems is counterproductive, costly, and time-consuming.

However, all personnel conflicts should be *recognized* and dealt with in some way. Dealing with a conflict may occasionally mean ignoring it or watching for awhile to see if it resolves itself; many times maturity wins out, and it goes away on its own. If some intervention is indicated, it should be done as soon as possible. Allowing problems to brew for weeks may ultimately double the work involved in resolution. Emergency care is stressful enough without expending the energy necessary to remember not to speak to someone.

Differentiating between minor and major problems is a skill that is learned only with time. There are no magic formulas or graphs that will guide that decision. The best monitoring device is your own sensing, your knowledge of the people involved and prior history. If you know that the people involved are inclined to bear grudges, or if this is the ten thousandth time this minor complaint has surfaced, it is necessary to address it directly and immediately.

CONFLICT RESOLUTION. This discussion of conflicts is related to those performance problems and personality-related issues that inevitably crop up in any working environment: "Laura is too abrupt," "Sharon doesn't restock her room," "Jeff is lazy," "Bill left early," "Elaine let 14 people stay in the trauma room, and there was so much confusion," "The night shift doesn't . . . ," "The day shift always . . . ," and so on. This discussion is not related to major problems. Staff members who hit patients, steal narcotics, or make gross clinical errors should be dealt with directly and rapidly.

There are many approaches to dealing with personnel conflicts and much controversy over what constitutes the best approach. Everyone has to decide for herself what methods work best, but the suggestions below may be helpful. New conflicts become known by means of three mechanisms: (1) someone comes into the office to complain directly, (2) there is some gossip about the incident or person, or (3) there is a sensing of something awry. In each of these situations, some decisions have to be made about how much attention the situation warrants, but for the purposes of this discussion, it is assumed that the decision is made. What follows is a list of helpful hints.

DON'T OVEREMPHASIZE THE PROBLEM. Comments such as "How could she be so stupid" or "He is such a jerk" do not help the situation. Comments such as, "Does this happen often?" "Can you give me more specifics?" or "I'm surprised. That's really out of character for him" may add some perspective. If you haven't been directly approached, but are trying to investigate, it's better to start out with "I heard there was a problem Saturday night" than "Jeff really blew again, huh?" Try to remain neutral, objective, and add some perspective rather than taking sides.

CLARIFY THE ISSUES. When discussing the conflict, be sure the *real* problems are identified. What appears to be laziness may be a lack of understanding of what the duties are; what appears to be a lack of caring may be a momentary preoccupation with personal problems or a previous patient; failure to restock a room could be the result of an unusually busy shift; abrupt-

ness may be the result of adjusting to a new role and the stresses involved. Review the issues carefully before deciding about intervention.

LEAVE THE RESOLUTION DECISION WHERE IT BELONGS. Once a problem has been identified, ask the *people who identified it* what they think should be done about it. Are they simply in your office to blow off steam (perfectly appropriate by the way, if *not* spread throughout the department), or do they feel some intervention is indicated? The answer to the "what do you think should be done" question is often surprising. When the decision is presented to them, often they feel that discussion is sufficient and wish to leave it at that, or wait to see if the problem recurs. Most people are not anxious to hang their colleagues.

ENCOURAGE CONFRONTATION. Once it has been decided that intervention is indicated, ask what the "complaining party" wants to do about it. Staff members are not children, and they should not be allowed to run to mommy or daddy and send them to tell Johnny to quit throwing sand. Most of them are capable of dealing directly with the problem themselves. Yes, it is uncomfortable and difficult at first, but having to say "you" and "I" will deescalate the subjective nature of the "he did, she said" conversations. Confronting someone directly forces one to see the other as a real person with assets, liabilities, and feelings.

Clearly there are times when the leaders must get involved. Chronic problems and performance problems that may result in discipline should be handled by the appropriate supervisor, but most conflicts are best worked out on a one-to-one basis.

SUMMARY. Establishing and maintaining a teamwork atmosphere is not easy. It requires diligence and commitment to the goal, but the benefits are obvious. If there is a teamwork problem, direct, emphatic confrontation with a goal of *resolution* is the recommended approach.

BIBLIOGRAPHY

Gellerman, S.: Motivation and productivity, New York, 1963, AMACOM, a division of American Management Associations, Inc.

Fulcher, J, K.: Personal communications, 1976-1980.

Herzberg, F.: Dual-factor theory of job satisfaction, Personnel Psych. Winter, 1967, pp. 369-389.

Maslow, A. H.: Motivation and Personality, New York, 1954, Harper & Row, Publishers, Ch. 5.

McClelland, D.: That urge to achieve, Think Magazine, 1966.

Smith, H. P., and Brouwer, P. J.: Performance appraisal and human development, Reading, Mass., Addison-Wesley Publishing Co.

Vroom, V.: Work and motivation, New York, 1964, John Wiley & Sons.

SUGGESTED READINGS

Drucker, P. F.: People and performance. In The best of Peter Drucker on management, New York, 1977, Harper's College Press.

Glassman, A. M.: The challenge of management, New York, 1978, John Wiley & Sons, Inc.

Hampton, D. R.: Behavioral concepts in management, Encino, Calif., 1972, Dickenson Publishing Co.

Mager, R. F., and Pipe, P.: Analyzing performance problems, Belmont, Calif., 1970, Fearon Publishers, Inc.

Mager, R. F.: Goal analysis, Belmont, Calif., 1972, Fearon Publishers, Inc.

CHAPTER 6

Triage

Triage is one of the most important and challenging roles in the emergency department. Two years ago, the cover of a leading nursing journal depicted the triage nurse as one sitting on a time bomb with phones ringing all around her and people yelling at her from all directions. There is much stress in triaging. It is a critical position, because it sets the pace and tone of the entire department and establishes priorities for patient care. It requires the person filling the position to possess much common sense, a good deal of intuition, medical knowledge, administrative knowledge and perspective, technical skills, communication skills, and leadership. He or she must possess the ability to respond quickly to possible life-threatening illnesses or injuries.

Most medical personnel can recognize the emergent status of an obvious multiple trauma patient or one in full cardiopulmonary arrest. But it requires great skill to accurately assess the patient whose illness or injury is far less obvious or one whose actual life-threatening problem may be masked by his chief complaint. Some of the skills of triage are intuitive, but many are learned.

DEFINITION

The formal definition of triage, taken from the French, is "to sort into three groups." It is the process of deciding the priorities for therapeutic intervention of a given individual or individuals and the place where these interventions should occur.

There are generally three categories of triage: Class I or emergent, Class II or urgent, and Class III or delayed. A Class I or emergent patient is one who has a life-threatening emergency and will die if immediate therapeutic intervention does not take place. A Class II or urgent patient is one who will require therapeutic intervention within 5 to 60 minutes. A Class III or delayed patient is one whose care may be delayed from 4 to 6 hours. A fourth class, Class IV or clinic patient, has been added to the triage categories to accommodate those patients who would normally be referred to a clinic as nonemergency patients.

In most emergency departments there is some form of triage, no matter how small or large the department. The type of triage system may vary depending on the needs and capabilities of the facility. Triage is one step toward a way to care for patients effectively and efficiently. Although the role of triage is filled by various individuals around the country, from the clerk to the physician, the trend appears to be toward registered nurse triage for both good patient care and cost effectiveness.

WHO SHOULD BE A TRIAGE NURSE?

A triage nurse should have extensive experience in dealing with emergency patients. Much of the background for triage nursing is drawn from good common sense, which usually is acquired from years of clinical experience and decision making, a collection of medical knowledge, and a working knowledge of the emergency department and its personnel and policies.

Requirements of a triage nurse

The triage nurse must:
- Be able to function well under stressful situations.
- Be able to make accurate assessments regarding patient care.
- Have a working knowledge of the internal operations of the emergency department.
- Know intradepartmental policies.
- Be able to make rapid and sound decisions.
- Have firm convictions.
- Possess good communication skills.
- Be able to offer emotional support to others.
- Be able to think ahead.
- Be able to supervise others.
- Be an on-the-spot teacher.
- Be able to control traffic flow.
- Possess good crisis intervention skills.
- Have a working knowledge of the prehospital care system.
- Be able to avoid conflict and loss of temper.
- Represent the hospital and the emergency department to the public.
- Assist in discharge planning.
- Be able to handle telephone triage.
- Be able to deal with patient communication problems such as patients who have expressive aphasia, the intoxicated patient, the belligerent patient, and those who are deaf or do not speak English.

Qualifications of a triage nurse

In order to function in the role of triage nurse, one must:
- Possess a valid state registered nurse license.
- Be certified as a mobile intensive care nurse (if that certification is available).
- Be certified in basic cardiac life support (and, preferably, advanced cardiac life support).
- Have a minimum of 2 years of critical care nursing experience, with at least 6 months of this being in the emergency department.
- Have at least four training shifts in the triage position with a senior triage nurse.
- Have at least three evaluation shifts in the role of triage.

Special considerations

Triage should be performed in a well-lighted central area with easy traffic flow, some privacy, and from which all patient care is initiated (or continued, as in the case of a patient arriving by ambulance from the prehospital care setting). The triage nurse's main responsibility is to accurately assess a patient and establish priorities for that patient. This includes not only therapeutic intervention, but also assignment to an acceptable place for treatment, considering other patients already in the department or

	Medical	**Administrative**
Temporal	Must be seen early for a life-threatening emergency; requires certain basic knowledge.	Logistical situation; may be a "quick" disposition, such as a police case, where one would not like to delay the police from their routine duties; the patient may also be a noisy psychiatric patient or a belligerent patient whose rapid disposition would be a benefit to all.
Spatial	Should be near the proper equipment (for example, the slit lamp, x-ray); best to put same types of patients in the same treatment area for better patient care (that is, surgical patients should be together in a surgical area; may have special requirements for care).	Makes logistics easier for ancillary personnel; noisy patients, rape victims, police patients may require a quiet, private place.

about to enter the department, the department staff, the physical set-up of the department, and the patient flow pattern.

There are four factors to consider when triaging*
1. Medical needs
2. Administrative needs
3. Temporal needs
4. Spatial needs

An example of what is meant by each is found on p. 91.

EVALUATING THE CHIEF COMPLAINT

The general approach to triaging a patient is to evaluate the chief complaint. *Do not make a diagnosis!* Do not focus solely on the obvious (for example, a fractured ankle) and overlook the not-so-obvious (for example, the syncopal episode that caused the patient to fall off the ladder and fracture his ankle).

Use your eyes, ears, nose, hands, and brain. First of all, *look* at your patient. He may be telling you that he doesn't have chest pain, but at the same time he is grimacing, clenching his fists, and having difficulty breathing; his neck veins are grossly enlarged. You will be able to learn a lot by simply looking at a patient. You will be able to see such things as fear, anxiety, respiratory problems, obvious bleeding, deformities, changes in skin color, and vascular perfusion along with a host of other things. Develop a habit of being a keen observer.

Keep your nose open to smells; you may be able to smell ketone bodies, alcohol, marijuana, incontinence, and purulent infectious processes. You may be able to tell what a child ingested by identifying an odor on his breath.

Use your ears to hear what the patient is saying and *what the patient is not saying.* Use your ears to hear gross rales, a cough, a raspy voice, or shortness of breath.

Touch the patient. Take a pulse. Besides being able to assess heart rate and cardiac output (roughly) you will be able to assess skin temperature and moisture and capillary per-

fusion. Touch and feel for crepitus, a deviated trachea, or "where it hurts."

Notice that you have done all of this without any invasive monitoring or elaborate laboratory tests. While you are doing this, ask the patient (if he is able to respond to your questions) about his chief complaint. "Well, Mr. Richfield, what brings you to the emergency department today?" Once a chief complaint is established, one may elect to use any one of many assessment formats. I prefer the age old mnemonic, which is taught at Los Angeles County Paramedic Training, of *PQRST,* in which:

P = provokes
What makes it (the pain) better? What makes it worse?

Q = quality
What does it (the pain) feel like? If the patient cannot describe the pain, perhaps some suggestions such as "burning," "stabbing," "crushing," "tearing," would be helpful.

R = radiates
Where is the pain? Where else does it go? Is it in one spot? Is it in many spots? Show me where it is.

S = severity
If we gave pain a number from one to ten, with one being the least severe and ten being the worse pain you could imagine, what number would you give this pain?

T = time
How long have you had this pain? When did it start? When did it end?

By using your eyes, ears, nose, hands, and brain (PQRST), you should be able to have a fair idea about if this patient requires immediate care. Remember: *do not make a diagnosis; make a triage decision.*

If you wish, you may also elect to employ the Larry Weed system of problem-oriented medical records to triage, in which:

S = subjective
Collect data about what the patient is telling you.

O = objective
What are you actually seeing?

A = assess
Assess the situation using subjective and objective findings.

P = plan
Establish a plan for the patient.

---

*Adapted from a lecture given to the Brotman Emergency Department Staff in May 1978 by James K. Fulcher, MD.

Example

S = *subjective*

"I ran into a telephone pole while jogging and hit my head."

O = *objective*

There is a 4-inch laceration across the forehead; patient is conscious and having no difficulty breathing.

A = *assess*

This patient has a laceration that will require suturing; he will probably also require a quick neurological examination.

P = *plan*

Triage the patient to the surgical area for suturing.

Example

S = *subjective*

"I have indigestion. I just ate a pizza. My wife insisted that I come to the emergency department. I'm really not sick."

O = *objective*

Patient is having difficulty breathing. His neck veins are elevated, he is grimacing, his skin is cold and clammy, he has a tachycardiac irregular pulse. His lips and nail beds are cyanotic.

A = *assessment*

This patient is sicker than he thinks. His objective findings indicate that something more than indigestion is taking place.

P = *plan*

Triage the patient immediately to a medical bed for acutely ill patients for immediate evaluation and therapeutic intervention.

Be familiar with the chief complaint and the appropriate questions to ask for each. Develop protocols or algorhythms for chief complaints.

Often the triage nurse is the individual who is directed to interact with the public. It is his or her responsibility to keep up to date on all that is happening within the emergency department. He or she should be able to answer such questions as, "Why is it taking so long?" or "How much longer will it be?" He or she must deal with the angry, anxious, frightened, intoxicated, belligerent, hysterical, pushy, or manipulative patient. He or she sets the tone for the entire department. He or she must remain calm and outwardly in control at all times.

If the nurse assigned to triage is having the proverbial "bad day," he or she should not be placed in the triage role. If, during his or her role as triage nurse, the stress becomes overwhelming, he or she should request to be replaced in that position. The entire atmosphere in the department is set by the first person the patient encounters in the emergency department. Triaging *can* be like sitting on a time bomb—and no one would send in other than an expert to dismantle the bomb. Triage is not a place for the inexperienced or the untrained. To be a good triage nurse is to be a skilled, astute, compassionate practitioner with a great deal of common sense and intuition. It is one of the *ultimate* challenges in emergency nursing.

EXAMPLES OF TRIAGE SITUATIONS

Situation 1

A private ambulance brings an elderly patient with a history of "he fell and broke his hip."

ASSESSMENT: The triage person assesses for the possibility that syncope may have occurred before the fall and asks about chest pain, palpitations, orthostatic dizziness, symptoms of gastrointestinal bleeding, and so on.

PLAN: If there are no medical problems, triage directly to the x-ray section of the emergency department. If the patient answers "yes" to questions concerning medical problems, triage for a rapid medical evaluation before having a surgical evaluation. If pulses are diminished or absent in the distal extremity, triage for immediate surgical evaluation.

Situation 2

A paramedic ambulance brings a 23-year-old woman with a history of a grand mal seizure that resulted in a fall. The victim struck her head and has a large, heavily bleeding occipital laceration.

ASSESSMENT AND PLAN: If she is still having seizures, triage for medical evaluation and treatment. If she is postictal, triage for rapid medical evaluation. If awake, alert, and oriented (times 4), triage for a rapid medical evaluation in the surgical area and a rapid repair of the laceration.

Situation 3

A family brings their 89-year-old grandfather to the emergency department with a chief complaint of rectal bleeding.

ASSESSMENT: Assess the patient and assure that airway, breathing, and circulation are intact. Does the patient have a history of hemorrhoids? Is it painful for the patient to have a bowel movement? Does he complain of a sore rectum? Is there blood streaking in the stool?

PLAN: If the answer to any of the above questions is "yes," the patient should be triaged to the surgical area. If the answer is "no," the patient should be triaged to the medical area.

Situation 4

A patient is driven to the emergency department in a private automobile. He is complaining of abdominal pain.

ASSESSMENT AND PLAN: If pain is less than 48 hours old, triage to the surgical area. If pain is more than 48 hours old, triage to the medical area. A woman with lower abdominal pain should be triaged to the gynecological area.

Situation 5

Two patients, a child with a possible drug ingestion and a man with an allergic reaction, arrive at the emergency department at the same time.

ASSESSMENT: The child is alert and oriented (times 4), playing with his mother's car keys; his vital signs are normal. The man has urticaria and is wheezing.

PLAN: The man should be triaged to the medical area immediately for evaluation and therapeutic intervention.

Triage the child to a bed as soon as one becomes available. If possible, have the physician do a rapid evaluation of the child after he has seen the man with the allergic reaction. The mother may sit with the child in a chair in the treatment area. If a rapid evaluation is performed, the physician may choose to write an order for Ipecac. This may be given with the child on his mother's lap in the hallway, away from the waiting area where the patient is in view of the nurse.

Situation 6

Five patients appear in the emergency department at the same time.

Patient 1: A 60-year-old construction worker is bent over, holding the area of his lower back. He states that he is in a great deal of pain and cannot stand up straight.

Patient 2: A 76-year-old woman with a history of a syncopal episode and a reported episode of hematemesis is brought in by the paramedics.

Patient 3: A 16-year-old boy in gym clothes hops in on one foot with the aid of his friends. His ankle is swollen and discolored. He has good distal neurovascular status.

Patient 4: A 5-year-old girl with a lacerated chin is awake, alert, and oriented; her mother states that she never lost consciousness. The laceration is not bleeding at present.

Patient 5: A 27-year-old jogger in respiratory arrest. The paramedics are ventilating him via an esophageal obturator airway. He has a sinus tachycardia with a rate of 144. He does have pulses present.

ASSESSMENT: Decisions must be made rapidly in this situation. There is not time to do a thorough evaluation of each of these patients. The patients should be triaged and ranked in order of treatment priority in accordance with their problem(s).

PLAN: Patient 5 is most critical. He is classified as a Class I or emergent patient. His problem is life-threatening, and he must be treated immediately.

Patient 2 is classified as Class II or urgent. She is pale. Her blood pressure is decreased, and her pulse has increased. One must assume that she is bleeding and not tolerating this blood loss well. She should be seen as soon as possible following the patient in respiratory arrest. Patient 1 is classified as a Class II or urgent patient because of the subjective assessment of "great pain." His problem does not appear to be a life-threatening one, but urgent triage would be a very thoughtful consideration to the patient. Patient 4 is in no apparent severe distress. The laceration is not bleeding and she is awake and alert. She is classified as a Class III or delayed. She can wait for 4 hours if necessary, even though such a situation is not desirable. Patient 3 is stable. He has no pulse deficits. He, too, is classified as a Class III or delayed patient and can wait more than 4 hours to be treated if necessary.

General classifications for triage

Class I—Emergent: patients with critical, life-threatening injuries or illness require immediate evaluation and therapeutic intervention, for example:

Cardiopulmonary arrest

Chest pain, pressure or discomfort, that is either a new pain or different from previous pain

Certain dysrhythmias

Respiratory distress

Bleeding

Hemorrhage from a wound

Hematemesis/melena/hematochezia

Epistaxis (severe)

Profuse vaginal bleeding
Severe trauma
  Victims of
    Automobile accidents
    Motorcycle accidents
    Automobile/pedestrian accidents
  Head trauma (unless obviously minor)
  Large open wounds
  Chest trauma
  Elderly patient who has fallen and is unable to walk
Drug overdose
Attempted suicide
Altered mental status
Those having seizures
Most ambulance patients
Any patient who, according to your instinct, looks sick, seems sick, acts sick
Class II—Urgent: Patients with major illnesses or injuries that should be treated within 20 minutes to 2 hours, for example:
Cardiovascular accidents or transient ischemic attacks
Obvious fractures with vascular compromise
Abdominal pain less than 36 hours in duration
Headaches that are described as sudden, severe, different
Open wounds (does not include minor lacerations)
Blood from any orifice (small amount)
Vomiting
Fever, chills (especially small children)
Palpitations less than 48 hours in duration
Jaundice
Class III—Delayed: Patients with minor injuries who are usually ambulatory, for example:
Minor burns
Sprains and strains
Closed fractures

Special classification

Patients with the following conditions should be triaged at least as Class II (urgent) patients, no matter how insignificant the complaint, because they may be at risk to greater problems than others:
Patients with artificial heart valves
Patients with organ transplants
Patients on renal dialysis
Patients with cancer (especially leukemia and lymphoma)
Patients who are paraplegics or quadraplegics
Patients who are insulin-dependent diabetics
Patients with lupus erythematosis
Patients with severe kyphoscoliosis (hunchback)

BIBLIOGRAPHY

Barber, J., and Budassi, S.: Mosby's manual of emergency care: practice and procedures, St. Louis, 1979, The C. V. Mosby Co.
Budassi, S.: The treacheries of triage, The J. Emergency Care **1**:40-43, Spring 1979.
Cowan, W.: Triage and how it works, Emergency Product News, April 1976, pp. 124-125.
Estrada, E.: Advanced triage, J.E.N. **5**:5, 1979.
Landon, B.: Triage: how to set priorities for patient care. In Giving emergency care competently, Nursing Skillbooks Series, Horsham, Pennsylvania, 1979, Intermed Communications.
McLeod, K. A.: The transformation of the ED nurse. Part I. Learning to take the trauma out of triage, R.N. **38**:22-27, July 1975.
Mills, J., Webster, A., Wolfsy, C., Harding, P., and others, Effectiveness of nurse triage in the emergency department of an urban county hospital, J.A.C.E.P. **5**: 11, November 1976.
Richards, R.: Making the telephone work for you, J.E.N. **2**(3):18, 1976.
Shields, J.: Making triage work, J.E.N. **2**(4):37-41, 1976.

CHAPTER 7

Patient assessment

Joan Kelley Simoneau

The spectrum of events that constitutes an emergency varies considerably with each individual patient. In recent years the number of patients utilizing the emergency department has increased markedly, and in the hectic environment thus created it becomes crucial that there be a continuous effort to identify patients with critical or potentially critical conditions. Often the responsibility of the initial evaluation falls upon the emergency nurse, who is frequently the first professional to encounter the patient.

Although the degree of assessment and intervention will be different for each patient, the process is a dynamic one. It is often of singular importance to the establishment of management priorities. Development of accurate decisions for action depends to a large degree on whether the nurse employs an organized and systematic approach to the assessment process. Although tools are helpful in the physical examination, the initial observations that serve to focus the assessment require no equipment whatsoever. During this period of time, the most important tools are the senses of sight, touch, smell, hearing—common sense! To be sure, much depends on the skill of the observer to interpret what significance the information collected has in the clinical situation.

It is essential to appreciate that the potential for deterioration exists for any patient in the department. If subtle changes are overlooked or ignored, this deterioration is not only possible, but it may become rapidly irreversible even

if recognized and treated vigorously later. If, for instance, we were to place each patient at an arbitrary point of relative wellness or equilibrium (point A), we can plot out a path based on timeliness of intervention. If we recognize the patient's physiological and emotional needs at that point and move to provide intervention, we will either serve to maintain his equilibrium or improve his condition. If, however, intervention is delayed or absent, the patient will move down a curve to point B. Point B is that place on the path at which a great deal of effort and skill must be expended in order to halt and reverse the descent. If the patient does not receive appropriate intervention at point B, he will progress further down to point C, or death.

In essence, all our efforts must be directed toward the arrest of any downhill descent at whatever point we receive the patient, whether sitting up and comfortable with only shoulder pain, or obtunded and gravely ill. The primary purpose of nursing assessment is to utilize the scientific method of collecting patient information, implementing nursing intervention based on a reasonable interpretation of signs and symptoms, and thus preventing deterioration and death.

The focus of this chapter is to identify the practical aspects of nursing assessment. Specific disease assessments are avoided in favor of presenting them within the individual chapters that deal with each system. Rather, an overview is provided that serves as a helpful guideline for the emergency nurse to use in the day-to-day situation. Potential barriers to assessments by nurses are also presented in order to build a respect for the obstacles that may hamper or destroy efforts to assess patients. Equipment and steps of assessment are covered in detail. With this information, perhaps more nurses will get involved with one of the most important and satisfying functions that the emergency nurse can perform: nursing assessment of the emergency patient.

BARRIERS TO PATIENT ASSESSMENT

If assessment of the emergency patient is such a vital aspect of emergency management, why is it that nursing assessment is not routinely performed in every department? The fact is that there are barriers to effective and consistent assessment that, if recognized and reduced or avoided, may have less impact on the process. Cosgriff and co-workers categorized the most common barriers into three groups: professional, institutional, and patient-related. These same groups are discussed in more detail in this chapter.

Professional barriers to assessment

Traditionally, patient assessment and management have been felt to be solely a physician's responsibility. Evaluating signs and symptoms, interpreting collected physical data, developing a working diagnosis of the cause of the abnormalities discovered, and initiating treatment were all considered to fall within the physician's purview; nurses were not expected to become involved with this process. Even today, the word "diagnosis" is considered to be a medical term, and many physicians and more traditional nurses are alarmed by the growing use of this term in the nursing vocabulary.

As emergency medicine, and indeed critical care, grew more sophisticated and as larger numbers of patients were seeking care within the emergency department, reality dictated that there were not sufficient numbers of physicians in each unit to provide timely evaluation for every patient. The on-duty physician began to rely on those nurses who had integrated knowledge with judgment for information about the status of patients within the department. These nurses became adept at aiding in the establishment of management priorities. Within recent years a growing awareness has been developing relative to the fact that not only are many nurses functioning actively in assessing patients and developing a nursing diagnosis through which they are fairly accurate in providing initial stabilization and intervention, but also that this function is a very important element in providing for the immediate needs of a large number of patients. Within the larger facilities particularly, there now exists a healthy respect for the fact that nursing professionals within the emergency department have become the pivot upon which optimal treatment can be made available for each patient.

Unfortunately there are still many facilities that continue to expound the traditional philosophy—hospitals in which the terms "nursing assessment," "physical assessment," and "nursing diagnosis" are not acceptable. Many older physicians have spent years practicing under the assumption, generally taught them in medical school, that they are the only professionals with the ability to evaluate a patient, develop a working hypothesis of the cause of the patient's problems, and extend the correct treatment. To be sure, the years of medical school training provide the physician with the knowledge and judgment necessary to treat a broad range of ills and injuries. But the concept that a physician is able to rely on nurses for valid information on patient condition and for appropriate intervention in emergencies when the physician is not available is a new one. Attitudes that relegate emergency nurses to a position of active involvement in undressing patients and obtaining their vital signs but inactive involvement in assessment of presenting signs and symptoms are frustrating to nurses who have been trained to do more than simple patient hygiene. Moreover, such conditions fail to use the health care team in the department effectively. On the other hand, in order to develop confidence in their abilities, emergency nurses must use their skills and knowledge wisely and not consider themselves surrogate physicians. Attitudes that are steeped in tradition retard the development of a solid team within the emergency department, particularly in environments where there is a failure to perceive that assessment of patients is a necessary function of the emergency nurse. If assessment is not considered part of the nursing obligation, evaluation of patients will be inconsistent and most likely performed only by those nurses who have a strong sense of identity and have been able to receive the necessary education to do assessments correctly.

Finally, if assessment is not considered a nursing role, or if other health professionals are threatened by such a role, the nurses involved will very quickly lose their motivation to develop and consistently use assessment skills.

The key to overcoming this barrier may well lie in stressing that assessment is part of the standard of emergency nursing and in actively seeking both formal and clinical training to develop the skills necessary to the function. If these skills are developed and used wisely, attitudes toward nursing involvement will continue to become more constructive and less restrictive.

Many states have begun to enhance more progressive attitudes by establishing nursing practice acts, which allow for the performance of expanded role functions. However, until nurses themselves become more comfortable with the responsibility for performing nursing assessments and initiating appropriate therapy, and until they assertively seek support from the medical community for the development of such skills, this barrier will continue to exist and undermine assessment efforts.

Institutional barriers to assessment

Multiple nurse contact. Contact of several nurses with one patient may be a significant barrier to effective assessment and intervention. In departments in which it is common that nursing personnel work without benefit of specific patient assignments, the resulting confusion and lack of communication regarding patient status (particularly in busy times), result in inconsistent or delayed intervention. Consider what may happen if one nurse triages a patient, another prepares him for examination and takes his vital signs, another enters the cubicle to complete the assessment process, another carries out treatment orders, and still another discharges him! Either perfect and consistent communication must take place or one can imagine that significant gaps or errors in management of the patient throughout his emergency department visit may occur.

The only way to reduce this barrier to effective assessment and intervention is to implement a system of staff assignment, specific not only to areas of the department but also to treatment beds. Such assignments will help establish responsibility and accountability for nursing assessments and nursing management. Additionally, it is important to reinforce the concept that when a nurse is assigned to a particular bed or area, that nurse is the primary nursing clinician for that patient(s). No other nurse should intervene in the patient care plan that is thus established unless appropriate communication is carried out between the two nurses.

Float nurse staffing. Using nurses from other areas to help staff the emergency department may become a significant barrier if a nurse in question serves infrequently as an emergency department nurse or has never received training in assessment in the emergency setting. Others who are working in the unit may errantly assume that the nurse in question is providing equivalent evaluation when in fact this may not be the case.

Each individual facility must determine, with input from the nurses in the emergency department, whether the benefits outweigh the risks of using float or registry nurses in their department. The qualifications and capabilities of such personnel, if they are used, must be clearly identified to the regular department staff, including the physician on duty, to prevent misconception and potential patient compromise. In addition, it is recommended that all float and registry nurses receive an orientation to the department before they are expected to perform without supervision.

Imbalance of staff versus patient volume. If the number of nurses does not allow sufficient time and contact with each patient, a barrier may develop. Nursing staff ratios should be calculated on known and anticipated volume, and the percentage of critically ill patients anticipated within that volume as determined by past experience and distribution studies. Identification of peak load through study and evaluation may be time-consuming, but it can be of tremendous value in setting realistic staffing equivalents and patterns.

Particularly in very busy departments, insufficient staffing may promote a dangerous situation wherein priorities are not established consistently and symptoms that require prompt intervention might be overlooked or patient flow into treatment areas disrupted. The additional danger of insufficient staffing is that although the minimum coverage may allow for the assessment process to be carried out under normal circumstances, unexpected volume peaks or depletion of existing staff through illness or break times may contribute to the same end results as were noted above. These factors are uncontrollable, but the institution must allow for sufficient staff to handle potential volume through careful evaluation of peak load trends.

Obviously there are times, such as disaster situations, when even careful planning and sufficient staff will not be adequate to meet the need. During these times, assessments must necessarily be limited to the essentials, but they are no less important, and each nurse must make effective decisions regarding the extent of evaluation that is appropriate under the circumstances. It is of tantamount importance, however, that during these situations frequent assessments be performed to prevent, or to recognize and treat, life-threatening conditions.

One of the most devastating effects of inadequate staffing is the eventual burn-out that occurs with the nurses who continue to provide effective assessments even though short-handed and stretched thin over an increasing caseload. Continuation of such efforts requires a motivation that often wears out unless administrative attention is given to the problems caused by lack of sufficient nursing staff per patient volume.

Lack of appropriate staff resources for assessment. A lack of language interpreters, multisystem laboratory facilities, social service or psychiatric support, and radiology services can significantly affect not only nursing assessment, but also physician assessment and management. Both categories of personnel are affected when the resources with which to perform thorough evaluations are not available.

One of the most underrated resources is the language interpreter. It is extremely difficult to adequately assess a patient who cannot speak or understand the same language as the health professional. If a language interpreter is not available, the entire patient history may be unattainable. Although behavioral clues may be interpreted and integrated into the assessment, vital subjective information is lost. This may contribute to misinterpreting or missing physical symptoms that otherwise might have helped establish a cause of the patient's condition. Sometimes, however, it is difficult even to establish a primary patient complaint upon which to base the assessment.

Accessible laboratory and radiological services make a great deal of difference in the quality of the physical assessment that is performed. A major element of the physical data base is lacking or delayed if the laboratory and x-ray service are located remotely from the emergency department, if they are closed during peak load hours, or if they are not available at all.

Environmental barriers. Within the institution, environmental barriers include poor lighting, excessive ambient noise levels, and lack of patient privacy. Poor area lighting interferes with critical observations such as skin color and wound status. High ambient noise levels interfere with the interpretation of auscultated sounds, if indeed they can even be heard. Lack of privacy may prevent adequate evaluation of the patient's body, and may also prevent collection of all the personal information that the patient may be embarrassed by giving without adequate privacy. We have all had experience with the gynecological examining table that was placed strategically so that when the door of the examining room was opened (whether by accident or on purpose), the patient and examining physician were exposed to full view of everyone in the vicinity!

The most effective way in which to reduce the impact of environmental barriers is to recognize them if they exist and take appropriate steps to improve the situation. Provide extra lighting if necessary, using focus lighting for the evaluation of wounds and skin color and for illuminating an area before any procedure. Take steps to reduce the noise level in the treatment areas by encouraging only appropriate and necessary conversation. Apply acoustical tile to ceilings, and padded linoleum to floors if there is any possibility of doing so. Reduce traffic flow of unnecessary personnel and visitors through the treatment areas to provide for privacy during examination and treatment.

Institutional barriers are not usually insurmountable, yet they tend not to be addressed because they often require money if significant changes are necessary in order to reduce or alleviate them. Hospital administration, aided by the objective input from nurses working in the unit, can do a great deal to effect change. If there are difficulties in identifying existing problems to those who are remote from the situation, rational and organized evaluations of the problems with alternatives for change may help those with the authority to make changes set priorities for doing so.

Patient-related barriers

By their very nature, patient-related barriers to assessment are unpredictable and present the greatest challenge. It is difficult to present a straightforward listing of all of the potentials, since there is often an overlapping that occurs.

Language barriers. Language barriers were discussed earlier, yet it is not merely the non-English speaking patient who may not receive adequate assessment, it is also the deaf, deaf-mute, and retarded patient who may not receive adequate assessment because of a language barrier. In more subtle fashion, when

there is a significant difference between the medical jargon used and the patient's level of understanding of this jargon, there may also be an effect on the assessment process. For example, Mr. Jones, who is obviously alert and oriented, enters the department complaining of pains in his abdomen. Mr. Jones is asked about his past medical history, what medications he is currently taking, and who his private medical doctor is (among a long list of questions). Should he manage to understand what is being asked of him and feed back the appropriate answers, he is taken into a treatment room and asked to undress and put on a gown, climb up onto a gurney, and wait to have his vital signs taken. If he is not totally bewildered by this alien environment, he will have more opportunity to become bewildered, because he will be expected to have the language tools to describe his symptoms and the ability to interpret what he is expected to do when he is asked to go into the restroom to collect a clean-catch urine.

This example identifies a few very important points. It is extremely difficult to know when a patient understands what is being said to him and when he does not. The best-dressed, most sophisticated in mannerisms, most alert patient might be the one patient who has not the slightest idea what "radiation of pain" means, or any other technical jargon for that matter! It is folly to make the assumption that any patient will be able to integrate what we consider logical and comprehensible. Nor should we assume that the myriad of tests or methodologies of assessment will not cause apprehension that will interfere with the patient's ability to make sense of it all.

To prevent inaccurate or misleading information from being exchanged, watch the patient's face and behavior carefully to identify whether he is able to synthesize what is happening, what you are saying to him, and what is expected of him. Although he may not understand the events, he will want desperately to give the information you are seeking to obtain so that he will receive what he hopes will be the correct treatment, and therefore he may not tell you that he is confused. Use simple and direct language even while attempting not to sound patronizing. Lack of understanding medical jargon is widespread but unpredictable, and there is the occasional patient who may be insulted by a patronizing tone or expression.

Interference by family members. In the process of history taking or examination, family interference may on occasion be hilarious but more often becomes extremely disruptive in the flow of information between patient and nurse. Such intrusion usually occurs when a family member insists on answering questions for the patient even though he may be quite capable of doing so himself. An example is the overprotective mother who will not allow her 20-year-old son to describe his symptoms and who insists on being present during examination so that she can make absolutely certain that her son "doesn't forget anything." Much more palatable, but certainly just as disruptive, is the elderly husband and wife team. After hours of arguing, Mrs. Smith finally talks her husband into coming into the department for his indigestion, and then she proceeds to interfere with the triage process by giving information that she feels her husband is forgetting or by arguing with the patient when she feels that his story is incorrect.

Whenever possible, obtain the patient's history from the patient himself. Use language that he can understand, and question him when anything he says does not make sense to you. State clearly what assistance you wish from any family member who might be present, where you wish them to be during the examination process, and what behavior you are not willing to tolerate. To avoid embarrassment of the patient and potential conflict or irritation between staff and family, family members should not be present during the physical examination portion of the assessment when the patient is capable of cooperating.

Emergency staff attitudes. Attitudes of the emergency staff are extremely important. The attitude of the nurse undertaking the assessment may make or break the quality of the relations thus established and subsequently interfere with patient compliance throughout and beyond his visit. If your attitude is one of haste, indif-

ference, or irritation, even if such attitude is not directly related to the situation currently at hand, the patient will sense it and respond either accordingly or by becoming agitated. He may be so afraid of answering questions "incorrectly" or of antagonizing you further that he will likely forget important elements to tell you or may even falsify the situation in order to smooth the interaction. Or, he may react with hostile behavior, beginning a cycle of resistance and counterresistance that is lethal to the assessment process. Remember that each patient who enters the department will be extremely sensitive to the fact that he is placing himself completely in the hands of complete strangers, even though it may be difficult to feel comfortable in trusting them with his life or health. If he senses that he is a burden, or is made to feel that he is stupid, or is treated with disrespect, the situation may become entirely too much for him to cope with, resulting in anxiety, fear, panic, or uncooperative behavior.

Prejudgment of the patient. Prejudging may be manifest in a variety of ways, all of which will somehow adversely affect the assessment process. One of the surest ways to produce defensiveness is the use of "why" questions when taking a patient's history or when triaging him upon his arrival at the triage desk. Questions such as "Why did you wait 6 months to come in if you have been having back pain for that long?" imply that the patient is misusing the department or is too stupid to take appropriate care of himself. Other "why" questions that are counterproductive to the interview are those directed at why the patient did or did not do this or that. "Why did you stop taking your seizure medicine," or "Why did you leave the bleach out where Johnny could get hold of it?" are examples of questions that will surely put the patient on the defensive and interfere with the smooth exchange of information. "Why" questions can be asked much more gently and supportively, and tone and expression play a significant role in how the patient may perceive the questions being asked of him. When you ask him the reasons for not taking prescribed medication, for example, if the question is asked with an accepting expression and a gentle tone, a potentially flammable situation may be turned into a healthy exchange of information.

A much more disturbing type of prejudgment is the premature determination that the patient is nonemergent based on inadequate or faulty data. The tendency to prejudge the patient is often influenced by the patient's attitude ("She doesn't act as if she has just been raped"), the number of visits that the patient has made to the department ("This is the third time this week that Jane has come in with the same complaint, and there is never anything wrong"), the presentation of history or symptoms that do not seem to correlate with the clinical picture on casual observation, and a variety of other factors. The unfortunate result of prejudgment by health professionals is that the patient ultimately bears the burden of proving that he has an emergency. In addition, prejudgment may result in collection of only that information that supports the prejudgment, thus causing errors in assessment or intervention.

It is extremely important to listen to the patient describe his history and symptoms no matter what the circumstances may be, unless he is comatose. All the while the patient is describing his situation, compare what he looks like with his report and history. Make every attempt not to jump to conclusions or to force the interview into the direction that you think correct. Above all, do not stop collecting information when you have only that which supports your subjective analysis of the patient's status. If you feel judgmental, try to determine why this has happened. Verify your conclusions with someone else before taking action, or more important, *not* taking action. Finally, recognize that prejudging a patient is a trap that may lead you into unnecessary error unless you are willing to concentrate on information contrary to your original snap diagnosis.

Patient attitude and appearance. The attitude and appearance of the patient may influence the assessment process. If the manner in which a patient responds to questions and directions is derogatory, the attitude of those around him and of those having to deal with him may be adversely affected. It is indeed difficult to be kind and gentle to everybody who comes into the department, especially on a busy shift during which you are barely able to maintain an empathetic attitude. The tenuous hold on your composure may indeed be threatened by an obstreperous, overbearing patient, especially when you might find it hard to get along with such behavior even on your good days! Resistance to directions, hostility that appears to have no legitimate basis, and mental confusion (particularly when caused by substance abuse) may alienate the staff and reduce effective interaction and assessment. It is most helpful to avoid personalizing antagonistic behavior, which often is an attempt on the part of the patient to cope with feelings of helplessness. Keep in mind that the most positive action that can be taken is to reassure the patient through empathetic and professional behavior and to let him know that he will be taken care of. When you feel that you cannot cope with the situation, get someone else on staff to take over for you. Most of all, recognize that you can help the patient regain control of his behavior only when you refuse to take it personally; and when he feels back in control of himself, his inappropriateness will no doubt subside.

The more difficult patient for most nurses is the dirty, foul-smelling, unkempt patient with layers of insect-infested clothing on. The patient with poor personal hygiene may be exposed to delays in assessment while the staff determines who is willing to touch him. In these situations, it is likely that the patient will receive only hasty or incomplete evaluation and may never even be completely undressed! Some facilities have showers that can accommodate a stretcher, and the patient can be wheeled into the stall fully clothed and washed down while he is being undressed. Whatever the method used to deal with the situation, this patient should receive the same meticulous and systematic assessment given to any other, albeit more desirable, patient.

Patient's age. The age of the patient may present unexpected problems. It is difficult to conduct an assessment on the very young or the very old patient who cannot describe symptoms or express discomfort appropriately. Elderly patients do not sense pain as acutely as younger patients, and in addition they are often confused and forgetful. In the pediatric patient even the mother may not be able to accurately describe the events relative to the child's illness or injury.

Neurological, cardiac, and respiratory parameters are different in the pediatric and geriatric patient, and it takes time and practice to develop the skills necessary to identify subtle signs and correlate them into a meaningful picture. With a basic understanding of common pediatric and geriatric disease and trauma, and with practice under the supervision of someone skilled in pediatric and geriatric assessment, the job of evaluating patients in these age ranges becomes easier. It is necessary, however, to respect that these patients are different from the young and middle-aged adult, and that care must be taken to evaluate them carefully in order to avoid error.

Summary. All the barriers to patient assessment exist in one form or another in departments all over the United States. They hamper and retard some professional emergency nurses, and they are resolved and worked around by others. The only possible way in which to lessen their potential impact on our daily operation and their interference with effective patient assessment is to be familiar with their many faces, to recognize that they exist, and to make every effort to provide optimal evaluation for every patient in spite of the barriers. When there are barriers that we can reduce, taking the opportunity to determine how best to do so will lessen their effect on our performance.

DOCUMENTATION OF NURSING ASSESSMENT AND INTERVENTION

Information collected through the assessment process and action taken during the intervention phase must be documented in such a manner that others who are concerned with the care of the patient will be aware of the events that have taken place. Not only is recorded information valuable for continuity of care, but it also serves as a helpful tool for audit and teaching purposes.

Many facilities utilize separate nursing flow records in the emergency department, whereas others use the face sheet of the patient's emergency department record. Often, however, the face sheet does not contain enough space for the documentation of serial nursing assessments. The form used for nursing documentation must be left to the discretion of the individual facility, but the method of documentation must be clearly understood by everyone involved in the management of the patient and should not vary significantly within the department. If several different methods are used in one department, information cannot be abstracted from the record quickly, and fragmentation of care, duplication of effort, and deletions in assessment are more likely to occur.

It is equally as vital for nurses to chart their findings as it is for physicians to document theirs. An organized method of charting facilitates patient management and contributes to the development of an individualized plan of action. Problem-oriented charting is one of the most effective modes; it is based on the problem-oriented medical record (POMR) format, which was developed by a physician who wished to have a tool that would aid in the organized management of all known and potential patient problems. The system includes the following four elements.

1. Data base: records the history, physical findings, and diagnostic test results
2. Problem list: lists the problems that can be identified as well as those that can conceivably be anticipated, and separates them all into active and inactive (resolved) categories
3. Plan: identifies a written plan for addressing each of the active problems on the list
4. Action: provides a record of the plans that are to be implemented, those that have been implemented, and an evaluation of their effectiveness

This method of documenting information provides for a "closed loop," wherein one step leads into another until each of the problems has been addressed and resolved. If an action has not been effective in resolving a problem, evaluation of the action naturally progresses back to the first step, where further data can assist in the development of further action.

Although a most effective method of documenting patient management over a long-term (inpatient) period, the POMR is being more frequently used in the emergency department when dealing with a single patient problem that might have numerous smaller problems associated with it. When the POMR is used, none of the problems can be overlooked, even though some may appear to be inconsequential relative to the entire picture. For instance, suppose the plan of action for a victim of a head injury is to discharge him home. If the original problem list that naturally develops from the history, physical, and diagnostic tests reveals that the patient lives alone, is elderly, and has some coordination difficulty physically, one could not discharge him home with head injury instructions before arrangements are made to have a friend or relative remain with him overnight. If no one is available to do so, then the problem must be resolved in a different manner, perhaps by admitting the patient overnight for head injury observation, even though under other circumstances such action might not have been necessary. Were the POMR not used in this case, personnel in a busy department might have overlooked a potentially dangerous situation fraught with legal liability.

The SOAP process, which is used in problem-oriented charting, is a simple and valuable framework for documentation in the emergency department. The mnemonic SOAP is merely an abbreviation for the successive recording of *s*ubjective information, or the information that the patient states about himself in answer to questions; *o*bjective information, or that which is elicited through examination and diagnostic tests, *a*ssessment of the information that has been gathered through the history and physical (working diagnosis), and *p*lan of action in order to resolve the problem. The SOAP process can be used effectively for documentation of the nursing assessment on nursing flow sheets. An example of charting follows.

S: 31 y/o cauc female c/o S.O.B. × 2 hrs. States dyspnea onset while brushing teeth. Onset associated c̄ sharp pain (L) midscapular line radiating through to anterior chest. Now "hurts to take a deep breath." Pain now intermittent, on inspiration, and of moderate severity with no relief on position change.

O: Alert, oriented ×4. Appears anxious. Skin moist, cool, pale. Although pain is intermittent, unable to find comfortable position when experienced. Neck veins flat @ 30° elevation. Respirations 30, regular, shallow, symmetrical chest rise. Breath sounds diminished (L) apex anteriorly, otherwise vesicular c̄ I > E @ posterior bases. 0 abnormal lung sounds. Peripheral pulses equal bilat., reg rate & rhythm. Monitor → SVT @ 130. BP 120/80. Heart sounds reg. Abd. nontender, flat. No calf tenderness.

A: Respiratory distress, moderate. SVT per monitor.

P: O_2 @ 5 l/cannula.
Cardiac monitor continuous Lead 2.
Blood specimens drawn, sent for CBC, lytes, hold for further tests. 1,000 cc N/S via #18 angiocath and reg. tubing started in dorsum R hand. ABGs drawn from L radial artery before O_2 therapy, Allen's test positive for ulnar circ.

Properly completed, the SOAP system can be an extremely effective tool for recording the patient assessment process and intervention followed by either nurses or physicians. Such a system emphasizes recorded data rather than memory, and reflects an orderly thought process. The system also lends itself to progressive audit; faulty documentation or thinking practically jumps off the page at the reviewer! Even if the evaluation of the patient is abbreviated because of the gravity of the situation, the examiner is not likely to forget anything if the SOAP process of recording is used from the outset.

Whatever method of recording is used, the essential point is that some reasonably straightforward method must be used, and whatever method is utilized must be clearly understood and preferably used by all the nurses and physicians. Many nurses complain that their charting is never read by anyone other than themselves. There is certainly more likelihood that such will be the case if they continue to use narrative styles of recording that reflect disorderly thought processes, or if they chart nothing of more significance than "Mr. Jones is complaining of pain."

Memory, verbal reporting, and cryptic notes recorded in small areas of the patient's face sheet or on the bed linen are not acceptable processes to use in documenting patient care. The qualititative recording of history and physical findings is necessary to a systematic thought process, and is becoming more important than ever before in legal reviews of patient records. In addition, documentation must be legible, accurate, and complete in order to be of most value. Problem-oriented charting, using the SOAP process, rapidly and readily reveals the thoroughness or sloppiness of the person recording the information. And both systems depend on the judicious use of abbreviations, which if not universally understood, may prove more a detriment than an aid to patient care.

SETTING PRIORITIES FOR ASSESSMENT

Many times during discussions of nursing assessment, a protest is made that not every patient who comes to the department requires the thorough assessment promoted in many textbooks. Some hospitals filter clinic cases through the emergency department when clinics are not available. Others have such a tremendous volume of cases that serial assessments seem ideal at best. There can be no hard and fast rules made either for assessment of each patient or for how the assessments must be done when time permits. However, when the caseload is heavy, skilled nurses adopt effective methods of assessment if the motivation, education, and support are there; therefore, heavy volumes are no excuse to neglect the process in most cases. Further, in departments that have a light emergency department caseload and therefore may not staff a 24-hour physician on duty, it is vital that nurses who are on duty perform nursing assessments in order to identify life-threatening conditions and treat them.

The individual nurse in each department must determine what extent of assessment is appropriate to each patient situation. Unfortunately, those patients who carry a label of "clinic patient" are almost automatically considered nonemergent and are infrequent benefactors of even the most cursory assessments. This is a dangerous practice; it is nearly always appropriate to perform at least a general overview and primary survey and to collect historical and subjective information from the patient in order to set reasonable priorities for his care. Even though he is labeled a clinic patient because he brought his clinic card with him or told someone that he belongs to a clinic, it cannot be assumed that he has no significant health emergency until someone makes an objective evaluation of his current situation.

It is precisely when caseloads are heavy, or when a department repeater comes in, or when a patient with a clinic label comes in, that the assessment process can establish unanticipated and potentially critical problems and avert a major catastrophe. Nursing assessment should not be reserved for the critical patient. If intelligent judgments are made regarding the extent of assessment warranted by each patient, nursing assessment can be made available for everyone who comes to the department for care.

STEPS IN ASSESSMENT

Following organized steps will help the assessment be maximally effective even when some of the steps must be delayed to allow for intervention. Although the steps presented in this section are in flow format, they will tend to vary depending on the individual circumstances; therefore, the format described is intended as a guide to the vital elements of the assessment process. The environment within the emergency department often dictates that the process be adapted to the situation at hand, and probably the most important concept for the nurse to understand is that she or he must develop and use consistently the approach that is most meaningful to the individual using it. Flexibility can be developed if the nurse is thoroughly familiar with the steps of assessment and is meticulous in follow-through. Proficiency is maintained by constant practice of the skills of assessment.

Primary assessment

The priorities of nursing assessment are always the respiratory and cardiovascular systems. Upon initial contact with the patient, determine the status of the airway, and respond to priorities for intervention. Visually observe for patency of the airway and adequacy of ventilation based on skin color, respiratory effort, and tidal volume, and use of accessory muscles in breathing. Determine the level of consciousness in terms of whether or not the patient is able to respond. Check the pulse simultaneously while observing for ventilation.

The primary assessment is mandatory for every patient with whom you come in contact, regardless of his presenting status. Also referred to as the "primary survey," this observation should take barely 30 seconds to complete. Obviously if a patient does not have a patent airway, or has inadequate ventilations, or is pulseless, intervention in these life-threatening instances supercedes further assessment. But the same holds true if there are variables that also may be life-threatening, such as cardiac dysrhythmias that are first noted while checking the pulse and appear to be hemodynamically significant. Under such circumstances, elements of the assessment process, such as history, are delayed or conducted simultaneously while intervention is implemented.

General survey

The general survey proceeds beyond the primary considerations of the ABCs to a more systematic observation of the patient. This observation should include:

- Affect and mood (including thought organization)
- Quality of speech (normal, slurred, silent, unable to speak)
- General appearance (manner of dress and hygiene, color of skin, facial expression)
- Posture and motor activity (upright posture should be observed if possible; motor activity should be observed while patient walks, sits, undresses, and so on)
- Odors (breath, skin)
- Evaluation of degree of distress (based on all of the observations preceding this determination)

The general survey can be conducted simultaneously with the primary survey. It becomes easier to combine the two with practice. Both the primary and general surveys also can be combined with the interview for historical information on many occasions; the determining factor will be the patient's condition at the time. If immediate or unanticipated problems arise, the interview may be delayed and completed either during the physical examination or after the patient has been stabilized.

History

The chief complaint is the focus of the historical interview in the emergency department, and the questions, although open-ended, should be directed at that complaint. The key to obtaining information about the chief complaint (the reason why the patient came into the department) is to listen to what the patient says as he tries to tell you what is wrong with him. What the patient tells you is by definition subjective, and therefore demands an objective assessment. The chief complaint should not be recorded as a diagnosis ("possible fractured left arm"), but exactly as the patient describes his problem (fell from stepladder, now pain and swelling L arm).

If the patient initially comes to the triage area and is physically able to proceed through that process, the history can be completed there. If, however, the patient enters the department by ambulance or other vehicle and cannot process through the triage area, it is generally the responsibility of the nurse managing him in the treatment area to collect historical information and to obtain whatever information the prehospital personnel may have regarding status or treatment before the patient's arrival at the department. If the patient can respond to questions, any history obtained from others should be validated with him. Often, when the anxiety of the transport into the department diminishes, the patient remembers information that he had not been able to recall previously. Whoever collects historical information should tell the patient who she is, and attempts should be made to prevent the patient from having to retell his story several times to different people.

There are times when a patient cannot describe his symptoms and reason for coming into the department. When this occurs, attempts to reach someone who can relate the history of the present complaint should be made. If the patient is unresponsive and there are no historians available, treating the patient becomes a much more difficult, time-consuming process, yet treatment must not be delayed until a history is available.

When you are obtaining information from the patient, the following elements should be addressed:
- History of the present illness or injury
    How and when the injury or illness first occurred
    Influencing factors
    Symptom chronology and duration
    Related symptoms
    Location of pain or discomfort
    What, if anything, the patient has done about his symptoms
- Pertinent past medical history
    Has this problem ever occured before? If so, was a medical diagnosis made and what was it?
    Has the patient ever had surgery? If so, for what and what was the result?
    Is there any familial medical history that may influence the patient's present complaint?
    Does the patient have a private doctor (obtain full name, if possible)
- Current medication (prescribed and unprescribed)
- Allergies
- Age and weight
- Tetanus immunization history if an injury is involved
- Last menstrual period date if female

In recent years, the mnemonic, PQRST, has been used to great advantage in assessing the complaint of pain or dyspnea. The PQRST helps define the complaint by focusing on essential elements of provoking factors, quality and severity, location and radiation, and the timing in terms of onset and duration.

P *(Provoking factors):* Ask the patient what, if anything, provokes the pain or discomfort. Is there anything that makes it worse or relieves it? What was the patient doing when it began?

Q *(Quality of the pain):* Ask the patient to describe the pain in his own words. It is particularly important to avoid "feeding" descriptive terms to him; instead use open-ended questions to allow him to use his own unique description. (Can you tell me how your pain feels to you?)

R *(Region or radiation):* Ask the patient to point to the area of his pain or discomfort if he can. Ask him if it travels anywhere or if he has pain any place else. Ask him if his pain has moved from the region of onset. There are times when a patient may not be able to isolate a single area of pain, particularly if the pain is visceral as opposed to cutaneous. In this case, ask if he can identify the general area for you. Do not touch him while he shows you where his discomfort is, as this may obscure his answers and provide you with incorrect information.

S *(Severity):* Ask the patient to describe the severity of his pain. It is sometimes helpful to use the scale of 1 to 10. On this scale 1 is equivalent to no pain at all, whereas 10 is the most severe pain the patient has ever experienced. Ask him if the pain has affected his normal activity and if so, how it has affected the activities of daily living. Watch him while he moves or undresses, and assess the degree to which the pain compromises his activities.

T *(Time):* This section deals with the time of onset and constancy or duration of symptoms. It is also helpful to ask if the patient has ever had the symptoms before, what they were related to, and how they were treated.

Case example

A 32-year-old Mexican-American woman arrives at the department with abdominal pain. Using the PQRST, the nurse obtained and recorded the following information.

32 y/o ♀ c̄ gradual onset RUQ pain that "comes and goes," increases p̄ meals but tolerable remainder of day. Does not awaken her @ noc. Pain has increased past 2 days and remains colicky. θ̄ vom-

iting or diarrhea/constipation, but nauseated when pain is at its peak. Position changes not helpful, also do not provoke. 0 radiation. Pt. has noted increase in skin temperature in past day, did not take temperature. No past hx of this or similar problems. LMP 7/9, -0- abnormality noted, Gravida VI para VI, last child now 2 y. No recent weight gain or loss, current wt. 160#.

Based on this history, a reasonably reliable working hypothesis can be formulated, particularly in determining the relative urgency of this patient's problem. Without the history, however, such a hypothesis would be necessarily delayed until the physical examination and extensive laboratory and x-ray studies could be employed to determine the possible cause of the pain.

Although the circumstances of the department may dictate compression of the interview into a few pertinent questions, the most important ones should be asked. Those that are most important will be relative to the individual patient presentation. Regardless of the time frame in which the history is obtained, every attempt should be made to collect as much history as is available and in some cases, to track down even that which is not immediately available when the patient arrives. There are adjuncts to the history that are sometimes available, such as a Medical Alert bracelet, personal medical information written on papers and hidden in a wallet, or the "Vial-of-Life," which is a new concept. The "Vial-of-Life" is a small vial into which a preprinted questionnaire, answered by the patient and containing vital medical history, is placed. The vial is then placed in the patient's refrigerator at home (only because it is less likely to become lost in that location), and a small seal identifying that the vial is inside is placed on the refrigerator door. Paramedics have been advised to look on the refrigerator door when responding to the home of a patient, particularly if the patient is elderly, infirm, or unconscious.

PHYSICAL EXAMINATION

It has been said that 80% of the time a good history will give enough information to establish a diagnosis, but the physical examination remains important to the adequate evaluation of the emergency patient, particularly when not much else is known about him. Physical examination is often abbreviated to the situation, with a great deal of skill and judgment necessary to determine what physical information is vital and appropriate and what does not need to be evaluated under the circumstances. The routine health examination that we have all experienced is not appropriate to the emergency department, but some routines do exist that are considered the appropriate standard of evaluation in courtroom deliberations. For instance, the minimum acceptable evaluation for a patient with a head injury is mental status and level of consciousness, assessment of posture and motor movements including reflexes, evaluation of eye movements and pupil status, and evaluation of gross focal neurological deficit. The physical exam is then supported by special diagnostic aids as appropriate: skull and cervical spine x-ray studies; EEG, and EMI scan. Depending on the cause of the head injury, other body systems might be examined as well, but the evaluator would have to determine the further extent of examination appropriate unless specific audit guidelines specify what those other parameters of examination will be in every case of head injury.

Nurses can and should perform physical examinations on patients under their charge; however, the main purpose in an emergency department with physicians on site is to recognize and treat life-threatening emergencies and to collect enough data to enable the nurse to establish priorities of care within a busy environment. Generally the nursing examination is performed briefly and rapidly, and therefore it is mandatory that you be well versed in normal findings in order to be able to interpret abnormal ones quickly and accurately. This art can be developed through persistence in performing examinations and utilizing adequate clinical supervision while learning to integrate your findings.

Probably the most important aspect of the examination is the establishment of a therapeutic and professional rapport with the patient. Here also is the potential for abruptness or prejudgment to disrupt the process and adversely affect the nurse-patient relationship. Remember to provide privacy and to use touch before the start of the examination to establish contact with the patient. Of course, if the patient is unconscious there is less opportunity to connect with him before evaluation, but explaining what you are doing before doing it is considered appropriate even under these circumstances.

Organizing yourself is also a significant aspect of performing a patient examination. Anticipate what tools you will need before beginning so that you do not have to leave the bedside for any reason. You may not use the full gamut of tools for each exam; however, it is helpful to be aware of what you may need so that you can select appropriately.

Tools for examination

The tools used in the nursing examination of a patient in the emergency department are not as numerous as those that are used in the health screening exam in a well-adult clinic or for specialized exams for neurology or cardiology. The major items used in the emergency department are described, and a short listing of other tools follows.

Stethoscope. The most common stethoscope is the binaural acoustic instrument that has both a bell and a diaphragm. Ideally, the stethoscope should be lightweight, have two large lumen tubings that are approximately 12 to 14 inches long, have metal sidepieces and flexible earpieces, and have a rubber or plastic rim around the bell and the diaphragm to reduce ambient noise interference. Not all stethoscopes sound alike, and different individuals have different desires regarding the type of instrument they feel most comfortable with. Try to select one that is not only well constructed, but that fits comfortably (particularly in the external ear) and has the features necessary to the situations in which you will be functioning.

Common problems encountered with stethoscopes include cracking of the diaphragm, tubing, or earpieces, inability to evaluate low-pitched sounds because of lack of a bell piece,

and poor transmission of sounds because of overly long tubing between the head of the instrument and the earpieces.

Care of the stethoscope is important to prolong the life of this vital piece of equipment. Cleanse the earpieces after each use, particularly if someone else has used the stethoscope. It is preferable that you own your own stethoscope, one that fits your unique ear canal angle. If you lend it out, be certain to protect yourself against cross-contamination by cleansing the eartips with alcohol before you use it. Check the tubing routinely along with the diaphragm, bell, and earpieces to detect cracks. These parts can be cleansed with a mild soap solution but must be dried completely with a soft clean cloth. Folding the tubing will predispose it to cracking, particularly if you fold it tightly. A well-fitted, well-designed, and well-constructed stethoscope will assist you in auscultating breath, heart, and bowel sounds. It will not amplify sounds, but will transmit them to your ears effectively by eliminating most ambient noises.

Otoscope/ophthalmoscope. Skills in diagnosing EENT disorders are not necessary for the emergency nurse; however, it is appropriate that you know how to use these instruments to evaluate loss of vision, nasal occlusion or bleeding, and presence of foreign bodies where necessary.

The otoscope is designed with a handle that is either portable and battery-operated or portable and recharged between use by a counter- or wall-mounted charger base. The instrument has an otoscope head attachment and usually can also accommodate an ophthalmoscope head when the other is removed.

The otoscope head attaches with a clockwise twist and snap-on motion. The head has a round ring for the attachment of an ear or nasal speculum, and also has a small ring magnifier that can be lined up with the distal opening of the speculum. There is also a light for the purposes of illuminating the inspection site. When using the otoscope in examining the ear, hold the scope handle firmly between the thumb and fingers of one hand and tilt the patient's head away from you. Grasp the auricle and pull it upward and backward in the adult or downward and back in the child. This maneuver will straighten the canal, and if tenderness is elicited with such an action, it should be noted. The fingers of the hand that is extending the ear canal should also steady the patient's head. Once this position is obtained, turn the scope light on and guide the speculum gently into the canal, inspecting the walls visually as you enter. If difficulty is encountered while advancing the speculum, pull slightly on the auricle to obtain more straightening of the canal, or increase the tilt angle of the patient's head.

The ophthalmoscope is used most commonly in the emergency department by nurses for pupil checks or to identify corneal or conjunctival foreign bodies. Few nurses have the time or skill necessary to conduct a more complete eye evaluation. Yet the ophthalmoscope can prove helpful in examination of external eye structures, evaluating pupillary response and accommodation, and evaluating the anterior chamber. As you become more familiar with the instrument and more comfortable with its use, practice identifying internal ocular structures such as the retinal wall, vessels, macula, and optic disk. It is, of course, more expedient to practice viewing normal structures until you establish skill.

The ophthalmoscope head is basically a simple instrument that has a small aperture through which you view the eye. It also projects a narrow beam of light and has a set of at least 22 lenses, depending on the model being used. These lenses can be rotated into the aperture by turning a lens wheel located on one side of the head. The lenses are used to focus on different structures within the eye, but they can also adjust to accommodate for myopia or loss of accommodation in either the examiner or the patient. When you turn the lens wheel, a clockwise turn will provide lenses with a shorter focus (these lenses are referred to as "plus diopters"), and a counter-clockwise turn will provide you with lenses that have a longer focus (these are referred to as "minus diopters"). A diopter is a unit that measures the power of a lens to converge or diverge light rays on an object.

The light beam can be adjusted from wide to narrow; generally the wide setting is easier to use. In addition, the light setting can be changed to a narrow slit or to a red-free filter. By passing the light beam through the refractory structures to the retina, you can evaluate the clarity of these normally transparent structures when the beam of light bounces back into your eye. The light also illuminates the fundus.

When using the ophthalmoscope in examining the eye, seat yourself direclty in front of the patient. If either of you has a history of astigmatism, that person should wear corrective lenses during the exam if they are available. The room can be dimly lit; there is no need for it to be completely dark. Ask the patient to focus on an object directly above and at some distance behind your head, which will enlarge and steady the pupil. Holding the ophthalmoscope handle firmly, place the head against your cheek and your eye directly behind the aperture. Place your index finger on the lens wheel and set the scope at '0' diopters, a setting that will neither converge or diverge light rays. Using your right eye, examine the patient's right eye while holding the scope in your right hand. Reverse this position when examining the patient's left eye. During the examination, keep your thumb on the patient's brow and your palm and fingers on his head to steady it and keep him from moving.

The eye examination should begin with the scope held approximately 12 inches away from the patient and approximately 15° lateral to his field of vision. In this position, identify the red reflex of the eye, which is the reflection of the light bouncing off the retinal wall. Following this reflection, move forward until the hand holding the scope nearly touches the patient's cheek. Keep your eye relaxed and identify the retinal wall by its pinkish color. Look for the optic disk, which is a pale pink with variations located to the nasal side. If you cannot locate it initially, find a blood vessel and follow its pathway centrally until you see the disk itself. Arteries appear light red, whereas veins appear dark red in the fundus of the eye. (The veins pulsate, whereas the arteries do not.) By turning the lens wheel, you should be able to bring the disk into sharp focus to evaluate its margins and depth. Look next for the macula, which is located about 1.5 disk diameters (DD) from the disk toward the temporal side and is slightly darker than the retina (the retina ranges in color from pinkish-yellow in fair-skinned people to brown in darker-skinned individuals). The sequence of examination recommended by most experts follows.

1. Assess pupil equality, size, shape, and reaction to light.
2. Identify the red reflex.
3. Evaluate the disk.
4. Evaluate the vessels.
5. Evaluate the retinal wall.
6. Evaluate the macula.

The otoscope/ophthalmoscope can also be used for nasal inspection by attaching the otoscopic head and a short, wide speculum to the round ring. Place the patient's head in a neutral position and first visualize the inferior nares bilaterally. Then, tilt his head backward and visualize the superior nares. Also evaluate the nasal mucosa, septum, turbinates, and middle meatus between the turbinates.

REFLEX HAMMER. The reflex hammer is a triangular-shaped rubber tip attached to a metal handle, which is narrow at the neck and at the distal end and wide at the middle. It is used to evaluate muscular contraction that results when a tendon is stretched suddenly by the force of the reflex hammer striking it. The hammer should be held between the thumb and fingers of one hand at the handle base. Position the patient's limb to produce a slight stretch of the muscle to be evaluated. Strike the tendon with a brisk but light and rapid tap of the hammer, controlling the movement of the hammer yet allowing it to move in an arc with your wrist as a fulcrum. The muscles most frequently evaluated in this manner are the biceps, triceps, brachioradialis, and quadriceps. Hyperreflexia and hyporeflexia are evaluated in context with the patient's norm and considered in context with the clinical situation; most commonly reflexes are recorded on a scale of 0 to 4:

4+ Brisk; hyperactive
3+ Brisker than normal but not necessarily pathological
2+ Normal

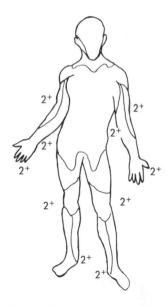

1+ Hypoactive
0+ Absent

The handle of the reflex hammer is also used to evaluate plantar reflexes and abdominal and cremasteric reflexes.

• • •

Other tools used in patient examination are self-explanatory and include:

1. Pocket flashlight
2. Thermometer, sphygmomanometer, and watch with second hand
3. Tongue depressor
4. Safety pins or cotton swabs for evaluation of nervous sensation
5. Flexible tape measure to compare size of extremities, size of skin lesions, size of masses, and circumference of an infant's head.

All necessary items for examination should be collected and kept close at hand before your examination begins so that you do not have to interrupt the process.

Techniques of physical examination

There are four essential techniques involved in the physical examination of any patient. The pattern of utilization may vary depending on the system being evaluated, but the sequence and organization of the approach used should be directed at minimizing patient movement and utilizing the time with the patient efficiently.

Inspection. This technique is perhaps the most vital of all of the examination techniques, because the observations obtained from the visual inspection of the patient as a whole and each system in particular help integrate what he says with what his physical appearance manifests. Inspection must always precede any of the other techniques, and although it may be difficult to master at first, continual practice will ease your discomfort in simply *looking* at the patient. Keep in mind what you are looking for so that your observations have purpose and organization.

Evaluate the patient's general appearance. Is he unkempt, malnourished, well kept, overweight? Does he appear to take good care of himself, or does he appear to have poor hygiene? These observations will help you get a flavor of the patient as a person, and to relate his general appearance to his illness. These observations do not need to be documented in the emergency department, although often the physician will note the patient's nutritional status. Look at the condition of the mucous membranes for information about oxygenation and hydration. Observing body movement and posture will provide you with information about pain, mental status and mood, as well as clues to degree of debilitation. After this general "quick look," your observations should become specific based on the presenting complaint and/or the specific system that you are evaluating first. Respiratory excursion and chest symmetry of expansion, apical thrust, and comparison of extremities for size and shape are all examples of observations that you will want to make routinely.

Palpation. Your hands become very important tools when used to palpate skin temperature, skin texture, vibrations and pulsations, masses or lesions, muscle tenseness or rigidity, and deformities. Different aspects of the hand are better equipped to feel different sensations. The dorsum of the hand is more sensitive to temperature changes, whereas the palm is more sensitive to vibratory sensations. The fingers are very sensitive to touch, but because this sensation can be diminished by increasing the pressure on the fingertips, light palpation is preferred to deep palpation as a general rule. However, pressure changes are utilized to palpate and distinguish one organ from another or to define the borders of organs. In fact, on examination of the abdomen, light palpation is generally followed by deep palpation in the process of identifying abdominal contents.

The preferred method of light palpation is to use the fingertips of one hand to distinguish hard from soft, rough from smooth, and muscle tone. The preferred method of deep palpation is to place the fingertips of one hand over and slightly forward of the fingertips of the other hand, which is placed over the area to be palpated. Both hands are then used to press firmly and deeply over the area. Palpation with both hands can also be employed to fix an organ in place with one hand while palpating its borders with the other, or by using one hand to entrap the organ between the fingertips.

Ballottement is a form of palpation in which light bouncing of the fingertips is performed along the surface of the skin. A sense of tenseness or resistance in abdominal organs or an increase in pressure within an organ or cavity may be appreciated with the use of ballottement. Ballottement utilizes light palpation in conjunction with rapid increases and decreases in pressure against the examiner's fingertips, thus increasing their sensitivity to touch.

When utilized properly, the technique of palpation will help confirm information obtained through observation. The technique is very helpful in identifying areas of pain or tenderness and in evaluating where the maximum point of pain or tenderness is located.

Percussion. Percussion is the technique of eliciting vibrations that can be heard and felt when a portion of the body is struck with the examiner's hand or fingers. The extent of the vibration varies depending on the density, position, and size of the tissue underlying the area being percussed. This technique is helpful in outlining the borders of an organ, identifying pain and tenderness within an area of the body, identifying fluid within an organ or cavity, and evaluating lung fields for consolidation, fluid, or air.

Percussion notes are difficult to describe, because the discrimination of sounds is relative to the amount of practice the examiner has had and to the patient himself when areas of his body are compared with one another. Generally, sounds are described in terms of pitch, duration, intensity, and quality. The pitch is determined by the speed with which vibrations travel through the body, strike an organ, and bounce back to the examiner's fingers. If the organ is close to the skin surface, the pitch will be high (not to be confused with *loud*) and is a result of the vibrations being returned rapidly to the examiner. The sound heard is dull sound: for example, the sound made if you were to strike your thigh, which is fairly dense and does not transmit vibrations at all. The duration is the length of time the vibration lasts, and is dictated by the distance of the organ from the skin surface and thus the amount of time available for the vibration to exist. A fairly solid tissue transmits a sound of short duration, whereas a hollow organ transmits a sound of reasonably long duration. The intensity of the sound is relative to the loudness or softness of the sound heard when an area is percussed. A solid organ will transmit a soft sound when percussed because the vibrations are traveling little if at all. The quality of the sound defines what type of organ is making the sound; in other words, the quality of sound that a musical instrument makes will give the listener a clue as to what the instrument is. For example, when the chest is percussed, a certain sound is set up if the lungs are normal and the alveoli are inflated with air. This sound is called "resonant," and has a different quality than would be heard if, for instance, the hemithorax were filled with bowel instead of normal lung.

It is the art of putting the different characteristics of vibratory sound together to come away with an awareness of abnormal pathology that makes the technique of percussion so valuable. It is not at all a helpful technique if one cannot interpret the findings. As a matter of fact, it becomes an exercise in futility unless the sounds are translated into meaningful terms. Most nurses do not feel comfortable with percussion because they are unable to interpret their findings. But it is a guaranteed fact that you will never learn to do this unless you percuss normal tissue and abnormal tissue and areas of the body having different density, in order to learn the different sounds. No amount of didactic lecture will provide you with that information.

Percussion notes are obtained through either direct means (striking the patient's skin with the fingers of only one hand), or indirect means (using fingers of both hands). The indirect method is most often employed, and it is performed by placing the middle finger of the left hand firmly against the patient's skin and striking the distal phalange with the tip of the middle finger of the other hand. The finger placed directly on the patient is called the pleximeter finger, and the striking finger is called the plexor finger. The pleximeter must be placed firmly to avoid damping the sound. No other part of the hand must come in contact with the skin because of the muffling or distorting effect that the other fingers or parts of the hand may cause. Sounds are produced most effectively by striking the pleximeter finger with short, brisk taps, exerted through the motion of the plexor wrist. The lightest percussion force that produces a sound should be used, although there are times when any striking force will be uncomfortable for the patient.

Because bone produces a flat percussion note, percussion is not usually carried out in areas where bone overlies cavities or organs. In addition, the deeper the organ lies beneath the surface, the more tissue lying above it will transmit the sound instead of the organ you are trying to evaluate. Therefore, it is generally not helpful to try, for instance, to evaluate a kidney using the anterior approach to percussion. A rule of thumb is that an organ that lies more than 5 cm below the surface is generally not detectable by percussion.

Finally, always compare the patient's body from side to side when eliciting percussion notes. It will be much easier to recognize normal sounds for each particular patient, and it will help you distinguish changes in quality from organ to organ. Particularly if sounds are subtle, moving from side to side will help you distinguish and differentiate what you are hearing.

Auscultation. Auscultation is the method of transmitting sound from an organ or area of the body to the examiner's ear either through placing the ear directly on the body or by using a stethoscope. The presence or absence of sounds, or the deviation from normal in sounds heard, assist in the development of a diagnosis. Remember that the stethoscope does not amplify sounds; instead it transmits sounds to your ear while reducing external noise interference. The diaphragm is useful when auscultating high-pitched sounds, and the bell is useful when auscultating lower-pitched sounds. However, the bell can be converted into a diaphragm if too much pressure is exerted against it, drawing the skin taut under the bell piece.

Like percussion sounds, auscultation sounds are described in terms of their pitch, intensity, duration, and quality. Those systems that are routinely auscultated during examination are the respiratory, cardiovascular, and gastrointestinal systems.

AUSCULTATING LUNG SOUNDS. Lung sounds should be auscultated for their relationship to the inspiratory/expiratory cycle as well as for the four elements listed above. There are three basic types of normal sounds that, depending on their location, may indicate a pathological condition.

VESICULAR SOUNDS. Normally heard in the lung periphery, these sounds indicate normal distension of alveoli with air. Their intensity is soft and their pitch is low; many liken the sound to rustling leaves. Their relationship to the inspiratory/expiratory (I:E) cycle is 1.5/1, because the last half of the normal, passive expiratory phase cannot generally be heard in the healthy adult. When the chest is *observed,* however, the expiratory phase should appear to be about one and a half times longer than the inspiratory phase, the extra half being the postexpiratory pause, during which the pressures within the alveoli have fallen and the diaphragm is completely relaxed.

BRONCHOVESICULAR SOUNDS. These sounds are the result of normal air flow in the larger airways other than the trachea and should normally be heard only over the mainstem just inferior to the clavicles anteriorly and between the scapulas posteriorly. As indicated by the name, these sounds are made up of two components: the movement of air through the mainstem bronchi, and the inflation of alveoli. In addition, these sounds are associated with a fairly equal inspiratory/expiratory cycle with a slight pause in between. When heard in the chest periphery, bronchovesicular sounds indicate early pulmonary consolidation or compression.

BRONCHIAL SOUNDS. If you place your stethoscope directly over the trachea, you will hear very loud, high-pitched, raspy sounds, which are the result of air moving through the trachea and are referred to as "bronchial" or "tubular" breath sounds. The expiratory time is longer than the inspiratory time, generally on a 1:2 ratio. If these sounds are heard anywhere on the chest besides directly over the trachea, they indicate pulmonary consolidation or compression, such as may be caused by pneumonia, edema, or tumor.

Breath sounds may change dramatically, depending on the degree of involvement of pulmonary tissues and the time span within which a pathologic condition has existed. The size of the chest may dampen sounds; a very obese or muscular chest may exhibit reduced lung sounds. When listening for the normal sounds described above, determine whether or not normal sounds are reduced, distant, or absent, and whether abnormal sounds are present.

ADVENTITIOUS SOUNDS. These include two general categories of sounds: rales and ronchi. The use of different descriptive names for these sounds is somewhat controversial; many dictionaries group all adventitious sounds under the heading "rales." Sometimes adventitious sounds are characterized as "crackles and wheezes." To facilitate your understanding, however, we describe adventitious sounds in this text according to the two general categories of rales and rhonchi.

Rales result from fluid collection in the tracheobronchial tree, generally starting in the alveolar sacs because of gravitational forces on the fluid; when air moves through this fluid a sound is produced.

• Fine rales are heard as soft clusters of

sounds with varying intensity and pitch. They are discontinuous and correlate most often with end-inspiration, since this is the point at which air has moved through the larger airways and entered the alveoli.

- Medium rales are slightly louder than fine rales but have more of a crackling sound, much like the fizz of a carbonated beverage. They are the result of fluid collection affecting the bronchioles and therefore can be heard in midinspiration, since this is the point at which air moves past the small bronchioles toward the alveoli. The sound will be extended through to end-inspiration because the alveoli are involved also; therefore, the true distinction of whether the rales are fine or medium is based on where in the cycle the sound is heard. Usually the distinction of fine or medium is not nearly as important as describing where in the phase you hear the sound.
- Course rales are often referred to as rhonchi, primarily because the fluid collection has now extended to the large airways. The sound is continuous as opposed to discontinuous as the other types of rales were; this sound is also rattling, bubbling, or gurgling and can be appreciated throughout the inspiratory/expiratory cycle. Another name for this sound is "death rattle," because it is frequently heard in the moribund patient when he is unable to clear his airway.

Rhonchi are sounds produced as a result of air passing through mucous or narrowed passages in the larger airways. Their pitch is medium to low, with a louder intensity than rales. In addition, rhonchi are generally heard on expiration.

- Course rhonchi are described above.
- Sibiliant rhonchi are also called "wheezes," and have a musical, whistling, or hissing quality. This sound results from the passage of air through narrowed bronchioles and is heard on expiration. The pitch and intensity of sibiliant rhonchi are medium; most of us know this sound as the musical, continuous noise heard in the asthmatic patient.

The *pleural friction rub* is also classified as an adventitious sound. It is an interrupted, coarse, grating sound that develops over an inflamed pleura or over an area where there has been a loss of lubricating fluid within the pleural "space." The clue to this abnormal sound is that it is usually unilateral and localized, whereas rales and rhonchi are usually not. The rubbing sound may be heightened if the patient is positioned toward the involved area, because this action brings the involved area closer to the stethoscope. Friction rub is a more difficult sound to distinguish until one has had a great deal of practice in auscultating lung sounds.

Adventitious sounds are often associated with changes in the I:E ratio simply because, in the case of rales and rhonchi, a pathologic condition exists that disrupts the normal movement of air through the tracheobronchial tree. Wherever the normal decrease in intraluminal diameter of the airways during expiration is accentuated during that phase, the phase will be prolonged; in emphysematous patients the I:E ratio may appear as 1:3, 1:4, or even 1:5 in severe cases.

Although auscultation of breath sounds takes practice, there are a few hints to help you feel more inclined to put your stethoscope on chests and begin to develop your skill in this technique. When listening to breath sounds, listen for the normals and for changes in the normals before attempting to identify "extra sounds." Begin anteriorly, preferably with the patient in a sitting position and breathing quietly through his mouth. Nose breathing tends to produce more turbulence, which may prove confusing, and deep breathing through the mouth tends to produce a bronchovesicular or even bronchial sound because it increases the velocity of air flow through the airways and mimics the sound heard over the trachea if the breathing is deep enough.

Whenever possible, examine the lungs in a quiet environment and have the chest completely exposed so that you can observe as well as listen. If the patient cannot sit up, place him in a semi-Fowler's position to listen to the anterior chest, and roll him from side to side to listen to the lateral and posterior walls. Under these circumstances it will be much more difficult and impractical to attempt a side-to-side auscultation as you move down the posterior chest. If help is available, have someone help you sit the patient forward while you listen to the posterior wall.

Always attempt to auscultate from side to side in order to compare what you are hearing, and use the interspaces, where sounds are more easily discernible. Anteriorly, you should begin at the apex of the lungs and work side to side and down the chest. Because of the lung topography, the upper lobes can be auscultated anteriorly, whereas the right middle lobe can be auscultated anterolaterally. Listen also on the lateral chest walls for the lower lobes. Proceed to the posterior chest and, again starting at the apices of the lungs, auscultate side to side and downward, ending at the lung bases. It is important to specifically listen for rales with the patient in a sitting position; often these sounds cannot be distinguished unless gravity is used to facilitate collection of the fluid in the alveoli of the lower lobes. In addition, fine rales may only be heard posteriorly, since it is in this area that the lower lobes are more closely approximated to the chest wall.

AUSCULTATING HEART SOUNDS. Although somewhat more difficult to analyze than lung sounds, heart sounds are nevertheless an important element in the chest examination and can provide a great deal of information about the integrity of the heart valves, the ventricular and atrial muscle, and the conduction system. Because many of the cardiac sounds have a low pitch, it is helpful to have a bell available. The goal of listening to heart sounds should be to identify changes in intensity of the normal sounds, changes in the timing of the normal heart sounds, and the presence of extra sounds or murmurs and their relationship to the cardiac cycle.

The process of events that occurs in the cardiac cycle can be graphically presented in steps:

1. Blood flows into the atria during diastole; pressure within the atria begins to slightly exceed that within the ventricles.
2. The atrioventricular (AV) valves open, allowing access of blood to the ventricular chambers and hence ventricular filling.
3. Ventricular contraction begins, and the pressure within the chambers exceeds that within the atria; the AV valves close.
4. As ventricular pressure continues to rise, it exceeds the pressure in the aorta and pulmonary artery, forcing the aortic and pulmonic valves open.
5. As the ventricles eject their blood, the intraventricular pressure again begins to fall; once it falls below that within the aorta and pulmonary artery, the aortic and pulmonic valves close.
6. The atria again begin to fill with blood, and the cycle begins again.
7. This entire sequence takes just 1 second at 60 beats per minute!

Heart sounds are the result of vibratory energy that is produced by the changes identified above. As the valves grow taut, as the ventricular chambers fill, and as blood is ejected into the great vessels, sounds occur that can be related to the cardiac cycle and even superimposed onto a phonocardiogram to show their relationship to electrical events. Normally, each cardiac cycle produces two sounds, the first and second heart sounds (S_1 and S_2).

The first sound is due to several events but is generally attributed to mitral and tricuspid (AV valve) closure after ventricular filling has completed. The first sound signals the onset of systole, and is approximately synchronous with the onset of the apical thrust and the carotid impulse. It is heard loudest at the mitral and tricuspid auscultory areas.

The second heart sound is referred to as the closure of the aortic and pulmonic valves, but also consist of sounds made by late atrial filling and early ejection of blood into the ventricles through the AV valves. The pitch of this sound is slightly higher than the first sound, and it has a snappier quality. It is heard loudest at the pulmonic and aortic auscultory areas at the base of the heart, and begins the diastolic phase of the cardiac cycle.

The period of time between S_1 and S_2 is cardiac systole; this period of time is shorter than the period of time between S_2 and S_1, or diastole. It is important to discriminate systole from diastole in order to differentiate extra sounds from normal sounds (S_3 and S_4 are *diastolic* sounds) and murmurs. The diastolic phase is affected by tachydysrhythmias, and is difficult to discern unless the cardiac thrust is used to identify systole and correlate with the heart sound heard at the same time.

Abnormalities of S_1 are primarily confined to changes in intensity as a result of mitral stenosis or conduction defects. Remember, S_1 should be louder than S_2 over the *apex* of the heart.

Abnormalities of S_2 are primarily confined to abnormal splitting or changes in intensity of S_2 between the aortic and pulmonic auscultory areas. Splitting of the heart sound is not always abnormal, however, as it may normally be appreciated because of the difference in timing between closure of the aortic valve and closure of the pulmonic valve. Normally, the aortic valve closes slightly earlier because pressures within the aorta are greater than pressures within the pulmonary artery; if you recall from the steps of the cycle, it is these pressures after ventricular contraction that close the aortic and pulmonic valves at the onset of diastole. A splitting sound can best be described as the difference in sound between the word "spit" and the word "split." When "spit" is spoken three times in succession and then "split" is spoken three times in succession, you will be able to appreciate how a split sound may sound. The abnormalities of S_2 splitting include a reversal of closure of the valves, resulting in a soft and then slightly louder sound; a prolonged delay in the closure of the pulmonic valve resulting in a wide split; and a fixed time interval between closure of the two valves resulting in a "fixed" split. In the physiological splitting of the aortic and pulmonic valves, the two sounds usually coincide during expiration but more apart during inspiration as a result of changes in intrathoracic pressure. For a more in-depth review of splitting, ejection clicks, and opening snaps, the reader is referred to a textbook of cardiac physiology and cardiac examination. These phenomena are difficult to evaluate and are not generally of isolated concern within the emergency department.

The third heart sound is a diastolic sound that may be normal in young children and women in the third trimester of pregnancy and pathological in the other adult. The mechanism for both is essentially the same: a low frequency sound that results from vibrations in the ventricle as the outward motion suddenly stops during early diastolic filling. Also called a "ventricular gallop," S_3 may occur in cardiac failure, increased preload, and abnormally slow rates.

The fourth heart sound is a diastolic sound that actually falls presystolic and is caused by poor distensibility of the ventricles as the atria contract and force blood into them. S_4 is often referred to as an "atrial gallop." If both S_3 and S_4 are heard in the diastolic phase, the sound is called a "summation gallop" and is clearly an abnormal finding that must be acted upon, in context with the clinical setting, as soon as possible.

MURMURS. Murmurs are sounds produced by several different mechanisms:

1. Turbulent flow across a partial obstruction such as a stenotic valve
2. Turbulent flow across a valvular irregularity but without obstruction
3. Turbulent flow into a dilated chamber
4. Turbulent flow out of a high pressure chamber through an abnormal passage
5. Increased flow through normal passages
6. Regurgitant flow across an incompetent valve or defect

The sounds that result in murmurs can be described either as a raspy or harsh sound, or as a sound with a blowing or musical quality; raspy being the sound most often heard over a stenotic valve and blowing being the sound most often heard over regurgitant valves or dilated chambers (much like the bruit heard over a dilated aortic aneurysm). Murmurs are conveniently divided into systolic and diastolic, and although there may be innocent or benign systolic murmurs, diastolic murmurs are almost without exception pathological.

The common scale used to describe the intensity of a murmur is the Levine Scale:

Grade I   Very faint, may not be heard in all positions

Grade II	Quiet but heard immediately upon stethoscope contact with the chest wall
Grade III	Moderately loud, but not associated with a thrill (tactile sensation associated with the sound)
Grade IV	Loud, usually associated with a thrill
Grade V	Very loud, may be heard without placing the stethoscope completely on the chest
Grade VI	Extremely loud, may be heard without placing the stethoscope on the chest at all

It is necessary to record murmurs according to the scale used to measure their intensity (for example, grade V/grade VI).

Some cardiac sounds have both a systolic and diastolic component, such as those heard with *pericardial friction rubs and venous hums.* Identifying these sounds can become somewhat confusing if they overlie other extra sounds in the cycle. Probably the most important to learn is the pericardial friction rub that may develop in inflammation of the pericardial sac and can herald tamponade. The elements of this sound are related to cardiac movement, most notably atrial contraction, ventricular systole, and ventricular diastole. Therefore, the sound has a short component that falls between S_1 and S_2, another that falls directly after S_2, and yet another that occurs immediately before S_1. If you think that you hear a friction rub, the sound should increase in intensity if you sit the patient forward and listen during expiration (the quieter of the two respiratory phases). The pericardial friction rub can best be described as scratchy and high-pitched.

Evaluation of heart sounds is difficult for the new practitioner; however, repeated practice can be enormously successful in recognition of normal and abnormal findings. The techniques of examination that will help you develop skill follow.

1. Use a quiet environment with the chest exposed.
2. Approach the patient on his right side and identify the auscultory areas.
3. Count the cardiac rate, and identify the rhythm.
4. Place your stethoscope over the aortic and pulmonic areas, and concentrate on the second heart sound. Note its intensity, and listen for splitting.
5. Move your stethoscope to the mitral and tricuspid auscultory areas, and concentrate on the first heart sound; note its intensity, and listen for splitting (splitting of the first heart sound is not generally appreciated because of its soft intensity).
6. Now concentrate on the time interval between S_1 and S_2; note any extra sounds in terms of timing, intensity, and pitch.
7. Listen to the diastolic phase; remember that it will be longer in duration than systole. Note any extra sounds in terms of their timing, intensity, and pitch.
8. Listen for systolic murmurs, and identify whether early, mid, or late systolic, location of the sound on the chest, radiation if any, intensity using the Levine Scale, pitch, and quality.
9. Listen for diastolic murmurs, and identify the characteristics as shown above.
10. Finally, listen for murmurs or other cardiovascular sounds that have both a systolic and diastolic component (pericardial friction rubs).

VITAL SIGNS AS AN ASSESSMENT PARAMETER

As an important element of the assessment process, vital signs deserve much more than the casual attention that they usually receive. The pulse rate, respiratory rate, blood pressure values, and body temperature can provide valuable information that, when combined with the remainder of the physical examination, can greatly affect the nursing diagnosis. In addition, when signs and symptoms conflict with one another and/or with values of the vital signs, it is imperative to pay meticulous attention to all elements of the physical examination to determine the cause of the conflict. In the hospital, the emergency department is the only unit where there is no prior exposure to each patient and therefore no opportunity to evaluate the presenting condition in terms of yesterday's laboratory tests or physical findings.

Vital signs are indicators of the patient's present condition and must be obtained serially in order to have any impact on the identification of trends or developments in the clinical situation. Because the vital signs reflect the activities of compensatory mechanisms within the body, they also provide information regarding the failure of these mechanisms. Variations from normal and from the patient's own normal must be explained clinically. Subsequent readings should be considered in light of the therapeutic interventions initiated.

Temperature

There are several new electronic and paper thermometers currently available with which to obtain a patient's temperature. There is no particular advantage of the glass thermometer over these newer tools. In fact, electronic thermometers are believed to have greater accuracy when used properly.

When taking oral temperatures, take the time to place the tip of the thermometer in the pocket of tissue at the base of the tongue against the sublingual artery. Temperatures across the buccal cavity change significantly depending on the distance from this artery. The sublingual site is not only easily accessible in the majority of patients, but also easily replicable, as opposed to the rectal and axillary sites where it is difficult to take repeated temperatures from the same place each time.

The rectal route has been proclaimed to be the only effective route to obtain accurate temperatures in the patient who is mouth-breathing because of pain or dyspnea. It is not necessarily accurate in all cases, however, for the following reasons:

1. The rectum is not known to have thermoreceptive elements and is distant from the central nervous sytem.
2. The rectum does not reflect early changes in temperature as rapidly as the sublingual site.
3. The presence of stool may impair accurate readings; if the stool is hard, the thermometer may not reach the suggested 3-inch depth and if soft, the tip of the thermometer may become imbedded in the stool and never contact the rectal wall.
4. The rectal site is not easily accessible and may be embarrassing to adults and older children.
5. It is not easy to replicate the exact site used, and rectal temperatures may vary with placement of the thermometer tip at different sites.

The axillary site is used more frequently in neonatal units where air flow and ambient temperature are carefully controlled. However, it is a safe and fairly accurate site when the proper precautions are taken to avoid environmental influence. These precautions include leaving the thermometer in place for at least 10 minutes, ensuring that the thermometer is resting against the axillary artery, and maintaining contact by keeping the arm tightly enfolded over the thermometer the entire time the instrument is in place.

In cases where core temperature is desired, it is possible to obtain readings by utilizing a probe, which is placed against the tympanic membrane, measuring the urine temperature, or measuring the temperature in the nasal turbinates.

Pulse

In this world of electronic sophistication, a habit has developed that is occurring with alarming frequency. This habit is a reluctance on the part of paramedics, nurses, and physicians to palpate all peripheral pulses as part of their assessment of the patient's status. When we are given pulse rates from the field in a prehospital situation, it is very likely that we are being told only what the monitored rate is. This information gives no indication of the quality and characteristics of the pulse. Equally important, rhythm disturbances may not be identified unless these changes are seen on the portable monitor. Irregularities of rhythm can be missed on a portable scope if they derive from premature beats or are irregularly irregular. Yet premature beats can be felt on palpation as either missing beats or beats with less amplitude from those preceding them, and irregularly irregular rhythms can be felt as a chaotic rhythm even if they tend to be subtle.

In addition to describing the rate and rhythm of the pulse, the quality should also be described as bounding, normal, weak and thready, or absent. If the pulse is parodoxical, as in the sensation under your fingertips of a rising and falling amplitude in concert with respirations, this should be recorded. If the pulse is unusually snappy and full, as in a "water-hammer" pulse, this information should be recorded. There are other characteristic pulse qualities that should be solicited in the cardiovascular assessment of patients by the actual palpation of all peripheral pulses.

Put in context with other physical findings, the pulse is an important indicator of cardiac function. Often, changes in the pulse rate are the first sign that compensatory mechanisms are being invoked in order to maintain homeostasis. Frequently in early volume depletion, a healthy individual with an intact autonomic nervous system may retain normal pressures with only one subtle change: a slight increase in the pulse rate and amplitude. Any deviation from the normal range for the patient's age that cannot be related to psychological or environmental factors should be considered an indication of a pathologic condition until proved otherwise.

Respirations

Performing a thorough respiratory assessment is not a time-consuming process. In fact, in most cases this entire system can be assessed, to the extent necessary in the emergency department, within 1 or 2 minutes. The objective of assessing respirations as a part of evaluation of the patient's vital signs is to identify impairment of ventilatory function, attempt to isolate the cause, and provide timely intervention. In collecting vital signs, one should not simply count the respiratory rate without completing respiratory evaluation. This should hold true for all emergency patients, not only the critically ill ones. The other factors besides respiratory rate and rhythm that should be assessed follow.

Signs of respiratory effort, such as tracheal tugging, nasal flaring, use of accessory muscles, or retractions. Generally a healthy individual will not make extra efforts to breathe; there will be no airway noise, the trachea will be fixed in midline, the nasal cartilage is quiet, and there is no utilization of the sternocleidomastoid or intercostal muscles to help lift the chest cage. In addition, there is no suprasternal, intercostal, or substernal indrawing on inspiration to indicate an increase in the work of breathing.

Chest contour. An increase in anteroposterior diameter can generally be seen on casual observation, and indicates that chronic alveolar distension is present. Other changes in chest contour are those that are seen in funnel chest, pigeon chest, kyphosis, and kyphoscoliosis. These particular anatomical changes in contour may interfere with normal lung inflation and may complicate or exacerbate the effects of respiratory pathologic conditions.

Symmetry of chest expansion. When the healthy individual inspires, the chest expands symmetrically on both sides. When pulmonary or chest wall pathologic conditions exist, the chest may rise asymmetrically during ventilation; this asymmetry can often be observed with the chest exposed. The asymmetry can also be palpated during inspiration.

Depth of ventilation. The patient's tidal volume can be estimated by observing the rise and fall of his chest during ventilation or by standing behind the patient and placing your hands around his chest cage with your thumbs placed parasternally. When palpating in this manner, your thumbs will be displaced laterally on inspiration and then will move back toward each other on expiration. The depth of ventilations is described as shallow, normal, or deep. A normal adult will move 300 to 500 cc air at rest, and will move up to 2,000 cc during exercise, with a corresponding increase in rate. When evaluating depth, remember that a fast rate is not necessarily moving increased volume, nor is a slow rate moving less volume.

Breath sounds and inspiratory/expiratory ratio. Simply counting the respiratory rate is not substantial; all these parameters must be evaluated when assessing respirations as a vital sign. The days of rapidly calculating a 15-second rate are long over for the critical care nurse in an intensive care unit or emergency department.

Blood pressure

Because the blood pressure varies with numerous factors, including patient condition, age, and sex, it is not the most reliable indicator of physiological changes. It is, however, vital information when considered with the pulse and respiration and in light of the clinical situation. The systolic pressure is a parameter of pump integrity, and the diastolic pressure is a parameter of vascular status. One cannot be fooled by normal pressures in the emergency department, because this is no indication that all is well. As mentioned previously, a healthy person may not exhibit signs of low circulating volume until all compensatory mechanisms have been exhausted. The patient may have only to change his position to cause a precipitous drop in his pressure. It is for this reason that anyone suspected of volume depletion by history or clinical findings should be evaluated for postural vital sign changes. Also known as "orthostatic vital signs" or the "tilt test," postural vital sign evaluation should be done on patients who have experienced syncopal events, those who appear dehydrated, and those who have a history of volume loss, as in prolonged vomiting, diarrhea, sweating, diuretic therapy, gastrointestinal bleeding, burns, or obvious blood loss, among other entities. Contrary to the neurological tilt test, which is used to test the integrity of the autonomic nervous system (ANS) it is not correct to provide a 5-minute period of time after a change in position when obtaining postural vital signs. The purpose of the test is to establish whether there has been a significant loss of volume that has necessitated the use of compensatory mechanisms inclusive of severe peripheral vascular constriction, not to test whether or not the ANS is functioning properly. Therefore, immediately after obtaining a pulse and blood pressure and writing them down while the patient is lying flat, elevate him to a full sitting position and retake the pulse and the blood pressure. Significant changes include:

1. Subjective feelings of dizziness or blurring of the vision
2. A decrease in pressure of 20 mm Hg or more
3. An increase in pulse rate of 20 beats/min or more

If these findings occur with a change to the sitting position, the test is considered positive for significant blood loss, and fluid replacement must begin with volume expanders such as lactated Ringer's solution, normal saline, or whatever other solution is appropriate for the situation. In addition and most important, the site of bleeding must be sought and the bleeding controlled. If the sitting portion of the postural vital sign exam is positive, the standing portion may be deferred, since it will not yield much of note under the circumstances and may prove detrimental to the patient. If there are equivocal changes from the lying to the sitting position, or no changes at all, the patient should be moved to a standing position if there is no contraindication to doing so (for example, a fractured leg), and the pulse and blood pressure retaken and recorded. Positive findings are the same as described for the sitting position.

Whenever evaluating the blood pressure, consider your findings in relationship to the patient's history; if he is undergoing antihypertensive therapy, the values obtained during his emergency department visit may represent a significant deviation relative to his "normal" pressure. Consider also the pulse pressure (the difference between the systolic and the diastolic pressures), which represents the approximate stroke volume when all other variables are constant. Peripheral vascular resistance and elasticity of the vessel walls are also critical determinants of the pulse pressure, and therefore approximating the stroke volume by measuring the pulse pressure is more qualitative than accurate; however, the pulse pressure will provide you with information about the status of the pump and peripheral vessels and indicate otherwise subtle hemodynamic changes.

Blood pressure recordings can be obtained either on the arm using the brachial artery, the thigh using the popliteal artery, or the calf using the "flush method." The flush method is performed on neonates or young infants to obtain the mean arterial pressure. The patient's foot is elevated above his heart and the blood is massaged out of the limb. A cuff is applied (infant cuff) around the calf and pumped to approximately 130 mm Hg. The foot is then lowered and the pressure in the cuff released in 5-mm increments until the foot flushes with blood; the pressure at which the foot flushes is the mean arterial pressure.

Both the auscultated method and the palpated method can be used, depending on the patient's condition and the environment, but the palpated method will not provide you with information about the diastolic (and thus the peripheral vascular system) pressure. Be certain to communicate which method has been used so that others who obtain the pressure use the same method or correlate their findings by another method. A single blood pressure recording yields little to no information; it is necessary to take serial pressures to monitor the hemodynamic status. In fact, all the vital signs must be taken and evaluated serially; the patient's condition in the department is a dynamic continuum that can be assessed only through continuous monitoring. Any time that therapy is instituted, all the vital signs should be evaluated in order to assess the efficacy of the treatment. Also, the vital signs should be repeated once more before a decision is made about the disposition of the patient from the department, whether he is discharged, admitted, or transferred to another facility.

Level of consciousness

Level of consciousness is one of the most vital of all the vital signs, because it is an indication of the status of cerebral perfusion and function. One of the more specific ways in which to describe the level of consciousness is to use the stimulation/response method, stating exactly how the patient responds to a specific stimulation. The stimulation/response method requires judgment, interpretation, and specific documentation to communicate the information to others who may also be evaluating the level of consciousness.

It is helpful to assess the consciousness in the order with which it may deteriorate. If the cerebral hemispheres are intact, well oxygenated, and functioning normally, the patient will be able to respond with purpose to your normal speaking voice. He will be able to answer questions readily and will remain awake during the interview and exam. In short, he will be fully conscious. If he is conscious, evaluate his degree of orientation, beginning with the one thing he is least likely to forget—his name. Progressively he should be asked where he is, what day or time it is, and what happened to him. Allowing for confusion relative to the stress of the situation or literally not having been told what hospital he was being taken to, assess his answers to evaluate whether he is oriented to person, place, time, and situation (orientation times 4). These four areas of orientation are also lost in a progressive order, beginning with disorientation to the situation, or amnesia for the situation. As a patient becomes less responsive, you will often find that he also becomes less oriented.

As the cerebral hemispheres become dysfunctional for any reason, the level of consciousness and degree of orientation will begin to deteriorate, but the changes may be extremely subtle early on, and unless the same stimulation is given, these changes may be overlooked until they become obvious. The following example of progressive changes reveals how these changes can be identified without the use of confusing labels such as "lethargic," "semiconscious," or "obtunded."

1. Mr. Jones is awake, responds to my voice by turning to look at me, and is oriented times 4.
2. Mr. Jones is sleepy but becomes awake and alert when I call his name. Follows all directions and answers questions appropriately when aroused. Oriented times 4.
3. Mr. Jones is drowsy but arouses when I shake his shoulder. Oriented times 3. When stimulation is removed, he drifts to sleep again.
4. Mr. Jones is sleeping most of the time, arouses sluggishly when his shoulder is shaken firmly, cannot follow more than

---

Types of painful stimulation

1. Supraorbital compression: Pressure over the supraorbital rim just medial to the midline (of the eye) will trap the nerve against the bony skull prominence and cause pain. This is useful in several ways. First, it should provoke a reaction in all but the most deeply comatose patient. Secondly, it may help to demonstrate a motor deficit on one side of the body or the other.
2. Sternal compression (rub): "Knuckle rub" causes pain but can leave tell-tale bruises, especially in older people. Again, here is a reminder to *describe the painful stimuli,* for example, "The patient responds to sternal compression with purposeful movement."
3. Interdigital compression: Trapping the digital nerves against a pencil, for example, placed between the fingers or toes is useful to determine if the patient will withdraw his limb, if you suspect hemiparesis.
4. Trapezius pinch: This pinch is painful, can bruise.
5. Calf pressure: This pressure is quite painful.

---

one direction at a time, and drifts back to sleep readily.

5. Mr. Jones is sleeping most of the time, arouses only to trapezius pinch and pushes my hand away. He is inarticulate when aroused and drifts back to sleep immediately.
6. Mr. Jones responds only to firm trapezius squeeze and evidences decorticate posturing without arousing.
7. Mr. Jones responds to firm trapezius squeeze with decerebrate posturing.
8. Mr. Jones responds to firm sternal rub with increase in pulse and respiration only; does not respond to any other stimulation.
9. Mr. Jones has no physical response to deep painful stimulation.

Placed in context with other neurological assessments including eye changes, respiratory changes, and motor movement and posturing, this stimulation/response method is very informative. The pain stimulations used to assess the level of consciousness do not need to be barbaric; begin with light pain such as pressure on the nailbeds, supraorbital nerve pressure, and interdigital pressure with a pencil. Deep pain can be applied by a firm pinch or squeeze of the trapezius muscle, the inner aspect of the thigh, or the inner aspect of the upper arm. Or deep pain can be applied with a firm sternal rub with your knuckles, although this method

may result in bruising of the sternal skin. Either the patient responds to deep pain, or he does not, and there is no need to become sadistic about applying more severe stimulation. If he is unarousable to anything other than deep pain, however, the objective of applying the painful stimulation is not to keep him awake, because if there is a significant intracranial pathological condition, nothing can do so until the condition is treated. Therefore, apply the noxious stimulation briefly and at intervals as opposed to constantly.

If the level of consciousness begins to deteriorate, follow through with an assessment of the pupils, respiratory rate and pattern, and muscle reflexes and tone.

Skin vital signs

Because it is the largest organ in the body, and because it is external, the skin is an excellent mirror of physiological changes that are occurring within the body. The dermis is well supplied by an extensive capillary system that is sensitive to changes in the autonomic nervous system. Sympathetic overactivity results in the release of endogenous catecholamines into the circulation, with a resultant increase in heart rate and blood pressure. The skin reflects these changes by becoming cool, moist, and pale. This sympathetic overactivity is frequently a response to pain, stress, or reduction in cardiac output. Parasympathetic overactivity may be

Table 7-1. Color changes in skin

Color	Cause	Location
Brown	Generic	Generalized
	Sunlight	Exposed areas
	Pregnancy	Localized to nipples, face, linea negra, vulva
	Addison's disease and some pituitary tumors	Local (exposed areas palmar creases) or generalized
Gray brown or bronze	Hematochromatosis	Exposed areas, genitalia, scars; may also be generalized
Reddish	Polycythemia	Face, conjunctiva, mouth, hands, feet
	Excessive heat	Generalized
	Sunburn, thermal burn	Exposed areas
	Increased visibility of normal oxyhemoglobin due to vasodilation as a result of fever, blushing, alcohol, inflammation	Localized
	Decreased oxygen utilization in skin, as in cold exposure	Exposed areas
Yellow	Increased bilirubinemia caused by liver disease, red cell hemolysis	Sclera in initial stages then generalized
	Carotenemia caused by increased carotene pigment as a result of myxedema, hypopituitarism, diabetes	Exposed areas although may be generalized; *not* seen in sclera or mucous membrane
	Chronic uremia	Exposed areas although may be generalized; *not* seen in sclera or mucous membranes
Blue	Hypoxemia	Central (lips, tongue, nailbeds)
	Decreased flow to skin because of anxiety, cold	Localized, peripheral
	Abnormal hemoglobin as a result of combination with methylene or sulfa	Central
Pale or white	Obstructive shock, hemorrhagic shock, distributive shock, cardiogenic shock	Generalized
	Renal failure	Generalized
	Fear or pain	Generalized and self-limiting

reflected in the skin by ruddiness due to relaxation of peripheral vasculature, increased temperature, and dry skin. The changes in skin color, moisture, and temperature can be assessed by evaluating the status of these skin vital signs. *Skin color* changes depend on many factors, including the size of surface vessels, the content and depth of melanin and carotene, the amount of oxyhemoglobin or reduced hemoglobin, and the lighting of the environment coupled with the skill of the evaluator (Table 7-1). Inspection of the skin for color changes should follow an organized pattern; note whether any changes seen are localized or generalized, then inspect for changes in areas that characteristically have the least amount of pigmentation that could obscure or confuse findings. These areas are the buccal mucosa, lips, nailbeds, earlobes, palms, and soles. Inspect the palms and soles while the patient is lying flat to prevent gravity-induced changes. In addition, the sclera and conjunctiva may reflect changes when pallor or jaundice exist (they take on a grayish hue in pallor and a yellowish hue in jaundice). The critical color changes to evaluate are cyanosis and pallor, because both require rapid intervention to reverse the cause. Cyanosis is not always evident in poorly ventilated patients or those who have less than 5 g circulating reduced hemoglobin. It is also difficult to see cyanotic changes in highly pigmented skin. If you are unsure whether the cyanosis that you see is central or peripheral, massage a small area of skin with your finger. Peripheral cyanosis disappears on massage, whereas central cyanosis will not. If skin color suggests blood loss or cardiovascular dysfunction, perform a capillary blanching maneuver to help substantiate your suspicion; a decrease in filling is seen after pressure is applied and released suddenly if your suspicion is correct. Patients who have a decrease in hemoglobin content due to anemia also appear pale, but the vasomotor tone is still good, and the capillary filling test will be normal.

Skin moisture should be evaluated by palpating the texture and turgor of the skin. Grasp a small section between your thumb and forefinger and evaluate whether the skin is thin and dry, inelastic or elastic, or thick and mushy (as in the patient with myxedema). If the water content of the skin feels excessive, check to see if pitting is present, and if it is, where it is located. Remember that a patient who has been confined to bed may not exhibit dependent edema of the lower extremities; instead, check the sacral area for pitting edema. And finally, check to see if the skin is dry, damp, or wet. Overactivity of the sympathetic nervous system may produce diaphoresis that may range from light to excessive.

An increase of blood flow through the capillaries under the skin will result in radiation of heat from the surface of the skin, whereas a decrease in flow will be manifested by coolness to touch. Evaluate the *skin temperature* by palpating the skin surface with the dorsum of your hand, which is most sensitive to temperature changes. Identify whether temperature changes are localized or generalized. Skin temperature is also affected by changes in the diameter of capillaries under the skin; dilated vessels will produce more heat from the skin surface, whereas constricted vessels will produce cool skin. All the skin vital signs should be evalu-

ated in concert with one another. If the findings do not correlate with one another, investigate why.

EVALUATION OF PAIN

Whenever a patient states that he is having pain, it is incumbent upon us to believe him. Pain is an extremely subjective sensation, and although an illness or injury may initially trigger the sensation, the manner in which the patient perceives his pain, and thus behaves, is uniquely his own. Cultural influences, past experiences in a health care setting, previous experiences with pain, individual coping mechanisms, and the gravity of the current situation all contribute to a patient's individual reactions to pain.

A patient's response to pain is also very much affected by the nature of the pain itself; chronic pain is more difficult to deal with than an acute episode. Whereas acute pain tends to generate anxiety, chronic pain tends to generate depression and the feeling that nothing can be done to relieve the pain. The patient with acute pain is much more likely to cooperate with treatment and the inevitable delays in treatment. The chronic sufferer is not, even though he wants very much to be relieved.

In the evaluation of pain, use open-ended questions to allow the patient to describe just what sensation he is experiencing in term that are most meaningful to him. Watch his face as he expresses how the pain feels to him, and watch his behavior as he attempts to deal with the situation in which he finds himself and with the anxiety of the emergency department setting. Often this setting aggravates discomfort and fear, and much of the time a great deal of pain relief may be engendered by your empathy and support. Depending on the particular pathological cause, the patient's ability to cope, and his age, pain may be described in many different ways (older patients often have diminished pain sensation and may not use the term "pain" at all in their description). It is helpful to have the patient rank his pain on a scale of 1 to 10. A "1" on the scale refers to a complete absence of pain, whereas a "10" on the scale refers to excruciating, unremitting pain.

When using this scale, ask the patient to rank this episode of pain in comparison with other painful experiences in his life. Find out what experience he is using to compare this situation with. Have the patient point to the painful area or place of maximum discomfort, if he can. Visceral pain, as opposed to superficial or cutaneous pain, is diffuse and difficult to pinpoint. Often it radiates to other areas of the body because it follows different dermatomes, or tracks of nerves. Thus, visceral pain will be more difficult for the patient to pinpoint. However, he can identify areas that are *not* painful, or indicate the general area of his pain.

The PQRST mnemonic is helpful in identifying the character, location, and intensity of the pain. Depending on the presenting complaint, physical maneuvers or palpation of the area of discomfort can help identify specific painful areas and intensity. Before palpating an area, however, inspect the site to be palpated. In the case of abdominal pain, auscultate for bowel sounds before palpating the belly, as palpation may change the nature of bowel action. In the case of posttraumatic spinal injury, do not move the spine to identify pain or tenderness before spinal films are taken. One can palpate for paraspinal muscle spasm before films are taken, but motion is strictly prohibited to prevent cord damage.

Do not rely on sympathetic nervous changes to substantiate a patient's report of pain. Reflex parasympathetic activity may interrupt common sympathetic findings of cool, clammy, and pale skin, which is often seen in severe pain. Continue to assess the patient's subjective description of the level of his pain, and allow him to react in his own way without making judgments about whether pain is present or whether it is incapacitating. There are few instances where some type of medication cannot be given; this medication might be a mild sedative to relieve anxiety and enable the patient to regain effective coping behavior. In some cases, medication given for pain has other beneficial effects, as is often the case with morphine sulfate in acute pulmonary edema. Although there are times when a patient may use complaints of pain to manipulate others for the purpose of obtaining drugs, this is really a rare situation and can usually be identified by the careful use of the PQRST mnemonic in combination with a physical examination.

LABORATORY ANALYSIS

The laboratory data base is an essential ingredient in the assessment of patients in the emergency department. Expensive at best, laboratory tests should not be ordered indiscriminately, but should follow an interview and examination process that indicates the appropriate testing requirements for each individual case.

A fair number of laboratory tests are utilized frequently within the emergency setting. In some departments it is a nursing responsibility to order routine tests when their need is established, whereas in other departments such orders are carried out by the physician on duty. In either case, a working knowledge of the common tests and the types of containers used to collect them is necessary for the nurse involved (Table 7-2).

Table 7-2. Tubes for drawing blood

Tube	Preservative or anticoagulant	Test
Red top	None	Serologies, chemistry panels, routine chemistries
Lavender top	Ethylenediaminotetraacetate (EDTA)	Hematology, lipoprotein electrophorophesis, acid phosphotase
Blue top	Sodium citrate (0.5 gm)	Coagulation studies
Gray top	Sodium fluoride	Blood glucose, blood alcohol, drug screens and tests that are not going to be run for some time.
Green top	Sodium heparin	Special procedures

Complete blood count. A complete blood count is a routine hematological screening test on serum; it includes hemoglobin, hematocrit, total red blood cell (RBC) count, white count and differential, and mean corpuscle cell volume, (MCV), mean cell hemoglobin concentration (MCHC), and mean cell hemoglobin (MCH). Elements of this test may on occasion be ordered separately, which will save the patient money. Five milliliters of venous blood are generally required.

Urinalysis. A urinalysis should always be a clean catch or catheter specimen collected in a sterile, dry container and examined within 2 hours. The standard examination includes appearance, pH, specific gravity, glucose and ketones, protein semiquantitation, and microscopic exam of the sediment for casts, crystals, RBCs, and bacteria.

Blood glucose. Venous blood for glucose levels should be obtained as a clot specimen in patients suspected of abnormalities in glucose metabolism. Collect the specimen before starting IV solution infusions or administering dextrose. Two to three milliliters are necessary to perform the exam. Record the conditions under which the blood was drawn (that is, fasting, last meal approximate time, time of last meal unknown, and so on).

Blood urea nitrogen. The blood urea nitrogen (BUN) test measures the amount of circulating urea in the blood, which is the end product of protein metabolism and is normally excreted in the urine. An elevation of the BUN may indicate renal failure, renal hypoperfusion, obstructive uropathy, and so on. One milliliter of venous blood is required.

Serum electrolytes. The venous specimen should be withdrawn from a vein and collected in a specimen container in as atraumatic a procedure as possible to avoid hemolysis. Hemolysis will result in a false elevation of the serum potassium. Electrolytes include potassium, chlorides, and carbon dioxide content. Although each of these elements can be tested individually, the implications of the result may change depending on the values of the other electrolytes in concert with one another.

Serum creatinine. The serum creatinine test evaluates renal function by measuring creatinine, a waste product of creatine that is found in skeletal muscle and is usually filtered by the renal glomerulus. The serum creatinine may be elevated in acute renal failure. Three milliliters of venous blood are required.

Cardiac enzymes. Tests for cardiac enzymes include creatine phosphokinase (CPK), lactic dehydrogenase (LDH), serum glutamic-oxaloacetic transaminase (SGOT). Levels may be elevated in cardiac muscle infarction, but can also be present in acute muscle injury or multiple injection patients. Therefore, cardiac isoenzymes are usually evaluated also, specifically those that are known to elevate in cardiac muscle infarction (LDH fraction 1 and CPK-MB). Five milliliters of venous blood are required.

Toxic screen. A toxic screen may be ordered specific to a certain drug or as a screen for sedatives, hypnotics, narcotics, and so on. It measures the specific amount of circulating drug per volume of plasma. This is a very expensive test and it takes a great deal of time to run (most facilities send the specimen out to a bioanalysis laboratory, which delays receipt of the results because of transit time). Five milliliters of venous blood are required.

Serum drug level. A serum drug level is generally ordered specific to one drug such as digoxin. It measures the concentration of drug in the blood at the time the level is drawn. Two to five milliliters of venous blood are required.

Serum amylase. Serum amylase is generally evaluated in patients with upper abdominal pain. The test measures the amount of circulating amylase, which is a digestive enzyme for carbohydrates and is elevated most notably in acute pancreatitis. Three milliliters of venous blood are required.

Arterial blood gases. Arterial blood gases are analyzed from arterial specimens collected in heparinized tubes or syringes. Elements include serum pH, P_{CO_2}, P_{O_2}, and bicarbonate levels. Results help determine the acid-base status of the internal environment and the degree of oxygenation of the tissues. Most test results include the percent of oxygen saturation of the red blood cells. Three milliliters are the minimum specimen required, which is collected under aseptic conditions.

White blood count and differential. A white blood count (WBC) and differential may be ordered instead of a CBC when an infection is suspected. However, both of these elements must be ordered and evaluated together, since the WBC may not be elevated even in severe infections whereas the differential will be. Mild to moderate leukocytosis may indicate an infectious process that is bacterial in origin. The differential is an evaluation of the different types of leukocytes that are found in the serum: neutrophils (56% of the total), eosinophils (2.7% of the total), basophils (0.3% of the total), and lymphocytes (34% of the total). Neutrophils are also called "polys" or polymorphonucleocytes, and "segs" or segmented cells. Monocytes are nongranular leukocytes and may be seen in chronic inflammatory conditions in small numbers. "Bands" are new neutrophils that are formed in response to overwhelming bacterial invasion that taxes the older neutrophil population. Such a condition is referred to as a "shift to the left." The WBC and differential are collected in a clot tube devoid of preservatives or anticoagulants, and 3 to 5 ml venous blood are required.

Coagulation studies. Various elements of the coagulation series evaluate the different stages of clotting. The studies include protime, partial thromboplastin time, platelet count, Lee White clotting time, and prothrombin consumption time.

PROTHROMBIN TIME. This test identifies defects in Stage III of coagulation. A calcium binding anticoagulant is added to the patient's serum, and the time between addition of this element and the formation of a fibrin clot is measured.

PARTIAL THROMBOPLASTIN TIME. This test identifies defects in Stage II of coagulation. It measures factors XII, XI, X, IX, VIII, V, II, and I; thus, it measures the clotting time of plasma when elements of the clotting process are added to calcium-free and platelet-poor plasma in a predetermined sequence.

PROTHROMBIN CONSUMPTION TIME (PCT). This test measures prothrombin utilization time. It identifies defects in Stage I and II of coagulation. PCT is also used to elevate coagulation of blood.

PLATELET COUNT. This test identifies the number of platelets in a peripheral smear and confirms defects in Stage I of coagulation.

LEE WHITE CLOTTING TIME. This test measures the time it takes for a fibrin clot to form in venous blood and identifies defects in Stage IV of coagulation.

Summary

For a complete listing of laboratory tests, the reader is referred to current texts on the subject. This review was intended as a quick guide to those tests commonly utilized in the emergency department and with which you will likely come into contact often during your career in that unit. Normal values will vary depending on the facility conducting the tests; check with the laboratory of your hospital to determine what the values are in your location.

PUTTING IT ALL TOGETHER

The goal of nursing assessment in the emergency department is to assess all pertinent parameters rapidly but thoroughly to establish priority needs and prevent death or decompensation. The process is more a question of emphasis on the patient's chief complaint and his subjective symptoms rather than what specific exclusions are appropriate in each case; therefore the process of assessment will change to meet the needs of each individual patient.

The following outline presents a workable flow upon which you may base your own assessment process. Whatever your approach, try to keep it practical, concise, and organized.

1. Primary survey
   ABCs
   - Is the airway patent? If not, clear the airway by suction or positioning, and maintain patency. Any airway noise indicates an airway obstruction that must be found and removed.
   - Is the patient breathing? Is he exchanging an adequate amount of air based on your observation of chest excursion and skin color? Apply supplemental oxygen to any dyspneic patient.

- Is the patient perfusing? Feel the patient's feet and fingers and palpate the pulse of a major artery (carotid or remoral). Establish cardiac massage if pulses are absent. If the patient is shocky, venous blood samples should be drawn and an IV solution started immediately.
- Is there obvious bleeding? Apply direct pressure if the site is accessible. Consider use of the Medical Anti-Shock Trousers if the bleeding is intraabdominal and therefore inaccessible until the patient can be moved to surgery.

2. General survey
   - Observe general state of health and nourishment.
   - Observe manner of dress and hygiene.
   - Observe for obvious signs of distress as manifested by behavior and facial expression.
   - Observe level of consciousness, awareness, mood, mannerisms, and behavior.
   - Note posture, motor activity, and gait.
   - Note speech for clarity.
   - Note odors such as alcohol, urine, chemicals, ketones, and drugs.

3. Vital signs
   - Count the rate of respirations; evaluate the rhythm, depth, and symmetry of chest expansion.
   - Palpate all peripheral pulses for rate, rhythm, quality and characteristics. Place the patient on a cardiac monitor if there is any indication of a dysrhythmia.
   - Evaluate skin moisture, color, temperature, and turgor.
   - Auscultate the blood pressure. Perform postural vital signs if appropriate.
   - Take oral, rectal, or axillary temperature.

4. Head-to-toe exam (performed relative to the patient's chief complaint and presenting clinical status)
   a. Head
      (1) Inspect
         - Is there any obvious injury present?
         - Perform a pupil check for size, equality, reaction. Perform a visual acuity test if appropriate. Check to see if both eyes move together in all directions; evaluate whether the patient can raise both eyebrows and open his eyes against resistance.
         - Is there any discharge from the natural orifices of the head? Perform the target test on any nasal or ear discharge in the postrauma patient; test the discharge for sugar with a Dextrostix. Perform test for cerebrospinal fluid on drainage from nose or ears in conjunction with Dextrostix evaluation. Allow drainage to drop directly on paper towel. Blood forms a sound ring; clear fluid, which is less viscous, spreads out away from blood.
         - Perform a fundoscopic and otoscopic exam if appropriate.
         - Check the oral mucosa for color, hydration, inflammation, and bleeding.
         - Evaluate the jugular veins for distension.
      (2) Palpate
         - Scalp for lacerations, contusions, and cranial contour
         - Facial bones and front sinuses for pain and tenderness
         - Neck for tenderness and stiffness; glands for enlargement or pain
         - Trachea for tenderness, crepitus, deviation
      (3) Auscultate
         - Carotid arteries for bruits
   b. Chest
      (1) Inspect
         - Chest contour
         - Obvious deformities of the chest wall
         - Obvious injury: contusion, open wounds, abrasions, discolorations
      (2) Palpate
         - Clavicular, sternal, shoulder, rib regions for pain, tenderness, crepitus
         - Point of maximum impulse; identify ventricular heave (accentuated thrust on systole)
         - Tactile fremitus in the chest periphery
      (3) Auscultate
         - Breath sounds for increase, decrease, absence
         - Adventitous sounds
         - Heart sounds for change in timing, intensity, pitch, quality; identify murmurs and/or extra sounds
      (4) Percuss
         - Chest periphery for normal resonance
   c. Abdomen
      (1) Inspect
         - For signs of trauma: discoloration, wounds
         - For distension, asymmetry beyond normal range, increased vascularity
         - For hernias, masses, rashes, scars
         - For pulsations, peristalsis

- For bulging flanks
(2) Auscultate
    - For bowel sounds in all four quadrants for at least 1 minute; are bowel sounds increased, decreased, or absent?
    - For bruit over the abdominal aorta
(3) Palpate
    - Beginning away from the site of any identified pain, palpate lightly for pain, tenderness, rebound, guarding.
    - Establish point of maximum tenderness.
    - If hernia was seen on inspection, palpate the mass. Can a thrust be felt as the patient coughs or strains?
    - Palpate both femoral arteries simultaneously. Are they equal in intensity?
    - Are both pulses present?
    - Press on the symphysis pubis gently, and inward on the ishial wings. Is pain elicited by this action? If so, where is the pain felt? Does it radiate?
    - Place your stethoscope on one knee and auscultate through the diaphragm while tapping firmly on the other knee; can you hear the sound transmitted to your ears? If not, suspect a fractured pelvis.
    If deep palpation is indicated:
    - Is tenderness or pain elicited in any quadrant?
    - Can the aorta be palpated in the epigastrium? Try to feel the lateral borders with two fingers of each hand; does the aortic pulsation push your fingers apart laterally, or anteriorly? Estimate the approximate size of the aorta (normal is 2 cm in the epigastrium).
    - Is the liver firm and smooth, or is it soft and tender? How far below the costal margin does it extend? (Normal is 2 cm below.)
    - Can the spleen be felt? Unless it is enlarged more than three times its normal size, it usually cannot be felt.
(4) Percuss
    - If the flanks were observed to be bulging on inspection, test for fluid motion by placing one hand on one flank and striking the other flank with your other hand with a tapping motion while another person places the ulnar surface of his hand at midline. If the bulging is caused by fluid and not fat, you will see and feel the fluid wave transmitted across the belly.

- Percuss side to side and top to bottom in all quadrants. Note any shifting dullness, location of tympany, and normal dullness over the liver.
d. Extremities
    (1) Inspect
        - Compare for symmetry, edema, discoloration, masses, deformities, and open wounds.
        - Are there needle marks present?
        - Are clubbing or nicotine stains evident on the fingers?
        - Do the veins of the hand remain elevated when the extremity is elevated above the heart?
        - Are ulcers or rashes present?
        - Can the patient move his fingers and toes without effort?
    (2) Palpate
        - Compare pulses and skin temperature in all extremities. Mark the location of the pulse in an injured extremity.
        - Evaluate lower extremities for clonus (support knee in partially flexed position, dorsiflex foot, and observe for rhythmic oscillations).
        - If edema is present, press thumb firmly against the edematous area for 5 seconds; evaluate for pitting.
        - Compare calves for tenderness, increased firmness, tension.
        - Gently palpate any enlarged, tender, or cordlike veins for size and quality.
        - Evaluate distal sensation on all extremities. Ask the patient if he can tell you where he is being touched. Evaluate his subjective ability to discern sharp from dull.
        - Ask the patient to squeeze your fingers; evaluate for equal strength.
    (3) Percuss
        - Deep tendon reflexes: biceps, triceps, patellar, Achilles, plantar.
e. Back
    (1) Inspect
        - Is there any deformity or abnormal curvature?
        - Are there obvious signs of injury?
        - Are there masses, rashes, or evidence of sacral edema?
    (2) Palpation
        - Is there tenderness or pain along the bony processes or paravertebrally?
    (3) Percussion
        - Strike the costrovertebral angles with

the ulnar aspect of your closed hand. Is tenderness or pain elicited?

SUMMARY

This chapter has discussed the essential elements of nursing assessment within the emergency department: purpose, barriers, tools, and components of the physical examination. In many departments there are more professional nurses in contact with the patients than there are physicians, and priority setting through knowledgeable assessment and appropriate intervention contributes significantly to decreasing mortality and morbidity. This is particularly so for the early moments of the patient's visit, but it is also valid for the entirety of the patient's stay in the department.

Because of traditional philosophies on the nursing role and responsibilities, many emergency nurses have never received proper training and supervision in systematic assessment. Thus, it is frequently by empirical judgment that intervention is provided; judgments that often are associated with high error rates. On the other hand, interventions that are implemented based on a scientific knowledge base and a rational therapeutic framework predispose patients for a much more favorable outcome.

Nursing assessment may either be very brief and confined to a narrow parameter, or it can be a reasonably rapid and efficient evaluation of all systems that may be affected by the current illness or injury. The extent of the evaluation is uniquely the decision of the nurse and is based on the patient's condition at the time, his chief complaint, and environmental factors. For those nurses who have been practicing logical and complete assessments, we believe that the information presented here will reinforce current practice. For those nurses who have never been trained to initiate assessment, we hope to have stimulated the desire to obtain appropriate education and direction. For those nurses who have been performing assessments but have fallen prey to undesirable behavior, whether because of existing barriers or other factors, we hope to have stimulated a change in attitude toward this most essential of nursing responsibilities within the emergency department.

BIBLIOGRAPHY

Abels, L. F.: Mosby's manual of critical care, St. Louis, 1979, The C. V. Mosby Co., Chapter 2.

Alexander, M., and Trown, M.: Physical examination, part I, Nurs. '73 **3:**7, July 1973.

Anderson, D., and Cosgriff, J.: The practice of emergency nursing, Philadelphia, 1975, J. B. Lippincott Co.

Assessing vital functions accurately, Nurs. '77 Skillbook Series, 1977, Intermed Communications, Inc.

Balinger, V., Rutherford, R., and Zuidema, G.: Injuries of head and spinal cord. In The management of trauma, ed. 2, Philadelphia, 1973, W. B. Saunders Co.

Bates, B.: A guide to physical examination, Philadelphia, 1974, J. B. Lippincott Co.

Beaumont, E.: Product survey: stethoscope, Nurs. '78 **8:**33-37, November 1978.

Block, D.: Some critical terms in nursing: what do they mean? Nurs. Outlook **22:**689-694, November 1974.

Bookman, L., and Simoneau, J.: The early assessment of hypovolemia: postural vital signs, J.E.N. **3:**43-45, September/October, 1977.

Cosgriff, J., and Anderson, D.: The practice of emergency nursing, Philadelphia, 1975, J. B. Lippincott, Co.

Friedman, H.: Problem-oriented medical diagnosis, Boston, 1975, Little, Brown and Co.

Groër, M. E., and Shekelton, M. E.: Basic pathophysiology: a conceptual approach, St. Louis, 1979, The C. V. Mosby Co.

Jarvis, C.: Vital signs: how to take them accurately and understand them fully, Nurs. '76 **6:**31-38, April 1976.

Jarvis, C.: Perfecting physical assessment, part I, Nurs. '77 **7:**28-38, May 1977.

Jarvis, C.: Perfecting physical assessment, part 2, Nurs. '77 **7:**38-46, June 1977.

Karch, A.: Nursing assessment, Crit. Care Update **3:**5-15, December 1976.

Lanros, N.: Assessment and intervention in emergency nursing, Bowie, Md., 1978, Robert J. Brady Co., Section I.

Lehman, J.: Auscultation of heart sounds, Am. J. Nurs. **72:**1242-1245, July 1972.

McConnell, E.: The nursing process, Crit. Care Update **5:**14-22, May 1978.

Secord, B.: Emergency care update: emergency assessment—the physical examination, part 2, Crit. Care Update **6:**29-31, January 1979.

Sitzman, J.: Nursing assessment of the acutely ill respiratory patient, Crit. Care Update **4:**20-31, September 1977.

Sherman, J.: Guide to patient evaluation, New York, 1976, Medical Examiner Publishing Co.

Sweetwood, H.: Bedside assessment of respirations, Nurs. '73 **3:**50-51, September 1973.

Tilkian, S. M., Conover, M. H., Tilkian, A. G.: Clinical implications of laboratory tests, ed. 2, St. Louis, 1979, The C. V. Mosby Co., Chapters 1 to 3.

Walraven, G., and others: Manual of edvanced prehospital care, Bowie, Md., 1978, Robert J. Brady Co.

Warner, C.: Emergency care: assessment and intervention, ed. 2, St. Louis, 1978, The C. V. Mosby Co.

CHAPTER 8

Basic and advanced life support

Myocardial infarction is the cause of death in over 650,000 people in the United States each year. Of these, over 350,000 people die in the first two hours of the infarct, usually before hospitalization. In an attempt to alter these statistics, many counties in the United States have developed sophisticated prehospital care systems, where early medical care is brought to the patient at the scene of the incident. Most prehospital care personnel are trained to administer basic life support if indicated and many have been trained to provide advanced life support as well.

Standards for cardiopulmonary resuscitation were drawn from the conference on cardiopulmonary resuscitation and emergency cardiac care sponsored by the American Heart Association and the National Research Council in 1973. The classic article, "Standards of Cardiopulmonary Resuscitation and Emergency Cardiac Care," published in the *Journal of the American Medical Association* was a result of this conference.

Basic life support courses are offered both by the American Red Cross and the American Heart Association to all interested persons. The American Heart Association also offers courses in advanced cardiac life support to medical personnel. For more information regarding these courses, the reader is referred to both of these agencies.

BASIC LIFE SUPPORT

Basic life support is one component of advanced life support. In basic life support, the rescuer is taught to recognize unconsciousness, establish a patent airway, assure adequate breathing, and provide circulation if it is not present. These maneuvers are known as the ABCs: airway, breathing, and circulation, or cardiopulmonary resuscitation (CPR).

Airway

The basic airway maneuver in an unconscious patient is the head tilt maneuver (Fig. 8-1). If there is a suspected cervical spine injury, the jaw thrust maneuver is used, where the head is left in a neutral position and the jaw is thrust forward with the thumbs and fingers (Fig. 8-2). Both maneuvers serve to pull the tongue away from the posterior pharynx. The tongue is the greatest cause of an obstructed airway in the unconscious patient. When either of these maneuvers is performed, the maneuver may be just enough to open the

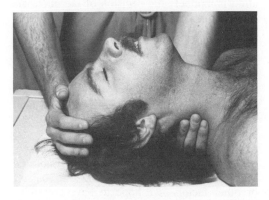

Fig. 8-1. The head tilt maneuver. (Photo by Richard Lazar.)

airway and allow for spontaneous respirations to begin without further assistance. One must remember, however, that it is essential to maintain an open airway until the patient is either intubated esophageally or endotracheally or the patient can maintain his own open airway. The only exception to this rule is when the rescuer is performing one-person CPR and it becomes necessary for him to leave the airway in order to perform chest compression.

Breathing

Once an airway has been established, one must check to see if breathing is present. If spontaneous breathing is present, simply continue to maintain an open airway. If spontaneous breathing is *not* present, one must breathe for the patient. The simplest and most common method is to provide mouth-to-mouth breathing, where the victim's nose is pinched shut, and the rescuer places his mouth over the victim's mouth and breathes into the victim's mouth (Fig. 8-3). Breathing is initiated by giving four quick breaths, in stair-step fashion, without allowing for exhalation. This method allows for a "loading dose" of oxygen to be administered before proceeding to the next step in CPR. When breathing into the victim's mouth, the rescuer should see the victim's chest rise (Fig. 8-4). If it does not rise, reposition the airway and try again.

Mouth-to-nose breathing is employed when there is some reason that mouth-to-mouth breathing cannot be used, such as in severe trauma to the mouth. When mouth-to-nose breathing is employed, the rescuer holds the victim's mouth shut with one hand, covers the victim's nose with the rescuer's mouth, and breathes into the victim's nose.

In mouth-to-mouth breathing, the rescuer must remember to remove his mouth from around the victim's mouth to allow for passive

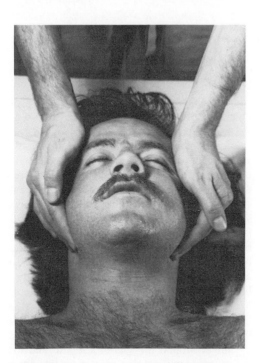

Fig. 8-2. The jaw thrust maneuver. (Photo by Richard Lazar.)

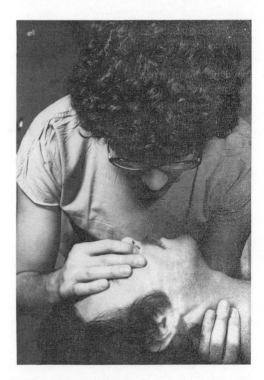

Fig. 8-3. Mouth-to-mouth breathing. The victim's nose is pinched shut and the rescuer places his mouth over the victim's mouth. (Photo by Richard Lazar.)

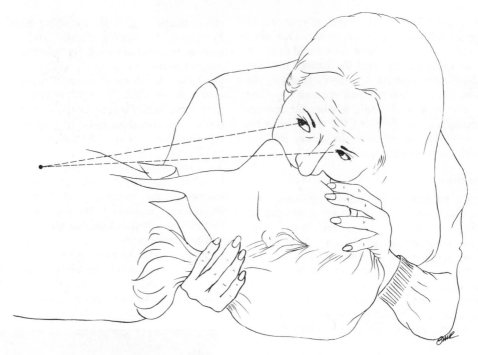

Fig. 8-4. Mouth-to-mouth breathing. Blow into the victim's mouth, observing the chest rise. (From Barber, J. M., and Budassi, S. A.: Mosby's manual of emergency care, St. Louis, 1979, The C. V. Mosby Co.)

exhalation. When performing mouth-to-nose breathing the rescuer must remember to open the mouth after each breath into the nose to allow for passive exhalation. The process of breathing for the victim should take place every 5 seconds until spontaneous respirations are resumed or until resuscitation efforts have ceased.

If the victim has a laryngectomy or a tracheostomy, the rescuer should perform mouth-to-stoma breathing, by sealing off the nose and mouth and breathing directly into the stoma.

When performing mouth-to-mouth breathing on an infant, the rescuer should cover the infant's mouth *and* nose with his mouth (Fig. 8-5). Other than that modification, breathing is performed essentially the same way, allowing for smaller breaths in accordance with the size of the child, at 3-second intervals. It is important to remember not to hyperextend the

neck of an infant. Infants' necks are very pliable, and hyperextension may actually block the airway posteriorly (Fig. 8-6).

Airway obstruction. Should attempts to ventilate the victim meet with resistance, one must perform a series of maneuvers to attempt to open the airway. The first maneuver is to reposition the airway. Sometimes, in the intensity of the rescue effort, good airway position is lost. Once the head and neck are repositioned, once again, attempt to give four quick breaths. If repositioning the head and neck was unsuccessful the presence of a foreign body is likely. Turn the victim to one side and attempt to manually clear the airway by using the cross-finger technique to open the mouth, and follow that by sweeping the index finger and the middle finger around the victim's mouth and into the posterior pharyngeal area in an attempt to locate the obstruction.

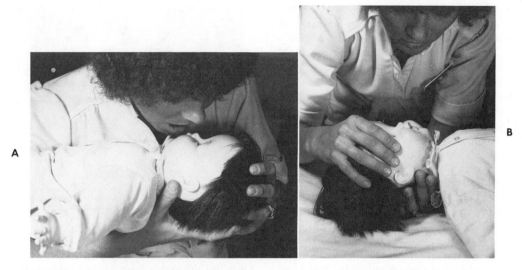

Fig. 8-5. Infant mouth-to-mouth breathing. **A,** The rescuer should cover the infant's mouth and nose with her mouth. **B,** It is important to remember not to hyperextend the neck of the infant. (Photo by Richard Lazar.)

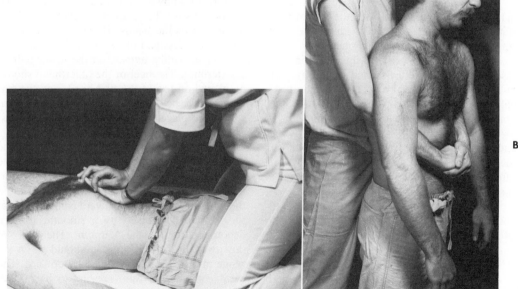

Fig. 8-6. A, Heimlich maneuver, lying. **B,** Heimlich maneuver, standing. (Photo by Richard Lazar.)

If this method is unsuccessful, one should then attempt to roll the victim on his side and administer four sharp blows to the victim's back, between the scapulas, with the heel of one's hand. Return the victim to the prone position and repeat the sweep of the victim's mouth to remove any foreign body that may have been dislodged by the back blows. Again, repeat attempts to breath mouth-to-mouth.

If this method, too, proves to be unsuccessful, one should attempt to dislodge the foreign body by employing the abdominal thrust maneuver (also known as the Heimlich maneuver). If the victim is in a prone position, straddle the victim and face his head. The rescuer should place the heel of one hand on the victim's abdomen at the point halfway between the xiphoid process and the umbilicus. The rescuer's other hand should be placed on top of the first hand (Fig. 8-6, *A*). The maneuver is then carried out by administering a quick inward and upward thrust of the hands in an attempt to increase intrathoracic pressure and dislodge the foreign body. This maneuver may be repeated three additional times. If the airway continues to remain blocked, one should repeat the entire procedure for the blocked airway.

The abdominal thrust (Heimlich) maneuver may also be administered with the victim in a standing or sitting position, with the rescuer standing behind the victim and placing his arms around the victim's waist. In this position, the rescuer should make a fist, and the fleshy part of the fist should be placed on the abdomen, halfway between the xiphoid process and the umbilicus. The other hand is placed on top of the first hand (Fig. 8-6, *B*). A quick inward and upward thrust is carried out. This maneuver may be repeated three more times before returning to the original methods of removing a foreign body.

The entire sequence should be repeated until an open airway is obtained or until advanced life support procedures are available.

Circulation

Attempts to assess circulatory status should be performed *only after adequate breathing has been established,* for circulation of unoxygen-

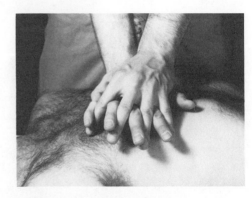

Fig. 8-7. Hand position for chest compression: no weight on fingers. (Photo by Richard Lazar.)

ated blood is essentially a useless procedure. Once the airway has been established and artificial breathing is initiated, the circulation should be checked by the carotid or femoral pulse. If a pulse is not evident, one must begin chest compression to provide artificial circulation. If a pulse is evident, one should be sure to continue to maintain an open airway and adequate breathing status.

When performing external cardiac compression (also known as cardiac massage), one should always be extremely cautious about placement of the hands. Be sure to locate the xiphoid process and place the heel of one hand two finger widths higher, on the lower half of the sternum. The heel of the other hand should be placed on top of the first hand, and the fingers should be ''locked'' together (no weight should be placed on the chest by the fingers) (Fig. 8-7).

The rescuer should be kneeling with the knees slightly separated and up as close to the victim as possible with the elbows in a straight, locked position (Fig. 8-8). The rescuer should then begin a smooth, downward compression of the sternum, followed by a smooth, upward decompression of the sternum. The ratio of downward to upward motion should be in the range of 50% downward and 50% upward. The ideal compression ratio appears to be 60:40. It is important to remember *not* to administer sharp, quick compressions, as this will only

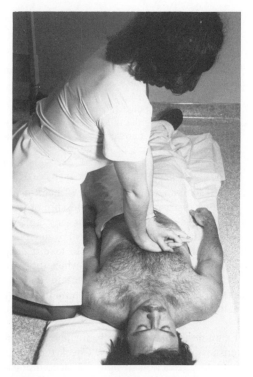

Fig. 8-8. Body position for CPR. The rescuer should be kneeling with the knees slightly separated, and the elbows in a straight locked position. (Photo by Richard Lazar.)

serve to contuse the myocardium and will not provide a cardiac output adequate to maintain life.

The depth of compression on an adult is approximately 1½ to 2 inches, although compression depth may vary from individual to individual. Chest compression performed in the proper fashion may provide one fourth to one third the normal cardiac output and may generate a systolic blood pressure of 100 mm Hg, which is compatible with life.

Chest compression should be repeated 80 times per minute when one-person rescue is taking place (to allow for compressions lost while the rescuer is ventilating the victim). The person performing one-person rescue should provide 15 chest compressions followed by two quick breaths, and then repeat the entire cycle over and over until additional help arrives or

until the rescuer is too exhausted to continue.

In a two-rescuer effort, chest compression should occur 60 times per minute, with a breath being interjected on every fifth upstroke.

There are two items that are absolutely essential to remember when performing CPR: (1) Be sure that the victim is on a firm surface when providing chest compression, *and* (2) artificial circulation should *always* be accompanied by artificial breathing.

When one is resuscitating infants and children, the 5:1 ratio of chest compression to breathing should be maintained. When compressing the chest, use either the index and middle finger on an infant and the heel of one hand on a larger child. Compression is applied over the center of the sternum at a depth of ½ to 1½ inches, depending on the size of a child. Compression rate should be 80 to 100 compressions/minute.

It is important to remember that *most* arrests in children are respiratory (airway-related) and that the child will continue to have pulses for a while. It is absolutely essential to maintain an open airway and adequate breathing throughout the resuscitation effort.

PHASES OF CARDIOPULMONARY ARREST
Prearrest phase of myocardial infarction

The most common prodrome to cardiac arrest is myocardial infarction. As was previously stated, over 650,000 people die in the United States each year as a consequence of coronary artery disease, many of these from myocardial infarction. Fifty to sixty percent of deaths due to myocardial infarction occur outside of the hospital. Many of these occur without much warning. Some, however, have the classic warning signs of crushing substernal chest pain, radiation of the pain down the left arm and up into the left jaw, nausea and vomiting, diaphoresis, or a variety of other atypical presentations.

Public education on the importance of contacting the prehospital care team at the onset of these signs and symptoms is essential in order to reduce the risk of death from myocardial infarction. Upon the arrival of the pre-hospital care team, intervention, both prophylactic and palliative, must begin in the early critical moments of the infarction.

When one deals with a victim of a possible myocardial infarction, it is essential to treat the victim as though he were actually having an infarction, even before it has been proved that it has actually occurred. One of the most important therapeutic interventions is to communicate with the patient and act in a calm, reassured manner. Anxiety does much to aggravate an already unstable condition. Let the victim know what you are doing, why you are doing it, and how you are going to carry out a procedure. At the same time, remember to provide information to the family about what is occurring.

If a person is suspected of having a myocardial infarction, one should administer oxygen by nasal cannula at 6 liters/minute. Have the victim sit up and attempt to find a position of comfort (usually a semi-Fowler position). Obtain a baseline blood pressure reading as well as pulse, respiratory rate, and temperature. Auscultate the lungs.

Any patient complaining of chest pain should be monitored for dysrhythmias and treated according to the appropriate protocol. When monitoring, if possible, monitor on lead II or lead MCL_1 (Fig. 8-9). One should avoid monitoring on lead I, as it often does not pick up atrial dysrhythmias.

Consider the fact that this patient may require pharmacological intervention rapidly. In order to provide for an immediate entry into the circulatory system, start an intravenous lifeline (IV). The solution of choice is usually dextrose 5% and water (D/5/W). The IV should be initiated, whenever possible, in a peripheral puncture site. When selecting the appropriate cannula to use, consider using a cannula with a gauge that provides for rapid injection of medications (at least an 18-gauge needle or cannula whenever possible).

Using the *PQRST* mnemonic, one should be able to obtain a brief but pertinent history:

P = provokes
   What provokes the pain? What makes it better? What makes it worse?

Q = quality
   What does it feel like? Is it burning? Crushing? Tearing?
R = radiates
   Where does it radiate to? Does it go into your arms? Your jaw? Your back?
S = severity
   How severe is the pain? If you gave pain a number, with one being the mildest and ten being the most severe, what number would you give this pain?
T = time
   When did the pain start? How long did it last?

Ask if the patient has a history of heart problems, lung disease, high blood pressure or liver disease. Also ask if he is taking any kind of medications, such as heart pills or water pills. Also ask the patient if it hurts to take a deep breath and what he was doing when the pain started. The clinician can ascertain the answers to these questions while initiating oxygen therapy and monitoring and initiating the IV.

Examine the patient briefly for level of consciousness and mental status. Check the pupils for equality, reaction to light and accommodation, keeping in mind that 10% of people have unequal pupils. Examine the neck veins for distention, and check the trachea with your fingers for midline position. Note skin vital signs (temperature, turgor, and moisture).

One of the major problems in myocardial infarction is pain, which causes anxiety, increased heart rate, and increased oxygen consumption. One of the keys in treatment of myocardial infarction is early pain relief.

One method of attempting to relieve pain is the administration of *nitroglycerin*. Nitroglycerin is a therapeutic measure to institute in both angina and myocardial infarction. It dilates the peripheral venous circulation, which causes a decreased venous return to the heart, a decreased cardiac output, a decreased myocardial workload, and decreased myocardial oxygen demand. An added benefit of nitroglycerin administration is that it dilates coronary arteries. Nitroglycerin may cause a drop in blood pressure. If the hypotension is significant, elevate the victim's legs to increase venous return. If this does not improve the hypotensive state, one must consider a fluid challenge or application

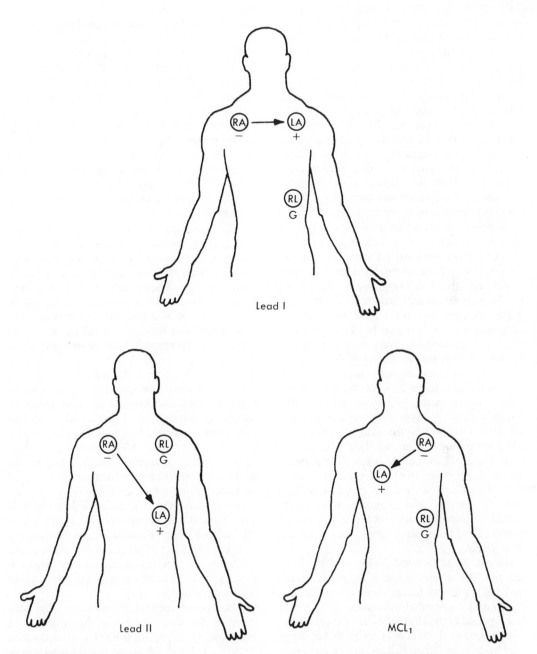

Fig. 8-9. Monitoring on three-lead ECG monitor. Leads II and MCL_1 are best leads to monitor for dysrhythmias. (From Barber, J. M., and Budassi, S. A.: Mosby's manual of emergency care, St. Louis, 1979, The C. V. Mosby Co.)

of the antishock trousers, or both. Nitroglycerin should not be administered to a patient whose systolic blood pressure is less than 100 mm Hg.

If the first attempt to relieve chest pain with nitroglycerin is unsuccessful, one may repeat the nitroglycerin dose, provided that the systolic blood pressure remains above 100 mm Hg. If the victim tells you that he has taken several of his own nitroglycerin tablets without obtaining relief, it may be that the victim's medication has become impotent. It would be wise to attempt an additional try with a nitroglycerin tablet taken from the medical team's supply.

If attempts to relieve pain with nitroglycerin have been unsuccessful, the next drug of choice is morphine sulfate, which decreases the pain of acute myocardial infarction, decreases preload, decreases myocardial oxygen demands, and relives anxiety. If the blood pressure is normal or elevated, give 3 to 10 mg slow IV push (over 2 or more minutes) until pain relief is obtained. If this amount does not relieve the pain, an additional *slow* IV push may be given, provided that the total amount given does not exceed 15 mg. If the patient becomes hypotensive following morphine administration, the same steps should be taken as when the patient becomes hypotensive following nitroglycerin administration. If respiratory distress occurs, naloxone (Narcan) is the drug of choice. It is a narcotic antagonist and should be administered in a 0.4 to 0.8 mg bolus. One can anticipate a response from naloxone in 4 minutes. It is, therefore, mandatory that one support the airway and maintain respirations should respiratory distress occur as a result of morphine administration until the naloxone takes effect.

Nitrous oxide (a combination of 50% oxygen and 50% nitrous oxide) is experiencing increasing popularity for its usefulness in relieving pain in myocardial infarction. Its use was first reported in the United States medical literature by Lown of Boston in 1976. It has been used widely in Great Britain and is currently under investigation at University of California at Los Angeles by Stern and McElroy.

When nitrous oxide (Entonox) is administered, it should be given as a 50% oxygen,

50% nitrous oxide mixture at a flow rate of 4 liters/minute by self-administered mask. As the nitrous oxide mixture takes effect, the mask will fall away from the patient and there will be no danger of overadministration of the gas. Nitrous oxide has been shown to effectively relieve pain without causing hemodynamic deterioration or dysrhythmias.

Management of dysrhythmias in the pre-arrest phase. The most common dysrhythmia seen in the patient experiencing myocardial infarction is premature ventricular contractions (PVCs, VPBs, PVBs). This dysrhythmia is observed in approximately 85% of myocardial infarction victims. Classically, premature ventricular contractions have been treated with lidocaine (Xylocaine). Currently, many articles recommend lidocaine as a prophylactic measure in those victims experiencing possible myocardial infarction, with or without ectopy. Whether one chooses to administer lidocaine to treat ectopy or as a prophylactic measure, the goal of lidocaine therapy is to reduce or prevent ectopy by decreasing ventricular irritability. This may be accomplished by maintaining adequate blood levels of lidocaine. If lidocaine is selected, it should be given in repeated bolus form, in bolus and drip form, or by rapid injection technique. If the repeated bolus method is selected, it should be given as 1 to 2 mg/kg bolus IV slowly over 1 to 2 minutes). If lidocaine is given too rapidly, seizures may result. In the average 70-kg man, administer 75 mg of lidocaine. Follow the initial bolus by an additional bolus of 50 mg lidocaine after 5 minutes. This bolus should be followed by additional 50 mg boluses every 10 minutes, up to, but not to exceed 325 mg. This method is particularly useful in the prehospital care setting where it is difficult to maintain a constant drip rate in a moving vehicle.

The second method of administering lidocaine is by administering an initial bolus of lidocaine, 1 to 2 mg/kg followed by a lidocaine "drip" of 2 gm lidocaine in 500 ml D/5/W running at a drip rate of 1 to 4 mg/minute to maintain a constant effective blood level of lidocaine.

The third method of administering lidocaine

if an IV route is unobtainable is by rapid injection technique. With this method, lidocaine is injected into the deltoid muscle in a 300-mg bolus by a specially designed rapid injector known as a LidoPen.

Studies have indicated that a significant number of patients experiencing myocardial infarction develop ventricular fibrillation without the warning dysrhythmias preceding. The exception to the administration of prophylactic lidocaine is in those victims who are demonstrating third degree infranodal block.

If the patient gives a history of liver disease and requires lidocaine therapy, the dose of lidocaine should be reduced to half, or an alternate antiarrhythmic drug should be considered.

It is important to remember that, if a bolus of lidocaine is given, it should be followed by additional boluses or a lidocaine drip to maintain a therapeutic blood level. If a bolus is given without additional boluses or a drip, the therapeutic blood level of lidocaine (2 to 5 mg/ml) will diminish in 5 to 15 minutes. If, on the other hand, a lidocaine drip is initiated without the benefit of a loading dose, one will not reach a therapeutic blood level in the first half hour of treatment.

If lidocaine is unsuccessful or the victim is allergic to lidocaine, one should consider an alternate antiarrhythmic drug, such as procainamide (Pronestyl). It should be given in a dosage range of 250 mg to 1 gm IV bolus and should not exceed 50 mg/minute.

Besides premature ventricular contractions, the next most common dysrhythmia to be seen in the victim experiencing myocardial infarction is bradycardia (a rate of less than 60 beats/minute). This dysrhythmia is seen in 65% of patients with an acute myocardial infarction, particularly those sustaining inferior wall infarctions. Therapeutic intervention includes administration of the parasympatholytic drug, atropine sulfate, in bolus form at a dosage of 0.5 to 1 mg by IV push if the heart rate is less than 60 beats/minute and there are associated PVCs that are probably rate-related. Atropine is also given if the heart rate is below 45, even if there are no PVCs present. It is also given if there is a heart rate of less than 60 beats/minute and there is associated hypotension. It is important to remember that atropine should not be given in less than 0.3 mg IV, as this may cause a paradoxical decrease in the heart rate. One should also be alert to the fact that greater than 0.6 mg given by IV push may cause tachycardia.

Arrest phase of myocardial infarction

Victims of many types of illnesses and injuries may suffer cardiopulmonary arrest. The primary dysrhythmias leading to cardiopulmonary arrest are ventricular tachycardia, ventricular fibrillation, and asystole. With the onset of any of these dysrhythmias, basic life support is an essential part of the therapeutic intervention. Although basic life support is essential, it may not be enough, and one may be required to use the skills, maneuvers, and medications employed in advanced cardiac life support, such as adjuncts for airway maintenance, circulatory assist devices, cardiac monitoring, dysrhythmia recognition and treatment, drug therapy, defibrillation and cardioversion, and special transportation maneuvers before moving the victim to a facility where further therapy will be provided. Besides advanced cardiac life support implementation, one must also be on the alert for signs and symptoms that will offer clues to the cause of the cardiopulmonary arrest. Some examples of this are distended neck veins, diminished breath sounds, and a deviated trachea, indicating that perhaps there is a pneumothorax present. A cardiopulmonary arrest is also possible following an automobile/pedestrian accident where there are indications that there has been an excessive amount of blood loss. In these instances, the cause of the arrest must also be treated (for example, placement of a needle into the anterior chest wall to relieve the tension pneumothorax or application of the antishock trousers and rapid volume replacement to correct hypovolemia).

Primary drugs in cardiopulmonary arrest are sodium bicarbonate and epinephrine (Adrenalin). Sodium bicarbonate is given to correct the acidotic state caused by apnea, in which carbon dioxide retention occurs and the body experiences respiratory acidosis and anerobic metabolism, which causes the body to produce lactic acid and go into a state of metabolic acidosis.

An acidotic state causes a decreased fibrillation threshold, excitability of ectopic foci, decreased myocardial contractility, and decreased effectiveness of both intrinsic catecholamines and those administered parenterally. Sodium bicarbonate, a base, is given to combat both the respiratory and metabolic acidosis. The initial dose should be 1 mEq/kg of body weight followed by half the initial dose every 10 minutes thereafter until ventilations are stabilized. If it is possible to measure blood gas levels rapidly, one should administer sodium bicarbonate in accordance with the protocol for a given pH. The ideal pH in a cardiopulmonary arrest situation is 7.30 to 7.35. One of the greatest problems in the cardiopulmonary arrest resuscitation effort is the tendency to administer too much sodium bicarbonate and to place the victim in a state of iatrogenic metabolic alkalosis. One of the many complications of an alkalotic state is that catecholamines are rendered ineffective. Alkalosis also impairs oxygen release to the tissues. The administration of sodium bicarbonate may also cause a severe sodium overload, as one ampule (44.8 mEq) contains the same amount of sodium chloride as 300 ml of normal saline solution.

Another classic drug that is commonly used in the cardiopulmonary arrest scenario is epinephrine, which is an endogenous catecholamine containing both alpha and beta adrenergic properties. Its primary use in cardiac arrest is to increase the force of the myocardial contraction (inotropism) increase the heart rate (chronotropism), increase blood pressure by increasing peripheral vascular resistance, increase the automaticity and spontaneity of ventricular contractions, and increase perfusion pressure generated form chest compression.

Although epinephrine is an excellent drug to employ in the cardiopulmonary arrest situation, it also offers many risks, such as the development of deteriorating tachydysrhythmias, PVCs caused by increased automaticity, and increased myocardial oxygen consumption, which may lead to myocardial ischemia and necrosis, caused by an increased cardiac workload.

The recommended dosage of epinephrine in the cardiopulmonary arrest situation is 0.5 to 1.0 mg IV, followed by an additional 0.5 mg every 5 minutes as required. If the IV route for administration is not available, epinephrine may also be given by the intracardiac route or the endotracheal route.

AIRWAY MANAGEMENT

Besides the head tilt and jaw thrust maneuvers used in basic cardiac life support, there are several airway adjuncts which may be used in advanced cardiac life support.

Oropharyngeal airway

The simplest airway adjunct is the oropharyngeal airway (Fig. 8-10). It is a curved tube that is made of either plastic, rubber, or metal. It is placed by inserting it into the mouth upside down and rotating it 180° until the curve fits comfortably over the tongue with the open-

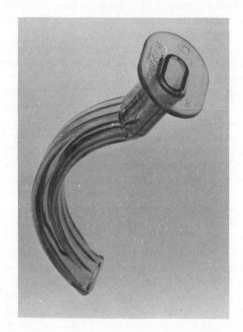

Fig. 8-10. Oropharyngeal airway. (Photo by Richard Lazar.)

ing extending into the posterior pharyngeal area. It prevents the tongue from slipping back into the posterior pharyngeal area. It may also be inserted by moving the tongue to one side with a tongue blade or other such piece of equipment and placing the airway with the opening extending into the posterior pharyngeal region (Fig. 8-11). It is essential that this piece of equipment be placed properly, as improper placement may actually block the airway. This

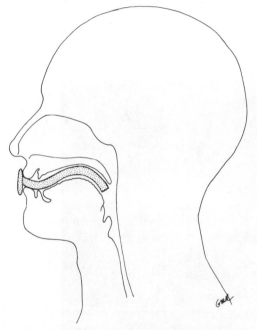

Fig. 8-11. Oropharyngeal airway in place. (From Barber, J. M., and Budassi, S. A.: Mosby's manual of emergency care, St. Louis, 1979, The C. V. Mosby Co.)

airway cannot be used in the conscious victim, as it may induce vomiting. Rather, it should be used in those patients who are unconscious but who continue to have adequate respiratory effort. Once the airway is in place, one must continue to maintain the head tilt or jaw thrust position to maintain a patent airway.

Nasopharyngeal airway

A nasopharyngeal airway (trumpet tube) may be used in the alert, conscious victim when there is a need for some sort of assistance in maintaining the airway (Fig. 8-12). It is a soft rubber tube that is inserted through a nostril after being lubricated with an anesthetic lubricant. It extends to the posterior pharyngeal area behind the tongue (Fig. 8-13). One must again remember to maintain an open airway by using either the head tilt or jaw thrust maneuver in conjunction with this airway.

Esophageal obturator airway

When a victim is apneic and unconscious, a means of providing positive pressure ventilation is necessary. One method of providing this is via the esophageal obturator airway (EOA) (Fig. 8-14). This airway is a piece of equipment that can be inserted by personnel untrained in inserting an endotracheal tube. It requires very little technical skill to place this airway, and training takes just a few minutes. The airway is composed of a *mask,* which is used to seal off the nose and the mouth, the *tube* with a blocked distal end and perforations in the area of the posterior pharynx, and a *balloon* that, when inflated, allows for little or no air passage into the stomach and prevents aspiration of vomitus. Sealing off the nose and the

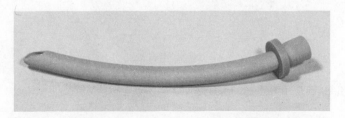

Fig. 8-12. Nasopharyngeal airway. (Photo by Richard Lazar.)

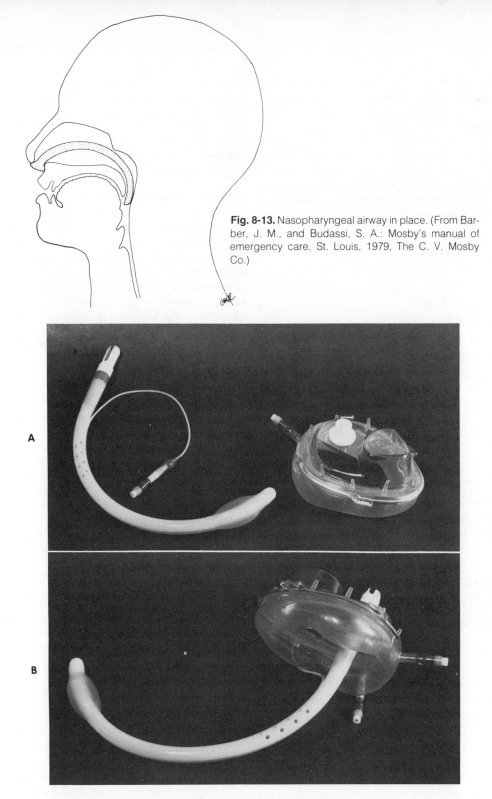

Fig. 8-13. Nasopharyngeal airway in place. (From Barber, J. M., and Budassi, S. A.: Mosby's manual of emergency care, St. Louis, 1979, The C. V. Mosby Co.)

A

B

Fig. 8-14. A, Esophageal obturator airway and mask separated. **B,** Esophageal obturator airway and mask, connected. (Photo by Richard Lazar.)

Fig. 8-15. Esophageal obturator airway in place. (From Barber, J. M., and Budassi, S. A.: Mosby's manual of emergency care, St. Louis, 1979, The C. V. Mosby Co.)

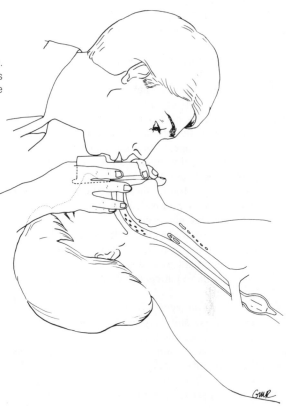

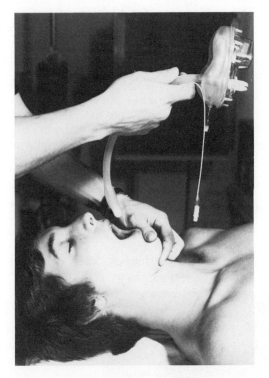

Fig. 8-16. To insert the EOA, grasp the lower jaw with one hand and lift it forward. (Photo by Richard Lazar.)

mouth, blowing air into the tube with a blocked distal end, and inflating the balloon ensure that the only other pathway for the air to follow is out of the perforation holes, into the posterior pharyngeal area, and into the trachea. (Fig. 8-15).

To insert the EOA, grasp the lower jaw with one hand and lift it forward (Fig. 8-16). Advance the lubricated tube into the posterior pharyngeal area with the tip pointing upward. Gently rotate the tube 180° and advance it carefully behind the tongue, into the posterior pharyngeal area, and down into the esophagus. When the mask reaches the face, press the mask firmly against the face to obtain a tight seal. Then, blow into the end of the tube. If the tube is in the proper position, the chest should rise. If the chest does not rise, the tube should be removed immediately, as it may have accidently passed into the trachea.

If, after blowing into the tube, you see the chest rise, auscultate the chest bilaterally on subsequent ventilatory efforts to assure that both lungs are being ventilated adequately. Once adequate ventilation is established, inflate the balloon with 35 cc air using a syringe and pushing it through a one-way valve. Continue to ventilate the patient until other means of ventilation are prepared, until the victim resumes spontaneous respirations, or until resuscitation efforts are ceased.

If the patient is unable to maintain his own respiratory efforts and a method of long-term ventilation is necessary, the patient should be endotracheally intubated, followed by removal of the esophageal obturator airway.

If the victim begins to have spontaneous respirations, the EOA must be removed. It is necessary to follow these instructions carefully for the EOA removal: Turn the victim on his side (this is not necessary if an endotracheal tube has been placed). Deflate the balloon and withdraw the airway. Be sure to have suctioning equipment available, as it is not uncommon for these patients to vomit following EOA removal.

The advantages of the EOA are that it is easy to use and easy to train someone to use. It may be used in those victims who have suspected cervical spine fractures and who are having difficulty managing their own airway, because the EOA may be placed with the head in a neutral position. Endotracheal tube placement is generally easier to accomplish with the EOA in place. The EOA also prevents aspiration of stomach contents and prevents air from entering the stomach. It allows for greater amounts of air to be distributed as compared with the bag-valve-mask system, and air intake is found to be equal to that found in endotracheal intubation.

The EOA *cannot* be used in the conscious or semi-conscious victim. It also, in its present size, cannot be used in infants and children (although there are pediatric sizes currently being developed). It is contraindicated in those victims with a history of caustic poison ingestion, esophageal disease, or current history of foreign body in the trachea.

The EOA may be accidently passed into the trachea, which is easily correctable if proper attention is paid to the placement procedure. There have been a few reported cases of perforation of the esophagus, but this occurrence is relatively rare.

Endotracheal intubation

In *endotracheal intubation,* a tube is passed directly into the trachea. An endotracheal tube is a tube that is open at both ends. It has a standard 15 mm adapter that can be used with a bag-valve-mask device or other type of resuscitation/ventilation equipment. It also has a balloon (cuff) located at the distal end of the tube (Fig. 8-17). Endotracheal intubation generally requires a great deal of technical skill, particularly in the prehospital care setting where conditions such as lighting and patient position are not always ideal.

To intubate the trachea, insert a laryngo-

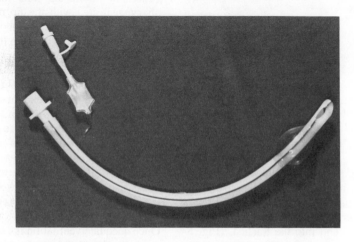

Fig. 8-17. Endotracheal tube. (Photo by Richard Lazar.)

scope, with either a curved blade or a straight blade attached, into the mouth along the left side (the blade will be in the midline position). The laryngoscope should be advanced until one can visualize the glottic opening by placing the curved blade into the vallecula or by placing the straight blade under the epiglottis. Lift the lower jaw with the laryngoscope—do not pry the upper teeth. Holding the laryngoscope in your left hand, advance the endotracheal tube with your right hand into the mouth and down into the trachea. Once the endotracheal tube is in place, inflate the balloon and blow into the

end of the tube to assure that the airway is in the trachea (once again, you should see the chest rise when you blow into the end of the tube). Auscultate the lungs at the same time to assure that both lungs are being ventilated (Fig. 8-18). If only one lung is being ventilated (most likely, the right), pull the endotracheal tube back slightly and reassess tube placement.

Once assured that the endotracheal tube is in place, remove the esophageal obturator airway if it was placed previously by deflating the balloon on the EOA and withdrawing it.

Attach the end of the endotracheal tube to a

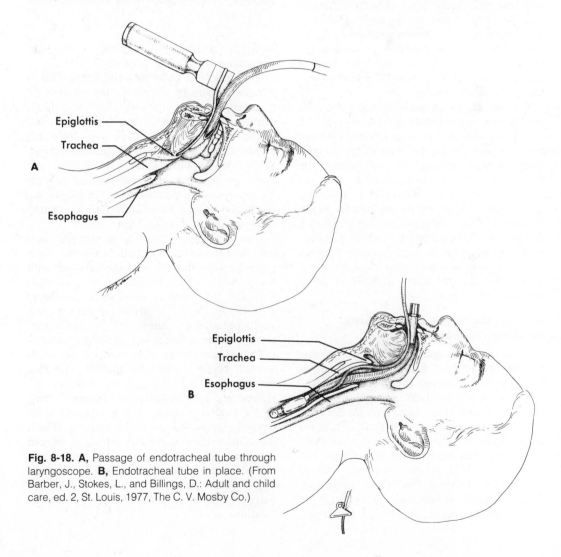

Epiglottis

Trachea

A

Esophagus

Epiglottis

Trachea

Esophagus

B

Fig. 8-18. A, Passage of endotracheal tube through laryngoscope. **B,** Endotracheal tube in place. (From Barber, J., Stokes, L., and Billings, D.: Adult and child care, ed. 2, St. Louis, 1977, The C. V. Mosby Co.)

bag-valve-mask device or some type of ventilator device. Be sure to secure the tube to the victim's face using tincture of benzoin and adhesive tape.

Once the patient is being ventilated with the endotracheal tube, assure that the tube is in the correct position by obtaining a portable anterior-posterior chest radiograph.

If the patient has spontaneous respirations for 8 hours and arterial blood gases are at an acceptable level, one may elect to remove the endotracheal tube. This is accomplished by suctioning the patient's nose and mouth and posterior pharyngeal area. The cuff should then be deflated and the airway withdrawn. Never withdraw the airway without first deflating the cuff. Be prepared to suction the patient should he vomit. Also, be sure to monitor the patient for cardiac dysrhythmias during the extubation procedure.

The advantages of endotracheal intubation are that one can maintain good control of the airway and protect it from aspiration. One can also ventilate the patient with 100% oxygen under positive pressure. One can suction the trachea using the endotracheal tube. With the tube in place, gastric distention is minimal.

The disadvantages of the endotracheal tube are that it is easy to pass into the esophagus during initial passage and it requires a skilled technician to place it. It may cause hypoxia if insertion is prolonged, and chest compressions must be interrupted while it is being inserted.

Surgical techniques/procedures for airway management

If neither the esophageal obturator airway nor the endotracheal tube can be placed, or if attempts at placement have been unsuccessful, one is obligated to attempt additional methods of obtaining access to the airway. This is particularly true when there is massive facial trauma or where there is a foreign body present that has blocked the airway and has not been removed by other methods such as the abdominal thrust (Heimlich) maneuver. Other methods of obtaining access to the airway are by means of surgical techniques

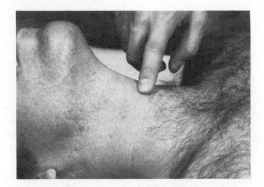

Fig. 8-19. Location of cricothyroid membrane. (Photo by Richard Lazar.)

such as transtracheal catheter ventilation, cricothyrotomy, or tracheostomy.

Transtracheal catheter ventilation. This is a rapid means of access to the airway via a catheter passed through the cricothyroid membrane. In this procedure the cricothyroid membrane is located—it extends from the cricoid cartilage to the thyroid cartilage (Fig. 8-19). One should palpate it by placing one finger on the thyroid membrane and moving the finger downward about 2 cm or by placing the finger on the cricoid cartilage and rotating the finger upward about 2 cm.

Once the area is located, prepare the skin with some sort of antiseptic solution. Then perforate both the skin and the cartilage with the catheter, which is attached to a syringe, directing the catheter downward (caudally) at a 45° angle. While advancing the catheter, apply negative pressure to the syringe plunger. When the catheter has perforated the cricothyroid membrane and is in the trachea, air will begin to enter the syringe. Advance the catheter over the stylette. Remove the stylette and syringe from the catheter. Attach an IV extension tubing that is attached to an oxygen release valve, to the catheter. Then, press the release valve and introduce oxygen into the trachea (Fig. 8-20). If the procedure has been successful, one should see the chest rise. When chest rise is seen, release the valve and allow the air to escape (passive exhalation).

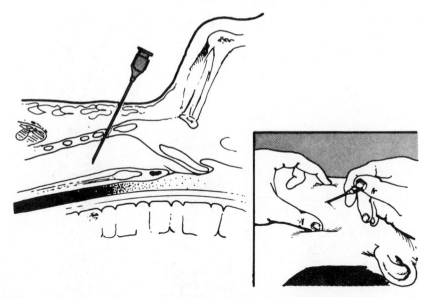

Fig. 8-20. Technique for performing needle cricothyrotomy. (From Stephenson, H. E., Jr.: Cardiac arrest and resuscitation, ed. 4, St. Louis, 1974, The C. V. Mosby Co.)

The advantages to this procedure are that it can be accomplished without interrupting chest compression, it is quick and, once it is in place, endotracheal intubation or tracheostomy can be performed while the patient is being continuously ventilated.

One must be careful, however, in that it may cause hemorrhage, perforation of the thyroid, perforation of the esophagus, subcutaneous emphysema, and mediastinal emphysema.

Cricothyrotomy. Cricothyrotomy is another method of rapid access to the airway. It can be performed by using a scalpel or other such sharp instrument to perforate the cricothyroid membrane. It is also performed by locating the cricothyroid membrane and preparing the skin with an antiseptic solution. The overlying skin should be spread to make it taut. One then should make a small incision over the cartilage through the skin. Once the skin has been invaded, make a horizontal puncture hole into the cricoid cartilage. At this point there may be a slight amount of bleeding, but it should not be excessive. Rotate the scalpel 90° to spread the cartilage (Fig. 8-21). Once

the opening is large enough, insert a small tube, such as a No. 6 tracheostomy tube, to maintain the opening. If a tube is not available, use whatever means necessary to maintain the airway. Supply oxygen to the victim through the opening. If the patient is apneic, place a cuffed tracheostomy tube and employ positive pressure breathing.

The advantages to cricothyrotomy are that there is rapid entry into an obstructed airway, one has the ability to rapidly place a cuffed tube in the apneic victim, and an endotracheal tube can be placed while the victim is being continuously ventilated.

The disadvantages to this technique are that hemorrhage is a possibility, one may inadvertently lacerate the esophagus, there may be false passage of the tube, and subcutaneous emphysema and mediastinal emphysema may result. Later complications include tracheal stenosis.

Tracheostomy. The third method of surgical intervention for a blocked airway is *tracheostomy*. Tracheostomy should be performed only after other methods of ventilation have failed and one has been unable to

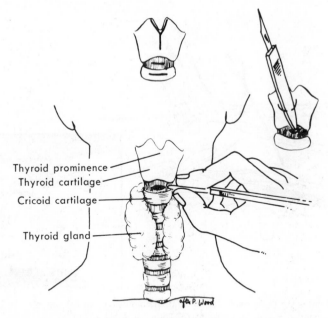

Thyroid prominence
Thyroid cartilage
Cricoid cartilage

Thyroid gland

Fig. 8-21. Cricothyrotomy incision, frontal view. (From Miller, R. H.: Textbook of basic emergency medicine, ed. 2, St. Louis, 1980, The C. V. Mosby Co.)

obtain control of the airway (usually because of laryngeal edema, foreign bodies, or tumors).

This procedure is performed by placing the patient on his back with a pillow under his shoulders with his neck in extension. The patient should be ventilated using an endotracheal tube, cricothyrotomy, or other method meanwhile. The skin should then be prepared and the patient draped. Make an incision into the skin at about the third or fourth tracheal ring (in an adult). Once an incision has been made, dissect down through the subcutaneous fat and platysma muscle. The midline muscles should then be retracted to expose the tracheal rings. Local anesthesia should be injected into the tracheal lumen to decrease the cough reflex. Create a stoma by removing 1 square centimeter of cartilage. Continue to suction the victim to remove any blood or secretions. Insert a tracheostomy tube, and check for air movement. Attach the end of the tube to the ventilation device. Auscultate the lungs. If the tube is function-

ing adequately, inflate the cuff. The corners of the incision should then be loosely sutured and the tube secured with tracheostomy tape. Dress the wound, and obtain a chest x-ray film.

The advantages to tracheostomy are reduced physiological dead space, prolonged positive pressure breathing, and direct access to the respiratory tract for the removal of secretions.

Complications of tracheostomy include inaccurate tube placement, laceration of arteries and nerves, hemorrhage, pressure necrosis from the cuff, perforation of the esophagus, subcutaneous emphysema, and mediastinal emphysema.

BREATHING

There are several different devices available for the delivery of oxygen to a patient. One should be familiar with the various types and be able to select the proper one for an individual patient's needs (Table 8-1).

Nasal cannula. The nasal cannula is the

Table 8-1. Summary of oxygen assist devices

Type of breathing device	Oxygen flow rate	Oxygen concentrations	Advantages	Disadvantages
Nasal cannula	2-6 liters/min	25%-40%	No rebreathing of expired air	Can only be used on patients who are breathing spontaneously
Face mask	10 liters/min	50%-60%	Higher oxygen concentration than nasal cannula	Not tolerated well by severely dyspneic patients; can only be used on patients who are breathing spontaneously
Oxygen reservoir mask	10-12 liters/min	90%	Higher oxygen concentration than nasal cannula or face mask	Must have tight seal on mask; can only be used on patients who are breathing spontaneously
Venturi mask	4 liters/min 8 liters/min	24%-28% 35%-40%	Fixed oxygen concentration	Can only be used on patients who are breathing spontaneously
Pocket mask	Expired air to 10 liters/min	18%-50%	Avoids direct contact with patient's mouth; may add oxygen source; may be used on apneic patient; may be used on child	Rescuer fatigue
Bag-valve-mask	Room air 12 liters/min	21% 40%-90%	Quick; oxygen concentration may be increased; rescuer can sense lung compliance; may be used on both apneic and spontaneously breathing patients	Air in stomach; low tidal volume
Oxygen-powered breathing device	100 liters/min	100%	High oxygen flow; positive pressure	Gastric distention; overinflation; standard device cannot be used in children without special adapter

*From Barber, J. M., and Budassi, S. A.: Mosby's manual of emergency care, St. Louis, 1979, The C. V. Mosby Co.

most commonly used oxygen delivery device. It can be used on the patient who is spontaneously breathing. If one adjusts the oxygen flow rate to 6 liters/minute, one can achieve an oxygen concentration of 25% to 40%.

Face masks (Fig. 8-22). Face masks are tolerated fairly well in most individuals except those who are experiencing severe dyspnea, where the face mask may make them feel as though they are suffocating. This device must also be used on the spontaneously breathing patient. At a flow rate of 10 liters/minute one can achieve an oxygen concentration of 50% to 60%.

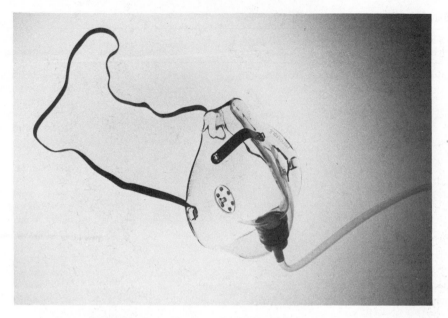

Fig. 8-22. Oxygen face mask. (Photo by Richard Lazar.)

Oxygen reservoir mask (Fig. 8-23). The oxygen reservoir mask is equipped with a plastic bag reservoir that fills with 100% oxygen while the patient is exhaling. Then when the patient inhales, with the liter flow at 10 to 12 liters/minute, the patient may receive a concentration of about 90% oxygen, provided the mask has a tight seal. This piece of equipment must also be used on the spontaneously breathing patient.

Venturi mask. If a victim gives a history of chronic obstructive lung disease and is currently experiencing respiratory distress, one should consider using the Venturi mask, which allows for delivery of a fixed concentration of oxygen by adjusting the oxygen flow caps on the device (Fig. 8-24). With a 4-liter oxygen flow one can obtain a 24% and 28% oxygen delivery. By turning the oxygen flow up to 8 liters and changing the oxygen flow cap, one can obtain an oxygen delivery of 35% to 40%. The proper method for using this device is to initiate the flow at the 24% oxygen concentration setting and observe the patient closely. If respiratory depression is not present, one may elect to increase the oxygen concentration to 28% and repeat the observation, continuing to increase the oxygen concentration as long as the patient tolerates the previously lower concentration well.

Pocket mask. A pocket mask may be carried by the rescuer and used when other forms of artificial ventilation are not available (Fig. 8-25). The pocket mask allows for mouth-to-mask breathing. The mask fits snugly onto the victim's face, covering the nose and the mouth. The victim's head should be tilted back and the jaw pulled forward, with the victim's mouth slightly open. The rescuer can then blow into the opening in the top of the mask (Fig. 8-26). One can add supplemental oxygen by attaching an oxygen source to the one-way valve located at the bottom of the mask. If the oxygen flow is regulated at 10 liters/minute, one can achieve a delivered oxygen concentration of about 50%. For pediatric use, the mask may be turned upside down, with the wide end at the top of the child's head and the narrow end just below his mouth.

Bag-valve-mask. A bag-valve-mask device

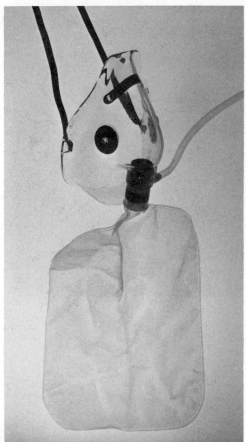

Fig. 8-23. Oxygen reservoir mask. (Photo by Richard Lazar.)

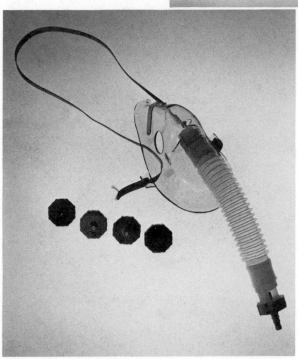

Fig. 8-24. Venturi mask and oxygen regulators. (Photo by Richard Lazar.)

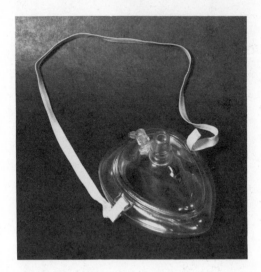

Fig. 8-25. Pocket mask. (Photo by Richard Lazar.)

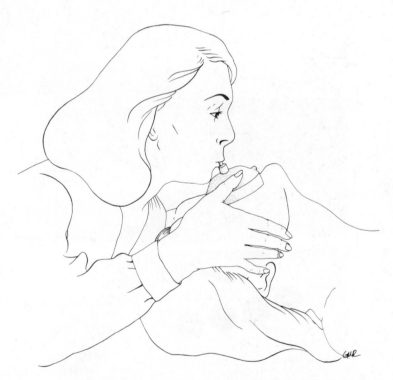

Fig. 8-26. Blowing into pocket mask. (From Barber, J. M., and Budassi, S. A.: Mosby's manual of emergency care, St. Louis, 1979, The C. V. Mosby Co.)

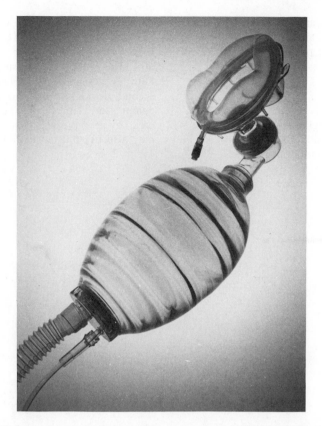

Fig. 8-27. Bag-valve-mask device with oxygen reservoir. (Photo by Richard Lazar.)

can deliver 21% oxygen (room air) to a victim. By adding an additional oxygen source of 12 liters/minute, one can achieve an oxygen concentration of 40%. By adding a plastic cap and a 3-foot corrugated tubing reservoir (Fig. 8-27) with an open end, one can obtain about a 90% oxygen concentration.

The mask of the bag-valve-mask unit is applied in the same way as the pocket mask, obtaining a tight seal around the nose and the mouth. It is appropriate to use an oropharyngeal or nasopharyngeal airway in conjunction with the bag-valve-mask device.

Although there are many brands of bag-valve-mask devices on the market, a transparent device is recommended so that one may observe and intervene rapidly should emesis occur.

Oxygen-powered devices. Oxygen-powered devices can deliver 100% oxygen at a

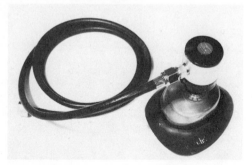

Fig. 8-28. Oxygen-powered breathing device. (Photo by Richard Lazar.)

rate of 100 liters/minute (Fig. 8-28) to a pocket mask, an attached mask, an esophageal obturator airway, an endotracheal tube, or a transtracheal catheter insufflation device. Timing and length of oxygen delivery are left up to the operator. This device should *not* be used in children under 12 years of age unless a special pediatric adapter is available.

CIRCULATION

When performing chest compression, assure that the victim is lying on a firm surface to allow for compression of the ventricles between the sternum and the vertebrae.

There are currently two types of chest compressors on the market. The first is a cardiac press, hinged device that is operated manually. The plunger is adjusted so that the sternum is compressed 1½ to 2 inches. The second device is an automatic gas-powered compressor. This device has a plunger powered by compressed gas. This compressor may also be adjusted to compress the sternum 1½ to 2 inches.

Text continued on p. 186.

Cardiac dysrhythmias
DYSRHYTHMIAS ORIGINATING IN THE SINUS NODE
Normal sinus rhythm

Rate	60 to 100 beats/minute
Rhythm	Regular
P waves	Present
QRS complexes	Present; normal duration
P/QRS relationship	P wave preceding each QRS complex
PR interval	Normal

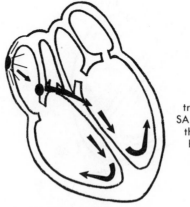

Impulse travels from SA to AV node through His bundle to Purkinje fibers

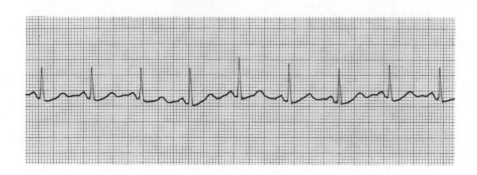

Significance: The SA node is the normal pacemaker of the heart; it is influenced both by the parasympathetic and sympathetic branches of the autonomic nervous system.

Intervention: None required.

Sinus tachycardia

Rate	>100 beats/minute but seldom >160 to 180 beats/minute
Rhythm	Regular
P waves	Present
QRS complexes	Present, normal duration
P/QRS relationship	P wave preceding each QRS complex
Pr interval	Normal

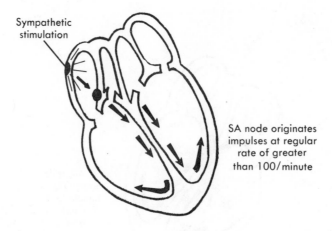

Sympathetic stimulation

SA node originates impulses at regular rate of greater than 100/minute

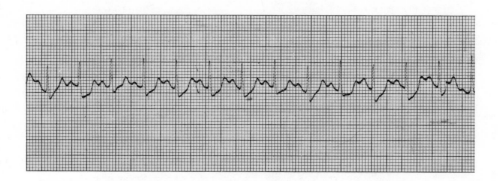

Significance: The normal pacemaker of the heart is firing at an increased rate because of anxiety, fever, pain, exercise, smoking, hyperthyroidism, heart failure, volume loss, specific drugs, or other reasons that may cause increased tissue oxygen demands. This condition may also be caused by decreased vagal tone (parasympathetic decrease), which allows the sinus node to increase its rate.

Intervention: Treat the cause; there is no specific drug given for sinus tachycardia except in the face of congestive heart failure; then digitalis is usually the drug of choice. If sinus tachycardia is the dysrhythmia seen following cardiopulmonary arrest, a Swan-Ganz catheter should be placed and the wedge pressure should be maintained at 15 to 18 mm Hg.

Sinus bradycardia

Rate	<60 beats/minute, but seldom <30 beats/minute
Rhythm	Regular
P waves	Present
QRS complexes	Present; normal duration
P/QRS relationship	P wave preceding each QRS complex
PR interval	Normal

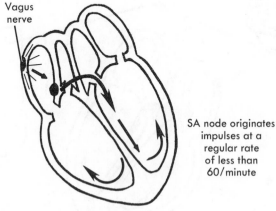

Vagus nerve

SA node originates impulses at a regular rate of less than 60/minute

Significance: The normal pacemaker, the SA node, is slowed by increased vagal tone (parasympathetic stimulation); causes include sleep, a normal athletic heart, anoxia, hypothyroidism, increased intracranial pressure, acute myocardial infarction, vagal stimulation (such as vomiting, straining at stool, carotid sinus massage, or ocular pressure), and specific drugs.

Intervention: Observe the patient for symptoms such as a decrease in blood pressure, a decreasing level of consciousness, syncope, shock, or acidosis.
1. Stop digitalis administration and concurrently administer oxygen.
2. Treat with atropine (0.3 to 0.6 mg IV push) or isoproterenol (Isuprel) or a pacemaker.

Sinus dysrhythmia

Rate	60 to 100 beats/minute, but this may increase with inspiration and decrease with expiration
Rhythm	Irregular
P waves	Present
QRS complexes	Present; normal duration
P/QRS relationship	P wave preceding each QRS complex
PR interval	Normal

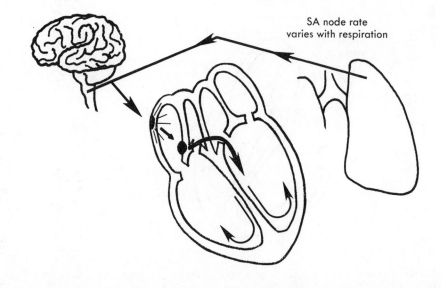

SA node rate
varies with respiration

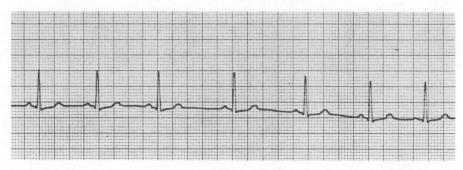

Significance: This dysrhythmia is a normal finding in children and young adults in whom there is a variation of vagal tone in response to respirations. As an abnormal finding, it may be found in patients with mitral or aortic valve problems or as a response to intracranial pressure or to specific drugs. For this variance to be considered a dysrhythmia, the variation must exceed 0.12 seconds between the longest and shortest cycles.

Intervention: Observe the patient, and document findings. If the dysrhythmia is not related to respiratory problems, treat the underlying cause.

DYSRHYTHMIAS ORIGINATING IN THE ATRIA
Premature atrial contractions (PACs, extrasystoles)

Rate	Usually 60 to 100 beats/minute
Rhythm	Usually regularly irregular
P waves	Present, but premature P wave may appear different in configuration (because it did not originate in the SA node)
QRS complexes	Present; normal duration
P/QRS relationship	P wave preceding each QRS complex
PR interval	Usually normal

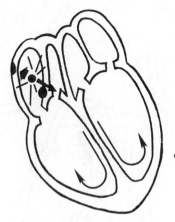

Atrial origin of abnormal impulse

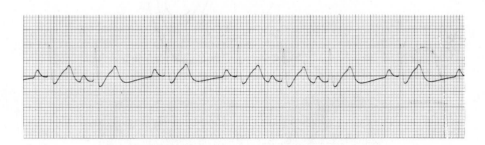

Significance: PACs are the result of an irritable ectopic focus that may be caused by fatigue, alcohol, coffee, smoking, digoxin, congestive heart failure, or ischemia; sometimes the etiology is unknown. They may be a prelude to atrial fibrillation, atrial flutter, or paroxysmal atrial tachycardia.

Intervention: Treatment is usually unnecessary, but should be given if more than six PACs occur per minute and the patient is becoming symptomatic. Oxygen should be the drug of choice, followed by quinidine, procainamide, or digitalis. If alcohol, coffee, or smoking is the cause, advise the patient to eliminate it.

Wandering atrial pacemaker

Rate	Usually 60 to 100 beats/minute
Rhythm	Usually regular or slightly irregular
P waves	Present; configuration varies
QRS complexes	Present; normal duration
P/QRS relationship	P wave preceding each QRS
PR interval	Normal

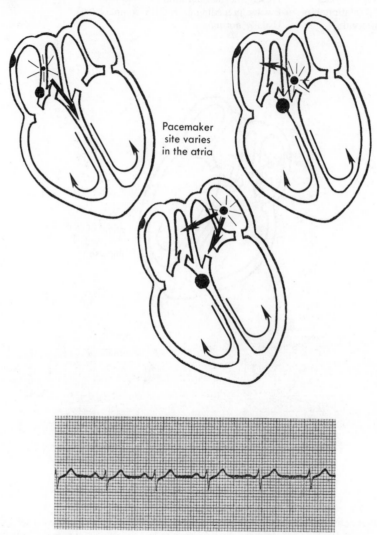

Pacemaker
site varies
in the atria

Significance: Either the SA node is suppressed or other atrial foci become excited and take over the pacemaker function of the heart. This dysrhythmia may be caused by specific drugs, inflammation, or COPD.

Intervention: Treatment is usually unnecessary. If the patient is receiving digitalis, it may be wise to withhold the digitalis and obtain a serum digoxin level. When treatment is necessary, treat the underlying cause.

Paroxysmal atrial tachycardia (PAT)

Rate	>160 beats/minute
Rhythm	Regular
P waves	May be hidden in T wave of previous beat
QRS complexes	Present; normal duration
P/QRS relationship	P wave preceding each QRS complex, but it may be difficult to see; if there is PAT with block, there will not be a QRS complex following each P wave
PR interval	Normal

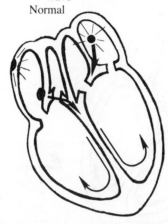

Irritable
focus in
atrial wall
beats regularly
at rate of
160-240/minute

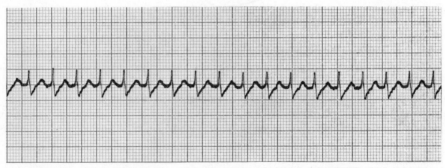

Significance: The onset of this dysrhythmia is usually sudden, as is the cessation. A pacemaker cell in the atrial wall becomes irritable and fires at a rate of 160 to 240 beats/minute. The danger of this dysrhythmia is that continuous rapid firing could lead to decreased ventricular filling and therefore decreased coronary artery perfusion. This is an extremely dangerous event for those who have a history of coronary artery disease, as a myocardial infarction may occur. It may also cause pulmonary edema, congestive heart failure, and shock associated with left ventricular failure. Common causes of this dysrhythmia are digitalis toxicity, alcohol, smoking, COPD, heart disease, anoxia, hypoglycemia, and pulmonary embolism.

Intervention: Treatment consists of oxygen, IV D/5/W TKO, and vagal stimulation (carotid sinus massage, Valsalva maneuver, or facial immersion in ice water). One may also elect to try an IV bolus of edrophonium chloride (Tensilon) or drip of metaraminol (Aramine). If these maneuvers fail and the patient is becoming symptomatic and hemodynamically compromised, he should receive synchronous cardioversion. If synchronous cardioversion is ineffective, atrial pacing may be initiated, or drugs such as digoxin, quinidine, propanolol, or hypertensive agents may be administered to induce reflex slowing caused by vagal stimulation by baroreceptors. The cause of the dysrhythmia should also be treated.

Atrial flutter

Rate	Atrial rate of 240 to 360 beats/minute
Rhythm	Regular or irregular
P waves	Saw-toothed pattern
QRS complexes	Present; normal duration
P/QRS relationship	Because of rapid atrial rate, ventricular response will vary; there may be a regular or an irregular response
PR interval	Irregular

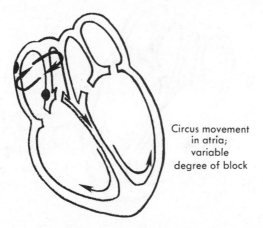

Circus movement
in atria;
variable
degree of block

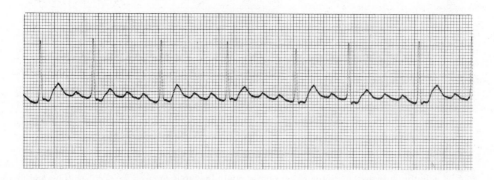

Significance: An irritable focus in the artia is responsible for this dysrhythmia. The atrial pacemaker fires at such a rapid rate that there is a variable block at the AV node, so that only every other, every third, or every fourth impulse reaches the ventricles. The ventricular response may be regular or irregular. Atrial flutter is a dangerous dysrhythmia in that ineffective atrial contraction may cause mural clots to form in the atria and consequently break loose, forming pulmonary or cerebral emboli. Atrial flutter may be seen in coronary artery disease, rheumatic heart disease, COPD, shock, anoxia, electrolyte imbalance, hyperthyroidism, and as a response to various drugs.

Intervention: Check the apical and radial pulses for perfusion. The treatment of choice is usually digitalization following synchronous cradioversion. Quinidine may be administered following reduction of the ventricular response by digitalis. Procainamide or propranolol (Inderal) may be given. Be sure to treat the underlying cause.

Atrial fibrillation

Rate	Atrial rate 400 to 800 beats/minute; ventricular rate varies
Rhythm	Ventricular rhythm *always* irregular
P waves	Irregular, rapid; appears like fibrillating baseline; P waves indistinguishable
QRS complexes	Irregular rhythm; normal duration
P/QRS relationship	Indistinguishable P waves; irregular ventricular response.
PR interval	Indistinguishable

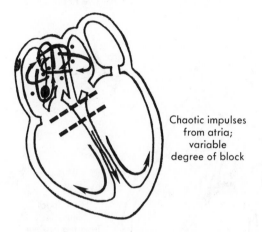

Chaotic impulses
from atria;
variable
degree of block

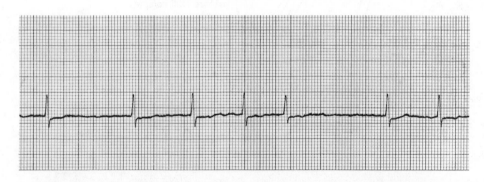

Significance: There is chaotic firing of multiple atrial pacemakers in rapid succession. The atria never firmly contract. The ventricles respond in an irregular fashion. Because of poor atrial empty- ing, there is danger of mural clot formation and embolism. Cardiac output drops because of lack of "atrial kick" (15% to 20% of cardiac output). This dysrhythmia is frequently seen in the pres- ence of coronary artery disease, rheumatic heart disease, hyperthyroidism, and, most commonly, digitalis toxicity.

Intervention: Check the ventricular response, both on the monitor and by checking peripheral pulses. Check the blood pressure. If the patient is severely symptomatic (syncope, altered level of consciousness, deteriorating vital signs, and chest pain), synchronous cardioversion should be administered. If the patient has been on digitalis therapy, a serum digoxin level should be ana- lyzed. If the patient has not been on digitalis therapy before the onset of this dysrhythmia, he may be treated with digitalis following successful synchronous cardioversion.

DYSRHYTHMIAS ORIGINATING IN THE AV NODE
Nodal (junctional) rhythm

Rate	Usually 40 to 60 beats/minute
Rhythm	Regular
P waves	May appear inverted or may not be present
QRS complexes	Regular; normal duration
P/QRS relationship	P wave may appear inverted before or after the QRS complex or may be entirely absent
PR interval	Less than 0.12 when P wave is present preceding QRS

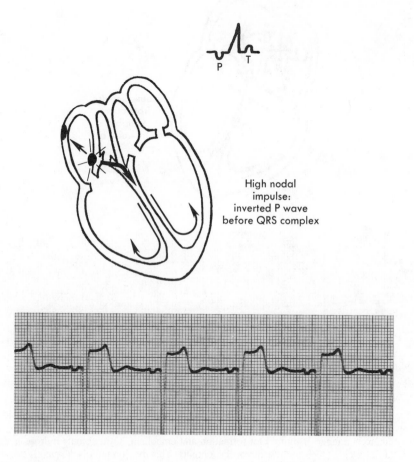

High nodal
impulse:
inverted P wave
before QRS complex

Significance: Usually when higher pacemakers in the atria fail, the AV node takes over as the pacemaker of the heart.

Intervention: If the patient has been on digitalis therapy, withhold the digitalis and obtain a serum digoxin level to check for digitalis toxicity. There is no specific therapy for this dysrhythmia. If the patient becomes symptomatic (syncope, altered level of consciousness, and chest pain) as a result of the slow heart rate, give atropine sulfate (0.4 to 0.6 mg IV push). If the atropine is found to be unsuccessful, isoproterenol would be the next drug of choice, given by IV drip. If both of these drugs are unsuccessful, pacemaker insertion is then indicated.

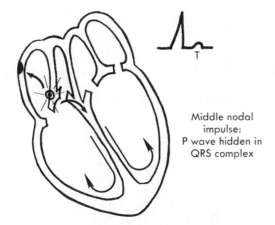

Middle nodal
impulse:
P wave hidden in
QRS complex

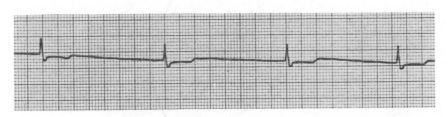

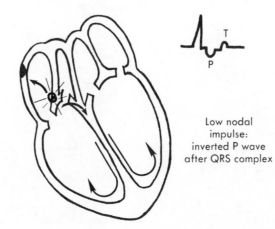

Low nodal
impulse:
inverted P wave
after QRS complex

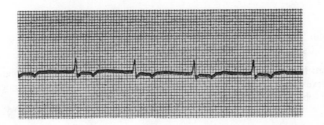

Premature nodal contractions (PNCs)

Rate	Usually normal or bradycardic
Rhythm	Irregularly irregular
P waves	May appear inverted or may not be present
QRS complexes	Regular; normal duration
P/QRS relationship	P waves may appear inverted before or after the QRS complex or may be absent; entire P/QRS complex is early
PR interval	Less than 0.12 when P wave is seen in premature beat

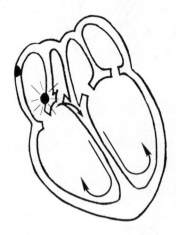

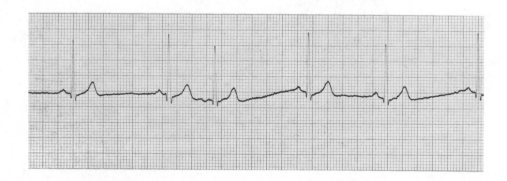

Significance: The AV junction is the pacemaker. This dysrhythmia is less frequently seen than PACs or PVCs; it may precede first, second, or third degree heart block.

Intervention: If the patient is on digitalis therapy, withhold digitalis and obtain a serum digoxin level. Observe closely. Pharmacological therapy may include quinidine or procainamide. Alcohol, coffee, and tobacco should be withheld from the patient's daily routine.

Nodal tachycardia (junctional tachycardia)

Rate	100 to 180 beats/minute
Rhythm	Regular
P waves	May appear inverted or may not be present
QRS complexes	Regular; normal duration
P/QRS relationship	P waves may appear inverted before or after the QRS complex or may be absent
PR interval	<0.12 when P wave is present

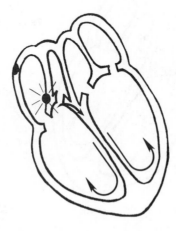

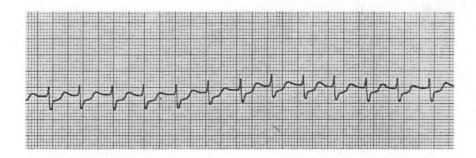

Significance: An irritable nodal focus takes over as the heart's pacemaker. Nodal tachycardia may be caused by heart disease, electrolyte imbalance, COPD, anoxia, or specific drugs.

Intervention: Check vital signs; if the patient is on digitalis therapy, withhold digitalis and obtain a serum digoxin level. Usually no other treatment is necessary.

First degree AV block

Rate	Usually 60 to 100 beats/minute
Rhythm	Usually regular
P waves	Present
QRS complexes	Regular; normal duration
P/QRS relationship	P wave preceding each QRS complex
PR interval	>0.20 seconds

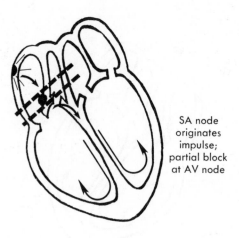

SA node
originates
impulse;
partial block
at AV node

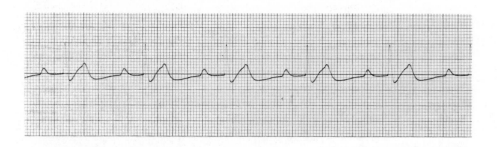

Significance: The SA node initiates an impulse that is delayed through the AV node. This may be caused by anoxia, ischemia, AV node malfunction, edema after open heart surgery, or digitalis toxicity.

Intervention: If the patient is on digitalis therapy, withhold digitalis and obtain a serum digoxin level. Administer oxygen and observe for progression to a higher degree of block. If the patient becomes symptomatic (syncope, altered level of consciousness, and chest pain), give atropine (0.4 to 0.6 mg IV). If atropine is unsuccessful, administer isoproterenol by IV drip. If isoproterenol is unsuccessful, prepare for pacemaker placement.

Second degree AV block—Mobitz type I (Wenckebach phenomenon)

Rate	Usually normal
Rhythm	Regularly irregular
P waves	One preceding each QRS complex except for regular dropped ventricular conduction at intervals
QRS complexes	Cyclic missed conduction; when QRS complex is present, it is of normal duration
P/QRS relationship	P wave before each QRS complex except for regular dropped ventricular conduction at intervals
PR interval	Lengthens with each cycle until one QRS complex is dropped, then repeats

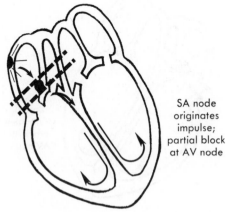

SA node
originates
impulse;
partial block
at AV node

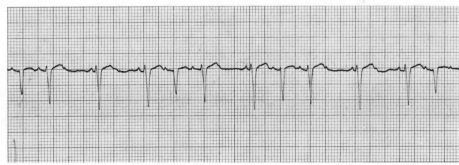

Significance: Each atrial impulse takes longer to travel through the AV node until finally a beat is dropped, and the entire cycle repeats itself. Although the etiology is not well understood, this dysrhythmia is commonly seen following inferior wall myocardial infarction.

Intervention: If patient is on digitalis therapy, withhold digitalis and obtain a serum digoxin level. Observe for further dysrhythmia development.

Second degree AV block—Mobitz type II

Rate	Atrial rate usually 60 to 100 beats/minute; ventricular rate usually slow
Rhythm	Regularly irregular (usually)
P waves	Two or more for every QRS complex
QRS complexes	Normal duration when present
P/QRS relationship	Two or more nonconducted impulses appearing as P waves without QRS complexes following
PR interval	Normal or delayed on the conducted beat; but remains same throughout the dysrhythmia

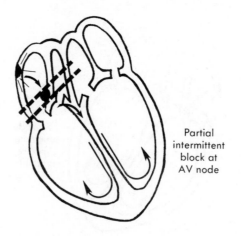

Partial
intermittent
block at
AV node

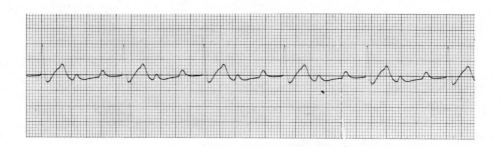

Significance: One or more atrial impulses are not conducted through the AV node to the ventricles. This may be a result of anoxia, digitalis toxicity, edema after open heart surgery, hyperkalemia, or anterior wall myocardial infarction.

Intervention: If the patient is on digitalis therapy, withhold digitalis and obtain a serum digoxin level. If the patient is symptomatic or in danger of developing a higher degree of block, administer 0.4 to 0.6 mg atropine IV. If atropine is unsuccessful, administer isoproterenol by IV drip. If isoproterenol is unsuccessful, prepare for pacemaker insertion. If hyperkalemia is the cause of the dysrhythmia, administer Kayexalate enema. Always give supplemental oxygen.

Third degree AV block—Stokes-Adams syndrome

Rate	Atrial rate 60 to 100 beats/minute; ventricular asystole
Rhythm	Irregular
P waves	Occur regularly
QRS complexes	Absent during episode
P/QRS relationship	P waves present; absence of QRS complex during episode
PR interval	None during episode

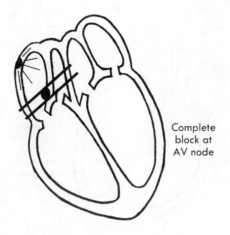

Complete block at AV node

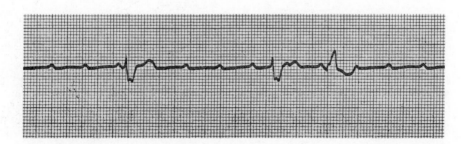

Significance: The SA node initiates an impulse that is not conducted through the AV node; the ventricles do not contract, and there is no cardiac output during the episode, resulting in poor peripheral perfusion and cerebral ischemia, which results in a syncopal episode. This syncopal episode may be followed by asystole if the temporary asystole lasts for more than just a few seconds.

Intervention: Take precautions against seizures; prepare to perform basic and advanced cardiac life support if asystole lasts for more than a few seconds. The patient should be treated with isoproterenol followed by pacemaker insertion. Also give an initial bolus of atropine while the isoproterenol drip is being prepared.

Third degree AV block—complete heart block

Rate	Atrial rate, 60 to 100 beats/minute; ventricular rate usually <60 beats/minute
Rhythm	Usually normal
P waves	Occur regularly
QRS complexes	Slow; usually wide (>0.10 second)
P/QRS relationship	Completely independent of each other
PR interval	Inconsistent

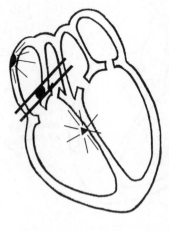

Complete block at AV node; may have nodal or ventricular independent pacemaker

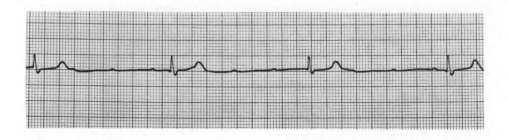

Significance: There is no conduction of SA impulse through the AV node. The ventricle begins to initiate its own impulse; the atria and ventricles beat independently of each other.

Intervention: If the patient is on digitalis therapy, withhold digitalis and obtain a serum digoxin level. Observe the ventricular rate closely. If the ventricular rate is slow, the patient will surely be symptomatic (syncope, altered level of consciousness, and chest pain) and cardiac failure may soon result. Placement of a pacemaker is indicated. Atropine and/or isoproterenol may be an effective temporary measure until the pacemaker is in place. Be prepared to perform both basic and advanced cardiac life support.

Rapid AV dissociation (isorhythmic dissociation)

Rate	May or may not be normal
Rhythm	QRS complexes regular
P waves	Vary; may be sinus, atrial, or nodal
QRS complexes	Usually regular; normal duration or wide
P/QRS relationship	SA node fires normally but does not conduct through AV node. AV node is also initiating impulses, but because the AV node is irritable, it may actually pass through QRS complexes, where retrograde conduction possibly occurs.
PR interval	Inconsistent

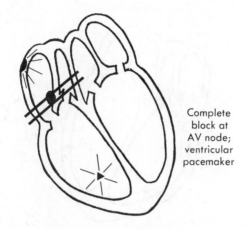

Complete block at AV node; ventricular pacemaker

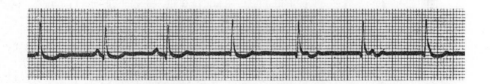

Significance: The sinus node initiates an impulse, but it is blocked by the AV node. The AV node also initiates impulses, as well as the ventricular pacemaker(s). The AV node is so irritated that the P wave may actually pass through the QRS complex and the impulse is conducted in a retrograde fashion.

Intervention: Observe the patient carefully. If he is symptomatic (syncope, altered level of consciousness, and chest pain) prepare for pacemaker insertion. Administer 0.4 to 0.6 mg atropine IV followed by isoproterenol by IV drip while preparing pacemaker equipment. Withhold digoxin preparations.

DYSRHYTHMIAS ORIGINATING IN THE VENTRICLES
Premature ventricular contractions (premature ectopic beats, extrasystoles, PVCs, PVBs, VPBs)

Rate	Usually 60 to 100 beats/minute
Rhythm	Irregular
P waves	Present with each sinus beat; do not precede PVCs
QRS complexes	Sinus-initiated QRS complex normal; QRS of PVC wide and bizarre, >0.10 seconds; full compensatory pause
P/QRS relationship	P wave before each QRS complex in normal sinus beats; no P wave preceding PVC; compensatory beats following PVC
PR interval	Normal in sinus beat; none in PVC

Single PVC

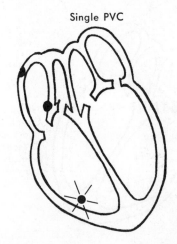

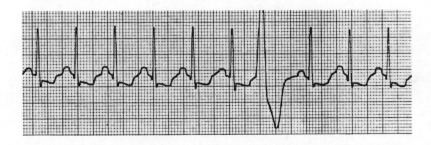

Significance: May indicate increasing ventricular irritability. PVC comes from an impulse initiated by a ventricular pacemaker cell. PVCs may occur as a result of hypoxia, hypovolemia, ischemia, infarction, coffee, alcohol, smoking, hypocalcemia, hyperkalemia, drugs, or acidosis.

Intervention: If the cause of the PVCs is known, remove the cause. Give lidocaine hydrochloride by IV bolus followed by additional boluses or lidocaine by IV drip (not to exceed 4 mg/minute). If the patient is hypoxic, administer oxygen. Other drugs that may be given are atropine (if PVCs are rate related), procainamide, quinidine, phenytoin (Dilantin), bretylium, and propranolol. If a serum electrolyte imbalance is the cause of PVCs, correct the electrolyte imbalance.

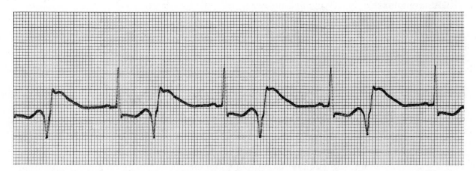

Ventricular bigeminy

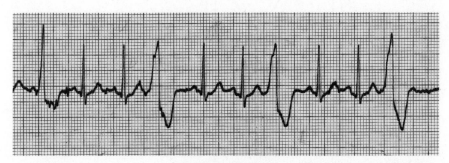

Ventricular trigeminy

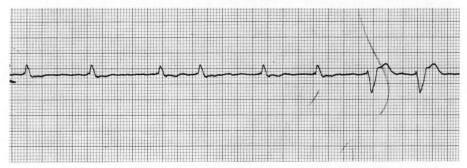

Couplet

Ventricular tachycardia (V tach)

Rate	150 to 250 beats/minute
Rhythm	May be only slightly irregular
P waves	Not seen
QRS complexes	Wide and bizarre
P/QRS relationship	None
PR interval	None

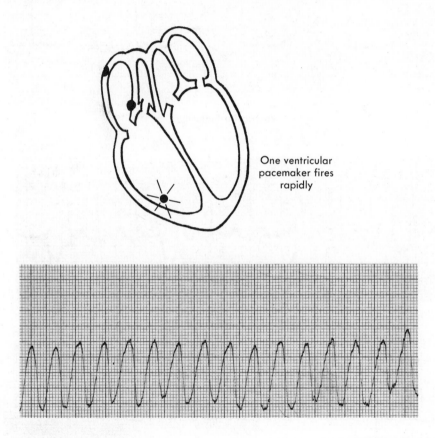

One ventricular
pacemaker fires
rapidly

Significance: This rhythm is actually several PVCs occurring consecutively. It cannot be tolerated for long periods of time. If it does not dissipate by itself, it will deteriorate to ventricular fibrillation. Because the ventricular rate is so fast, there is essentially little cardiac output, and cardiac arrest will soon result.

Intervention: If a defibrillator is close by, immediately defibrillate or synchronously cardiovert (opinions vary as to the dosage). If the patient appears to be tolerating the dysrhythmia relatively well, administer a bolus of lidocaine before defibrillation. Administer oxygen as well. If attempt(s) to defibrillate are unsuccessful and the patient becomes unconscious, pulseless, and apneic, immediately begin basic and advanced cardiac life support.

Ventricular fibrillation

Rate	Rapid, disorganized
Rhythm	Irregular
P waves	Not seen
QRS complexes	Sometimes not seen; other times extremely bizarre, wide patterns, appearing like baseline oscillations
P/QRS relationship	None
PR interval	None

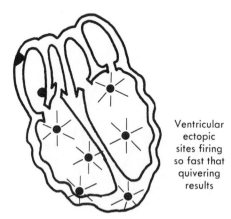

Ventricular
ectopic
sites firing
so fast that
quivering
results

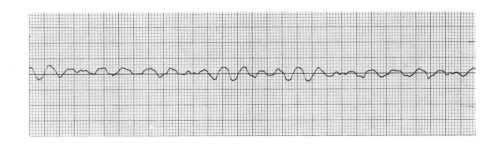

Significance: This is the most common dysrhythmia seen in cardiopulmonary arrest. It produces essentially no cardiac output; death will result if it is allowed to persist for more than 4 to 6 minutes.

Intervention: Begin basic and advanced cardiac life support immediately. Administer oxygen at 100% concentration under positive pressure; administer epinephrine IV (10 ml of 1:10,000 solution or 1 ml of 1:1,000 solution) and 2 ampules sodium bicarbonate IV. Allow the drugs to circulate for 90 seconds and reevaluate the rhythm—if it is the same, defibrillate the patient at 400 watt-seconds. If this is unsuccessful, the following treatments may be tried: (1) two electrical discharges in rapid succession, (2) increased paddle size, (3) anterior-posterior paddle placement, (4) atropine 1 mg by IV push (to decrease vagal tone), (5) calcium chloride, and (6) isoproterenol. If ventricular fibrillation is recurrent, you may give (1) atropine (0.6 mg IV), (2) 100 mg lidocaine (''slow bolus''), (3) procainamide, or (4) bretylium.

Idioventricular rhythm

Rate	Usually <20 beats/minute but it may be faster
Rhythm	Regular or irregular
P waves	None
QRS complexes	Wide and bizarre
P/QRS relationship	None
PR interval	None

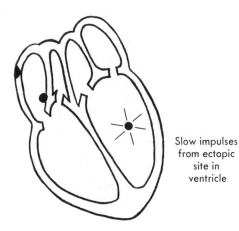

Slow impulses from ectopic site in ventricle

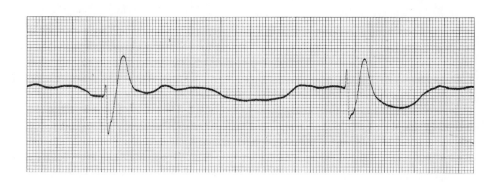

Significance: This dysrhythmia is associated with a poor prognosis; it probably indicates a large myocardial infarction with concurrent loss of a large amount of ventricular mass.

Intervention: Give atropine (0.6 to 0.8 mg IV push); repeat if unsuccessful. Give isoproterenol (2 to 20 mg/minute by IV drip titrated to a rate of 60 to 80 beats/minute). Administer a fluid challenge (200 ml IV over 2 to 5 minutes), pacemaker insertion, open chest massage, or 100 mg dexamethasone IV. If the patient is on dialysis, the rhythm may be caused by a severe electrolyte imbalance, and large amounts of sodium bicarbonate and calcium chloride should be considered.

Asystole (ventricular standstill)

Rate	None
Rhythm	None
P waves	May or may not appear
QRS complexes	None
P/QRS relationship	None
PR interval	None

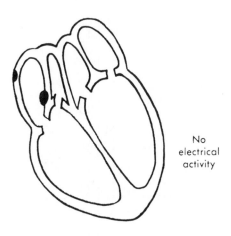

No
electrical
activity

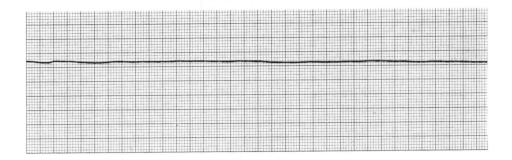

Significance: Asystole often implies that the patient has been in cardiopulmonary arrest for a prolonged period; mortality is high (>95%).

Intervention: Do *not* defibrillate. Give 100% oxygen under positive pressure, IV or intracardiac epinephrine, calcium gluconate or calcium chloride, and sodium bicarbonate IV; allow the first two drugs to circulate for 90 seconds. If this is unsuccessful, repeat the treatment and give atropine (to decrease vagal tone increased by myocardial infarction and maneuvers such as defibrillation and intubation). You may try isoproterenol by IV bolus or intracardiac or pacemaker insertion.

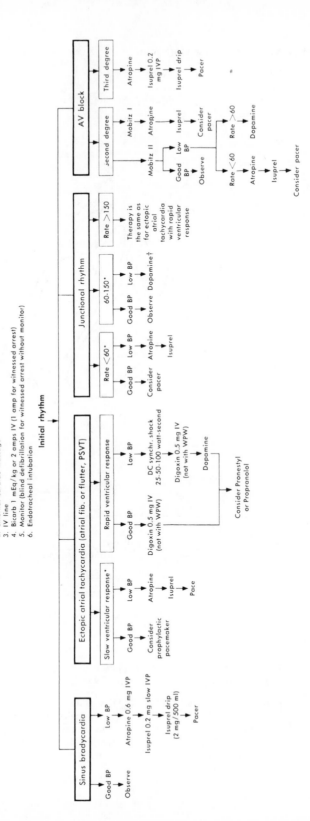

Cardiac arrest

1. Airway: mouth-to-mouth, bag, or esophageal airway
2. External cardiac massage
3. IV line
4. Bicarb 1 mEq/kg or 2 amps IV (1 amp for witnessed arrest)
5. Monitor (blind defibrillation for witnessed arrest without monitor)
6. Endotracheal intubation

Initial rhythm

Sinus bradycardia

Good BP → Observe

Low BP → Atropine 0.6 mg IVP → Isuprel 0.2 mg slow IVP → Isuprel drip (2 mg/500 ml) → Pacer

Ectopic atrial tachycardia (atrial fib. or flutter, PSVT)

Slow ventricular response*

Good BP → Consider prophylactic pacemaker

Low BP → Atropine → Isuprel → Pace

Rapid ventricular response

Good BP → Digoxin 0.5 mg IV (not with WPW) → Consider Pronestyl or Propranolol

Low BP → DC synchr. shock 25-50-100 watt-second → Digoxin 0.5 mg IV (not with WPW) → Dopamine → Consider Pronestyl or Propranolol

Junctional rhythm

Rate <60*

Good BP → Consider pacer

Low BP → Atropine → Isuprel

Rate 60-150*

Good BP → Observe

Low BP → Dopamine†

Rate >150

Therapy is the same as for ectopic atrial tachycardia with rapid ventricular response

AV block

Second degree

Mobitz I → Atropine → Isuprel → Consider pacer

Mobitz II →

Good BP → Observe

Low BP →

Rate <60 → Atropine → Isuprel → Consider pacer

Rate >60 → Dopamine

Third degree → Atropine → Isuprel 0.2 mg IVP → Isuprel drip → Pacer

Fig. 8-29. Algorithm for drug therapy of dysrhythmias in cardiac arrest. (Courtesy Charles R. McElroy, MD., and Marie K. Silver, M.D., Los Angeles, Calif.; modified from Crit. Care Q. **1:**23-25, 1978.

Initial rhythm

| Idioventricular | V tachycardia | V fibrillation | Electromechanical dissociation | Asystole |

Asystole
Precordial thump (for witnessed arrest only)
Epi 5-10 ml of 1:10,000
CaCl₂ 5 ml
No history or evidence of trauma → Repeat epi and CaCl₂ → Isuprel → Pacer → Consider aortic balloon, steroids

Electromechanical dissociation
Epi 5-10 ml of 1:10,000
CaCl₂ 5 ml
R/O tension pneumothorax — Chest tube (before CXR)
Flail chest or tamponade or possible aortic rupture → Open chest (4th ICS) Strip pericardium and clamp descending aorta

*Consider digitalis toxicity; if this is a possibility, give 2 gm MgSO₄ IV/10 minutes.
†If digitalis toxicity, give Dilantin in addition to dopamine.

V fibrillation
Epi 5-10 ml of 1:10,000
Defib. 400 watt-second

Persistent V fib.
CaCl₂ 5 ml epi 5 ml
Defibrillation
Atropine 0.6-1.0 mg
Lidocaine 100 mg
Defibrillation
A-P or "double defib."
Isuprel 0.2 mg
Pronestyl
Defibrillation
Bretylium

Recurrent V fib.
Lidocaine 100 mg
Defibrillation
Lidocaine 50-100 mg
Atropine 0.6-1.0 mg
Defibrillation
A-P or "double defib."
Pronestyl
Defibrillation
Bretylium

V tachycardia
Defib. 400 watt-second
Lidocaine 100 mg IVP 90 seconds
Defibrillation
Lidocaine 50-100 mg IVP
A-P or "double defib."
Procainamide
Defibrillation
R/O digitalis toxicity → Dilantin, MgSO₄, Bretylium
Propranolol → Bretylium

Idioventricular
Good BP → Pacer
Low BP → Atropine → Isuprel → Bretylium → Pacer and steroids

Drugs used in cardiac arrest

1. Atropine—0.4-0.8 mg IV push, may repeat dose in 5 minutes.

2. Bretylium—5-10 mg/kg IV in 50 ml D/5/W (usual initial dose for adults: 300-400 mg).

3. Bicarb—1 mEq/kg bolus initially, followed by half the initial dose every 10 minutes depending on the arterial pH; pH is not to exceed 7.30.

4. Calcium chloride—5 ml (½ ampule). Repeat if necessary, according to flow sheet or every 5-10 minutes, twice only.

5. Digoxin (Lanoxin)—0.5 mg IV as initial dose.

6. Phenytoin (Dilantin)—100 mg IV over 5 minutes; repeat until arrhythmia stops or 1000 mg has been given, or untoward effects develop.

7. Dopamine (Intropin)—1 ampule (5 ml containing 200 mg) in 250 ml D/5/W (contains 800 μgm/ml). Run at 10 μgm/kg/minute; increase to 15-20 μgm/kg/minute as needed (for 70 kg man, begin at 50 μgm/minute) until BP is controlled.

8. Epinephrine—0.5 mg IV according to flow sheet, every 5 minutes (5 ml of 1:1000).

9. Isoproterenol (Isuprel)—0.2 mg IV bolus, followed by 2 mg/500 ml D/5/W, run at 1-4 μgm/minutes (15-60 μgm).

10. Lidocaine—100 mg IV push over 2 minutes (50 mg/minute) or 2 mg/kg (followed by a drip of 4 mg/minute); may repeat dose up to 225 mg total.

11. Magnesium sulfate (MgSO₄)—2-4 mg IV (4.8 ml of 50% solution) over 10 minutes.

12. Procainamide (Pronestyl)—100 mg every 5 minutes, given slowly over 2 minutes to the following end points: (1) a total of 1 gm, (2) cessation of the arrhythmia, or (3) development of untoward effects; followed with drip at 1-3 mg/minute. (May give loading dose more rapidly during arrest.)

13. Propranolol (Inderal)—1-3 mg every 5 minutes until the arrhythmia stops, until 10 mg has been given, or until pulse drops below 80.

Fig. 8-29, cont'd. For legend see opposite page.

Name plate

Time	BP	P/R	Pupils R/L	IV type and place	CPR closed /open	ECG rhythm	Defib (w/s)	Amount and route Epineph-rine	Bicarb.	Lidocaine	Atropine	CaCl.	Miscell. (Drugs & IV)	Airway type	pH	PO₂	PCO₂	NA HCO₃	Notes and comments

Date _____
Time _____
Age _____
Sex _____
Weight _____

Arrest history _____

Medication history _____

Time arrested _____
CPR initiated in field _____ Yes/No
Time/By whom _____
Defibrillator type _____
Portable/Standard _____

Paramedic sq. _____
Time of arrival in ED _____
Outcome _____
Expir./Admit./Ward _____

Nurse's signature _____

Pupils
Key: • Constricted   NR = Non-reactive to light
     ● Dilated   R = Reactive to light
     M = Midpoint

Fig. 8-30. Cardiac arrest flow sheet. (From Barber, J. M., and Budassi. S. A.: Mosby's manual of emergency care, St. Louis, 1979, The C. V. Mosby Co.)

Table 8-2. Drugs in advanced life support

Drug	Dosage	Administration
Sodium bicarbonate	1 mEq/kg initially followed by 0.5 mEq/kg; may be repeated every 10 min during arrest period	Administer according to pH when blood gas results are available
Epinephrine (Adrenalin)	1.0 mg by IV bolus (10 ml of 1:10,000 solution or 1 ml of 1:1,000 solution); may be repeated every 5 min	If IV route is not available, administer 0.5 mg intracardiac
Lidocaine (Xylocaine)	50 to 100 mg slow IV bolus followed by lidocaine drip (2 gm lidocaine in 500 ml D/5/W at 1 to 4 mg/min	May also be administered as a 50 to 100 mg slow bolus IV followed by 50 mg slow IV bolus after 5 min, followed by a 50 mg slow bolus IV every 10 min until the victim reaches a stable environment where a lidocaine drip can be administered If IV route is not available, may be administered IM rapid injection technique at a dosage of 300 mg
Atropine sulfate	0.5 to 1.0 mg IV bolus; may be repeated at 10-min intervals	
Calcium gluconate	10 ml of 10% solution given by IV bolus; may be repeated every 10 min	
Isoproterenol (Isuprel)	2 mg in 500 ml D/5/W IV run at rate of 2 to 4 μg/min	May be given IV bolus at a maximum dosage of 0.2 mg; may also be given at the same dosage intracardiac
Metaraminol (Aramine)	200 mg in 500 ml D/5/W IV at 0.5 to 1 ml/min (200 to 400 μg/min) titrated to desired blood pressure	May also be given IM at a dosage of 2 to 10 mg
Levarterenol (Levophed) (norepinephrine)	8 mg in 500 ml D/5/W at rate of 1 ml (8 μg)/min, titrated to desired blood pressure	
Dopamine hydrochloride (Intropin)	400 mg in 500 ml D/5/W, at an intermediate dosage rate of 5 to 10 μg/kg/min (350 to 700 μg/min for a 70 kg man)	See Appendix F for dosage chart
Propanolol (Inderal)	1 mg by IV bolus; may be repeated every 2 to 3 min not to exceed 3 mg	
Procainamide (Pronestyl)	100 mg slow IV bolus (over 2 min; wait 3 min and repeat until desired effect is seen; dosage not to exceed 1 gm	
Furosemide (Lasix)	40 mg by slow IV bolus (over 2 min)	

Defibrillation

When ventricular fibrillation occurs, if intervention does not take place in 4 to 6 minutes, biological death will occur. Basic and advanced life support is essential at this point. The most definitive therapy for ventricular fibrillation is defibrillation, in which an electrical impulse is passed through the myocardium, depolarizing all the cells of the myocardium at once, with the expectation that the depolarization will be followed by a spontaneous repolarization of all of the cells simultaneously. If this occurs, there is a possibility that one of the higher pacemakers, the SA or AV node, will resume function as the primary pacemaker of the heart, producing a life-sustaining rhythm.

Because the fibrillating heart is generally hypoxic, one should begin basic cardiopulmonary resuscitation immediately. If the initial defibrillation is unsuccessful, one should begin pharmacological intervention. The two drugs of choice in ventricular fibrillation are sodium bicarbonate and epinephrine. These should be followed by another attempt to defibrillate the myocardium, once sufficient time has been given to circulate the administered medications.

The defibrillation threshold is the amount of energy it takes to defibrillate the ventricles.

If a patient is particularly large and defibrillation attempts have been unsuccessful, one may elect to administer the next defibrillation attempt in an anterior-posterior paddle placement position (Fig. 8-31) and administer two defibrillation electrical charges in rapid succession in an attempt to decrease the defibrillation threshold.

When defibrillating, placement of the paddles of the defibrillator and resistance across the thorax are important factors to consider. The larger the size of the paddles used, the lower the resistance of the thorax. The anterior-lateral position for paddle placement is most commonly used (Fig. 8-32). A coupling agent should be used when defibrillating. One should never defibrillate without first applying a coupling agent. Saline-soaked 4 × 4s are an adequate form of coupling agent as well as the commercially available electrode jellies, pastes, prejelled electrodes, and jelled pads. Do *not* use alcohol-soaked pads as a coupling agent, as it is highly flammable and will ignite.

The recommended dosage for defibrillation varies greatly in the literature. We recommend a dosage of 2 watt-seconds/kg in a child, 3.5 to 6 watt-seconds/kg in a small adult (under 50 kg), and a total of 400 watt-seconds for an

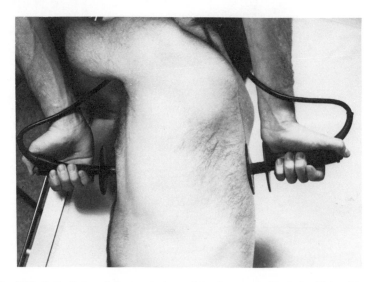

Fig. 8-31. Defibrillation. Anteroposterior paddle placement. (Photo by Richard Lazar.)

adult weighing over 50 kg. If the starting watt-second dosage in the pediatric patient is ineffective, the dosage should be doubled on the second attempt at defibrillation.

Ventricular tachycardia should be treated with synchronous cardioversion (see Ch. 16 for procedure). If the synchronous mode is not available on the equipment being used, one may elect to defibrillate if the patient is hemodynamically compromised. Atrial dysrhythmias that are producing a hemodynamic compromise, such as atrial fibrillation, atrial flutter, and atrial tachycardia, should be electrically treated with synchronous cardioversion.

Remember that electrical defibrillation may produce dysrhythmias as well as correct them. Therefore, one should be prepared to deal with the consequences of the event.

When defibrillating via the external route, one should first assure that the machine being used has a power source, such as a charged battery or a wall current source. Turn the machine on and place the "defibrillate/synchronize" switch in the defibrillate mode. Select the dosage level, and prepare the paddles with a coupling agent. Then place the paddles in the appropriate positions. At this point reconfirm the dysrhythmia by observing the oscilloscope. Once the dysrhythmia is confirmed, apply pressure to the paddles to assure good contact, be sure that the area around the patient is cleared of personnel and electrical equipment, and discharge the current from the machine via the paddles.

Once the current is delivered, interpret the rhythm immediately following. At the same time, assess the patient to see if pulses are present and if spontaneous breathing has resumed.

When internal defibrillation is chosen as the means of defibrillation, replace external paddles on the defibrillator with internal paddles. Use sterile saline as the coupling agent, and apply it to gauze sponges; place them over the internal paddles. The dosage level in internal defibrillation is usually between 10 and 50 watt-seconds in the adult. The procedure is then carried out as for external defibrillation.

Cardioversion

Cardioversion is used as an emergency measure in supraventricular tachycardia with aberrant conduction and in ventricular tachycardia. Synchronous cardioversion is the most rapid method of converting non-digitalis-induced ectopic tachycardias. It may also be used

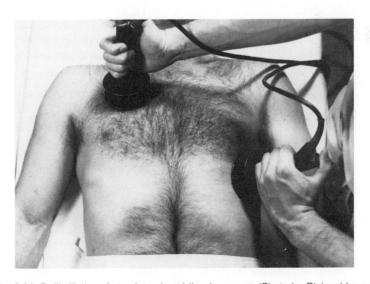

Fig. 8-32. Defibrillation. Anterolateral paddle placement. (Photo by Richard Lazar.)

in those patients with long-term atrial flutter or atrial fibrillation where the patient has become symptomatic because of these dysrhythmias. It is also used in non-digitalis-induced paroxysmal atrial tachycardia (PAT) with block.

Explain the procedure to the patient, and obtain written consent whenever possible and if time permits. If the procedure is nonemergent, the patient may be given a quinidine reaction test. If the patient is on digitalis, withhold it for 24 to 72 hours before the cardioversion (although this is not usually possible in emergency situations.) A safe digitalis level in atrial fibrillation may be a toxic level in normal sinus rhythm.

Whenever possible, give the patient nothing by mouth for at least 12 hours preceding the procedure to prevent the possibility of emesis and aspiration. Obtain a serum potassium level; hypokalemia predisposes the patient to ventricular fibrillation. Ask the patient to empty his bladder before the procedure and to remove his dentures.

If the procedure is an emergent procedure, give the patient a brief explanation of the procedure. If possible, obtain a consent from the patient or family; if not, responsibility for the procedure is assumed by two physicians. Remove the patient's dentures, and draw blood for a serum digoxin level. If the victim is known to be receiving digitalis, a lower watt-second setting should be used during the procedure.

Keep the area as quiet as possible. Have the resuscitation equipment readily available. Start an IV line with an 18-gauge or larger cannula. Diazepam (Valium) should be drawn and ready to administer in bolus form. It should be administered slowly by IV push at small increments until the patient reaches a light phase of unconsciousness. Assure that the victim is disconnected from all other electrical equipment *and oxygen*. Turn on the oscilloscope and synchronous unit. Connect the patient to a running ECG strip. Obtain precardioversion 12-lead ECG whenever possible. Be sure that the machine has been set in the synchronous mode and that the mode has been tested before this cardioversion attempt.

Set the energy level between 25 and 200 watt-seconds. Do a continuous recording of heart activity throughout the procedure. Remember to use a conduction medium between the patient and the paddles. Place the paddles in the anterolateral or anteroposterior position. Quickly check the area to assure that all other equipment is disconnected from the patient and that all personnel are standing clear of the area. At this point give a verbal command, and discharge the electrical impulse.

Observe the patient closely for respiratory rate and ECG rhythm. If the cardioversion attempt is unsuccessful, repeat the procedure using a higher watt-second setting. One may also elect to change to the alternate paddle placement position. If the attempt is successful, do a postcardioversion 12-lead ECG.

Once the cardioversion is completed, check vital signs every 15 minutes for 1 hour, then every 30 minutes for 2 hours, then every 2 hours. Monitor the cardiac rhythm and record any dysrhythmias. Tend to burns that may have been produced during the procedure. The patient should remain in the hospital for at least 24 hours following the procedure for observation. If there are no further problems, the patient may then be discharged from the hospital under a physician's care.

Complications of cardioversion include asystole, junctional rhythms, premature ventricular contractions, ventricular tachycardia, embolization, and reversion to atrial fibrillation or atrial flutter.

Open chest massage (open thoracotomy)

Open thoracotomy and open chest massage may be required in cases of penetrating wounds to the heart, pericardial tamponade, tension pneumothorax, crush injuries to the chest, or chronic lung disease in a patient with a barrel chest when other more conservative measures for chest compression in cardiopulmonary resuscitation have failed. This procedure is reserved only for the trained physician to accomplish.

The victim should be supine and have an esophageal obturator airway or an endotracheal tube in place. Place two large-bore IV lines in peripheral sites. Clean the area where the thoracotomy will be performed with a simple surgical soap solution, and keep surgical draping to a minimum. The physician makes an anterolateral incision in the fourth or fifth intercostal space on the left side of the chest. Spread the ribs by use of a rib retractor and introduce the gloved hand into the chest cavity. This trained hand will be able to note if the pericardial sac requires opening. Then massage the heart with the gloved hand. If possible determine the injury and do a repair. Once the repair is accomplished or the patient is "relatively" stabilized, transport the patient to the operating room as soon as possible for irrigation, repair, closure, chest tube placement, and so on.

Carotid sinus massage

Carotid sinus massage is the procedure usually chosen for patients who are experiencing paroxysmal atrial tachycardia. In carotid sinus massage, pressure is placed on the carotid bodies, which causes an increase in local blood pressure. This stimulates the carotid baroreceptors, which in turn stimulate the autonomic nervous system. This activates the vagus nerve via the parasympathetic system and causes a reflex drop in the blood pressure and heart rate.

The procedure is accomplished by placing the victim in a supine position and administering oxygen at 4 to 6 liters/minute by nasal cannula. Initiate an IV of D/5/W into a peripheral vein and monitor the patient closely. Before applying the actual carotid pressure, auscultate the carotid arteries for the presence of bruits. If a bruit is heard over one of the arteries, eliminate that artery as the site for the massage. Locate the carotid pulse of the victim (Fig. 8-33). Gently press the carotid artery between the fingers and the vertebral transverse processes. Apply the pressure in a small circular motion, rotating backward and medially. This motion should last for no more than 5 to 10 seconds—or less if a rhythm change is seen sooner. If the first attempt is unsuccessful, repeat the attempt. Be sure to always have resuscitation equipment standing by during the procedure. *Never* massage both carotid arteries

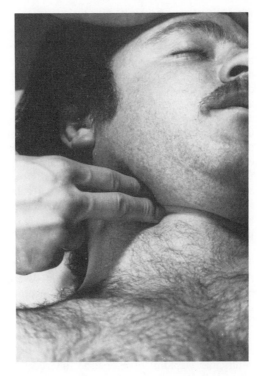

Fig. 8-33. Locate the carotid pulse. Gently press the carotid artery between the fingers and the vertebral transverse processes. (Photo by Richard Lazar.)

at once. If the carotid massage is successful, monitor the patient continuously for several hours following the procedure. Remember that successful conversion is often preceded by a short period of asystole followed by a few PVCs before normal sinus rhythm. If the patient is in atrial flutter, do not use carotid sinus massage, as this procedure may increase the block already present.

Complications of the procedure include further dysrhythmias (such as ventricular tachycardia, ventricular fibrillation, and asystole), cerebral occlusion (which leads to a cerebrovascular accident), cerebral anoxia, and seizures.

Other modes used to produce vagal stimulation in an attempt to decrease heart rate are drug therapy (with norepinephrine or metaraminol), the Valsalva maneuver, emesis, ocular pressure, and facial immersion in ice water.

Electrical mechanical dissociation

Electrical mechanical dissociation is a phenomenon in which ECG complexes are seen but there is essentially no cardiac output because there is no ventricular contraction, evidenced by the absence of a pulse. The patient appears in full cardiopulmonary arrest. Death almost always follows this event, although there are certain causes of electrical mechanical dissociation that may be treated if identified early during this process.

The causes of electrical mechanical dissociation may be divided into three general categories: (1) a decreased preload, (2) an increased afterload (or obstruction), and (3) a decrease in pump action.

A decreased preload may be caused by hypovolemia, cardiac tamponade, or atrial tumors. An increased afterload will be seen in severe pulmonic or aortic stenosis, tension pneumothorax, or massive pulmonary embolus. Decreased pump action can be caused by massive myocardial infarction, severe electrolyte imbalance, and ruptured papillary muscle or intraventricular septum. Therapeutic intervention is to apply therapy specific to the cause of the electrical mechanical dissociation.

Pacemakers

A pacemaker is a lifesaving device used to provide electrical stimulation at low voltage to the myocardium. All pacemakers have a source of electrical energy, usually a battery, and electrical impulse conductors, electrodes. Mercury batteries will last 3 to 4 years; lithium batteries may last up to 7 years. Nuclear-powered pacemakers will most likely be found to have a much longer time of usefulness than any of the other energy sources. There are four types of pacemakers: demand, fixed rate, atrial synchronous, and paired pacing.

Demand pacemaker. The demand pacemaker (Fig. 8-34) is generally used when there is some type of electrical conduction present. The pacemaker senses the patient's own QRS complexes and fires only if a QRS complex is not present after a fixed interval (usually 0.8 seconds). Problems with this type of pacemaker include false sensing of QRS complexes when near microwave ovens, electric razors, electric motors, or radar. It may also malfunction by initiating an impulse on the T wave of the patient's own cardiac cycle, which may lead to ventricular tachycardia. Electrical mechanical dissociation may also occur when a QRS complex appears on the monitor but no pulse is generated.

Fixed rate pacemaker. A fixed rate pacemaker is also known as a conventional pacemaker. It is set at a predetermined rate and fires at this rate no matter what the patient's underlying rhythm is. The problem with this type of pacemaker is that paced beats may compete with supraventricular beats, resulting in ventricular fibrillation.

Atrial synchronous pacemaker. An atrial synchronous pacemaker is used when the ventricles do not respond to the supraventricular pacemaker of the heart. This pacemaker fires after the P wave to cause ventricular contraction. The atrial synchronous pacemaker has a transthoracic placement.

Paired pacing pacemaker. A paired pacing pacemaker is also known as a paired coupling pacemaker. This pacemaker is used in tachycardia or in states of decreased myocardial contractility. It is set to fire at the absolute end of refractory systole so that there is no mechanical systolic response. The heart is unresponsive to this stimulus for a period twice as long as normal, causing an increased contractile force on the next contraction. A complication of this type of pacemaker is the possibility of causing ventricular fibrillation.

There are two methods of placing pacemakers, external and internal. External placement is used in emergency situations as a temporary measure. Electrodes are attached to the skin surface of the chest. This method of pacing is usually not very effective. Internal pacing requires interval implantation of the electrodes by one of two methods: transthoracic and transvenous.

Transthoracic (percutaneous) approach. This approach requires that electrodes be introduced directly through the chest wall and into the myocardium using a special cardiac needle; it is a temporary pacemaker indicated for use in emergency situations.

Transvenous approach. The transvenous

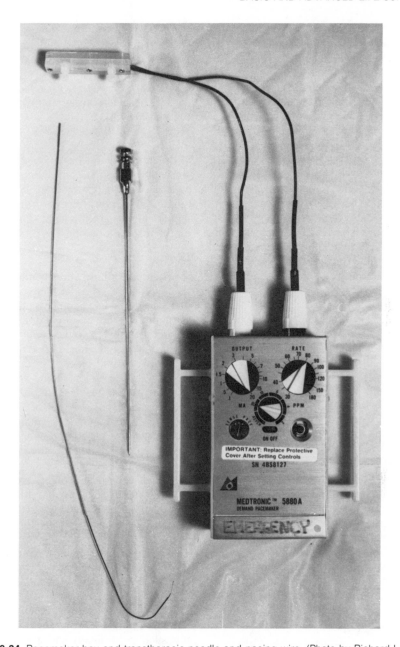

Fig. 8-34. Pacemaker box and transthoracic needle and pacing wire. (Photo by Richard Lazar.)

approach is accomplished with a cutdown. A bipolar electrode wire is introduced into the right antecubital vein or the jugular vein and fed into the right ventricular endocardial surface. This procedure is usually done under fluo-roscopy, or in emergent cases, by connecting the distal end of the pacer wire to the V lead of the ECG machine using an alligator clip. When the wire reaches the endocardium, a current of injury will appear on the ECG print-out. The rate of the transverse pacemaker is usually set at 60 to 70 impulses/minute. If the pacemaker is to be a permanent pacemaker, the batteries and the pacemaker pack are implanted in the subcutaneous tissue of the chest.

Dysrhythmias that may respond to pacemakers include atrial asystole, ventricular asystole, progressive heart block, complete heart block, recurrent bradycardia, and recurrent myocardial irritability.

Complications. If the batteries in a pacemaker wear down and are not replaced, the patient may develop bradycardia, syncope, or cardiac arrest. Other problems that may occur are dysrhythmias, dislodgement, perforation of the myocardium, thrombophlebitis, infection, hiccoughs, electrode fracture (which leads to a nonfunctional pacemaker), and generator failure (which leads to pacemaker failure).

Care. When caring for a patient who has a pacemaker in place, locate the pacemaker generator and check for trauma near the site. Then ask the patient when the batteries were last changed and what type of batteries they are (the patient should carry a card containing this information). Check both the central and peripheral pulses. Then record an ECG strip and observe for the location of a pacemaker spike.

CARDIOPULMONARY RESUSCITATION OF INFANTS AND CHILDREN

Although there are certain aspects of cardiopulmonary resuscitation that are unique to infants and children, it is important to remember that the basic principles of *A*irway, *B*reathing, and *C*irculation remain the same. In the majority of neonates, infants, and children, respiratory arrest is the primary factor in cardiopulmonary arrest, followed by cardiac arrest as the terminal event. It is therefore absolutely essential that airway be obtained and maintained meticulously throughout the resuscitation effort.

Medications are given on the basis of weight up to, but not to exceed, adult dosages. In order to administer the proper dosage of a medication in a neonate, infant, or child it is important to know, or be able to estimate, the weight of the child (see Table 22-1).

Airway

When attempting to maintain the airway of a pediatric victim, do *not* hyperextend the neck of an infant, as this maneuver may block the airway from the posterior aspect. The adult standard esophageal obturator airway should not be used on the child.

Breathing

Breathing should be accomplished by using small puffs of air in the infant and small child at a rate of 20 per minute. When mouth-to-mouth respirations are performed, the entire mouth and nose of the child should be covered by the rescuer's mouth.

Circulation

When performing chest compression to provide circulation, use the index and middle fingers of one hand and compress the center of the sternum on an infant. An alternate method is to use both thumbs to do the compressions. On an older child, use the heel of one hand to perform compressions and place it in the center of the sternum. Compression should be accomplished at a rate of 100 beats/minute; the depth of the compressions should be ½ to ¾ inch in a neonate and ¾ to 1 inch in a young child. Check the adequacy of the compressions by feeling for a pulse with each compression.

Defibrillation, when necessary, should be administered at 2 watt-seconds/kg of body weight initially, followed by double that dosage if the initial attempt is unsuccessful.

Neonatal resuscitation tips

When a neonate is born breathing spontaneously and the heart rate is greater than 100 beats/minute, the baby should be kept warm and dry.

If the baby's breathing is absent or labored, but the heart rate remains above 100 beats/minute, suction the airway and stimulate the infant. At this point, most infants will begin to breathe spontaneously. If the infant does not begin to breathe, begin mouth-to-mouth-and-nose breathing by giving four quick puffs of air or administer four quick units of air using the bag-valve-mask device. If the infant does not

Table 8-3. Pediatric drug dosages*

Medication	Dose	Route
Sodium bicarbonate	1 mEq/kg	IV, dilute 1:1 with D/5/W
Epinephrine	0.1 ml/kg of 1:10,000 solution	IV push
Calcium chloride	1.0 ml/5 kg of 10% solution	*Slow* IV push
Atropine sulfate	0.01-0.03 mg/kg	IV push; must give at least 0.1 mg
Lidocaine	0.5-2.0 mg/kg	Slow IV push
Isoproterenol	0.1-0.5 μg/kg/minute	IV drip, 1 mg in 500 ml D/5/W
Dopamine	2.50 μg/kg/minute	IV, titrated
Naloxone	0.01 mg/kg	IV push
Aminophylline	7 mg/kg loading dose, then 4 mg/kg every 4-6 hrs	IV, initial dose over 20-30 minutes

*Modified from Melker, R.: Crit. Care Q. **1:**49, May 1978.

breathe spontaneously at this time, continue breathing in the methods listed above, check for pulses, use supplemental oxygen when ventilating, and consider endotracheal intubation. Breathing should continue at a rate of 20 to 30 breaths/minute.

If breathing is absent and the pulse rate drops to less than 100 beats/minute, open and suction the airway and initiate artificial methods of breathing. If the respirations and the heart rate continue to decrease, continue ventilation by artificial means and begin external chest compression at a rate of 100/minute. At this point, consider pharmacological intervention. Medications are usually given intravenously, usually using the umbilical vein.

BIBLIOGRAPHY

Ayres, S. M., and Grace, W. J.: Inappropriate ventilation and hypoxemia as causes of cardiac arrhythmias, Am. J. Med. **46:**495-505, 1969.

Baskett, P. J. F.: The role of entonox in pain relief, British Operating Theatres, Publication No. 1 on British Health Care and Technology, September 1972.

Calvert, A., Lown, B., and Gorlin, R.: Ventricular premature beats and anatomically defined coronary heart disease, Am. J. Cardiol. **39:**627-634, 1977.

da Luz, P. L.: Hemodynamic and metabolic effects of sodium nitroprusside on the performance and metabolism of regional ischemic myocardium, Circulation **52,** September 1975.

Fitzgerald, R. T.: Crash cart drugs, Crit. Care Q. **1:**1, April 1978.

Helefant, R.: Nitroglycerine: new concepts about an old drug, Am. J. Med. **60:**905-909, 1976.

Kerr, F., and others: Nitrous oxide analgesia in myocardial infarction, Lancet **1:**63-66, January 1972.

Kerr, F., and others: A double-blind trial of patient-controlled nitrous-oxide/oxygen analgesia in myocardial infarction, Lancet **1:**1397-1400, June 1975.

Killip, T.: Arrhythmia, sudden death and coronary artery disease, Am. J. Cardiol. **28:**614-616, 1971.

McElroy, C. R.: Arrhythmias of arrest, Crit. Care Q. **1:**1, April 1978.

Pantridge, J. F., and others: The acute coronary attack, London, 1975, Pitman Medical Publishers.

Singer, J.: Cardiac arrest in children, J.A.C.E.P. **6:**198-205, 1977.

Standards for Cardiopulmonary Resuscitation (CPR) and Emergency Cardiac Care (ECC): Supplement to J.A.M.A. **227:**833-868, February 18, 1974.

Thornton, J. A., and others: Cardiovascular effects of 50% nitrous oxide/50% oxygen mixture, Anesthesia **28:**484-489, 1973.

Zito, R., Reid, P., and Longstreth, J. A.: Variability of early lidocaine levels in patients, Am. Heart J. **94:**292-296, 1977.

SUGGESTED READINGS

Attia, R. R., and others: Transtracheal ventilation, J.A.M.A. **234:**1152, 1975.

Cauthorne, C.: Coping with death in the emergency department, J.E.N. **1:**24-26, November/December 1975.

Chandra, N., Rudikoff, M., and Weisfeldt, M. L.: Simultaneous chest compression and ventilation at high airway pressure during cardiopulmonary resuscitation (CPR) in man, Circulation Pt. II **58:**203, 1978.

Chambers, W., Miles, R., and Stratbucker, R.: Human chest resistance during successive countershocks, Circulation 55-56, Supplement III, 183, 1977.

Chameides, L., and others: Guidelines for defibrillation of infants and children, Circulation **56:**502A-503A, 1977.

Chaoda, and others: Effects of atropine in patients with bradyarrhythmias complicating acute myocardial infarction, Am. J. Med. **63:**503-510, 1977.

Chopra, M. P. and others: Lidocaine therapy for ventricular ectopic activity after acute myocardial infarction: a double-blind trial, Br. Med. J. 3:668-670, September 18, 1971.

Collingsworth, K. A., Kalman, S. M., and Harrison, D. C.: The clinical pharmacology of lidocaine as antiarrhythmic drug, Circulation 50:1217-1230, 1974.

Criley, J. M., Blaufass, A. H., and Kissel, G. L.: Cough-induced cardiac compression self-administered form of cardiopulmonary resuscitation, J.A.M.A. 236:1246-1250, 1976.

Dahl, C. F.: Myocardial necrosis from direct current countershock: effect of paddle electrode size and time interval between discharges, Circulation 50:956-961, 1974.

Del Guericio, L. R. M., and others: Comparison of blood flow during external and internal cardiac massage in man, Cardiovasc. Surg. I:171-180, 1964.

Gillette, P. C.: Ventricular arrhythmias. In N. K. Roberts and H. Gelbands, editors: arrhythmias in the neonate, infant and child, New York, 1977, Appleton-Century-Crofts.

Glassman, E.: Direct current cardioversion, Am. Heart J. 82:128-130, 1971.

Gordon, A.: Improved E.O.A. and New E.G.T.A. In Safar, P.: Advances in cardiopulmonary resuscitation New York, 1977, Springer-Verlag.

Green, H. L., Heib, G. E., and Schate, I. J.: Electronic equipment in critical care areas: status of devices currently in use, Inter-Society Commission for Heart Disease Resources Report, Circulation 43:A101-A123, 1971.

Greenblatt, D. J., Gross, P. L., and Bolognini, V.: Pharmacotherapy of cardiopulmonary arrest, Am. J. Hosp. Pharmacol. 33:579-583, 1976.

Gutgesell, H. P., and others: Energy dose for ventricular defibrillation of children, Pediatrics 58:898-901, 1976.

Helmers, C.: Assessment of three year prognosis in survivors of acute myocardial infarction, Br. Med. J. 37:593-597, 1975.

Hodgkin, B. C., Lanbrew, C. T., Lawrence, F. H., III, Bonner, R. A., and Irish, J. A.: Improved aortic pressure and oxygenation by modified cadiopulmonary resuscitation, Circulation, Part II, 58:203, 1978.

Humphries, J. O.: Survival after myocardial infarction, Modern Concepts of Cardiovascular Disease 46:51-56, 1977.

Kezdi, P., Kordenat, R. K., and Misra, S. N.: Reflex inhibitory effects of vagal afferents in experimental myocardial infarction, Am. J. Cardiol. 33:853-860, 1974.

Koch-Weser, J.: Antiarrhythmic prophylaxis, N. Engl. J. Med. 285:1024-1025, 1971.

Koch-Weser, J., and others: Antiarrhythmic prophylaxis with procainamide in acute myocardial infarction, N. Engl. J. Med. 281:1253-1260, 1969.

Kouwenhovy, W. B., and others: Closed chest cardiac massage, J.A.M.A. 173:280, 1960.

Kübler-Ross, E.: Death, the final stage of growth, Englewood Cliffs, N.J., 1975, Prentice Hall, Inc.

Kübler-Ross, E.: On death and dying, New York, 1969, MacMillan Publishing Co., Inc.

Kuenzi, S.: Crisis intervention in acute care areas, Am. J. Nurs. 75:830-834, May 1975.

Lewis, A. J., Alshie, E., and Criley, J. M.: Pre-hospital cardiac care in paramedic mobile intensive care unit, Calif. Med. 117:1-8, 1972.

Liberthson, R. R., and others: Pre-hospital ventricular defibrillation, N. Engl. J. Med. 291:317-321, 1974.

Liberthson, R. R., Nagel, E. L., and Herschman, J. C.: Pathophysiologic observation in pre-hospital ventricular fibrillation and sudden death, Circulation, 49:790-798, 1974.

Lown, B.: Electric reversion of cardiac arrhythmias, Br. Heart J. 29:469-489, 1967.

Lown, B., Crampton, R. S., DeSilva, R. A., and Gascho, J.: The energy for ventricular defibrillation—too little or too much? Sounding Boards, N. Engl. J. Med. 298:1252, 1978.

Marks, M. J. B.: The grieving patient and family, Am. J. Nurs. 76:1488-1491, September 1976.

Melker, R. J.: The pre-hospital care of the pediatric patient. In Los Angeles County Paramedic Manuals, Los Angeles, 1977, Los Angeles County Paramedic Training Institute.

Melker, R.: CPR in neonates, infants and children, Crit. Care Q. 1: April 1978.

Melker, R.: Development of the pediatric esophageal obturator airway, Annual meeting, University Association for Emergency Medicine, San Francisco, May 8 to 20, 1978.

Merx, Q., Yoon, M., and Han, J.: The role of local disparity in conduction and recovery time on ventricular vulnerability to fibrillation, Am. Heart J. 94:603-610, 1977.

Miller, S. A.: Dealing with sudden death: the survivors, Crit. Care Q. 1:71-77, April 1978.

Morgan, M. T.: Ventricular defibrillation, Crit. Care Q. 1:43-47, April 1978.

Nieman, J., Rosbrough, J., Garner, D., and Criley, J. M.: The mechanism of blood flow in closed chest cardiopulmonary resuscitation. Abstract presented at the American Heart Association 52nd Scientific Session: Anaheim, California, November 1979.

Ohomoto, T., Miura, I., and Konno, S.: A new method of external cardiac massage to improve diastolic augmentation and prolonged survival time, Ann. Thorac. Surg. 21:284-290, 1976.

Oliver, C. T.: Open chest massage, Crit. Care Q. 1:67-70, April 1978.

Pansegrau, A. F.: Hemodynamic effects of ventricular defibrillation, J. Clin. Invest. 49:282-297, 1970.

Pantridge, J. F., and others: Electrical requirements for ventricular defibrillation, Br. Med. J. 2:313-315, 1975.

Pappelbaum, S., and others: Comparative hemodynamics during open vs. closed cardiac resuscitation, J.A.M.A. 193:659, 1965.

Peterson, B. L.: Morbidity of childhood near-drowning, Pediatrics 59:364-370, 1977.

Raizes, G., Wagner, G. S., and Hackel, D. B.: Instantaneous nonarrhythmic cardiac death in acute myocardial infarction, Am. J. Cardiol. 39:1-6, 1977.

Rudikoff, M., Tucker, M., Taylor, G., Green, H. I., and Weisfeldt, M. L.: Importance of compression rate during external cardiac massage in man, Circulation, **53-54:**225, 1976, Supplement II.

Saunamaki, K. I., and Pederson, A.: Significance of cardiac arrhythmias preceding first cardiac arrest in patients with acute myocardial infarction, Acta Med. Scand. **199:**461-466, 1976.

Schaeffer, W. A., and Cobb, L. A.: Recurrent ventricular fibrillation and modes of death in survivors of out-of-hospital ventricular fibrillation, N. Engl. J. Med. **293:** 259-262, 1975.

Sloman, G., and Pineas, R. J.: Major cardiac arrhythmias in acute mycoardial infarction: implications for long-term survival, Chest **63:**513-516, 1973.

Smith, R. B., and others: Percutaneous transtracheal ventilation, J.A.C.E.P. **5:**765, 1976.

Sodi-Polaris, D., and others: The polarizing treatment of acute myocardial infarction—possibility of its use in other cardiovascular conditions, Dis. Chest **43:**424, 1963.

Solomon, H. A., Edwards, A. C., and Killip, T.: Prodromata in acute myocardial infarction, Circulation **40:** 463-471, 1969.

Spencer, D. C., and Beaty, H. N.: Complications of transtracheal aspiration, N. Engl. J. Med. **286:**304, 1976.

Stephenson, H., Jr.: Cardiac arrest and resuscitation, ed. 4, St. Louis, 1974, The C. V. Mosby Co.

Taylor, G. J., Tucker, W. M., Greene, H. L., Rudikoff, M. T., and Weisfeldt, M. L.: Importance of prolonged compression during cardioulmonary resuscitation in man (Medical Intelligence), N. Engl. J. Med. **296:**1515, 1977.

Thompson, P. L., and Lown, B.: Nitrous oxide as an analgesic agent in acute myocardial infarction, J.A.M.A. **235:**924-927, 1976.

Todres, I. D., and Rogers, M. C.: Methods of external cardiac massage in the newborn infant, J. Pediatrics **86:**781-782, 1975.

Tacker, W. A., and others: Energy dose for human transchest electrical ventricular defibrillation, N. Engl. J. Med. **290:**214-215, 1974.

Tweed, W. A., Wade, J. G., and Davidson, W. J.: Mechanisms of the low-flow state during resuscitation of the totally ischemic brain, Can. J. Neurol. Sci. **4**(1):19-23, 1977.

Wasserberger, J., and Eubanks, D. H.: Pediatric Resuscitation Equipment and Techniques. In Advanced paramedic procedures, St. Louis, 1977, The C. V. Mosby Co.

Weaver, W. D., and others: Angiographic findings and prognostic indicators in patients resuscitated from sudden death, Circulation **54:**895-900, 1976.

Webb, S. W., Adgey, A. A., and Pantridge, J. F.: Autonomic disturbance at onset of acute myocardial infarction, Br. Med. J. **3:**89-92, July 8, 1972.

Willis, W.: Bereavement management in the emergency department, J.E.N. **3:**35-39, March/April 1977.

Winkle, R. A., Derrington, D. C., and Schroeder, J. S.: Characteristics of ventricular tachycardia in ambulatory patients, Am. J. Cardiol. **39:**487-492, 1977.

Winkle, R. A., Glanz, S. A., and Harrison, D. C.: Pharmacologic therapy of ventricular arrhythmias, Am. J. Cardiol. **36:**629-650, 1975.

Worthley, L. I. G.: Sodium bicarbonate in cardiac arrest, Lancet **2:**903-904, October 12, 1976.

Wyman, M. G., Lalka, D., Hammersmith, L., Cannom, D. S., and Goldryer, B. N.: Multiple bolus technique for lidocaine administration during the first hours of acute myocardial infarction, Am. J. Cardiol. **41:**313, 1978.

CHAPTER 9

Laboratory specimens and intravenous fluid therapy

Emergency personnel are responsible for frequent collection of laboratory specimens and initiation of intravenous fluid therapy. The principles and details of these procedures are vital information for the emergency nurse. Although the procedures themselves are not difficult to perform in most instances, they require attention to detail in order to be accomplished quickly, accurately, and without complications.

The site for venipuncture is determined by several factors, including the purpose, accessibility of a suitable vein, and anatomical variables attendant to the age or condition of the patient. These guidelines are useful in site selection for both blood sampling and fluid therapy and are addressed in relation to the specific procedures.

BLOOD SAMPLING
Vacuum tube system

Obtaining venous blood samples is a part of almost every patient's management in the emergency department. Laboratory analyses are useful to establish baseline values and to monitor trends of hematological indices as well as serving a distinct role in diagnostics. Some emergency centers draw routine blood samples on all patients, consisting of a complete blood count, and tests for hemoglobin and hematocrit, blood sugar, and electrolytes. Other studies frequently performed are cardiac enzymes, toxicology screens, drug levels, typing and cross-matching, coagulation studies, and cultures.

For new or acutely ill patients it is always wise to draw an additional tube or more of blood and refrigerate it in case the physician desires additional chemistry tests later in the course of clinical management. It is important that emergency nurses understand the special considerations in obtaining and handling specimens. If certain precautions are not taken with the sample, in some cases, the blood can be rendered useless for study or the results may provide either false or misleading data. These special procedural considerations are pointed out in relation to certain studies.

If feasible, explain to the patient what you are going to do and why. Although most adults have had earlier experience with venipuncture, it is important to relate the steps of the procedure as you proceed. Ensure their comfort by permitting them to lie down or sit down and by positioning and supporting the extremity. Extremely anxious individuals may have syncope, so anticipate this complication.

After the patient is positioned comfortably, wash your hands carefully before proceeding.

Site selection. Locate a large peripheral vein, preferably in the antecubital fossa (Fig. 9-1). Although the wrist, forearm, and back of the hand may be used, these sites are not as desirable, because the patient finds the areas more sensitive to pain and such veins may collapse more readily, especially when a vacuum device is used. Another consideration in site selection is to always reserve a desirable vein

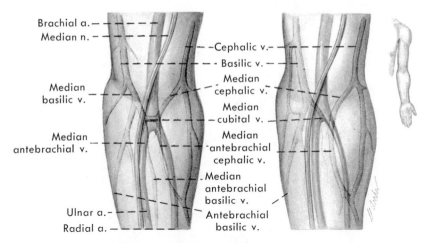

Brachial a.
Median n.

Median basilic v.

Median antebrachial v.

Ulnar a.
Radial a.

Cephalic v.
Basilic v.
Median cephalic v.
Median cubital v.
Median antebrachial cephalic v.
Median antebrachial basilic v.
Antebrachial basilic v.

Fig. 9-1. Relationship of superficial arteries and nerves illustrated by two common vein arrangements of antecubital fossa of left arm. (From Needle and cannula techniques, Chicago, 1971, Abbott Laboratories.)

for IV therapy. Occasionally in the emergency department an individual may have only one good vein because of chronic illness (for example, diabetes, atherosclerosis), previous venesections, IV drug abuse, scarring or tissue destruction from concurrent or previous trauma, or other factors. If such a case is noted, determine the need for IV fluids and collect the samples as the IV is initiated (see p. 203).

Procedure. The vein may be distended by applying a tourniquet or a blood pressure cuff. Palpate distal pulses to ensure that neither device has interfered with arterial flow by assessing for a palpable pulse. Allowing the arm to hang dependently or lightly slapping the site may help raise the vein for puncture. If these measures fail to distend the vein and circumstances permit, the tourniquet should be removed and warm towels applied for 10 or 15 minutes. This measure often will create venous engorgement sufficient for venipuncture. In more serious instances when time cannot be lost, antishock trousers may be used to distend veins of the upper extremity (see p. 247) or the vein may be entered surgically (see p. 209).

Assemble the vacuum device using a single or multiple-draw needle as appropriate. (The multiple-draw needle will prevent leakage of blood into the vacuum container or onto the patient's arm or clothing as tubes are changed. Its container end is rubber-covered, which essentially seals it off between tubes.)

When the vein has been distended and can be palpated, clean the puncture site with antiseptic solutions such as alcohol or povidone iodine. Be certain to check for iodine sensitivity before cleansing. Cleanse the area beginning at the proposed site of insertion and continue to 2 to 3 inches toward the periphery of the target. Use a firm circular motion. Allow the povidone iodine to dry. If the iodine-based solution has obscured the vein, it can be wiped off with alcohol. Do not directly touch the selected needle insertion site; rather, palpate the vein above the needle entry point to avoid recontamination. Alcohol is not immediately effective as an antibacterial agent but does remove desquamated epithelium, skin oils, and surface particles. (Povidone iodine is more effective when skin oils have been removed with alcohol before its application.) Since these agents may induce a counterirritant response and momentary venospasm, wait a minute to actually enter the vein, which will also permit the agents to dry. Instruct the patient to open and close his fist to aid in venous toning and distension that is caused both by pumping blood out of the muscle tissue and

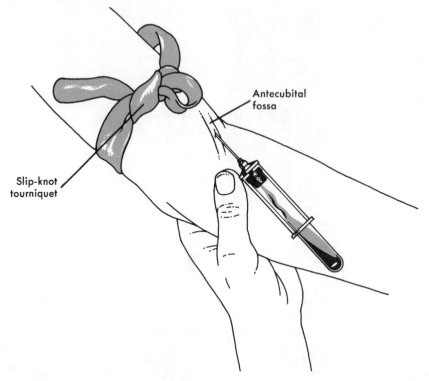

Fig. 9-2. Venipuncture using vacuum tube device. Note position of thumb to stabilize vein. (Right hand of nurse holding collection device has been omitted for visual clarity.)

by the trapping venous blood in the extremity below the tourniquet.

Stabilize the vein with your thumb, and draw the skin taut below the site to prevent the vein from moving as the needle approaches it (Fig. 9-2). Insert the vacuum tube device with the first sample tube attached (at about a 30° angle with the bevel up) into the skin next to the vein (Fig. 9-3). If the vein is quite small, direct the bevel downward (Fig. 9-4). With the vein still stabilized, enter it and remove the tourniquet, permitting the tube to fill. Be sure to allow the tube to fill completely since all chemical additives in the vacuum tubes are calibrated for a full tube sample. If a tube is filled only partially, the disproportionate amount of chemical will distort results in some instances. If a tube fails to fill or fills partially, try an alternate tube before abandoning the site since the problem may simply be a loss of vacuum in the tube or insufficient vacuum to attract the total sample.

If only one sample is needed, remove the tourniquet and then remove the needle, sealing off the site at once with a small, dry, sterile pressure dressing. Avoid using an alcohol wipe since the moisture retards coagulation and irritates the sensitive puncture wound. If the antecubital area has been used, instruct the patient not to bend his arm, because this may cause extravasation of blood into surrounding tissues. Maintain pressure over the site for 2 to 4 minutes to prevent hematoma. This time should be extended for patients with coagulation defects, blood dyscrasias, or those receiving anticoagulant medications.

Meanwhile, if there is an additive in the tube, gently mix it with the blood by inverting the sample eight or ten times. *Do not shake the tube vigorously,* because this action will cause hemolysis of cells, often rendering the blood useless for laboratory study.

Multiple tubes may be obtained using a

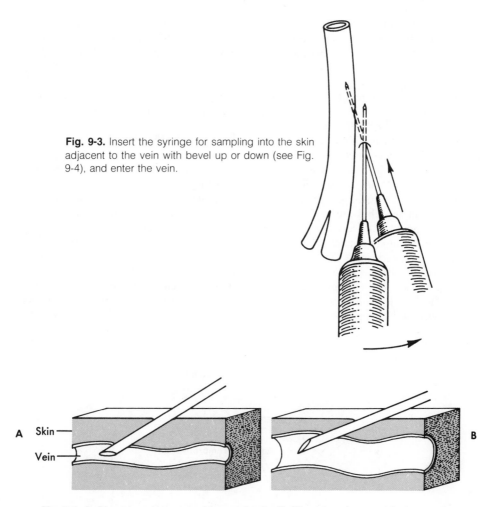

Fig. 9-3. Insert the syringe for sampling into the skin adjacent to the vein with bevel up or down (see Fig. 9-4), and enter the vein.

A Skin

Vein

B

Fig. 9-4. A, Direct bevel downward for small vein. **B,** Direct bevel upward for large vein.

vacuum system. It is imperative, however, to give strict attention to stabilizing the needle device while changing tubes to avoid accidental dislodgment or puncture of the opposite wall of the vein.

If a patient has veins that collapse easily (often the case if there is attendant dehydration), the vacuum system may not be useful in sample collecting. Instead, a syringe technique may produce better results.

Syringe technique

Select a large syringe with an 18- to 20-gauge needle for an adult (or a 19- to 23-gauge for a

child) and proceed with the vein preparation and entry as previously described. When the vein is entered, pull back gently on the plunger to aspirate the sample. Vigorous aspiration or application of undue pressure will cause hemolysis of cells and can induce vein collapse. When the desired sample is obtained and the tourniquet removed, it may be transferred to vacuum laboratory tubes. Do this quickly, before the blood begins to coagulate. Be sure to remove the needle from the syringe and the rubber stopper from the tube to facilitate transfer. *Do not force the blood through the needle.* Complete the transfer gently to avoid damage to cells or the creation of air bubbles, either of which could interfere with accurate results of studies. Replace the stopper and label the tubes carefully before transferring them to the laboratory. A small, dry, sterile dressing may be placed over the venipuncture site.

Pediatric blood sampling

Position and restrain the child as necessary (see p. 496) for a finger stick, heel stick, or regular venipuncture with a pediatric vacuum device. (The appropriate needle size for the collection ranges from 19- to 23-gauge, and 3 to 5 ml pediatric vacuum tubes are preferred.)

Finger sticks should be done on the tip of 4th (ring) finger on the nondominant hand. Avoid "cutting across" fingerprints. The site should be cleaned carefully before the stick and covered with a small, sterile dressing afterward.

All infant heel sticks should be done in the lateral, not medial heel to avoid vulnerable anatomical structures. A Lancet or No. 11 scalpel is used to pierce to a depth of at least 4 mm, and the necessary blood is milked from the site for pipette or slide collection. If the area should clot before all samples are obtained, flow can be reestablished with vigorous scrubbing using an alcohol wipe.

Femoral vein punctures (Fig. 9-5)

The femoral vein is a frequent alternative for venipuncture if superficial veins are not satisfactory. (The subclavian and internal jugular may also be used in extreme circumstances.) Femoral puncture, although a common emergency department procedure, may produce complications, such as thrombosis, pulmonary embolus, or accidental puncture of the femoral artery, resulting in hematoma, thrombus formation, or even gangrene. It is important therefore that emergency nurses be well versed on the technique in order to minimize risks.

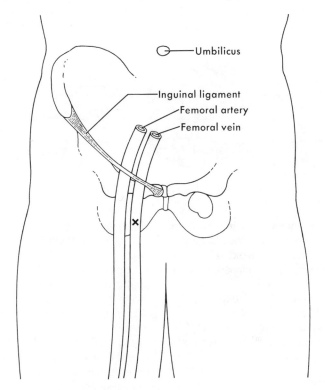

Fig. 9-5. Femoral vein puncture site.

The femoral vein lies medial to the femoral artery. One should therefore locate the pulsation of the latter vessel and make the puncture 1 to 2 cm medial to the pulsation. Although a vacuum device may be used, some clinicians prefer a large syringe for this procedure, because accidental arterial puncture would be more obvious in the nonvacuum system. If the blood is inadvertently arterial, be sure to provide the same care afterward as described on p. 388).

Sampling sequence

When multiple samples are required, the recommended sequence is as follows:

1. Blood cultures
2. Samples without additives
3. Coagulation studies
4. Samples with additives

In emergencies, however, it is suggested that the most urgent sample be obtained first. For example, if there is a questionable drug overdose, the toxicological study is done first; in severe hemorrhage posttrauma, the type and cross-match test is the highest priority. Even the experienced practitioner is sometimes confronted with a clinical situation in which it is almost impossible to get blood samples, so it is important for emergency nurses to set their priorities based on the potential that all samples may not be obtained.

Other considerations

Icing samples. Certain blood specimens require immediate icing to ensure laboratory accuracy. Although protocols for this will vary with institutions and depend largely on the time interval between collection and analysis, ordinarily the following tubes are to be placed in ice:

Lactic acid
Coagulation studies
Arterial blood samples

Infusion site. Sampling should not take place at or immediately above an infusion site unless no other site is available. The infusion could affect hemoconcentration, blood sugar content, and electrolytes, depending on the fluid being administered. If the infusion site must be used,

be sure to note this on laboratory slips and on the chart.

Alcohol levels. It is recommended that a cleansing agent besides alcohol be used when drawing blood to determine an alcohol level. Although there is no evidence that the alcohol wipe affects results, it can later be legally argued that the cleansing agent influenced the test outcome, as opposed to ingested alcohol. Nurses should note on the laboratory slip that alcohol was *not* used to clean the skin.

Zinc levels. Use an ordinary sterile tube and cork stopper for blood drawn to determine zinc levels instead of the typical vacuum tube, which can affect zinc levels because the rubber stoppers contain a considerable amount of zinc.

Ammonia levels. Do not ask patients to open and close their fists, since this activity reportedly affects ammonia levels in the blood.

Blood cultures

In order for blood cultures to have any merit in diagnostics, they must be collected with considerable care. Several important guidelines are essential to follow in order to produce meaningful results.

1. Label the laboratory slip with the time, body temperature, and any antibiotics that the patient is receiving (or has received within a week) in addition to the usual identifying data.
2. Aerobic, anaerobic, and fungal cultures each require a separate sample and bottle type. At least 5 ml blood are required.
3. Change the needle each time a culture medium is inoculated. The amount of blood should yield a 1 : 10 dilution of blood to media.
4. The stopper of the culture medium tubes, the venipuncture site, and the probing finger should be cleansed in an identical fashion. For example, use a 70% alcohol wipe, air dry; apply tincture of iodine, air dry; and use another alcohol wipe, air dry. (The final alcohol cleansing helps in site visualization.) Wipe dry with a sterile 4 × 4 inch gauze sponge before venipuncture. This three-stage process is one recommended method, but the emergency

nurse should ascertain what procedure is required according to laboratory policy. For example, some institutions request that the nurse wear a sterile glove to eliminate possible contamination with the probing finger.

SPECIMENS OTHER THAN BLOOD
Collection of spinal fluid

Three to five test tubes of spinal fluid are usually collected, depending of course, on the tests desired. It is crucial that the specimens be numbered serially during collection. Usually 1 to 2 ml is sufficient for each study. If a problem is encountered during the procedure and only one tube is collected, it should be sent at once to the microbiology laboratory. Under aseptic conditions the specimen should be divided for other hematological and chemical analyses *after* necessary cultures are obtained. Cerebrospinal fluid should always be transported promptly to respective laboratory areas after the lumbar puncture, because a delay may invalidate selected studies.

Urine specimens

Although collection of urine is a routine procedure for most nurses, there are several considerations that the emergency clinician must take into account in order for certain test results to be meaningful.

Urine specimens should be obtained by clean midstream catch, catheterization, or percutaneous bladder tap (see p. 512) as indicated by the clinical condition of the patient. (The exception is the sexually assaulted patient whose urine should be collected without cleansing the genitalia [see p. 483]). Of course, the container should be dry and sterile for cultures and at least dry and clean for other studies. It is highly desirable to split routine urinalysis specimens and refrigerate one portion for later requests such as culture and sensitivity. Do not permit urine specimens to remain at room temperature for more than 30 minutes, because chemical changes begin to occur that affect test results.

In the emergency department it is important to note on the laboratory slip any drugs (or suspected toxic substances) that the patient has taken, because there are many agents that affect test results. Any suspected heavy metal intoxication should be noted, too, because it will speed up laboratory process. At least 20 to 40 ml urine should be collected for toxicological screening.

See pp. 480-482 for genitourinary samples that relate to venereal disease.

Percutaneous fluid or pus specimens

Fluids aspirated from body cavities or wounds should be collected in a sterile syringe and immediately transferred to a test tube or bottle. Anaerobic specimens should be collected before irrigating the cavity or wound. Any air bubbles should be eliminated from the syringe to increase anaerobic conditions. (Many hospitals use an anticoagulant such as heparin in the collection receptacle, because clots tend to trap bacteria.) Note any use of heparin, antibiotics, or steroids on the laboratory slip along with the time of collection. Double-package any specimen suspected of containing virulent organisms, and clearly mark the fluid with an appropriate warning to protect transportation and laboratory personnel.

Emesis and gastric lavage washings

All emesis should be saved for quantitative and qualitative studies.

If gastric lavage has been done, save the initial aspirate from the quantitative specimen. Send all lavage results to the laboratory for analysis.

Be sure to list symptoms and suspected poison on the laboratory slip. Often this information can help the toxicologist delimit his analysis and avoid the prolonged complete toxicology screen.

Stool specimens

Freshly evacuated warm stool is the specimen of choice for culture. Transfer a small sample from the bedpan into a sterile container and send to the laboratory at once. Specimens obtained by rectal swabbing should exhibit visible particulate matter. Do not artificially incubate the specimen for parasites, because certain factors in the stool can be destroyed by heat, such as trophozoites. It is important that liquid stool be examined within 20 to 30 minutes since water can destroy some parasites. Cellophane tape (not frosted) can be used to trap pinworm larvae for microscopic detection when placed over the anus. This technique is usually an overnight routine and seldom falls into the realm of the emergency department.

Collecting throat and sputum cultures

Cultures from the throat or sputum may be needed to help assess respiratory problems. It is desirable for the emergency nurse to know how to obtain these specimens.

A throat culture may be obtained via the nasopharyngeal route (by using a fine, flexible, wire, cotton-tipped applicator), or the throat may be swabbed directly through the oral cavity. Since many patients experience a strong gag reflex during this procedure, the nurse should be prepared for a vomiting episode. This reflexive response can be minimized by accomplishing the task swiftly. The culture should be promptly transported to the laboratory in its designated culture tube.

Sputum should be collected directly into a dry sterile container or one with a fixative that stops autolytic cell changes. Either specimen must be promptly transported to the laboratory. To obtain a reliable sample of sputum, it must come from the deeper tracheobronchial tree. (Saliva is useless for analysis and should not be collected.) Instruct the patient to breathe deeply and cough in order to raise secretions.

Weak or unconscious patients will require tracheal aspirations to obtain the specimen. A commercial mucus trap in conjunction with a suction catheter is usually employed for this purpose.

Forensic specimens

Forensic specimens require special procedures for collection. See Chapter 4 for details.

ARTERIAL BLOOD GAS SAMPLING

Nurses in the emergency department are often required to obtain arterial blood for analysis. The several important steps in this procedure are discussed on pp. 384-388.

INTRAVENOUS FLUID THERAPY

The majority of patients who enter the emergency department as a result of either serious illness or trauma require intravenous fluid therapy. Not only are IVs employed as a mode of supplying volume, but they also serve as a means of rapid access to the circulation for IV drug administration and facilitate central monitoring (see pp. 254-259).

As with other venipunctures, the infusion site is selected based upon the condition of the veins, the purpose of the infusion, the expected duration of therapy, and the comfort of the patient. If possible, a large, straight, and easily accessible vein is preferred. If feasible, consider whether the individual is right- or left-handed, and place the infusion where it will least interfere with arm movement. Avoid the antecubital fossa and the wrist when possible, since either site could result in restricted motion if immobilization is required. It is wise to select the most distal vein on the forearm that is suitable for the infusion. If you encounter difficulty, you can always move more proximal to the antecubital fossa. However, if you spend the antecubital veins initially, lower veins in that arm are rendered virtually useless for venipuncture because of the course of venous blood flow. Lower extremities are seldom used except as a last resort because they tend to produce a number of complications, including thrombi, pulmonary embolus, and site necrosis, especially in the chronically ill or diabetic patient, particularly when irritating drugs are administered or IV therapy is used over an extended period of time. A scalp vein is ideal in infants, and the umbilical vein may be employed in neonates during the first 2 or 3 days of life.

If sclerosing or irritating drugs are to be administered, a large-volume vein should be used so that the substance is rapidly diluted and carried away from the infusion site. As noted earlier, lower extremities should be avoided if possible.

Several factors determine the equipment selected for IV fluid administration. The purpose and probable duration of the infusion and the condition and accessibility of suitable veins must be considered. Table 9-1 outlines some

Table 9-1. Selection of intravenous devices*

Type	Size	Indications	Remarks
Steel needle or butterfly	19-21	Older children or adults	Inexpensive; good for short term or single drug administration; less likely to cause thrombophlebitis even after long-term use; recommended for diabetics since steel is less likely to be irritating than plastic
	21-23	Younger children or elderly with fragile veins	
	25-27	Scalp vein	
Catheter over needle device (angiocatheter)	14-16	Blood or blood products	Device is well tolerated since it is flexible; infiltration is unlikely
	16-20	Crystalloid solutions or medication infusions	
Needle over catheter device (intracatheter)	14-16	CVP Monitoring via central lines or blood administration	Choice for CVP monitoring; excellent for long-term therapy or when large volumes are to be infused; infiltration is unlikely
	18-20	Crystalloid solutions or medication infusions; some blood administration	Flexible catheter can be used at joints without restricting mobility
			Since needle is larger than catheter, ensure that no leakage occurs around the puncture site before dressing is applied

*In the emergency department a large-bore device is generally recommended for trauma because of a high likelihood that blood or blood products may be necessitated.

general guidelines. Common sense is also pertinent. For example, one should not attempt to insert an infusion device that is larger than the vein selected. It may be appropriate, however, to attempt to distend a small vein to accept a larger device if blood component therapy necessitates the use of a large bore needle or catheter when a larger vein cannot be cannulated percutaneously.

Emergency personnel find the regular use of an anesthesia extension tubing helpful because it permits easy access to the needle or catheter for IV drug administration and makes any tubing changes less cumbersome. Of course, the added 8 to 12 inches is useful in preventing tension on the line during the several emergency transfers so common for the patient in the setting.

Needles and catheters

There are four basic types of needles and catheters for intravenous infusions.
1. Metal needle, including the scalp vein needle (butterfly) (Fig. 9-6)
2. Metal needle with mounted plastic catheters or catheter over the needle device (angiocatheter) (Fig. 9-7)
3. Needle over a catheter device (intracatheter) (Fig. 9-8)
4. Inlying catheter used for surgical entry into the vein

The techniques for installing these devices vary. The procedure for initiating an infusion via a scalp vein is discussed and modifications for other devices outlined.

Butterfly. The patient should be made as comfortable as possible and the procedure explained if circumstances make this feasible. Careful handwashing before initiating the infusion is extremely important.

All equipment should be assembled and within easy reach including the fluid, tubing, butterfly needles (always have a spare), antibiotic ointment,* skin cleansing agents, arm board, restraints, IV standard (pole), tape, and tourniquet. Start the flow to clear the tubing of all air and then clamp off the flow. Select the site. If the site is excessively hairy and if time permits, shave the area to improve visualization, reduce the chance for contamination, and

*The use of antibiotic ointment may not be advantageous, since it has been suspected to be a good medium for bacterial growth.

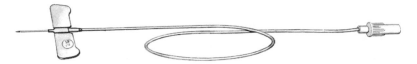

Fig. 9-6. Butterfly winged infusion device. (From Needle and cannula techniques, Chicago, 1971, Abbott Laboratories.)

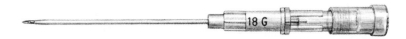

Fig. 9-7. IV catheter with Teflon (catheter over needle device). (From Needle and cannula techniques, Chicago, 1971, Abbott Laboratories.)

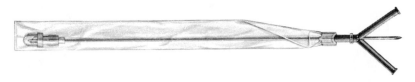

Fig. 9-8. Needle over catheter device. (From Needle and cannula techniques, Chicago, 1971, Abbott Laboratories.)

prevent discomfort later associated with removing tape adherent to hair.

For an adult, the veins on the back of the hand or the cephalic vein are prime choices because they do not roll readily and the infusion can be tolerated well, excepting complications. Avoid joints when using the nonflexible needle devices if possible, because arm boards to enforce immobility are poorly tolerated (see p. 208). The scalp is a suitable location for certain pediatric infusions (see p. 503).

Apply the tourniquet and cleanse the site as previously described (see p. 197). Hold the limb with one hand, and use the thumb to pull the skin taut and anchor the vein. Holding the folded wings, point the needle (bevel up) in the direction of the vein's course, maintaining an approximate 45° angle. Enter the skin to one side of the vein about ½ inch below the proposed site entry. *This is extremely important with a butterfly, because the subcutaneous tissue helps anchor the device.* Reduce the angle of the needle until it is almost parallel to the vein and enter the vessel's lumen. Rotate the needle 180° to prevent posterior vein wall puncture at this point. A backflow of blood should

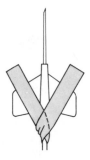

Fig. 9-9. Scalp vein taping.

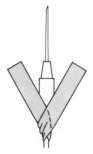

Fig. 9-10. Catheter over needle taping.

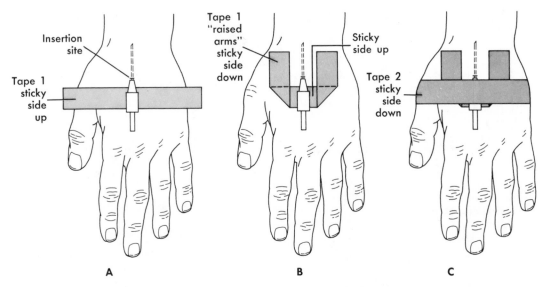

Fig. 9-11. Alternate method of taping. **A,** Tape 1, sticky side up. **B,** Tape 1 "raised arms" sticky side down. **C,** Tape 2, sticky side down.

be noted, and the needle advanced. (To prevent blood from leaking onto the arm or linens, compress the vein just above the needle tip until the tubing is attached.) Release the tourniquet, and relax tension on the site, while still holding the needle in place until the infusion tubing is attached and the device is secured with tape. Adjust the infusion rate and complete the care of the site, including antiseptic cleansing before application of the final sterile, dry dressing.

TAPING AND THE USE OF ARM BOARDS AND RESTRAINTS. It is neither necessary nor desirable to cover the IV site with large bulky dressings because they interfere with important observations of the site. The IV should be taped securely, but this does not mean that several pieces of 3-inch tape be wrapped around the extremity! A common problem of IV therapy is edema of the extremity, and if tape were applied encompassing the entire circumference of the arm and overlapped, a serious interference in blood flow could result.

The butterfly should be secured with ½-inch tape passed below the wings (adhesive side up)

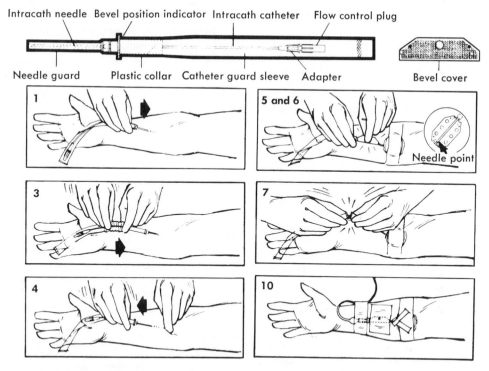

Intracath needle Bevel position indicator Intracath catheter Flow control plug

Needle guard Plastic collar Catheter guard sleeve Adapter Bevel cover

Fig. 9-12. Intracatheter insertion procedure. (Intracath is a registered trademark belonging to The Deseret Co., 9450 South State St., Sandy, Utah 84070. Courtesy The Deseret Co.)

and then the ends of the tape passed obliquely over the wings (Fig. 9-9). *Do not tape the wings flat because this causes the tip of the needle to elevate, which could obstruct fluid flow or even perforate the vein.* Loop excess tubing into a coil and secure all joints with chevron taping.

Catheter over needle devices (angiocatheter). The catheter over the needle device consists of a soft flexible catheter surrounding the venipuncture needle. As with the intracatheter, the needle is retracted along with its stylette after successful vein entry.

As soon as the vein is cannulated, advance the catheter and retract the needle in a smooth reciprocal motion. Discard the stylette, remove the tourniquet and attach the tubing. Using ¼-inch tape, secure the needle at the puncture site by taping the hub of the needle. Loop excess tubing into a coil, and secure all joints with chevron taping (Fig. 9-10). Fig. 9-11 illustrates an alternate taping method.

Needle over catheter devices (intracatheter). An intracatheter consists of a catheter inside a needle. The needle makes the puncture, the long catheter is threaded into the vein, and the infusion established after removal of the stylette. At this point, the needle is retracted, a needle guard placed, and the apparatus secured.

Use of the needle over catheter with adequate skin preparation and continued protection of the puncture site may reduce the incidence of complication often associated with venipunctures, particularly with prolonged use. (If the patient is restless or disoriented, proper restraints must be applied before venipuncture and catheterization are attempted.)

Directions for installing Deseret Intracath
(Fig. 9-12)

1. Prepare for venipuncture, remove needle guard, and make venipuncture in usual manner.
2. Blood flashback in catheter indicates placement of needle in vein. Further flow may be halted

by pressing flow control plug into catheter adapter.

3. To push catheter into vein, grasp lightly with one hand just back of collar. With other hand, grasp catheter ½ inch away and push catheter forward. Squeeze catheter with first hand and return other hand to position on catheter ½ inch away. Repeat procedure until catheter is placed desired distance into vein. CAUTION: If catheter placement is not successful, pull out needle and catheter together. Do not pull out catheter first, as sharp bevel edge of needle may cut catheter as it is being withdrawn.

4. Hold catheter in vein by digital pressure in front of needle. Carefully remove needle from vein and skin.

5. Cover puncture site with sterile pressure dressing, and secure with tape.

6. Place needle cannula completely in channel of bevel cover; make sure catheter is in channel; snap closed.

7. Grasp needle at hub, and with gentle pressure separate collar-sleeve from needle hub; carefully remove over catheter and adapter.

8. Firmly engage catheter adapter to needle hub by sliding needle back along catheter.

9. Remove plug (and stylet on applicable models); connect IV tubing.

10. Secure catheter to skin with chevron cross-over tape technique, between puncture site and needle (as illustrated) to prevent catheter movement. Press tape firmly to catheter. Complete taping procedure. (Used with permission, Deseret Co., Sandy, Utah 84070.)

Periodic inspection. All catheter placement sites should be inspected periodically for flow rate, placement, and security of dressing. Do not remove catheter dressing with scissors, because the catheter may be cut. If catheter extends across an area of flexion, immobilization should be considered to prevent mechanical irritation.

Arm board use

Arm boards may be useful to stabilize the arm. Avoid elbow extension over a prolonged period if possible. The wrist should be straight or slightly extended, however, and the fingers allowed to curl around the armboard or a hand roll, maintaining a position of function (Fig. 9-13).

Special sites for IV infusions

Subclavian vein catheter insertion. A subclavian IV line is useful for long-term infusion therapy and is often used to monitor central venous pressure. It is extremely important that emergency nurses be prepared to help prepare the patient through procedural explanation (if feasible) and positioning. Understanding the steps of the line insertion will facilitate smooth nurse-physician teamwork and improve the chances for a successful subclavian catheterization (Fig. 9-14).

Place the patient in a Trendelenburg (head down) position to engorge the superior veins if conditions permit. If time permits, drape the site of entry and prepare the area for surgery. Use a large-bore intracatheter (14- to 16-gauge) with a syringe attached to pierce the skin 3 cm inferior to midline of the clavicle. The needle is then advanced toward the sternal notch.* The needle must be deep to the clavicle, piercing a layer of fascia before the subclavian vein can be entered. At this point, blood can be aspirated with ease. (If the bevel is pointed toward the feet, a cannula can be passed through the needle into the subclavian vein and on into the vena cava without being damaged by the point of the needle.) At this point the needle is removed and the catheter is sutured into place. Antibiotic ointment may be used before the site is dressed. Complications include pneumothorax, hemothorax, IV infusion into the thorax, air emboli, thrombi, sepsis, and laceration of the subclavian artery. An x-ray film should always be taken to validate correct placement of the line and to rule out any untoward events in the thorax.

Internal jugular catheter placement. Prepare the equipment and skin as previously described, and turn the patient's head away from the selected internal jugular vein site. The needle should enter between the heads of the sternocleidomastoid muscle. Since the target

---

* A new approach to subclavian puncture is to locate a small tubercle by palpating along the inferior border of the clavicle to the medial aspect of the deltopectoral groove. This tubercle is the exact site for needle insertion. It is important for the needle to be held bevel down to avoid accidental catheterization of the jugular vein.

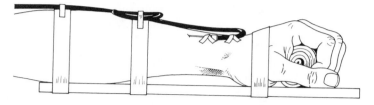

Fig. 9-13. Armboard use.

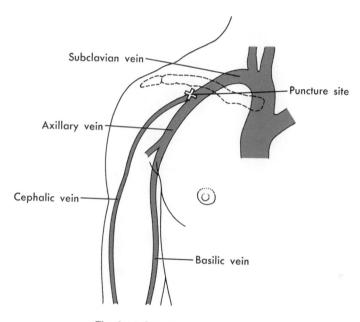

Subclavian vein

Puncture site

Axillary vein

Cephalic vein

Basilic vein

Fig. 9-14. Subclavian puncture site.

vein lies just beneath this point, the needle should be directed at a 45° angle to the skin toward the thoracic inlet between the clavicular and sternal heads of the sternocleidomastoid muscle. When blood can be aspirated, cannulation is confirmed. The catheter should be advanced and secured before dressing the site. Complications include accidental cannulation of the trachea or esophagus, carotid artery perforation, and the several others attendant to the subclavian line. An x-ray film should be taken to ensure proper location of the catheter (Fig. 9-15).

Venesection (venous cutdown). A vein may be surgically entered in dire circumstances to establish an intravenous route when percutaneous line placement is not possible. If antishock trousers are available, they should be used first to see if autotransfusion of lower body blood will adequately distend a vein for venipuncture. Veins of the upper extremity are preferred (cephalic or basilic veins) but the

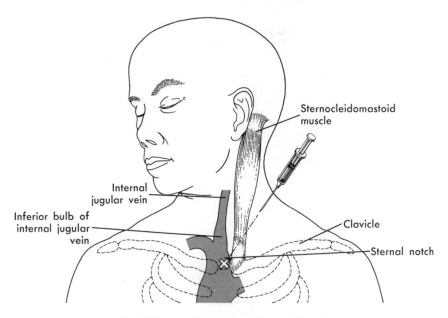

Fig. 9-15. Internal jugular vein cannulation site.

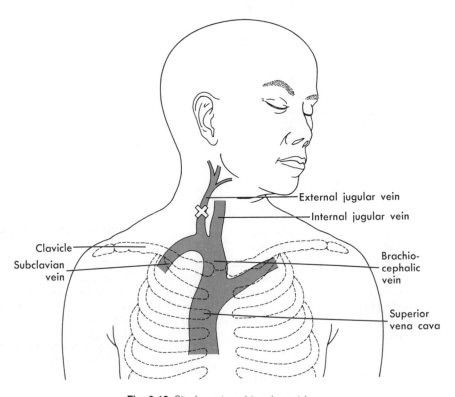

Fig. 9-16. Site for external jugular cutdown.

saphenous vein is also commonly cut down. Occasionally the external jugular (Fig. 9-16) or brachial veins are also used. When the lower extremity can be avoided, the risk of complications is severely lessened. If there is severe injury below the diaphragm, the venesection should be done in the arm to bypass the inferior vena cava and ensure that fluid actually reaches the upper central circulation.

Fig. 9-17 shows the steps of a venesection that can be accomplished in an emergency within a couple of minutes. Most hospitals have venesection trays prepared and shelved for this minor surgical procedure. If not, needed are drapes, a scalpel, one curved clamp, one or two mosquito hemostats, tissue and vascular scissors, No. 15 scalpel blade, 4 × 4 inch sterile sponges, 2-0 silk suture, and a venous catheter (a No. 5 to 8 infant feeding tube bevel cut to the desired length or a No. 3.5 umbilical artery catheter will suffice). The use of a tourniquet is optional. Of course, skin preparation and post-venesection dressing supplies will be required as with other infusion line placements.

Problems in establishing and maintaining an IV infusion

It is not uncommon to encounter difficulty in starting an IV in an emergency. The patient may already have compromised peripheral circulation, or concurrent activity makes the procedural circumstances less than ideal! It is advisable to start at the lowest site that seems practical and move up the extremity for subsequent attempts. Never use a lower point on an already traumatized vein except as a last resort. Use the opposite extremity if feasible.

"Blown" veins (hematoma). The "blown vein" is indicated by a rapidly developing hematoma at the venipuncture. If this should occur, abandon the site and apply firm pressure until hematoma expansion is controlled.

Occasionally, with precipitant or sudden, uncontrolled venipuncture, a vein will swell quickly because of rupture of its posterior wall. This happens most often with catheter over needle devices, which create more friction as they penetrate the skin. The installer may have a tendency to really "push," and with sudden penetration of the vein, both walls are punctured. The site may be saved in some instances by slightly withdrawing the catheter and its needle and attempting advancement once again. Resistance to catheterization of the vessel usually indicates that the device is being forced along a subcutaneous route. In such cases, it is probably advisable to abandon the site and find an alternate one. Firm pressure should be applied to a hematoma for a minute or two to limit its expansion.

Disruption of flow. If the flow of the solution stops, slows, or if edema is present, check for infiltration (see below) and consider that the needle may have "clotted off." Remove the dressings, and check the tubing for kinks. Move the needle or catheter slightly in the vein or withdraw it slightly. Change the position of the patient's arm. If none of these maneuvers is successful in reestablishing the blood flow, aspirate the needle or catheter to check for patency and remove any coagulated blood. *Never* irrigate the needle or catheter, because the flushing could force a thrombus into circulation.

In the rush of an emergency, several other questions should come to the nurse's mind if problems develop. Was the tourniquet removed at the time the IV was established? Is the flow clamp closed on either the main or extension tubing? Is the tape too tight? Is an arm board or restraint interfering with flow? Although these causes seem almost too obvious to consider seriously, they can easily occur in the rather chaotic environment of an emergency setting.

Infiltration. Occasionally the IV needle becomes dislodged from its original position and permits the infusing fluid to flow into subcutaneous tissue. If there is edema, difficulty regulating the flow rate, or if the dripping ceases, suspect infiltration. Infiltration can be verified by applying a tourniquet 4 to 6 inches above the site. If the IV is still infusing into the vein, the drip will cease. If the solution is flowing subcutaneously, the tourniquet will not alter the drip rate. An alternate method to detect infiltration is to lower the IV flask below the level of the puncture site and observe for a "flashback" of blood.

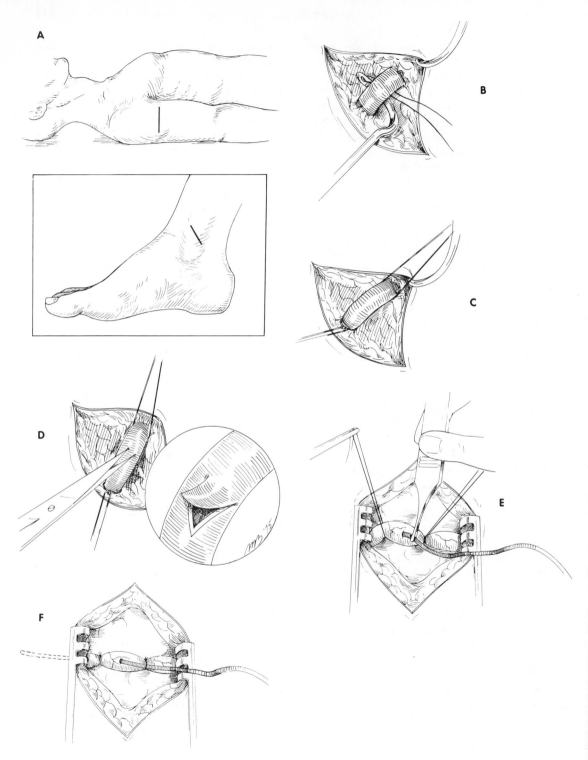

Fig. 9-17. Venesection. **A,** Common sites for venesection. **B,** Isolating vein. **C,** Tying off vein. **D,** Incising vein. **E,** Inserting plastic catheter for fluid infusion. **F,** Catheter sutured in place. (From Barber, J., Stokes, L., and Billings, D.: Adult and child care, ed. 2, St. Louis, 1977, The C. V. Mosby Co.)

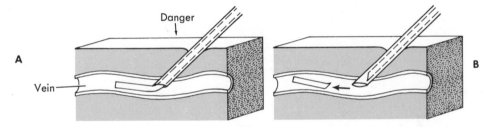

Fig. 9-18. If an intracatheter is removed by grasping the needle, **A,** the catheter may be severed and released into circulation, **B.**

Terminating the infusion

When terminating an IV infusion, proceed with the following steps: (1) stop the solution flow by clamping the tube; (2) remove all tape, arm boards, restraints, and dressings; (3) hold a dry, sterile gauze square over the needle site while removing the needle carefully; (4) apply pressure until all bleeding or seepage has stopped; (5) place a small dressing over the infusion site; and (6) record the amount of fluid absorbed and the time of discontinuation. Note the reason for termination.

Special caution should be exercised when removing an intracatheter. The needle and the catheter must be removed as a unit. Merely grasping the needle may sever the intracatheter, releasing a plastic embolus into circulation and thus creating a life-threatening complication (Fig. 9-18).

SUMMARY

This chapter deals with several common tasks that the emergency nurse must perform daily in order to assess and stabilize patients who are acutely ill or who have been victims of trauma.

Although collection of laboratory specimens and initiation of IV therapy become routine procedures within the nurse's role in the emergency department, continued attention to detail is imperative to maximize their benefit to the patient and to ensure both safety and efficiency in the clinical management.

BIBLIOGRAPHY

Herbst, C. A.: Indications, management, and complications of percutaneous subclavian catheters, Arch Surg. **113:**1421-1425, December 1978.

Kurdi, W. J.: Refining your IV therapy techniques, Nursing '75, November 1975, pp..41-47.

Milliam, D. A.: How to insert an IV, A.J.N. **79:**1268-1278, July 1979.

Needle and cannula techniques (Monograph), North Chicago, Ill., 1971, Abbott Laboratories.

Scranton, P. E.: Practical techniques in venipuncture, Baltimore, 1977, The Williams & Wilkins Co.

Snider, M. A.: Helpful hints on I.V.'s, A.J.N. **74:**1978-1981, November 1974.

CHAPTER 10

Patient teaching in the emergency department

Margaret Miller

RESPONSIBILITIES OF EMERGENCY DEPARTMENT NURSES

The opportunity for patient and family health education is as available in the emergency department as it is in any other hospital department or health agency. However, the rushed emergency department situation, the varied census, and the increased anxiety levels of patient and family place additional responsibilities on the emergency department nurse. These responsibilities include being familiar with the process of teaching and learning, being able to decrease the patient's anxiety levels to enhance the effectiveness of learning, and maintaining knowledge and skills regarding a large variety of health problems. Increased familiarity and use of any process involving knowledge and skill result in greater ease in use of this process and less chance of forgetting the essential steps in the process. For example, in the process of starting an IV infusion, our first attempts are rather awkward because of our unfamiliarity with the equipment and various sequential steps. However, after initiating numerous infusions, our skill proficiency improves to the point where communication with the patient can be maintained while the infusion is being started. It is evident that a high anxiety level inhibits learning. Therefore, the emergency nurse must use verbal and non-verbal means of decreasing the anxiety level of

the patients that we are teaching. There is probably not a single emergency department patient who does not feel increased stress while in an emergency department. Added to the health problem that caused them to come to the emergency department, the emergency department situation itself with the numerous stimuli of bright lights, unfamiliar equipment, strange sounds, and bustling personnel increases the patient's anxiety. In addition, listening to hospital jargon with numerous shortened phrases and long medical terms can cause the patient to feel uncomfortable. Emergency nurses can decrease the patient's anxiety by explaining in laymen's terms what they are going to do and the reason for the procedure either before or while doing it. Nonverbal communication of touch, facial expression and body language can be effective in reducing anxiety. Recalling what our mothers did for us as children when we were hurt or injured brings to mind the effectiveness of nonverbal communication. The simple acts of actively listening to what the patient is saying, staying with the frightened patient, or providing a personal item can decrease a person's anxiety level.

A major problem in providing effective patient teaching in the emergency department is the variety of health problems that people have in the emergency department. This fact places an additional responsibility on the emergency nurse: that of keeping current in knowledge and skills required for self-care for a large variety of health problems. The nurse in the coronary care unit or the orthopedic unit is usually concerned with a single health issue, whereas the emergency nurse must be prepared to teach self-care or home care measures necessary for patients with a multiplicity of health problems. As with most problems, there are several solutions available. Professional continuing education, either through in-service, continuing education programs, or self-instructional methods, is essential. In addition, individuals with expertise regarding the specific injuries or disease processes can develop teaching protocols for the various health problems to be used as a reference in the emergency department. There are numerous reasons for the increased emphasis on patient teaching. Foremost among them are cost consciousness, the promulgation of the Patient's Bill of Rights, and fear of malpractice litigation. The economic situation of increased costs for health care has resulted in the general public focusing on prevention of health problems. We are all well aware of numerous campaigns aimed at prevention of lung diseases, hypertension, and occupational hazards. Recent state and national legislation reflects an increased emphasis on preventive health education as evidenced by the establishment in 1971 of the Presidential Committee on Health Education and the 1974 HEW Health Planning Commission's listing of health education as one of the top ten priorities. Some states have initiated health maintenance organizations that focus on preventive health teaching. Locally, health planning councils are funding home health care departments that promote self-care or professional home care in preference to costly institutional care for persons with chronic health problems.

RATIONALE FOR PATIENT TEACHING

In 1972, the American Hospital Association defined the Patient's Bill of Rights, which includes the right of every hospital patient to be informed of procedures used in providing care and methods of providing self-care follow-ing dismissal from a health agency. In some health care agencies, this bill of rights is given to patients as they are admitted and has been widely reprinted in popular magazines. This has increased the general public's awareness of the responsibilities of health care professionals. In addition, numerous television programs with a health/illness/injury focus repeatedly emphasize that a "good" health care provider is also a health teacher.

During the 1970s the number of malpractice suits has increased dramatically. One of the major causes has been the public's increased awareness of their right to informed consent and knowledge of home self-care methods regarding medications, activity, and precautions necessary because of specific health problems. No longer do most people keep health care professionals on a pedestal and not question their methods. The increased level of public education and publicity regarding errors made by health care professionals have changed this situation. Because of these changes, the need for the preparation of health professionals to provide patient education is evident.

TEACHING/LEARNING PROCESS

To ensure effective utilization of the teaching/learning process, analysis of the sequential components is necessary. The seven components of the teaching/learning process follow.

1. Identification of the expressed or implied learning needs of the patient/learner
2. Assessment of the learner's readiness, capabilities, and motivation
3. Cooperative establishment of realistic learning goals
4. Selection and use of the appropriate teaching method based on the identified need, the content to be learned and the assessed individual characteristics of the learner
5. Provision for time and facilities to facilitate learning
6. Evaluation of the effectiveness of learning
7. Recording of the content taught and the learner's response

To be an effective teacher, the nurse must have knowledge and skills regarding the content area, communicate effectively, and be able to establish rapport with the patient.

Identification of learning needs

The initial step in the teaching process, identification of implied and expressed learning needs, is directly related to the patient's problem. If the patient has an arm fracture requiring a cast, the implied learning need is for methods to care for the casted arm that will promote healing and prevent complications. However, the patient may express his need for additional health education regarding a concomitant health problem or question the advisability of taking certain medications or taking part in various activities. Specific questions the patient asks identify expressed learning needs. If these questions are ignored, the patient may block the information you are attempting to provide regarding cast care. We are familiar with the concepts that unanswered questions are anxiety producing and even moderate levels of anxiety can block learning.

There are two general categories of home care learning needs: techniques or procedural needs and general supportive care learning needs. When technical or procedural care needs are identified, the nurse/teacher should include the following content: what has to be done and why, how to do it, when, the anticipated results of the procedure, a list of necessary equipment and instructions regarding care of the equipment, and situations in which professional help is necessary and whom to call. For example, a patient has a laceration on his finger, requiring sutures. The physician has prescribed antibiotic ointment application twice daily with reapplication of a sterile dressing. This procedure will require cleansing of the sutured and surrounding area, ointment application, and dressing changes. The nurse explains why this is necessary—to prevent infection—and demonstrates the method. In defining frequency, the nurse might relate this to mealtimes or simply morning and night. A verbal explanation of a noninfected sutured wound and possibly a visual aid is necessary to identify anticipated results. The same method can be used to de-

scribe or show an infected suture line that would necessitate professional help. Either providing the patient with the prescribed ointment and dressings or giving him a prescription for them is necessary. Many emergency departments now give the patient a card with the name and phone number of the health professional he should contact if further problems arise.

In the category of general supportive care, the nurse/teacher selects the appropriate content from a list of potential needs. Included in this broad category is pertinent information regarding: hygiene, rest requirements, nutritional and elimination needs, skin and pressure point protection, correct body alignment, necessary position changes, oxygenation and ventilation needs, range-of-motion and activity levels, safety factors, scheduling of medications and other therapeutic measures, as well as means of providing for emotional well-being. As we can see, the educational needs list can be very long, which requires knowledgeable selectivity on the part of the emergency nurse in identifying the specific learning needs of each patient.

Patients being transferred to another unit either within the agency or to another health care facility also have learning needs. Specifically, they need to know where they are going, how they will get there, and the rationale for their transfer. Explaining the rationale for and the logistics of the transfer can prevent higher anxiety levels and undesirable physiological responses to stress for the patient.

Assessment of learner

After identifying the probable learning needs of the patient, the nurse must assess the status of the learner regarding his readiness to learn, his capabilities, and his motivation. Numerous factors influence the patient's readiness to learn self-care measures, including age, educational background, socioeconomic and cultural influences, his present anxiety level, concomitant or previous health problems, treatment methods that have been instituted, and his self-concept. The nurse can obtain this information from a variety of sources. The patient's record indicates the patient's age and family status as well as his nationality, ability to finance health care, and possibly his economic/social grouping revealed by the location of his home. However, most of the necessary information is obtained by interviewing the patient and making pertinent observations. For example, we ask patients about allergies, medications taken at home, and present health problems during the admission procedure. The patient's method of speaking or answering questions may be an indicator of educational background. The patient's record will indicate diagnostic and therapeutic measures that have been or will be initiated. It is important to plan the time for patient teaching in order not to interfere with or counteract other therapeutic methods. To illustrate, if a patient has received a CNS depressant, the stimulus of initiating patient teaching might counteract the desired effect of the medication. Observation provides us with additional information. If the patient's basic physiological needs are not met, his readiness to learn is definitely diminished. When a person is experiencing hypoxia, dehydration, malnutrition, inadequate elimination or rest, or is in acute pain, initiating patient teaching is unproductive. These situations require immediate remediation. Patient behaviors or appearance that might indicate a poor self-concept are poor hygiene, lack of eye contact, or muffled voice quality. An inadequate self-concept can block learning.

In assessing the patient's capabilities to learn, look for physical limitations that would prohibit the learning of some skills. Physical wholeness and dexterity are prerequisites to learning some home care techniques requiring use of psychomotor skills. If the person has had previous experiences to which we can relate present learning, learning is much easier. By using similes and analogies to define or explain content, the new learning situation becomes much more meaningful. In assessing motivation level, we look for verbal, nonverbal, and behavioral clues. Verbal clues indicative of increasing motivation levels might be specific questions the patient asks or his initiation of discussion regarding home care of his condition. A less direct verbal clue of increased motivation is a statement such as "I'm going to have to learn how to do that" or general

observations regarding what the nurse is doing. Nonverbal clues might be changes in facial expression indicating increased interest in what the nurse is doing. Watching rather than looking the other way can be a clue. Observation of independent behaviors can indicate increased motivation. Small independent actions such as reaching for a tissue show a degree of independence indicative of increased motivation and a desire to change from the dependent, sick role. Physical behaviors and the degree of muscle tenseness can indicate excessive anxiety, which interferes with motivation and readiness to learn. Persons who are anxious may exhibit either excessive or decreased activity of voluntary muscles. Although one person may exhibit withdrawal behaviors such as maintaining a fetal position, covering the face, or lowering the eyes to decrease contact with others, the majority of anxious people exhibit overactive behaviors. They might tense arm, facial, and neck muscles, exhibit excessive oral behaviors, fidget with covers, or develop tremors when attempting purposeful motion.

Information regarding the patient's age can help us determine his ability to understand specific learning content or adhere to self-care measures. A two-year-old child is incapable of comprehending and does not have the refined motor skills necessary to change a bandage. Therefore, a parent or guardian is the person we would teach. An elderly person may have the learning capabilities but many times requires more time for comprehension.

With increased travel opportunities and the immigration to the United States of people of various cultural and ethnic backgrounds, language can present a problem. If the emergency department staff is unable to converse in the patient's language, a resource person must be obtained. Many hospitals now maintain a list of persons in the community who are willing to assist in these situations. Not only can they help with language but also with their knowledge of cultural factors that will either enhance or detract from adherence to home care measures we are teaching. In the teaching situation, we need to build on the assessed strengths and minimize or delete the factors that will inhibit learning.

Establishment of goals

The third step in the teaching/learning process is establishing realistic, individualized learning goals. Learning goals should be realistic in terms of the assessment data we have obtained and time constraints. For example, if the patient has a fractured leg and concomitant diabetes, a hangnail, and a cold, emergency department personnel would need to determine the paramount learning needs and not try to cover all the learning needs of this patient. Because of his diverse problems, the patient would probably not be able to comprehend all the information if you tried to ''cover the waterfront.'' A realistic focus might be on two of his needs. You might share with the patient the learning needs you have identified and ask him what he feels is most important to him, thereby cooperatively establishing his learning goals. Because you cannot meet all his needs, referral to community agencies or local groups such as the Diabetes Association clinics or health maintenance organizations is necessary. Local phone companies and public health agencies publish listings of resources available in various communities. This can be a handy reference for any emergency department.

To individualize the teaching/learning process, it is necessary to interview the patient to find out his work and home situation and to identify potential problems he might have in adhering to prescribed home care measures. To illustrate, a patient comes to the emergency department with acute back pain that occurred after 2 hours of sawing, lifting, and stacking logs for his fireplace. Following x-ray films, it is determined that he has strained his back, so he is given a muscle relaxant and taught proper lifting and bending methods. It would also be appropriate to find out this man's occupation. If he has a desk job, his return to work the next day would not interfere with his recuperation. However, if his job involved loading trucks, requiring much bending and lifting, return to work would be delayed until recuperation is determined. The taking of his medications should be correlated with his work schedule for maximum effectiveness. Remember that absorption of medication depends on metabolic rate. If the patient has a work schedule of 4 PM to 12 midnight, his schedule for taking the prescribed muscle relaxants will be different from a person working from 9 AM to 5 PM. Discussing the scheduling of taking medications is one component of the teaching process.

In addition to considering the patient's home/work situation, the nurse/teacher needs to identify individualized adaptations necessary because of a person's past experiences with self-care, potential job-related problems, and family or cultural taboos and expectations. If the person has had positive experiences with self-care, his attitude toward learning is more positive. It is advantageous to use methods and approaches that have been successful on previous occasions. For example, if a patient finds it is easy to remember taking prescribed medications related to mealtimes, that approach should be used. For some people, keeping a record is helpful in assuring that medications taken or treatments done are following the prescribed timing. After all, charting is the method a nurse uses to keep track of giving medications. By identifying why patients have not adhered to prescribed home care measures, you might be able to minimize a negative attitude toward learning as well as discover what approach to use in teaching. For example, many younger persons learn best using various types of audiovisual machines, whereas an older person may prefer discussion or demonstration. Occasionally, people will state the reason they did not follow through with home care measures is that they feel they could have learned something much easier if their ''favorite'' method had been used.

Some occupations, either because of the nature of the work or unusual hours, may cause problems with follow-through in home care measures. To illustrate, consider the needs of a long-haul truck driver who is treated for a bladder infection. The physician prescribes sulfisoxazole (Gantrisin) 500 mg four times daily. Recognizing the sulfa base of this medication, you will need to teach him the need for increased water intake to prevent formation of sulfa salt urinary stones. Because of the nature of his work, you will need to discuss methods of having fluids available, probably a thermos, as well as the kinds of fluids that produce the desired acid ash.

Occasionally the individual's or family's expectations for the person treated in the emergency department conflict with adherence to prescribed home care measures. Consider the workaholic patient who is treated for recurrent angina. Possibly because of either financial reasons or his role in his family, he states he is leaving the emergency department because he needs to get ''right back to work.'' Obviously we are not going to change this individual's culturally based life-style with a single teaching opportunity in the emergency department; however, we would want to seize this teaching opportunity to explain the causes and effects of angina, the anticipated results of the prescribed medications, as well as factors that may cause or precipitate the condition. To reiterate, our objective is to elicit data and adapt our approach in establishing realistic, individualized learning goals that will help the patient provide self-care and prevent complications.

Selection of teaching method

The fourth step in the teaching process is the selection and use of the teaching method appropriate to the content to be taught and the assessed capabilities of the learner. Many patients require only informal teaching, such as answering their specific questions or a quick review of previously learned content; an example is the person with numerous children, several of whom have had fractures requiring casts. Other patients, however, require a more structured teaching approach in which specific learning needs are identified and a planned learning experience is necessary. There are three types of learning: cognitive, affective, and psychomotor. Cognitive learning involves thinking and reasoning, which results in new understandings. Affective learning involves a change in attitude or values. This type of learning takes more time than either cognitive or psychomotor learning. To achieve a learning goal based on affective needs will most likely necessitate referral to a community health agency or health-related group such as the ostomy or stroke clubs, church groups working with drug abuse clients, and so on. Psychomotor learning involves matching brain and extremities to complete a task. Following demonstration of a skill, the person should have practice time before an evaluative return demonstration.

In general, the content and learning goal dictate the most appropriate teaching method. For example, if the patient needs to learn sterile dressing change, the most appropriate method is demonstration. However, explanation of the rationale and discussion regarding necessary equipment and potential problems is also necessary. Planning ahead regarding essential content, necessary equipment, and potential resources gives the nurse a feeling of self-confidence that is imparted to the patient. Advance planning also decreases interruption of the teaching/learning process.

The effectiveness of learning depends on several principles. A major tenant of adult learning is that active participation by the learner increases the meaningfulness of learning. This is the reason that a two-way discussion and demonstration followed by practice are more effective than a lecture of dos and don'ts. Incentives, physical and verbal, motivate learning. Physical types of incentives such as balloons, suckers, or a box of raisins are effective motivators for children. Adults, typically, respond to verbal and nonverbal positive reinforcement. Sincere statements accompanied by appropriate nonverbal behaviors usually stimulate the patient to learn more effectively and maintain desired behaviors. To increase internal motivation (a feeling of ''I need to know that''), we should explain the rationale and importance of self-care measures we are teaching. By using analogies and similes, we utilize another principle of learning: building on past knowledge or skills, thus increasing the ease and speed in learning new content or skills. Recalling the age-old statement that ''nothing succeeds like success,'' we attempt to provide successful, motivating experiences by starting with the easiest content and proceeding to the more complex concepts. This is the basis of education—learning words before sentences, adding before multiplication, and so on. An accepting, comfortable atmosphere motivates learning; however, a mild degree of anxiety promotes learning. We are all familiar with another basic principle: repetition strengthens learning. This is particularly true of psychomotor skills.

There are numerous teaching methods—discussion, demonstration, question and answer, visual aids, as well as the lecture—with which we are all so familiar. The advantage of lecturing or "telling" is speed, but the disadvantages far outweigh the advantages. Telling the patient violates all the principles of learning stated above. The advantages of the discussion method are that it involves two-way communication and allows for incorporation of the principles of effective learning. Using visual aids as an adjunct increases the sensory experience of the patient and gives meaning to abstract terms or concepts. For example, showing the patient with a fracture the x-ray film of his broken bone provides him with a graphic, realistic picture of his problem. A chart or picture showing the location of body parts can be a help in defining anticipated effects of prescribed treatment or in explaining the extent of trauma. Demonstration is the most effective method for teaching skills. You can spend 30 minutes explaining the technique of figure-eight bandaging, but a 5-minute demonstration will be more meaningful. When demonstration is used, it is essential that the patient have an opportunity for practice and to return the demonstration so that errors can be prevented. The question-and-answer method of teaching is the most direct, since the patient is requesting specific knowledge, and the nurse responds to his specific learning need. In reality, more than a single teaching method is used in each teaching/learning situation. The content dictates the appropriate methods to be used.

One requirement common to any teaching method is that the nurse-teacher must communicate effectively. Using our assessment data, we should speak at the level of the learner. Remembering that the goal of communicating is mutual understanding, we should use common, nontechnical words rather than multisyllable words. Because we are using health care terms, we must define words that the patient does not comprehend. We should avoid intermingling hospital jargon or medical term initials that are not intelligible to the layman. Matching our tone of voice, facial expression, and body language with what we are saying adds emphasis to our statements and prevents the patient from receiving conflicting messages from us. Learning takes time; hence, rushing our communication with the patient only serves to inhibit learning. Allowing time for the patient to restate, rephrase, or ask questions will enhance learning. We, as teachers, need to actively listen and become astute observers of both signs of understanding and expressions of fear or doubt. Proceeding with the teaching process in the face of fear and doubt is unproductive. Since we obviously cannot know all about every topic, we should not be afraid to say "I don't know." If a patient asks a question that we are unable to answer, it is necessary for us to find the answer and get it back to the patient. A humanistic approach to teaching is appreciated. To illustrate, sharing our own experiences in self-care with the patient can be beneficial. If you have developed a method for keeping track of taking medications, such as a calendar chart, share your successful method with the patient. Because enthusiasm in the learning situation is contagious, we should exhibit enthusiasm for teaching patients home care measures. To maintain our enthusiasm for teaching specific content, increasing the variety of teaching methods we use allows us creative expression. In addition, a variety of teaching techniques benefits the patient/learner, particularly when we use his "best way to learn."

Providing facilities and time

After our teaching plan is implemented, it is helpful to provide the patient with some time to practice newly learned skills and absorb the content you have taught. Lack of space in a busy or small emergency department can prove to be a problem. However, the patient does need a place to practice or reflect on potential questions or concerns. The possibility of using an adjacent office or conference room might be considered, because this would provide the proximity to allow the nurse to stop in and observe skills or answer questions as they arise.

Evaluation

Evaluation of the effectiveness of learning is the final step in the teaching/learning process. The content and teaching method dictate the evaluation method that should be used. For example, if discussion has been used to teach home care of a casted limb, you might ask the patient to restate or rephrase what he will do at home to prevent the cast from getting wet. If a visual aid has been used to show the figure-eight method of bandaging, you might ask the patient to identify, on his body, areas requiring the thickest part of the bandage. Following the demonstration of a skill and practice time, a return demonstration is the evaluative method of choice. Rephrasing in the patient's own words is more difficult than restating exactly what you have said. The ability to rephrase indicates a higher degree of comprehension than restatement. Another valuable evaluation method is asking "what if" questions. For example, if a patient is to be dismissed with an anticonvulsant medication, a question you might ask to evaluate the patient's understanding of the need for maintenance of consistent anticonvulsant blood levels might be: "What will you do if you have the flu and vomit your morning pill?" Incidental observations of behaviors indicating incorporation of new learning into the patient's repertoire of behaviors is another valid evaluation method. To illustrate, you have taught a patient with dependent ankle edema active range-of-motion exercises. As you pass the door of his room, you observe him doing the exercises without prompting. If a patient asks pertinent questions related to self-care in his family or work situation, this demonstrates his ability to correlate new learning with his real life situation. As we all know, there is no such thing as a dumb question! It is difficult to evaluate attitudinal changes in the rushed emergency department situation, but it is possible on occasion. For example, the uncontrolled or new diabetic says she will attend the local diabetes association's group meetings. This indicates an interest in self-help. More valid evaluation methods are follow-up phone calls to the association to ascertain if the referred patient did attend or a report-back system from referral agencies to the referring emergency department. Statistical data regarding patient readmission for the same health problem may be used to evaluate the effectiveness of learning.

Documentation

After completing the sequential steps in the teaching/learning process, documentation on the patient's record is necessary. Because of the JCAH criteria, it is essential for emergency department nurses to accurately document patient teaching done and the patient's response. It is just as important legally to record patient teaching as any other therapeutic measure. As with all other measures initiated, the nurse records specifically what content was taught and how, and the patient's response, as well as the time and nurse/teacher's name and status. To illustrate: "9:45 AM: Demonstration of hand bandage change. Correct return demonstration using sterile technique. Home care instruction sheet 'Bandage Changing' given to patient. M. Miller, RN." If someone other than the patient is taught, that person's name and status should be recorded in the patient's record.

HOME CARE INSTRUCTION SHEETS

Recalling that high anxiety levels decrease retention of newly learned content and skills, it is advisable to develop home care or self-care instructional handouts for the most common patient problems in your emergency department. Statistical data concerning your admissions can serve as a guide in setting priorities for the development of home care instructions. Who should develop them? Because emergency department personnel have traditionally worked cooperatively and all emergency department nurses will be using the handouts, it seems logical that the instruction sheets should be developed by the staff. The home care guides may be developed by individual nurses according to their special interests, but others in the department should have an opportunity for input. Because involvement begets commitment, the more group work there is, the more effective the outcome will be. It is important to use laymen's terms when developing home care guides. To illustrate, if your patient is to apply an ointment to his sutured finger in the morning and evening, stating "b.i.d." on the instruction sheet is inappropriate. Home care guides should be "short and sweet and to the point." Areas of content that should be included are specific care measures that you have taught and objective signs and subjective symptoms indicating that he should either call his doctor or the emergency department. The benefits of these home care guides are that they provide a checklist for the patient and they decrease the number of call-backs with questions on home care. Following development by either individual nurses or the staff, a constructive critiquing and a specified trial period should be instituted. This permits more input and allows the ED staff to refine the content or wording. Some agencies decide that color coding the various patient instruction sheets is an advantage in sorting and selecting the necessary sheet. It is essential to recall that the home care instruction sheets are only an *adjunct* to the individualized approach of the nurse/teacher.

Because of rotating staffs and the emergency department crisis-like situation, emergency department staff may forget to include important home care measures. To minimize this possibility, the staff can develop a patient teaching plan file for a handy reference in the department. Using a file card or loose-leaf book system, the staff can outline the following information: patient problem and diagnosis, potential resulting problems, therapeutic preventive and restorative home care measures, specific content and equipment lists, and suggestions regarding teaching and evaluation methods. The patient teaching plan file should be developed according to the same priorities as the home care instruction sheets—based on the statistical data regarding your patient census. To assure inclusion of patient teaching in patient care, an annual or semiannual in-service program on the use of the teaching plan file and the home care instruction sheets, and a

review of the teaching/learning process would be helpful for new as well as experienced staff. Including the patient teaching process in the orientation of new staff is essential.

Two assurances that patient teaching will be an integral part of emergency department patient care are inclusion of the teaching plans and home care instruction guides in the emergency department policy/protocol manual and incorporation of patient teaching into the staff performance appraisal form. The inclusion of patient teaching into the chart audit criteria of the JCAH has provided impetus to ensure the integration of patient teaching in the patient care plan.

CONCLUSION

To ensure adherence to therapeutic, restorative, and supportive self-care measures and prevent potential complications following treatment in the emergency department, it is the responsibility of the emergency nurse to provide effective, individualized instruction regarding home care measures. The emergency nurse must be familiar with the sequential steps involved in the process of patient teaching, as well as documentation of instruction given and patient's response. The process of patient teaching includes the following: identification of learning needs; assessment of the learner's readiness, capabilities and motivation; cooperative establishment of realistic learning goals; selection and use of the appropriate teaching method based on the assessment data; provision for time and facilities necessary for learning; and evaluation of the effectiveness of learning. The process is not complete until the content taught and the learner's response is documented on the patient record. Application of the principles of teaching and learning and effective communication are basic to instituting patient teaching plans.

To ensure the integration of patient teaching into each patient's plan of care, protocols and policies on patient teaching should be written and the process of patient teaching included in emergency department staff orientation and in-service programs, quality assurance audit criteria, and staff performance appraisal forms.

A tool that is helpful for both nurse and patient is the home care instruction sheet. These can be developed by the emergency department staff either individually or using group process based on the typical patients in the emergency department. Development of a patient teaching plan file provides the emergency nurse with an easily accessible reference. Since knowledge of home self-care measures is one of the rights of patients and will also benefit the department staff by reducing the number of call-backs or return visits to the emergency department, it is essential that patient teaching be considered as an integral part of emergency department patient care.

EXAMPLES OF AFTERCARE PROCEDURES

Home care for an overdose

1. Limited activity for 24 hours.
   a. No school for children.
   b. No work for adults.
2. Clear, cold, sweet liquids for 8 hours followed by reduced amounts of food for the next 24 hours. Force fluids by mouth.
3. Check level of consciousness, breathing, and pupils every hour for 12 hours, then every 4 hours for the next 12 hours.
4. In a small number of cases, signs of serious injury may appear later, so see your doctor for a check-up.
5. Appearance of any of the following signs means that you should consult your doctor immediately:
   a. Nausea and/or vomiting.
   b. Unusual sleepiness or difficulty awakening. (Wake up the patient every hour during the first night.)
   c. One pupil much larger or different from the other; peculiar movements of the eyes, or difficulty on focusing.
   d. Weakness, paralysis, or numbness of arms or legs; peculiar gait, stumbling.
   e. Mental confusion or disorientation. (Excessive drowsiness, change in personality, inattentiveness, incoherent thought, inability to concentrate, stupor.)
   f. Irregular or labored breathing.
   g. Persistent dizziness.

Head injury

You have been examined by the emergency room physician for a head injury. The physician does not feel you need hospitalization. However, in some cases something may happen after you leave the hospital. Read carefully the problems below, and call your doctor or the emergency unit if any of these develop:
1. Severe or continuous headache
2. Nausea or vomiting
3. One pupil different from the other, or if a light shown into the eye will not make the pupil smaller.
4. Excessive or increasing drowsiness, difficulty in arousing, or change in personality.
5. Weakness or numbness of arms or legs, peculiar gait, or stumbling.
6. Convulsion or "fit."

We also suggest you do not operate any moving equipment until you are feeling better.

Suggestions for care of back strain

1. Put boards under your mattress if it is not firm. Resting flat in bed is important. Usually it will feel better to put a pillow beneath the knees, so that they and the hips are slightly bent.
2. Apply heat to the painful area of your back, using a heating pad or warm water bottle. Wrap the heat source in a towel to protect the skin.
3. Take medications as follows:_____
_____.
4. No lifting or straining if at all possible.
5. If your symptoms persist, see your physician or return to the Emergency Department for further evaluation.

   The interpretation of your x-ray film as given to you by the physician in the emergency department is only a preliminary report. The x-ray specialist reviews these films, and if there is a change in the diagnosis, you and your doctor will be notified in 24 hours.

Suggestions for care of a sutured laceration

1. Keep the wound and dressing as clean and dry as possible. Change your bandage only if it gets wet or dirty.
2. If your laceration starts to bleed, press firmly over the dressing with your fingers. If this does not stop the bleeding, come back to the emergency department, or contact your private physician.
3. Watch for signs of infection:
   a. Swelling
   b. Excessive redness
   c. Drainage
   d. Pain
   e. Heat—either local or systemic as shown by a fever.

   If these symptoms occur, return to the emergency department or contact your private physician.
4. It is advisable to have your laceration examined

by your physician in 48 to 72 hours. He can detect early signs of infection.

5. Contact your private physician for an appointment for suture removal on _____.

Cast care

A cast is applied to a broken bone to maintain it in correct alignment. To safeguard the efficiency of a cast, follow the instructions below.

1. No bathing in shower or tub until the cast is removed. Do not try to cover your cast with plastic. This is not effective, and the cast is ruined when wet. You will have to take a sponge bath.
2. If your cast is made of one of the new plastic materials (not plaster), you may get it wet.
3. Do not put any sharp object down your cast to scratch. This may open the skin and cause infection.
4. Keep the casted limb elevated whenever possible.
5. Watch for swelling, coldness, and discoloration of fingers and toes. Contact your physician or return to the emergency department immediately if these signs occur.
6. If your ankle and foot are casted, always use your crutches as instructed. Do not put more weight on your cast than is ordered by your doctor.
7. Do not trim or cut the cast. Consult your doctor if you are having any problems such as swelling, sore areas under the cast, or foul odor coming from the cast.
8. Allow several periods during the day and

HOW TO TAKE A CHILD'S TEMPERATURE BY MOUTH

1. Shake the thermometer down.
2. Place the long, silver tip of the thermometer under the child's tongue.
3. Have the child close lips gently, being careful not to bite the thermometer.
4. Hold the thermometer in place for 3-5 minutes.
5. Remove the thermometer.
6. Rotate the thermometer until the wide silver line can be seen.
7. Read degree of temperature (exactly where the mercury stops). Read the temperature at the end of the silver line and write down the number.

CU/BMC 6-75

YOUR CHILD HAS A FEVER

102°

100.2°

98.6° Normal

Saint Joseph Hospital
Emergency Service

YOUR CHILD HAS A FEVER

Do not give Aspirin just because child does not "feel well." Give Aspirin only for —

1. Rectal temperature over 101°F. Child known to have had convulsions may be given Aspirin immediately for fever.

2. Oral temperature over 100°F. Child known to have had convulsions may be given Aspirin immediately for fever.

Baby Aspirin dosage —

One (1) "baby" Aspirin for each year of the baby's age up to 5 years of age.

If your child's rectal temperature is over 103°F even after you have given Aspirin or Tylenol sponge the child.

If your child is known to have convulsions with fever, sponging should be done at rectal temperature of 102°F or over.

Sponging Your Baby

1. Put the baby in cool water and sponge all over.
2. Do not add alcohol to water.
3. No alcohol sponge.
4. Sponge child 15-20 minutes.

Temperature may be checked after 25-30 minutes — your aim should be to bring it down to at least 102°F.

Do not be alarmed if child shivers while being sponged as this is a normal reaction. While you are sponging the baby, also offer cool drinks such as cool weak tea, water, 7-Up, etc. After you have taken the child from the bath tub, put on as few clothes as possible.

HOW TO TAKE A CHILD'S TEMPERATURE BY RECTUM

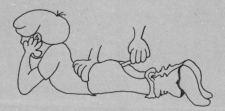

1. Shake the thermometer down.

2. Lubricate silver end of the thermometer.

3. Spread the buttocks so that the rectum can be easily seen.

4. Insert the thermometer gently into the rectum until the silver tip can no longer be seen.

5. Hold the thermometer in place for 3-5 minutes.

6. Remove the thermometer.

7. Rotate the thermometer until the wide silver line can be seen.

8. Read degree of temperature (exactly where the mercury stops). Read the temperature at the end of the silver line and write down the number.

HOW TO TAKE A CHILD'S TEMPERATURE

1. Shake the thermometer down.
2. **Oral Thermometer**
   a) Place the long, silver tip of thermometer under child's tongue.
   b) Have child close lips gently, being careful not to bite the thermometer.

Rectal Thermometer
   a) Lubricate silver end of the thermometer.
   b) Spread the buttocks so that rectum can be seen easily.
   c) Insert thermometer gently into the rectum until silver tip can no longer be seen.

3. Hold thermometer in place for 3-5 minutes.
4. Remove the thermometer.
5. Rotate the thermometer until the wide silver line can be seen.
6. Read degree of temperature (exactly where the mercury stops). Read the temperature at the end of the silver line and write down the number.

CU/BMC 6-75

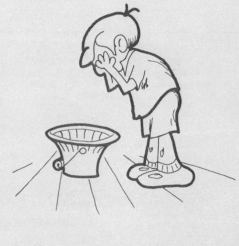

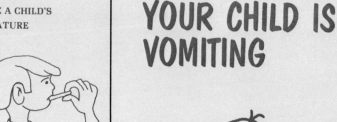

YOUR CHILD IS VOMITING

Saint Joseph Hospital
Emergency Service

night for elevation of the cast on pillows.
9. If it is raining or snowing, stay inside!
10. Remember to exercise the shoulder, hip, elbow, knee, toes, or fingers of the limb involved.

Suggestions for care of an upper respiratory tract infection or cold

1. Remain at home until you feel better, and get a lot of rest.
2. Drink plenty of fluids, and eat a light, well-balanced diet.
3. Use a cool vaporizer in the bedroom. This will keep the secretions more liquid.
4. Use disposable tissues to blow your nose, and cover your mouth when coughing.
5. Aspirin or acetaminophen (Tylenol) may be taken every 4 hours for pain and fever.

BIBLIOGRAPHY

Adair, L. P.: Patient education, Nurs. Care **9**(4):29-31, 1976.

Appelbaum, A. L.: Patient education seen as an integral part of patient care, Hospitals November 16, 1977. p. 115.

Carlton, B., and others: Defining a role for the health educator in the primary care setting, Health Education March/April 1978, p. 22.

Fralic, M. F.: Developing a viable inpatient education pro-

YOUR CHILD IS VOMITING

Persistent vomiting — If your child cannot keep down even plain water for more than half a day, contact your physician. Vomiting causes loss of body water resulting in dehydration.

Stop: All feedings
Rest the stomach
No milk
No solid foods
Nothing by mouth for at least an hour

Infants: Start feeding sugar water* or 7-Up in a bottle or with a spoon.

*Sugar water — Add 1 teaspoon of sugar to 4 ounces (½ cup) of boiled cool water.

Older Children: Feed small quantities of cold water or ice chips.

When: The child can keep water or ice chips down, then you may give several sips OR swallows every 15 minutes of:

a. Weak tea, kool aid, sweetened
b. 7-Up
c. Gingerale

When: The child can keep down gingerale, 7-Up, or tea, you can further add other liquids such as:

a. Clear broth
b. Fruit juices — apple, pineapple, or orange
c. Jello — liquid or solid form

Medication: Do not give any medications to stop vomiting, unless ordered by your doctor.

Do Not Give Aspirin: It may increase your child's vomiting.

If your child needs medicine for fever, you may use Tylenol or Tempra in liquid form

If: your child has not vomited for 8-12 hours and feels hungry, you may give the following foods:

First Day
1. Cereal — Rice, oatmeal, cooked cream of wheat
2. Mashed potato, soft cooked rice with butter
3. Dry toast, Soda crackers
4. Apple sauce, Jello
5. Mashed ripe bananas

Second Day
1. May start 2+ or skim milk
2. Lean meat suitable for age: Chicken or Beef
3. Vegetables — Green beans, peas, carrots, spinach cooked tender
4. Vanilla ice cream or puddings, or fruit — jello

gram—nursing director's perspective . . . Braddock General Hospital, Pittsburgh, Pennsylvania, J. Nurs. Admin. **6**(9):30-36, 1976.

Hicks, A. P., and Ashby, D. J.: Teaching discharge planning . . . Texas Women's University, Dallas, Nurs. Outlook **24**(5):306-308, 1976.

Jones, P., and Oertel, W.: Developing patient teaching objectives and techniques, Nurse Educ. **2**(5):3-13, 16-28, September-October 1977.

Kelly, L.: The patient's right to know, Nurs. Outlook **24**(1):26-32, 1976.

Levin, L. S.: Patient education and self-care: how do they differ? Nurs. Outlook **26**(3):170-175, March 1978.

Lewis, H. L.: Nurse practitioners in prevention and health education, Hosp. Prog. **59**(1):80-83, 1978.

Murray, R., and Zentner, J.: Guidelines for more effective health teaching, Nursing '76 **6**(2):44-53, 1976.

Murray, R., and Zentner, J.: Nursing concepts for health promotion, Englewood Cliffs, N.J., 1979, Prentice-Hall, Inc.

Pohl, M.: Teaching function of the nursing practitioner, Dubuque, Iowa, 1973, W. C. Brown Co.

Redman, B. K.: Guidelines for quality of care in patient education, Nurs. Digest **4**(9-10):25-26, 1976.

Redman, B. K.: Curriculum in patient education, Am. J. Nurs. **78**:1363-1366, August 1978.

Redman, B. K.: The process of patient teaching in nursing, ed. 2, St. Louis, 1980, The C. V. Mosby Co.

Reilly, M.: Let's set the record straight: preparing the discharge summary and the patient's instruction sheet, Nursing 79, Sept., 1979, p. 56.

CHAPTER 11

Wound management

WOUND MANAGEMENT

Wound management actually involves two basic principles: (1) decreasing the likelihood of infection and (2) promoting optimal wound healing. There are several factors one must consider when applying therapeutic intervention for a wound.

What kind of an injury is it?
How did it happen?
Where is the wound located?
What condition is the wound in?
Can the wound edges be approximated?
How old is the patient?
What is the occupation of the patient?
What type of physical condition is the patient in?
Does the patient have any current illness or any history of illness?
What is the patient's skin condition like?
When did the injury occur?
Has anything been done to the wound already?
What type of movement does the patient have distal to the wound?
Is vascular status intact?

Process of wound healing

Vasoconstriction occurs immediately as a response to an injury. This process causes sludging and then vasodilatation, which results in redness and swelling in the subepithelial layer of the skin. A day following the injury, epithelial cells begin to migrate. At the same time fibrin begins to form. This period is known as the proliferative period. During the next year, as the wound becomes older, collagen is being laid down at the areas that sustain the greatest stress. It is important to caution the patient that the tensile strength of a wound will be at its weakest on the third day following the injury.

General management of wounds

As with any other type of illness or injury, assure that airway, breathing, and circulation are maintained. Next, control the bleeding. Be sure to check for signs and symptoms of impending shock, and treat in accordance with findings. Check for chest wounds and other chest injuries (see Chapter 16). Check the wound for pain, pallor, pulselessness, paresthesia, and paralysis distal to the injury site. If there is evidence of possible fracture or dislocation, splint the area (see Chapter 19). If possible, determine the type of weapon used. If it was a gun, determine the caliber of bullet used and the distance from which the weapon was fired. If a wound looks suspicious, be sure to note it in your nurse's notes, and notify local police authorities.

If a wound looks infected or if it might be infected, culture it and send a specimen to the laboratory.

When cleansing a wound, be sure that the light source is good so that you can properly observe and care for the wound. When scrubbing the wound, do so after the patient is free of pain. This generally means that a local or regional anesthetic should be given before the wound is cleansed. Use a soft sponge, isotonic saline (not water), and a surgical preparation soap such as Betadine. Scrub the wound for approximately 5 minutes, longer if the wound is very contaminated. Use plenty of irrigating solution, because "the solution to pollution is dilution." Cleanse both the wound and the surrounding tissue. Remove all foreign material, especially cinders or dirt particles, as this has a tendency to form a "tattoo" as it ages. If the wound is a puncture wound, it should be soaked in a solution of warm saline and a surgical preparation soap for at least 10 to 15 minutes. If the area around the wound is particularly hairy, you should shave the areas near the border of the wound, except the eyebrows, which should never be shaved. All devitalized tissue should be debrided. The wound should then be sutured or packed with iodoform gauze, dressed with an antibiotic ointment, and covered with a nonadherent dressing.

Infection

Most wounds contain bacteria. One can then ask the question, "How many bacteria are too many bacteria?" As a general rule, any wound that is more than 8 to 12 hours old has "too many bacteria," and closure should be delayed until the wound can be debrided and cleansed. The exceptions to delayed closure are facial wounds, where the area is highly vascular and the chance of infection is low.

If a wound infection is going to occur, it will usually occur 2 to 3 days following the accident. It will appear as a swollen area that is erythematous and painful, with red streaks and possibly an exudate. The patient will have an elevated temperature and may have lymphedema and lymphangitis.

Therapeutic intervention for a wound infection includes culturing the wound to determine what the causative organism is, cleansing the wound with a solution of saline and a surgical preparation soap, soaking the wound three times a day, and placing the patient on an antibiotic regimen. You may wish to remove some or all of the sutures. These patients should be observed closely at frequent follow-up visits.

Types of wounds

There are six basic types of wounds with which you should be familiar: abrasions, avul-

sions, contusions, lacerations, punctures, and abcesses.

Abrasion. An abrasion is a wound caused by the skin rubbing against a hard surface. The friction caused by this event scrapes away the epithelial layer of the skin, exposing the epidermal or dermal layer. Physiologically it is similar to having a second degree burn. Therapeutic intervention for an abrasion is to cleanse the wound by scrubbing and irrigating it, remove any foreign bodies, and apply a topical antibiotic ointment and a nonadherent dressing. This dressing should be changed once a day until eschar forms. Be sure to tell the patient to avoid direct sunlight to this area for about 6 months, as it may be damaged by hypopigmentation.

Avulsion. An avulsion is a full-thickness skin loss in an injured area. Therapeutic intervention includes cleansing the wound by scrubbing and irrigating, debriding any devitalized tissue, repairing any injured muscles or tendons, providing a split-thickness graft or a flap, and covering the wound with a bulky dressing.

Contusion. A contusion is an extravasation of blood into the tissue. This type of injury usually results from blunt trauma. Therapeutic intervention includes application of a cold pack and analgesia if necessary; no dressing is necessary.

Laceration. A laceration is an open wound or a cut that may be minor or major. It extends at least into the deep epithelium and may vary considerably in length and depth. Therapeutic intervention includes controlling the bleeding with both pressure and elevation of the injured part, evaluating the distal neurovascular status, and applying local anesthesia so that the wound can be properly examined and cleansed. It should be cleansed by scrubbing and irrigation. At this time it is appropriate to remove any foreign bodies. The necrotic margins should be excised and the wound approximated and then closed, either using tape strips or sutures. Following closure, a mild antibiotic cream should be applied, and a dry nonadherent dressing should be placed over the wound. If the wound is very deep and there is suspicion or evidence of underlying structural damage, the patient may require surgery for repair of the wound.

Puncture wound. A puncture wound is made by a penetration of the tissue by a sharp or pointed object. A puncture wound may appear innocent, but may actually have resulted in severe damage to underlying structures. There also is the possibility of gross contamination. Puncture wounds seldom bleed. Therapeutic intervention depends on the depth of the penetration and the amount of the contamination. In general, soak the wounded part in a soapy solution twice a day for 2 to 4 days. If there is a foreign body that has been removed, remember to tape it to the chart. If the wound is known to be contaminated, it should be soaked, then anesthetized, cleansed, and inspected. If a foreign body is small and one is certain that its removal will not cause any further damage, one may do so. If there is necrotic tissue, it should be excised, the wound should be packed, and a drain placed. If the foreign body is very deep or if there is a possibility that its removal may cause further damage, the patient may require surgery to have it removed.

Abscess. An abscess is a localized collection of pus. Contrary to old practice, one should not wait for an abscess to "point." If it is suspected that there is an abscess, one should drain it with a needle and syringe. Therapeutic intervention is to anesthetize the area and drain the abscess in an independent position. An elliptical area should be removed. After the wound is cleansed, it should be packed loosely to allow it to drain. Apply a loose dressing, and have the patient return every 2 days until the wound is almost healed. If the patient is febrile, antibiotics should be administered.

Types of anesthesia for wound management

The most common type of anesthetic used for local anesthesia is lidocaine, which may be used with or without epinephrine. Epinephrine is usually used in an area of high vascularity where one wishes to control bleeding. Ounce for ounce, lidocaine is more potent than the other anesthetic agents; however, it is more toxic than the others. It is generally not very irritating and lasts longer than other anesthetic agents.

Other agents that are used for anesthesia are procaine, mepivacaine (Carbocaine), bupivacaine (Marcaine), and tetracaine (Pontocaine).

Besides local infiltration, an anesthetic agent may be used to produce regional anesthesia: that which is produced when an anesthetic drug is injected along the course of a nerve. This injection abolishes conduction of afferent and efferent impulses temporarily. The patient does not lose consciousness, although he may lose motor function temporarily.

Suturing

Suturing is the art of stitching two edges together in order to promote good wound healing with a minimal amount of scarring. Remember that suture material is a foreign body and that the human body will have a certain amount of inflammatory reaction to it. Always use the finest suture material available that will do the job. Also, use the minimal amount of tissue necessary to promote wound healing.

Types of suture material. There are two categories of suture material: absorbable and nonabsorbable. Absorbable suture removes tension from the surface of the wound and closes dead space. Dead space is the space beneath the wound that may fill with fluid and become a culture medium. Some of the types of absorbable suture are gut, chromic, Dexon, and Vicryl.

Nonabsorbable suture is generally used on the surface of the skin. Types of nonabsorbable sutures are silk, cotton, Dacron, nylon, dermal, and steel.

When to remove sutures. Where the wound is located and how well the wound is healing dictate when sutures are removed. Sutures are usually removed from the eyelids in 2 days; the face in 3 to 5 days; the trunk in 7 to 10 days; and the hands and feet in 10 to 14 days.

Penetrating trauma

If a person has been the victim of a penetrating trauma and the object is still in place, *do not remove the object*. It may be shortened to allow for transportation of the victim, but it should not be removed. Be sure that the penetrating object is stabilized and secured so that there is no chance of it being dislodged while the pa-

Stitches for suturing

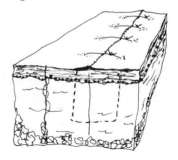

Simple interrupted sutures

Rationale: To bring skin edges together evenly; skin edges are slightly elevated and upon healing will flatten.

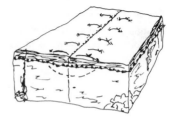

Vertical mattress suture

Rationale: Assures eversion upon healing.

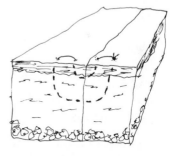

Horizontal mattress suture

Rationale: To closely approximate skin edges and have slight amount of eversion, especially in areas under tension.

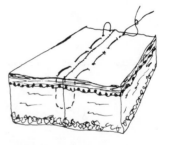

Half-buried horizontal mattress sutures

Rationale: Good to use in flaps or V-shaped wounds; also good in parallel lacerations.

Continued.

Stitches for suturing—cont'd

Subcuticular suture

Also known as a continuous intradermal suture.

Rationale: Good to use in wounds where sutures should be left in place for longer periods of time, as in wounds that are under a great deal of tension.

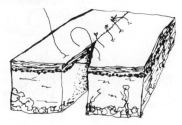

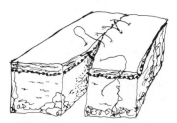

Continuous suture

Rationale: Good to use where suture marks probably will not show, as in scalp.

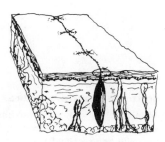

Buried suture

Rationale: To reduce dead space; to reduce tension in surface of wound.

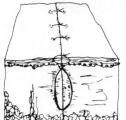

tient is in transit to the emergency department.

Any penetrating trauma to the head, including the eye, the ear, the nose, and the mouth, may result in intracranial injury.

High pressure paint gun injuries. High pressure paint gun injuries are increasingly frequent. This injury usually occurs when the victim has a cloth wrapped around the tip of his finger and is cleaning the end of a high pressure paint gun. The gun may release and a large amount of foreign material is pressurized into a closed space such as the finger tip and up into the hand and arm. This causes much tissue swelling, decreased circulation, and consequently, ischemia and necrosis. Signs and symptoms are a small puncture wound that looks relatively benign, induration, swelling, and a mottled look of the extremity. The patient will guard the extremity, as it will be very tender to touch and very cool. *Do not soak the extremity in warm or hot water, and do not inject local anesthesia,* because both of these may cause increased swelling, vasospasm, and increased ischemia. If the injected material is radiopaque it will show up on x-ray film.

Therapeutic intervention includes a tetanus toxoid booster as well as tetanus immune globulin. The patient should receive antibiotics, usually cephalothin (Keflin), taken to the operating room, and placed under general anesthesia; the wound is debrided, and a fasciotomy is performed.

Gunshot wounds. When a person is shot, the amount of trauma will depend upon the location of the wound and the mass, size, and velocity of the missile. If the missile struck a muscle mass, the damage will probably be severe, because muscle has a high density. If the missile struck bone, the direction of the missile may have changed and the bone fragments may actually act as missiles. A small entrance wound and a large, explosive exit wound indicate a high velocity missile fired at close range. The energy dissipated by a high-velocity missile is equal to the difference between the energy present when the missile enters the body and that left when it exits. It is therefore common to see a violent expansion of the missile track, which ruptures veins, arteries, and nerves and fractures bones.

A small entrance wound with no exit wound indicates a low-velocity missile that is retained within the tissue.

TETANUS AND TETANUS PROPHYLAXIS

Each year in the United States over 100 people of all ages contract tetanus. Of these victims, 50 die. So, although tetanus is not seen frequently in the emergency department, it should be readily recognized, as its effects may be devastating.

Tetanus is caused by *Clostridium tetani,* a gram-positive, spore-forming, aerobic bacillus. It is highly resistant to anything, including sterilization, because it is a spore former. Its incubation period is anywhere from 2 days to 2 weeks. It is found in soil, in garden moss, on farms, and anywhere else where animal and human excreta can be found. It enters the human circulation and attaches itself to cells within the central nervous system, where it depresses the respiratory center in the medulla and eventually causes death if untreated.

Signs and symptoms of mild tetanus are local stiffness in the joints and mild trismus. Moderate tetanus demonstrates itself as generalized body stiffness, moderate trismus, difficulty swallowing, and a decreased vital capacity. In severe tetanus, the patient will have severe trismus, pain in the back and the penis, seizures, opisthotonus, tachycardia, hypertension, dysrhythmias, and hyperpyrexia. The frightening fact is that the patient will remain alert throughout this process.

Therapeutic intervention includes assurance of the ABCs, oxygen at high flow, hyperalimentation, antibiotics, and good supportive nursing care.

It is important to note that even people who have contracted tetanus will require tetanus prophylaxis following recovery from the disease.

Tetanus prophylaxis

Initial immunization series

In an infant and young child, give diphtheria/tetanus/pertussis (DPT) injections:
0.5 ml at 2 months
0.5 ml at 4 months

0.5 ml at 6 months
0.5 ml at 18 months
0.5 ml at 5 to 6 years
For age 6 years to adult, give tetanus/diphtheria (TD) injections:
0.5 ml initially
0.5 ml 4 to 6 weeks later
0.5 ml 6 months to 1 year later
0.5 ml booster every 10 years

Tetanus prophylaxis for injuries*

Immunized	Prophylaxis
With a booster within 12 months	Meticulous wound care
Within past 10 years	0.5 ml absorbed tetanus toxoid
Booster more than 5 years ago (clean, small wound)	0.5 ml absorbed tetanus toxoid
More than 10 years age (clean, small wound)	0.5 ml absorbed tetanus toxoid
Within 10 years (wound severe or more than 24 hours old)	0.5 ml absorbed tetanus toxoid, 250 units tetanus immune globulin; antibiotics
More than 10 years ago or no immunization (clean, small wound)	0.5 ml absorbed tetanus toxoid (with follow-up instructions to complete initial immunization series)
More than 10 years ago or no immunization (moderate wound)	0.5 ml absorbed tetanus toxoid, 250 units tetanus immune globulin (with follow-up instructions to complete initial immunization series)
More than 10 years ago or no immunization (severe wound)	0.5 ml absorbed tetanus toxoid, 500 units tetanus immune globulin, (with follow-up instructions to complete initial immunization series)

HUMAN AND ANIMAL BITES

Any bite inflicted by a human being or an animal (wild or domestic) is a contaminated wound and should be treated accordingly. Other factors to consider when treating a patient with a bite are the age of the victim, the general physical condition of the patient, the location of the wound, the severity of the wound (location, size, depth, amount of contamination), the time elapsed since the bite, and what first aid, if any, has been given.

Complications of bites may include infection, cellulitis, abcess, septicemia, osteomyelitis, tenosynovitis, pyarthrosis, rabies, or loss of the injured part.

Any patient who has sustained a bite should be instructed to return to the emergency department or private physician if a fever develops, if the area becomes red or swollen, or if streaks appear. He should also return if the area becomes very hot, if there is increasing pain at the site, or if a foul odor develops and there is drainage. The patient should be instructed to keep the injured part elevated above the level of the heart for the first 24 hours if possible. Be sure to instruct him about anything specific he should know about prescribed medications.

Human bites

A human bite may be self-inflicted or inflicted by another person. A human bite is one of the most contaminated types of wounds a person can receive and may cause a severe infection. The human mouth contains more than 10^8 bacteria per milliliter of saliva. It contains the gram-positive organisms *Staphylococcus aureus* and *Streptococcus* and the gram-negative organisms *Proteus, Escherichia coli, Pseudomonas, Neisseria* and *Klebsiella*. A significant number of organisms are coagulase-positive, penicillin-resistant *Staphylococcus aureus*.

The most common location for a human bite is the long or ring finger at the metacarpophalangeal joint.

Signs and symptoms of human bites are a history of the incident (although the patient may be hesitant to tell you), and teeth marks or lacerations across the knuckles caused by a fist hitting the teeth.

Therapeutic intervention includes applying local anesthesia, obtaining a culture and gram stain, and then irrigating and scrubbing the

---

*Recommendations of the American College of Surgeons.

wound thoroughly. Any devitalized tissue should be debrided. These wounds are generally not sutured, except for facial wounds. Be sure to evaluate neurovascular status distal to the injury. Give the patient a broad-spectrum antibiotic, and check for currency of tetanus prophylaxis. These patients should follow a strict after-care regime.

Complications of human bites are abscess, cellulitis, osteomyelitis, pyarthrosis, and infection.

Dog and cat bites

Over 1 million people in the United States are bitten by cats and dogs each year. The organism present in the mouth of animals is most commonly *Pasteurella multocida*. The chance of infection increases if the patient is very young (under 4), older (over 50), if there is a prolonged period of time before medical help is sought, if the wound is located in a low vascular area, or if the wound is a puncture wound.

Common signs and symptoms of dog and cat bites are a history of a bite, puncture wounds, infection, pain, swelling and tenderness over the wound area, inflammation, regional adenopathy, and a low-grade fever.

Therapeutic intervention includes obtaining a culture and gram stain before irrigating and scrubbing the wound thoroughly and debriding any devitalized tissue. These wounds may be sutured. Assess distal neurovascular status, administer broad spectrum antibiotics, and assure current tetanus prophylaxis. The wound should be cleansed often and should be checked by a medical person every 2 days until it is healed. Application of a dressing is optional. Administer rabies prophylaxis if indicated.

RABIES AND RABIES PROPHYLAXIS

Rabies is caused by a virus found in the saliva of many mammals. This virus is highly neurotoxic. Its incubation period is anywhere from 10 days to several months. The patient with rabies will usually give a history of having been bitten by an animal. It is important to obtain a history as to what type of animal it was, the geographic region where the bite took place, and whether the animal was provoked.

The patient will tell you that he has had general malaise for 3 or 4 days. He will have a fever, headache, granulomatous lymphadenitis, photophobia, muscle spasm, and may lapse into coma.

Therapeutic intervention includes ensuring airway, breathing, and circulation, culturing the wound, irrigating and scrubbing the wound, debriding any devitalized tissue, and perhaps, suturing the wound (this is a controversial issue in the literature). The patient should be given antibiotics and tetanus prophylaxis.

The bite should be reported to the local health authorities. Rabies vaccine is given if there is reason to believe that the animal has rabies, if the animal becomes rabid while in quarantine (10 days), if the animal is wild such as a bat, skunk, wolf, fox, or raccoon, or if the animal is not found and information about rabies in that animal is not available.

The two types of rabies vaccine used are duck embryo vaccine (DEV) and human or equine serum. DEV is given over 2 to 3 weeks. Then, boosters must be given 10 to 20 days following the initial series. This vaccine is given alternately in the anterior abdominal wall (right and left sides) and the lateral aspect of the thighs. Equine serum or human serum is given when the suspicion of rabies infection is very high. It is given both directly into the wound site and into the buttocks.

BIBLIOGRAPHY

Callaham, M. L.: Treatment of common dog bites: infection risk factors, J.A.C.E.P. **7**:11-15, March 1978.

Committee on Trauma, American College of Surgeons: A Guide to Prophylaxis Against Tetanus in Wound Management, Bull. Am. Coll. Surg. **57**:32, December 1972.

Furste, W.: Four key ways to 100% success in tetanus prophylaxis, Am. J. Surg. **128**:616-623, 1974.

Parks, B., Hawkins, L., and Horner, P.: Bites of the hand, Rocky Mount. Med. J. **71**:85-88, 1974.

Scarella, J.: Management of bites: early definitive care of bite wounds, Ohio State Med. J. **65**:25-31, 1969.

SELECTED READINGS

Anast, G. T., Bliss, A., and Warner, C. G.: Emergency treatment of bites and stings, J.E.N. **1**:27-31, September-October 1975.

Anderson, H. W.: An open wound is a whole patient, Emerg. Med. **9**:127, November 1977.

Barber, J. M., and Budassi, S. A.: Mosby's manual of emergency care, St. Louis, 1979, The C. V. Mosby Co.

Boswick, J. A.: Wound care, Postgrad. Med. **55:**171, January 1974.

Bryant, W. M.: Wound healing. In Bekiesz, B., editor: CIBA clinical symposia, 29(3), 1977.

Chenoweth, S. R.: Forensic consideraitons in gunshot wounds. (Unpublished manuscript.)

Dushoff, I. M.: A stitch in time, Emerg. Med. **5:**21-43, January 1973.

Edsall, G., Elliot, M. W., Peebler T. C., Levine, L., and Eldred, M. C.: Excessive use of tetanus toxoid boosters, J.A.M.A. **202:**111, 1967.

Finegold, S. M., Bartlett, J. G., Chow, A. W., and others: Management of anerobic infections, Ann. Intern. Med. **83:**375-389, 1975.

Grabb, W. C., and Smith, J. W., editors: Plastic surgery, Boston, 1973, Little, Brown and Co.

Graham, W., Calabretta, A., and Miller, S.: Dog bites, Am. Fam. Physician **15:**132-137, 1977.

Harris, D., Imperata, P. J., and Oken, B.: Dog bites—an unrecognized epidemic, Bull. NY Acad. Med. **50:**981-1000, 1974.

Meislin, H. W., Lerner, S. A., Graves, M. H., and others: Cutaneous abcesses, Ann. Inter. Med. **87:**145-149, 1977.

Moritz, A. R., and Morris, C. R.: Handbook of legal medicine, ed. 2, St. Louis, 1975, The C. V. Mosby Co.

Nichol, T. D., and Cole, N. M.: Management of soft tissue injuries of the face to reduce scar formation, J. Ky Med. Soc. **71:**8, August 1973.

O'Reilly, R. J., and Blatt, G.: Injection by misdirection, J.A.M.A. **233:**533, 1976.

Peacock, E. E., Jr., and Van Winkle, W., Jr.: Surgery and biology of wound repair, Philadelphia, 1970, W. B. Saunders Co.

Quick, G., and Podgorny, G.: Penetrating wounds, Emerg. Med. Serv., March-April 1977.

Shields, C., and others: Hand infections, J. Trauma **15:** 235-236, 1975.

Vass, J. G.: Effects of antimicrobial soap on ecology of aerobic bacterial flora of the human skin, Appl. Microbiol. **30:**551-556, 1975.

Waltz, J. R., and Inbau, F. E.: Medical jurisprudence, New York, 1971, Macmillan Publishing Co., Inc.

Wolcott, M. W., editor: Furguson's surgery of the ambulatory patient, Philadelphia, 1974, J. B. Lippincott Co.

CHAPTER 12

Shock management

Rebecca Hathaway and Janet M. Barber

DEFINITION

Shock is defined as generalized tissue hypoperfusion. However, the shock syndrome is not as simple as the definition may seem. Shock has a variety of causes, multiple types, overlapping stages, numerous treatment modalities, and unpredictable outcomes. Shock then can more appropriately be defined as a syndrome, characterized by acute circulatory dysfunction at a cellular level that causes inadequate perfusion of vital organs and abnormal metabolism (Table 12-1).

PATHOPHYSIOLOGY
Cellular level

It is important when discussing the pathophysiology of shock and dealing with the patient in shock to focus on the cell. At the cellular level, nutrients are necessary to perform metabolic functions. Any decrease in oxygen supply, hypoxia, produces abnormal alterations in cellular metabolism.

Fig. 12-1 summarizes the factors that interplay in the oxygen needs of the cell and the mechanism of hypoxia. Hardy (1977) states that "the role of efficient circulation is to deliver oxygen and nutrients to the cell, and to remove metabolic products from the cell." Hypoxia results when the blood flow and available oxygen are reduced because of abnormalities in the cardiopulmonary unit, blood volume, or vascular circuit, including the microcirculation.

Ninety-five percent of energy production at the cellular level is accomplished through the mitochondrial electron transfer linked reactions. The mitochondria consume over 90% of the available oxygen provided by the microcirculation. Therefore, any alteration in oxygen supply to the tissue and mitochondrial energy production will greatly affect the ability of the cell to carry on aerobic metabolism. Additionally, when the cell is deprived of oxygen over extended periods, the cell membrane will become damaged.

Besides cellular membrane damage, there is a change in intracellular lysosomes in the shock syndrome. As the shock state progresses, the lipoprotein membranes of the lysosome break down, releasing proteolytic enzymes into the cell and then into the blood stream. The effect of proteolytic enzymes in the vascular system is vasodilation, a result of the conversion of inactive kinogens into vasoactive kinins.

Microcirculation

As a response to cellular injury during the shock syndrome, histamine is also produced. The histamine causes microcirculatory changes. Capillary endothelial damage occurs in the form of swelling and separation, with fluid moving through capillary membranes into interstitial spaces. Particles as large as protein molecules and red blood cells can pass through the capillary wall into the interstitium.

Intracellular edema also occurs late in shock.

Table 12-1. Compensatory hormonal mechanisms in hemorrhagic shock*

Initiating defect	Hormonal response	Desired hemodynamic effect	Clinical manifestations
Circulatory failure, trauma, hemorrhage	Secretion of *epinephrine* and *norepinephrine* from the adrenal medulla	Peripheral vasoconstriction Increased blood flow to heart, brain, and important organs Inotropic—increased heart contractility Chronotropic—increased heart rate Increased cardiac output	Maintenance of normal blood pressure Increased pulse Decreased pulse pressure Diaphoresis Cool skin
Kidney ischemia	Secretion of *renin,* which stimulates secretion of *angiotensin* I and *angiotensin* II	Peripheral vasoconstriction Increased blood flow to heart, brain, and important organs Increased cardiac output	Maintenance of normal blood pressure Increased pulse Decreased pulse pressure Diaphoresis Cool skin
Release of angiotensin II	Stimulates release of *aldosterone,* which causes sodium retention (and proportional water retention) in the kidney	Increasing circulating volume Increased cardiac output	Decreased urine output Hypercapnia
Stress, trauma, blood loss	Osmoreceptors in posterior pituitary release *antidiuretic hormone* (ADH), which causes water retention in distal tubules of the kidney	Increased circulating volume Increased cardiac output	Decreased urine output

*From Romano, T.: J.E.N. **4:**58, September-October 1978.

This is caused by an ineffective "sodium pump," which cannot function in an ischemic or damaged cell. Consequently, the cell takes on fluid from the extracellular compartment.

The combination of intracellular edema and capillary endothelial damage with subsequent increased interstitial fluid results in a significant intravascular volume deficit.

Hypotensive events

It is important to note that ischemic and cellular damage from hypotensive episodes sets up the chain of events summarized by a reduction in mitochondrial oxidation, a breakdown in lysosomes causing release of enzymes, changes in microcirculation from histamine production, and a decrease in intravascular volume from intracellular edema and increased interstitial fluid.

Hypotension can be caused by abnormalities in the heart-lung function, by blood volume alterations, and by changes in the larger vessels and microcirculation. Table 12-2 summarizes the potential causes of hypotension that can trigger the shock syndrome.

TYPES OF SHOCK

Characterized by inadequate tissue perfusion, the shock syndrome can vary in type. The four classic types of shock follow.

1. Septic (sometimes referred to as distributive): vasodilation causing an alteration in vascular circuit and decreased peripheral vascular resistance

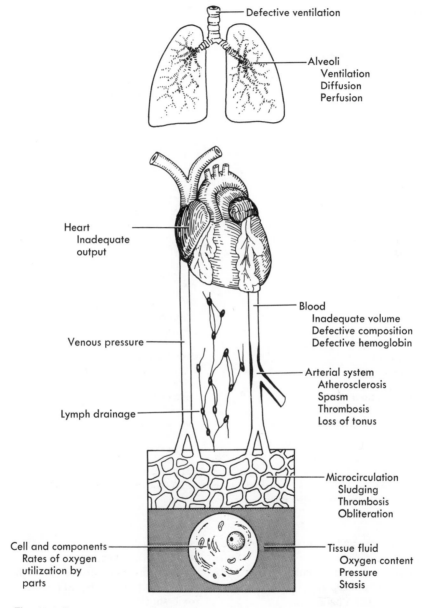

Fig. 12-1. Factors that affect cellular oxygen needs and the mechanism of hypoxia.

Table 12-2. Causes of hypotension*

Volume deficits
  Whole blood loss
  Plasma loss
  Interstitial fluid loss or shift
  Water deficit
Electrolyte deficits or excesses
  Na, K, Cl, Ca, Mg
Acid-base imbalance
  Respiratory acidosis
  Metabolic acidosis
  Respiratory alkalosis
  Metabolic alkalosis
Sepsis
  Septicemia
  Infection with fluid shift (peritonitis)
Respiratory insufficiency
  Hypoxia
  Hypercarbia
  Right-to-left pulmonary shunts (atelectasis, pneumonia, lung contusion)
  Pneumothorax
  Mechanical disturbances due to trauma (flail chest, tracheolaryngeal injury)
  Pulmonary embolism
Cardiac causes
  Cardiac arrest or fibrillation
  Coronary occlusion
  Pericardial tamponade
  Cardiac arrhythmia
  Myocardial failure
  Cardiac contusion
Central nervous system causes
  Brain injury
  Increased intracranial pressure
  Reflex vagal stimuli
  Psychic stimuli
  Brainstem and spinal cord injury
	Endocrine causes
	  Adrenocortical insufficiency
	  Adrenomedullary dysfunction (e.g., shock before and following resection of pheochromocytoma)
	  Thyroid crisis
	  Hyperinsulinism
	  Diabetic coma
	Shock during operation
	  Hypovolemia (from anesthetic vasodilatation and preexisting blood-volume deficit, or acute blood loss)
	  Heart failure
	  Hypoxia
	  Hypercapnia
	  Myocardial ischemia
	  Arrhythmia
	  Miscellaneous other causes
	Shock in recovery room
	  Hypovolemia
	  Cardiac failure
	  Hypoxia
	  Hypercapnia (due to inadequate ventilation)
	  Coronary insufficiency
	  Arrhythmia
	  Electrolyte imbalance
	  Endotoxin shock
	  Pulmonary embolus
	  Excessive medication
	Miscellaneous
	  Drug reactions
	  Transfusion reactions
	  Fat embolism
	  Hepatic failure
	  Anaphylaxis

*From Gurd, with modifications and additions. Adapted from Hardy, J. D.: Shock and cardiac arrest. In Hardy, J. D.: Critical surgical illness. Philadelphia, 1971. W. B. Saunders Co.

2. Hypovolemic: inadequate blood volume or preload
3. Cardiogenic: difficulty with or failure of the cardiopulmonary unit
4. Neurogenic (see Chapter 14)

SEPTIC SHOCK
Cause

Septic shock is a condition of inadequate tissue perfusion following a bacteremia most commonly a result of a gram-negative enteric bacilli. It has been described in the literature also under other names including bacterial shock, bacteremia, blood poisoning, and endotoxic shock.

Gram-negative bacilli, the most frequent cause of sepsis, include *Escherichia coli*, *Klebsiella pneumoniae*, *Proteus*, *Pseudomonas*, and *Serratia marcescens*. Gram-positive organisms such as meningococci, clostridia, viruses,

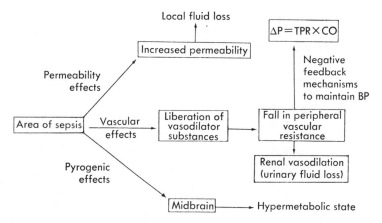

Fig. 12-2. Pathophysiology of septic shock. (From Hardy, J. D.: Textbook of surgery, ed. 5, Philadelphia, 1977, J. B. Lippincott Co.)

rickettsiae, and fungi may also precipitate septic shock.

Septic shock most frequently is iatrogenic, increasing in incidence in hospitals since 1935. The shock syndrome is more often fatal if precipitated by an organism contracted while in the hospital.

Predisposition

Septic shock is more common in men than women. This is because of the increased number of urinary tract infections in men. Women are most vulnerable following pregnancy. Except for neonates, septic shock is uncommon in children.

It is important for the emergency nurses to ascertain if the patient has had recent pelvic examination, appendectomy, Foley catheter insertion, or childbirth. These procedures are frequent methods for induction of causative organisms. Indwelling biliary tubes, intrauterine devices perforating the uterus, instrumented abortions, and peritonitis from a ruptured appendix, leaking anastomosis, or subphrenic abscess are also ways gram-negative bacilli may be introduced.

Septic shock is often seen after multiple system trauma. Other predisposing factors include prostatism with pyelonephritis, biliary tract obstruction from calculi, diabetes, cirrhosis, carcinomas, and long-term steroid therapy.

Pathology

Galen first considered sepsis when he described the phenomenon of local inflammation with classic pain, heat, redness, and swelling. In this example Galen was describing the effect of an infecting agent and the release of substances producing local vasodilation.

If the same phenomenon is magnified, the systemic effect of sepsis can be created. The mechanism and exact agent released that causes vasodilation is unknown. It is thought that there is a reaction between the products from the bacteria, probably endotoxins, and the polymorphonuclear leukocytes. In this reaction, an endogenous leukocyte protease is liberated having both vasodilator and pyrogenic effects.

The agents released from bacteria during sepsis are extremely important regardless of the exact reaction. The liberation of the substances creates three important systemic effects: (1) the midbrain and temperature control are affected to create pyrogenic effects, (2) vascular circuitry is affected, causing vasodilation and dramatic reduction in peripheral vascular resistance, and (3) permeability is increased, with subsequent fluid loss (Fig. 12-2).

In septic shock there is an increased production of catecholamines.

At a cellular level, septic shock is characterized by a significant increase in protein catabolism and by an increase in the rate of mitochondrial oxidation. Therefore a hypermetabolic state exists. As the catabolism and hypermetabolic state continues, cellular hypoxia ensues.

The spiking fever produced by pyrogenic effects of sepsis gives rise to chills and shivering. The shivering in turn causes an increased muscular activity and consequently an increase in heat production, sometimes as much as three times normal. Chills and spiking fever are taken seriously by emergency nurses and often alert them to impending hypotension.

It is not uncommon for patients to experience hyperdynamic changes with sepsis for several days up to several weeks.

The cellular hypoxia continues placing more demand on the cardiopulmonary system. Fluid loss concomitantly progresses; at the same time, there is vasodilation and reduced peripheral vascular resistance. Therefore, myocardial workload is markedly increased; however, the cycle is vicious because supply cannot meet demands. Shock progresses, and the cellular level changes ensue.

The continuous demand for oxygen and an increased cardiac output bring about myocardial fatigue and failure. Failure is thought to be caused by increased myocardial workload, depletion of myocardial catecholamines, and depressant effects on cardiac muscle from the endotoxins.

Effect on cardiovascular system/hemodynamics

During the early phase of septic shock, there is a normal to reduced central venous pressure or right atrial pressure because of the low to normal preload in the early hyperdynamic state. As mentioned earlier, the peripheral vascular resistance is reduced along with systemic arterial pressure in the presence of a widened pulse pressure. Cardiac output in the initial phase will be normal or increased depending on the degree of vasodilation and vascular capacitance.

As the septic shock syndrome continues, compensatory mechanisms are no longer effective and add additional work, becoming decompensatory. Cardiac failure follows, marked by an increase in vasoconstriction and peripheral vascular resistance (afterload). The cardiac output falls, as does stroke volume, signified by narrowed pulse pressure.

The goal in managing the patient in septic shock hemodynamically is to maximize the cardiac output by preloading using the Starling mechanism. This is accomplished by increasing the intravascular volume and selecting the appropriate fluid. This is discussed later in the chapter under Principles of Therapy.

Effect on pulmonary system

Systemic and/or pulmonary sepsis are major causes of respiratory insufficiency. Sepsis can initiate acute respiratory disease (ARD) (see also shock lung, pp. 259-260).

Often respiratory insufficiency is the fatal event for the patient in septic shock. Protection of the pulmonary system in the patient with septicemia includes sterile technique in suctioning, handwashing, strict asepsis when placing indwelling catheters, and preventing atelectasis.

Hyperventilation occurs early in the shock state as shown by an initial respiratory alkalosis. This is most likely the result of a decreased cerebral blood flow and a fall in arterial pCO_2. There is decreased blood flow to the lung with resultant hypoxia and carbon dioxide retention. Metabolic acidosis occurs in the later stages as a result of the increased lactate production.

Effect on renal system

During septic shock there is an intrarenal distribution of blood flow from the cortex to the medulla. As septic shock progresses, the glomerular filtration rate is decreased, leading to oliguria, decreased medullary sodium, and a decrease in the kidney's ability to concentrate urine effectively. As shock persists, vasoconstriction occurs; acute tubular necrosis and renal failure, azotemia, hyperkalemia, and acidosis may result.

Signs and symptoms

Signs and symptoms of early septic shock syndrome include fever, chills, and leukocytosis. Hypotension may follow even in the presence of warm skin. Urine output is normal very early. Tachycardia also occurs early. Signs and symptoms in the latest stages of septic shock include heart failure, pulmonary insufficiency, and metabolic acidosis.

Early signs and symptoms
Fever and chills
Hypotension (skin may be warm)
Tachycardia
Leukocytosis (WBC 15,000 to 30,000)
Changes in mental status
Tachypnea (respiratory alkalosis)
Late signs and symptoms
Hypotension
Cool pale extremities
Peripheral cyanosis
Oliguria (increased BUN and creatinine) (decreased creatinine clearance)
Heart failure (increased left-side pressures)
Respiratory insufficiency
Metabolic acidosis
Coma

Assessment parameters/baseline data

The assessment of the patient is important in terms of prevention, diagnosis, monitoring, and evaluating the therapeutic response. Thal (1977) suggests that the following baseline data are critical for adequate diagnosis and vital for effective management of septic shock.

1. Ventilation: effectiveness and amount of breathing effort, auscultation
2. Skin: color, turgor; presence or absence of diaphoresis
3. Hemodynamics*
   Heart rate
   Blood pressure (direct from method preferred)
   Right heart function: cardiac output or right atrial pressure with triple lumen pulmonary artery catheter
   Left heart function: pulmonary artery wedge pressure with triple lumen pulmonary artery catheter
   Adequacy of cardiac output: calculation of cardiac output using thermodilution Swan-Ganz catheter or AV oxygen difference

---

*See pp. 254-259 for details of hemodynamic monitoring.

4. Abdominal exam: rigidity, masses, distension, and fluid
5. Extremities: estimation of fluid loss, detection of fractures and soft tissue injury
6. Urine output and specific gravity
7. Laboratory tests: hematocrit, white blood count, electrolytes, blood urea nitrogen (BUN), creatinine, blood sugar, arterial blood gases (ABGs), bicarbonate and base excess
8. Chest film
9. Blood and urine cultures
10. Coagulation studies

The baseline data are useful in making a diagnosis. Once the diagnosis is underway, treatment modalities are in process. The assessment information is also important in the prevention of complications and the management of complications if they occur. For example, disseminated intravascular coagulation is a major complication of septic shock and can be more effectively managed with baseline coagulation studies.

Treatment

Principles of therapy for patients with shock syndrome are discussed later in the text. Treatment for patient in septic shock consists of any or all of the following.

• Maintenance of adequate ventilation; prevention of airway obstruction, atelectasis, or pulmonary edema. Oxygen therapy, intubation, assisted ventilation, and use of positive end expiratory pressure (PEEP) may be indicated. ABGs are monitored to guide maintenance to acid-base balance.

• Volume replacement based on the Starling mechanism. The choice of fluid is extremely important; the quantity of fluid is in excess of normal fluid volume. Electrolytes are monitored to prevent hypokalemia or hyperkalemia.

• Selected pharmacological agents:
   Digitalization may be used to enhance contractility (see p. 253).
   Beta-adrenergic blockers are sometimes used to control tachycardia; however, their use is rare since they will depress

myocardial function (for example, iso-proterenol, see p. 726).

Vasopressors and vasodilators such as dopamine are used to support systemic arterial pressure through vasodilator effect on peripheral and renal vasculature (see p. 721). Fluid volume is essential when using vasodilators.

Epinephrine may be used as myocardial catecholamines become depleted (see p. 723).

Furosemide may be considered for oliguria (see p. 724).

Steroids have been used experimentally to reduce inflammation, reduce peripheral vascular resistance, and treat cellular injury from endotoxins. Use of steroids in septic shock is still controversial, since they can cause an increased incidence of gastrointestinal hemorrhage and they have an immunosuppressive effect (see p. 254).

Antibiotics are instituted to cover most likely organisms, although cultures and sensitivities are not immediately available (for example, clindamycin [Cleocin], ampicillin, gentamycin). Care should be taken because of nephrotoxic characteristics of antibiotics.

- Urine output is carefully monitored.
- Surgical intervention may be needed in patients with septic shock caused by abscess, infected bowel, infected uterus, inflamed gall bladder, or perinephritis.
- Salicylates and cooling blanket are necessary to lower body temperature and reduce metabolic demands.
- Prevention of complications includes prevention by early detection of gastrointestinal hemorrhage, detection of arrhythmias, prevention of shock lung, and consideration and early detection of disseminated intravascular coagulation.

HYPOVOLEMIC SHOCK

Hypovolemic shock occurs when there is a deficit in intravascular fluid volume relative to vascular capacity. Wilson (1976) states that this is a 15% to 25% intravascular volume reduction.

Cause

A hypovolemic shock syndrome may be caused by any condition that precipitates a reduction in volume such as trauma causing blood loss, gastrointestinal hemorrhage, excessive vomiting or diarrhea, or severe dehydration. The literature also identifies hypovolemic shock as traumatic shock, hemorrhagic shock, wound shock, and oligemic shock.

Hemodynamics

Hemodynamically, hypovolemic shock is characterized by low filling pressure, normal left heart function, increased peripheral vascular resistance, and inadequate cardiac output.

Following trauma and tissue damage, shock may occur. Intravascular volume is not significantly reduced; however, the damaged cells take on large amounts of fluid, the vasoactive mechanism of shock is accelerated, and the lysosome changes occur rapidly. Consequently, a hypovolemic hemodynamic picture is seen. When fluid is administered in this situation the patient's condition improves. The hemodynamic picture and other signs and symptoms of hypovolemic shock are described below.

Hemodynamic picture
  Hypotension
    Increased pulse rate
    Decreased cardiac output or right atrial pressure
    Decreased pulmonary capillary wedge pressure (PCWP) or pulmonary artery diastolic pressure (PADP)
    Decreased cardiac output
    Increased peripheral vascular resistance evidenced by cold clammy skin.
Other signs and symptoms
  Inadequate perfusion
    Decreased mental status and obtundation
    Decreased urine output
    Peripheral cyanosis
    Acid-base imbalance
    Arrhythmias

Emergency management

The treatment of hypovolemic shock begins with a head-to-toe assessment, obtaining baseline data and determining the cause of the intra-

Table 12-3. Identification of degree of severity of shock*

Test or sign		Normal or average	Preshock state to mild shock	Degree of shock	
				Moderate	Moderately severe to severe
Sensorium	Orientation	Well-oriented Time/place/person	Oriented	Fairly well oriented	May be confused and disoriented
	Enunciation	Distinct	Normal—slurred words	Somewhat slowed and few slurred words	Slow and slurred to monosyllabic utterances and groans
	Content	Appropriate; structured sentences	Sentences normal	Slow sentences or phrases and words	Often incoherent
Pupils	Size	Equal (2 to 4 mm)	Normal	Normal	Normal to dilating or dilated
	Constriction with light	Rapid	Rapid	Rapid	Slow or nonreactive
Pulse	Rate	60 to 100/min	100 to 120/min	120 to 150/min	Maximal
	Amplitude	Full	Full amplitude to slight decrease	Variable: mild decrease	Thready
Blood pressure (mm of Hg)	Systolic	120 to 145	Normal or slightly low	Decreased—often 40 to 50 mm of Hg below usual BP	Less than 80 to unobtainable
	Diastolic	60 to 90	Normal or slightly low	Decreased, but less so than systolic	40 to 50 to unobtainable
	Pulse pressure	40 to 70	30 to 40	20 to 30	Less than 20
Jugular vein filling	Patient flat	Fills to anterior border of sternocleidomastoid muscle	Normal to trace of filling	Trace to no filling	No filling
			May be full in septic shock or grossly distended in cardiogenic shock		
Urinary output via catheter	ml/min	0.6 to 1.5	0.6 to 0.8	0.4 to 0.6	0.3 or less
	ml/10 min	6 to 15	6 to 8	4 to 6	3 or less

*From Flint, T., and Cain, H.: Shock: emergency treatment and management, ed. 4, Philadelphia, 1970, W. B. Saunders Co.

Continued.

Table 12-3. Identification of degree of severity of shock—cont'd.

Test or sign	Normal or average	Degree of shock		
		Preshock state to mild shock	Moderate	Moderately severe to severe
Tilt test—rapid lying to sitting position				
Pulse	Transient increase	Increased	Rapid	Already maximal
Blood pressure	Less than 10 mm decrease	10 to 25 mm decrease	25 to 50 mm decrease	Marked decrease to unobtainable
Symptoms	No "lightheadedness"	No lightheadedness	Lightheadedness	Unable to sit up
Therapeutic, if whole blood loss	—	Probably do not transfuse	Transfuse!	Transfuse!
Est. blood loss	—	To 750 ml	1,000 to 1,250 ml	1,500 to 1,750 ml or more
Est. % blood volume loss	—	15%	20 to 25%	More than 30 to 35%
Capillary blanching test				
Blanching of forehead skin with thumb pressure	Return of circulation to 1.25 to 1.5 sec	1.25 to 1.5 sec	More than 1.5 sec	Pallor before and after test
		Note: With hypercapnia, there may be almost instantaneous return		
Central venous pressure	Normal (3 to 8 cm of saline)	Normal / May be elevated in cardiogenic shock	Low	Extremely low

vascular deficit. Once the cause is ascertained, it can be treated with the appropriate therapeutic adjuncts.

1. Ensure an adequate airway. Intubate the patient if necessary. Administer 100% oxygen. If ventilatory assistance is required, use a volume-cycled respirator for delivery of 12 to 15 ml/kg. Maintain the inflation pressure below 40 cm of water to reduce the hazard of pneumothorax.

2. Position the patient flat and elevate the legs. Consider antishock trousers if the patient is hypovolemic. Do not place the patient in the Trendelenburg position except for placement of an IV line. (See p. 208).

3. Establish at least two large-bore IV lines—one for monitoring the CVP. Infuse Ringer's lactate* (2,000 to 3,000 ml) over 20 to 30 minutes. Warm all IV fluids after the first 2 liters. Perform fluid challenge:

   a. Give 200 ml Ringer's lactate over 10 minutes. If the jugular vein distends or if there is evidence of pulmonary congestion, temporarily withhold additional fluids except to maintain the IV infusion route.

   b. If there is no evidence of overloading, give additional 200-ml increments of Ringer's lactate over 10-minute periods until there is improvement or evidence of fluid overload.

4. Draw venous blood for testing: electrolytes, complete blood count, hemoglobin, hematocrit, cardiac enzymes, coagulation studies, and typing and crossmatching.

5. Obtain an arterial blood sample for baseline pH, pCO_2 and pO_2 measurement.

6. Correct fluid-electrolyte and acid-base problems.

7. Insert a Foley catheter to monitor urinary

---

*Use colloids cautiously until the fluid volume is stabilized. Avoid using colloids unless proteins are low. Low molecular weight dextran interferes with typing and cross-matching and increases bleeding from raw surfaces.

output. Measure the output every 15 to 60 minutes with a urinometer and record. Consider furosemide or mannitol (Osmitrol) challenge if it falls below 30 ml/hour. (See Chapter 12.)

8. Monitor the pulse pressure, ECG, CVP, and/or PWP. (See Chapter 12.) Remember that the CVP can be normal or elevated in shock states. The *trend* is the most important point to monitor.
9. Blood may be used to maintain the hemoglobin level at 12.5 to 14 gm/100 ml.* Monitor calcium levels since citrates affect calcium levels. Fresh frozen plasma will increase clotting factors but not platelets. Warm blood carefully to prevent ventricular fibrillation.
10. Consider pharmacological adjuncts:
    a. Steroids (after correction of hypovolemia): methylprednisone (Solu-Medrol), 30 mg/kg (p. 730); hydrocortisone (Solu-Cortef), 150 mg/kg; dexamethasone (Decadron), 6 mg/kg (p. 717).
    b. Digitalis (p. 720): If shock persists despite adequate fluid administration, rapid digitalization should be considered.
    c. Inotropic agents: dopamine, isoproterenol (p. 726), metaraminol (p. 728).
    d. Calcium (p. 716), 10 ml of a 10% solution for low cardiac output, especially for patients who receive massive transfusions of citrated blood.
    e. Furosemide (p. 724), 5 to 10 mg, doubling the dose every 15 minutes if there is an inadequate response, for shock unresponsive to fluid therapy.
    f. Antibiotics at the first sign of infection (after appropriate smears and cultures).

*If hypovolemia persists after administration of 2 to 3 liters of crystalloid and blood is not readily available, give colloids (5% albumin or plasma) to comprise at least one fourth of additional fluid therapy. Up to 50% of the additional fluids should be colloidal in cases of septic shock or prolonged shock states.

11. Consider autotransfusion (see p. 249).
12. Watch for complications of disseminated intravascular coagulation (DIC).

Antishock trousers. Antishock trousers are used on victims of major trauma who have signs and symptoms of hypovolemic shock. They are particularly useful for lower extremity or abdominal injuries but have other applications for trauma characterized by severe hypovolemia. There are three basic objectives in using the trousers:

1. To autotransfuse approximately 1,000 ml of blood within 1 to 2 minutes.
2. To decrease blood flow to the lower extremities
3. To immobilize injuries of the lower extremities and to reduce blood loss by application of direct pressure.

When the shock trousers are applied and inflated, the internal pressure redirects available circulating blood volume out of the lower extremities into the central circulation to support perfusion of the vital organs (Fig. 12-3).

Antishock trousers are merely to assist in initial stabilization and do not alter underlying problems.

APPLICATION OF ANTISHOCK TROUSERS

1. Assess the area for foreign objects that could puncture the suit (such as glass, needles, and rocks). Fold open the suit, open the stopcock valves, and attach the foot pump.
2. Position the trousers so that the top edge of the suit will be applied just below the lowest rib (Fig. 12-4, *A*).
3. Logroll the patient onto the suit.
4. Wrap the trouser legs around the limbs and fasten them (Fig. 12-4, *B* and *C*).
5. Position and secure the abdominal section (Fig. 12-4, *D*).
6. Inflate the suit to about 104 mm Hg or until air escapes through the release valves *or* until the patient's blood pressure is within acceptable limits. (Any or all chambers of the three-chambered suit may be inflated.)
7. Close the stopcocks; detach the foot pump.
8. Monitor the vital signs carefully. Antici-

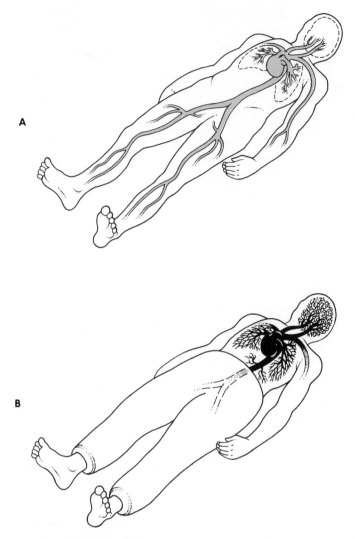

Fig. 12-3. In shock states perfusion of vital organs is greatly enhanced by application of antishock trousers. **A,** Before application; **B,** after application.

pate vomiting. Have suction at hand, or anchor a nasogastric tube.

9. Deflate the suit only after the patient is in the surgical unit or when cardiovascular stabilization has been assured. The following steps should be followed for deflation:

a. Deflate the suit chambers gradually. Each time the blood pressure drops 5 mm Hg, *stop* deflation, accelerate the flow of IV fluids, and wait until the blood pressure reaches the predeflation level.

b. Continue the cycle of deflating the suit 5 mm Hg, accelerating IV fluids, and stabilizing the blood pressure until the trousers are loose enough to remove easily.

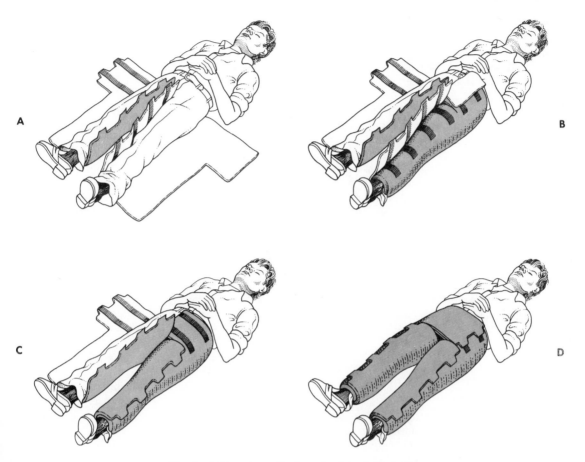

Fig. 12-4. Steps in application of antishock trousers.

10. Draw blood for measurement of the lactate level and arterial blood gases to determine the metabolic effects of the prolonged suit compression and hypovolemic compromise.

Autotransfusion. Autotransfusion is a technique for managing massive hemorrhage by the collection of blood shed by the patient and the return of this blood after processing (filtering and defoaming using an autotransfuser pump). Emergency candidates for autotransfusion include patients with:

Exsanguinating hemorrhage

Religious beliefs that oppose use of another individual's blood via transfusion

Hemorrhage in which banked blood is not readily available; that is, extremely urgent cases in which there is not time for pretransfusion laboratory tests or delivery of blood from a distant site

Difficult blood to type and cross-match in which no suitable banked blood is available

History of previous transfusion reactions

Contraindications include patients with:

Wounds more than 4 hours old

Gross contamination of shed blood by leakage of abdominal contents

Inadequate liver or kidney function

Autotransfusion requires that all members of the core emergency team be well versed in the use of the autotransfuser and understand the procedures involved in preparing both the patient and the equipment for the autotransfusion. Since the procedure is only an interim adjunct to management of shock from hemorrhage, surgery personnel should be alerted at once regarding this patient.

EMERGENCY MANAGEMENT

1. Prehospital personnel should alert the emergency department that they are enroute with a candidate for autotransfusion so that personnel can ready the equipment and supplies. (Other prehospital care is carried out as usual.)
2. Obtain a sample for urinalysis and venous blood for testing:
   PTT (partial thromboplastin time)
   Thrombin time
   Prothrombin time
   Fibrinogen level
   Fibrinogen split products
   Free plasma hemoglobin
   Potassium
   Calcium
   Creatinine
   BUN
   Complete blood count
   Platelet count
3. Draw blood for arterial blood gas testing.
4. Proceed with autotransfusion* after taking baseline vital signs and ensuring that basic life support needs have been met, including delivery of high-flow oxygen and regular administration of resuscitative fluids (that is, other than autotransfused blood, such as plasma protein fraction [plasmanate]). At least two IV lines must be established, and monitoring the CVP is recommended.
5. Record the approximate amount of shed blood collected and retransfused along with the type and amount of any anticoagulants. Note the source of blood collected.
6. Monitor the patient for complications.
   a. Air or fat embolus (p. 287)

---

*The procedure usually involves collecting blood via chest tubes. Details of the procedure vary with the bleeding site and the autotransfuser apparatus.

b. Bleeding caused by coagulation defects
   c. Hypothermia
   d. DIC (p. 259)
   e. Hemolysis of red cells
   f. Sepsis
7. After the transfusion, continue to monitor previously cited laboratory values and vital signs.
8. Consider the use of platelet transfusions and forced diuresis if indicated.

CARDIOGENIC SHOCK

Cardiogenic shock, commonly called ''pump failure,'' is a shock syndrome characterized by an abnormality in the function of the cardiopulmonary unit creating inadequate tissue perfusion.

Cause

Cardiogenic shock can be due to myocardial failure from myocardial infarction of a large portion of cardiac muscle.

Andreoli (1979) states that 15% of patients in the hospital because of myocardial infarction have a clinical picture of cardiogenic shock. Cardiac tamponade and pulmonary embolus may also impair cardiac performance causing cardiogenic shock.

Hemodynamic monitoring (see also pp. 254-259)

The most dramatic events of cardiogenic shock center around the cardiovascular system. These parameters are used for diagnosis, selecting the treatment regimen, and evaluating the patient's response to therapy.

Right heart function: Monitored with cardiac output (COP) or right atrial pressure (RAP). Right-side pressures will be normal early and increase following left-side pressure increases. Right-side pressures reflect filling pressure in right heart chambers.

Left heart function: Monitored with pulmonary artery end-diastolic pressure (PAEDP) or pulmonary capillary wedge pressure (PCWP). PCWP will be elevated above 12 to 15 mm Hg pressure. PAEDP closely approximates PCWP if wedge not available. Left-side pressures reflect filling pressure in left heart.

Cardiac output: Measured by using thermodilution Swan-Ganz catheter. Cardiac output will be low; normal, 4 to 8 liters/minute. Cardiac index is more accurately used to index cardiac output based on body size or body surface area. In cardiogenic shock, cardiac index will be less than 2.2 liters/minute/m^2, normal, 2.5 to 4.8 liters/minute/m^2.

Oxygen saturation: *Right atrial oxygen saturation* can be sampled using a triple lumen Swan-Ganz catheter. Right atrial oxygen saturation closely approximates mixed venous oxygen saturation. It will be reduced by ventilation perfusion abnormalities, diffusion abnormalities, or intrapulmonary shunting.

Arteriovenous oxygen saturation difference: The arteriovenous oxygen saturation difference is obtained by sampling arterial and mixed venous blood and determining oxygen saturation. If the difference is greater than 30%, then tissues are extracting more oxygen than normal. One can assume that cardiac output is inadequate to meet cellular demands.

Signs and symptoms

In addition to a hemodynamic picture of low cardiac output, elevated left-side pressures, and increased peripheral vascular resistance, the following signs and symptoms occur in cardiogenic shock.

Hypotension (less than 90 mm Hg systolic)
Impaired tissue perfusion evidenced by:
  Cool pale extremities; may also be cyanotic
  Diminished pulses
  Clammy skin
  Changes in sensorium
  Decreased urine output
Decreased stroke volume evidenced by narrow pulse pressure
Tachycardia (bradycardia if ischemia is posterior to left ventricle)
Increased peripheral vascular resistance evidenced by signs above of vasoconstriction
Baseline data are important to assess when patient is admitted to the emergency department, including those explained before in relation to septic shock, with the exception of urine and blood cultures.

Treatment

Andreoli (1979) states that current studies indicate an 80% mortality rate for the patient in cardiogenic shock. Aimed at increasing pump performance and improving the cardiac output, treatment includes the following.

1. Improve cardiac output by correcting or treating abnormalities in preload, afterload, heart rate, and contractility; this may include correcting arrhythmias if present
2. Maintain ventilation and acid-base balance, and decrease hypoxemia
3. Pharmacological agents
   Morphine sulfate to relieve pain (see p. 730)
   Atropine to treat bradycardia if present (see p. 715)
   Inotropic agents to improve contractility (see isoproterenol, dopamine pp. 726 and 721, respectively)
   Adrenergic agents to support blood pressure (see levarterenol [Levophed] p. 727, metaraminol [Aramine] p. 728)
   Mannitol to increase renal blood flow (see p. 728)
   Vasodilators/nitroprusside to decrease peripheral vascular resistance (see p. 738)
4. Hemodynamic monitoring and assessment of cardiac output
5. Monitoring renal status through use of Foley catheter, hourly urine output, and specific gravity.
6. Cardiac assist in the form of external counterpulsation or the intraaortic balloon pump may be used to increase myocardial blood supply and reduce afterload, therefore decreasing cardiac work.

ANAPHYLAXIS

Anaphylaxis (or anaphylactic shock) is an acute systemic allergic reaction that results from the release of chemical mediators after antigen-antibody interactions. The usual causes are penicillin reactions or responses to snake or insect venom. Anaphylaxis is usually immediate in onset, but it may be delayed for 10 to 30 minutes.

Signs and symptoms

Sudden anxiety, restlessness, and feeling of doom
Intense itching, especially of the feet and hands
Pounding headache
Coughing and difficulty breathing (for example, stridor with supraclavicular, suprasternal, and intercostal retractions)
Nausea, abdominal cramps, and even involuntary defecation
Seizures
Flushing of skin
Change in voice or loss of voice as a result of laryngeal edema
Dramatic hypotension
Urinary incontinence

Emergency management

The emergency nurse should take immediate steps to ensure basic life support. Intubation and positive pressure ventilation may be necessary. Aqueous epinephrine (1:1000) 1 to 2 ml is given directly IV or IC. (Epinephrine may be given IM [0.3 to 0.5 ml] if shock is not present; a 0.3 ml dose may be injected intradermally around the bite or sting or injection site to retard the development of anaphylaxis.) *Do not wait to establish an IV line* to administer epinephrine! The dosage may be repeated in 15 minutes if symptoms persist. In the meantime, initiate an IV of 1,000 ml D/5/W. Some physicians will choose to administer 100 mg hydrocortisone (Solu-Cortef) IV over 1 to 2 minutes. Metaraminol (Aramine) or levarterenol (Levophed) may be given via a titrated drip. Diphenhydramine (Benadryl) 50 to 75 mg may be ordered IV to help combat the intense allergic reaction.

All patients who have anaphylaxis in the emergency department should be admitted for at least 24 hours to ensure stabilization. Before discharge, it is important to instruct the individual about anaphylaxis and stress its prevention.

PRINCIPLES OF THERAPY FOR SHOCK

The management of a patient in shock involves attention to aspects of airway and ventilation; maintenance of blood volume, pressure, and circulation; and provisions to ensure cellular oxygen consumption and nutrition.

Airway and ventilation

All patients in shock deserve special attention to this factor, since even the most optimum airway and oxygen delivery falls short of compensating for perfusion deficits in the shock state. The natural airway should be ensured by proper positioning and suctioning (see p. 132), and supplementary oxygen at high flow rates should be initiated at once (that is, 15 liters by nasal cannula). A face mask, mechanical ventilatory assistance, or endotracheal intubation should be used if the airway is compromised.

The goal of therapy is to maintain an arterial pO_2 of 100 mm Hg during resuscitation. Never withhold oxygen for fear of oxygen toxicity, since this is not a valid concern in short-term therapy even for the patient with chronic obstructive lung disease.

If ventilator assistance is necessary, a volume-cycled type is most desirable to ensure tidal volumes of 12 to 15 ml/kg. This is approximately twice the rate for normal individuals in a nonshock state. Emergency personnel should not be reluctant to deliver this exaggerated amount! It should be noted that normal blood gas values often can be maintained with less, but that *high* tidal volumes are necessary for preventing and correcting congestive microatelectasis. The inflation pressure, however, is kept to less than 40 cm water pressure if possible to minimize the risk of pneumothorax. Water pressures over 50 cm may require the use of a "prophylactic" chest tube, particularly if there is evidence of pulmonary disease or chest trauma.

If high tidal volume fails to correct the problem, positive end expiratory pressure (PEEP) at 5 to 15 or more cm water pressure may be useful. Intermittent mandatory ventilation (IMV) can be used for spontaneously breathing patients who can tolerate lower tidal volumes and greater PEEP, up to 30 cm water pressure.

The respiratory therapy regimen is designed to maintain a respiratory rate of 12 to 16/minute to avoid a respiratory alkalosis that develops with tachypnea. Dead space of up to 300 ml may be required to maintain the pCO_2 within a range of 30 to 50 mm Hg without cutting back tidal volume.

Most clinicians avoid the use of any respiratory depressant or paralyzing drugs in shock states (for example, pancuronium (Pavulon), diazepam, or morphine and curare or succinylcholine, respectively), because they have deleterious effects in low pressure states.

Fluids

The initial fluid infusion therapy should consist of crystalloids, preferably Ringer's lactate. As soon as the ABCs of basic life support are assured, one (preferably two) large-bore IV line is started in a large vein. (The second line is desirable for measuring the CVP. See p. 256.) A device large enough to accommodate transfusion therapy is desirable, of course. When the initial IV is started, it is useful to employ Y-blood tubing with a filter to avoid a change later when colloid therapy is done.

Antishock trousers or a venesection may be required adjuncts to infusion therapy in the event of preexisting peripheral collapse (see p. 209 and p. 247).

Two to 3 liters of fluid are given over 20 to 30 minutes while carefully monitoring the hemodynamic picture (see pp. 254-259). If additional fluid is required to maintain the blood pressure, blood may be started to maintain the hemoglobin within a normal range (12.5 to 14 gm/100 ml. In the meantime, an aggressive search for occult bleeding should be under way if the site of blood loss is not obvious.

Plasma or albumin may be ordered if the serum protein levels are abnormally low in order to maintain oncotic pressure. However, it should be used with extreme caution in sepsis, because it tends to contribute to respiratory failure. Fresh frozen plasma is helpful in restoring essential clotting factors (except platelets) that are deficient in banked blood.

Low molecular weight dextran (LMWD) is often used, but it tends to increase bleeding from raw surface areas and may produce allergic reactions in selected patients. Furthermore, it will interfere with typing and crossmatching unless red cells are washed with saline.

The amount of fluid is largely determined by hemodynamic monitoring (see p. 254). The blood pressure, pulse, rate, urinary output, and condition of the skin and lungs are important parameters to scrutinize in addition to the CVP, pulmonary wedge pressure, or other more sophisticated indices.

Acid-base balance

The majority of acid-base problems can be corrected with the use of a good ventilatory regimen. Occasionally, sodium bicarbonate may be indicated. It is given with extreme caution to prevent alkalosis, which interferes with oxygen dissociation.

Digitalization

Many shock patients have accompanying heart failure and thus require an inotropic agent. Digoxin is usually administered in several small doses while carefully monitoring the ECG. Several hours may elapse before the digitalization effects are noted.

Dopamine (Intropin) may be given for its positive inotropic effect. The effects are variable depending on the dose rate, so it must be administered cautiously. A microdrip set is used, and it is titrated on a minute-to-minute basis.

Additional drug therapy

Ionized calcium must be available for cells in shock, and its mobilization tends to be impaired during this compromised state. It is an especially important adjunct for the patient who has had multiple transfusions. The nurse must be very cautious in giving calcium to digitalized patients, because it tends to contribute to the development of digitalis intoxication.

Other agents may also be useful in shock states, such as isoproterenol, metaraminol, norepinephrine, and phenylephrine. Their use is generally reserved for individuals who have been unresponsive to other therapy. It is important that fluid resuscitation be vigorous, however, before any pressor drugs are used, because their effects in low volume states can be devastating.

Steroids are still controversial for routine use in shock states, but some clinicians favor the administration of at least 200 mg of hydrocortisone for patients unresponsive to other standard therapy. The dramatic improvement seen in selected instances may be related to subclinical adrenal insufficiency. Some researchers have found it beneficial to give larger doses, and to trust that their early and aggressive use will stabilize the cell membranes and preserve organelles.

Vasodilators such as nitroprusside, diuretics such as furosemide (Lasix), and heparin may also be employed. Heparin is indicated for its role in intravascular coagulation (see p. 725).

Other nursing measures

The patient in shock should be flat or in the shock (not Trendelenburg) position with only the legs elevated. A head-down position (once favored) has been abandoned because it may cause the diaphragm to migrate upward, thus compromising ventilation.

A Foley catheter is a ''must'' to facilitate the recording of frequent outputs. The adult output should be maintained at least 30 ml/hour. The patient should be kept warm to prevent unnecessary utilization of oxygen in relation to heat production. Finally, it should be noted that if analgesics are required, they should not be given IM to the patients in shock because of erratic peripheral circulation. Verbal reassurance and local anesthesia for certain invasive procedures are important considerations, however.

Hemodynamic monitoring

Hemodynamic monitoring is ongoing assessment of cardiovascular functioning. There are both noninvasive and invasive ways to accomplish hemodynamic monitoring.

Noninvasive hemodynamic monitoring. Modes include many of the routine observations nurses make in relation to the patient in shock. The ECG and routine vital signs (pulse, blood pressure, respirations) reflect both cardiac and respiratory efficiency. Determining the level of consciousness and its trend provides information about how effectively the brain is being perfused and nourished. The character and rate of peripheral pulses furnish clues to the adequacy of cardiac output and the responsiveness of compensatory mechanisms such as vasoconstriction. Pulse deficits or extrasystoles may also be discovered. The routine observations about the skin condition (cyanosis, diaphoresis, coolness) and characteristics of the oral mucosa (dryness, dullness cyanosis) also reveal the efficiency of cardiac output and peripheral vasomotor reflex activity. The urinary output reflects the status of renal perfusion and the level of hydration, at least in part. Finally, the postural vital signs help detect hypovolemia by demonstrating the compensatory mechanics of blood volume dynamics to postural changes.

Noninvasive monitoring is a continuing process throughout the management of the patient's acute stage in the emergency department.

Invasive hemodynamic monitoring. Modes include monitoring arterial blood gases, systemic arterial pressure, central venous pressure (CVP), pulmonary artery (PA) pressure, pulmonary wedge pressure, cardiac output, and oxygen saturation (arterial and venous.) These methods are physiologically specific and provide more accurate data about the status of the cardiovascular mechanisms. They are used in the emergency department primarily for determining the mechanisms of the shock syndrome and for guiding shock therapy.

ARTERIAL PRESSURE. This monitoring method involves the cannulation of the radial or femoral artery and the use of transduction and amplification of arterial pressure to an oscilloscope (or a modified apparatus) (see Fig. 12-8). It is particularly beneficial to monitor the arterial pressure when the cardiac output is low and when vasopressor therapy is initiated. It also provides an access point for serial arterial blood gas measurements.

The visual arterial wave seen on an oscilloscope provides data about the function of the left ventricle. The upstroke indicates the ven-

Postural vital signs

Assessment

Indications: Postural vital signs should be assessed on all patients with (1) evidence of significant fluid loss through bleeding, vomiting, diarrhea, perspiration, or wound drainage; (2) unexplained tachycardia; (3) hypotension without tachycardia; (4) history or suspicion of chronic or concealed bleeding; or (5) blunt abdominal or chest trauma.

Contraindications: Postural vital signs are *not* indicated if other injuries or the patient's general condition preclude safe administration of the test.

Rationale for test: When a patient assumes a vertical position, gravity tends to cause sequestration (pooling) of blood in the capacitance vessels of the legs and trunk. Normally, individuals adapt readily to this postural change through rapid vasoconstriction of the vessels in which the blood tends to pool. This adjustment is not possible for the volume-depleted patient whose vasoconstrictor potential has already been maximally utilized.

Interpreting results: Postural changes (from lying to sitting or standing) resulting in a *decrease* of 20 mm Hg or more in the systolic or diastolic blood pressure *or increase* of 20 beats or more per minute in the pulse rate is a *positive* test result, and the patient should be considered *hypovolemic* until proved otherwise.

CAUTION! The patient may experience weakness, dizziness, visual disturbances, or fainting during the test. These symptoms are promptly eliminated in most instances when the patient lies down again. Be certain to protect the patient during the assessment of postural vital signs to prevent injuries.

Test*

1. With the patient supine, take and record the blood pressure and pulse as a baseline against which changes of both measures taken after position changes can be evaluated.
2. Have the patient sit up to a 90° position and again record the blood pressure and pulse.
3. Have the patient stand if possible, and again record the blood pressure and pulse. If significant changes occur, or if the patient's symptoms become acute during the sitting portion of the test, the third step may be eliminated and the results of the sitting portion considered positive.

Correct charting of the results is done in the following manner:

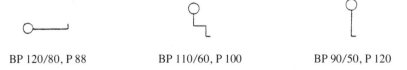

| BP 120/80, P 88 | BP 110/60, P 100 | BP 90/50, P 120 |

---

*From Bookman, L. B., and Simoneau, J. K.: The early assessment of hypovolemia: Postural vital signs, J.E.N. **3:**43, 1977.

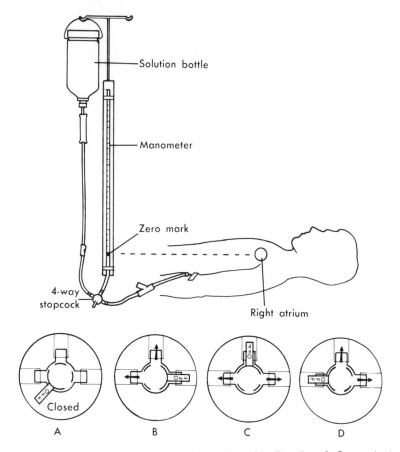

Fig. 12-5. Central venous pressure assessment is read at midaxillary line. **A,** Stopcock closed. **B,** Stopcock open to IV solution and manometer. **C,** Stopcock open to IV solution and patient. **D,** Stopcock open to manometer and patient. (From Barber, J., Stokes, L., and Billings, D.: Adult and child care, ed. 2, St. Louis, 1977, The C. V. Mosby Co.)

tricular ejection force, and the lowest point of the downstroke of the wave reflects diastole.

CENTRAL VENOUS PRESSURE (CVP). This conventional mode of hemodynamic monitoring involves placement of a catheter into a large vein through a percutaneous puncture or vensection. The CVP catheter can be used to assess right atrial pressure and right heart function. The changes in venous pressure reflect blood volume and venous return to the right heart.

Since left heart output depends on venous return, the CVP indirectly serves as an index of the left heart's activity. (It should be noted, however, that rapid or critical changes in the left side's functioning are not readily detectable by CVP monitoring.) The CVP is often used in the emergency department for guiding fluid replacement in hypovolemic shock states.

PROCEDURE (Fig. 12-5)

1. Place the patient in a supine (flat) position.
2. Measure at the midaxillary line (5 cm from the top of the chest) in the fourth intercostal space at the level of the right atrium.
3. Place the manometer zero reading at this point.
4. Fill the manometer from the attached IV solution (do not overflow) (Fig. 12-5, *B*).
5. Turn the stopcock on the IV line open to

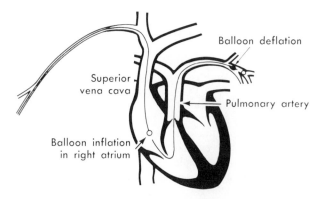

Fig. 12-6. Flow-directed, balloon-tipped (Swan-Ganz) catheter, showing inflation of balloon in right atrium and consequent "floating" of catheter through right ventricle and out to distal pulmonary artery branch. Balloon is deflated, advanced slightly, and reinflated to obtain PAW pressure. (From Schroeder, J. S., and Dailey, E. K.: Techniques in bedside hemodynamic monitoring, St. Louis, 1976, The C. V. Mosby Co.)

the patient and the manometer. The fluid level will fall and fluctuate (decreasing on inspiration and increasing on expiration) (Fig. 12-5, *D*).

6. When the fluid level appears stable, note where the top of the fluid column reaches.
7. Record this reading as the CVP.
8. Adjust the stopcock to close the manometer and open the IV line to the patient (make sure to readjust the IV solution) (Fig. 12-5, *C*).

The normal range of CVP is 4 to 10 cm of water pressure. A value greater than 10 cm may indicate tamponade, right heart failure, fluid overload, pulmonary edema, tension pneumothorax or hemothorax. A value below 4 cm may indicate hypovolemia, vasodilation, dehydration, septic shock, or drug-induced shock.

PULMONARY ARTERY WEDGE PRESSURE. The pulmonary artery wedge (PAW) pressure is measured by the use of a flow-directed, balloon-tipped catheter (Figs. 12-6 and 12-7). The catheter may be a double or triple lumen thermodilution catheter, such as a Swan-Ganz. The device allows for monitoring of CVP, pulmonary artery (PA) pressure, and pulmonary capillary wedge pressure (PCWP). The balloon tip serves both to guide the catheter to the pulmonary artery and to occlude a pulmonary capillary for pressure measurement. PCWP

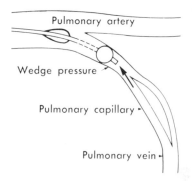

Fig. 12-7. During initial positioning of balloon-tipped catheter in pulmonary artery, balloon is deflated. Catheter is then advanced, and balloon is reinflated just enough to obtain PAW pressure. (From Schroeder, J. S., and Dailey, E. K.: Techniques in bedside hemodynamic monitoring, St. Louis, 1976, The C. V. Mosby Co.)

measures left atrial pressure and left heart filling pressure, thus, the performance of the left heart.

Emergency nurses may come into contact with the use of the thermodilution catheter in shock resuscitation. An increase in PA pressure, for example, signals left heart failure or volume overload.

The nurse who cares for the patient with a PA catheter must be alert to risks associated with

PA pressure monitoring. Among these are dysrhythmias, thromboembolism, infection, and infarction.

The thermodilution catheter is inserted with the benefit of fluoroscopy when feasible, but it may be floated into position using changes in pressure wave forms to identify its location within the structures.

Transduction and oscilloscope amplification are used to indicate the physiological events.

The Swan-Ganz catheter permits electronic monitoring of cardiac output and sampling of mixed venous blood.

PROCEDURE

1. Position the patient in the Trendelenburg position if insertion is into the internal jugular, external jugular, or subclavian vein.

2. Prepare a percutaneous insertion site by scrubbing with antiseptic solution and drying, or do a surgical cutdown (see p. 209) to gain access to a peripheral vein. Acceptable sites include:

   Internal jugular vein
   Supraclavicular or infraclavicular subclavian vein (infraclavicular approach has higher risk of pneumothorax)
   Brachial vein
   Antecubital vein
   Femoral vein

3. Enter the vein with a suitable needle and/or catheter introducer with spring guide, thin-walled sheath, and a tapered perforating catheter. When the catheter introducer is in place, remove the spring guide and perforating catheter, leaving the sheath in place, through which to advance the monitoring catheter. When this has been accomplished, withdraw the sheath over the catheter.

4. When the catheter is in the vena cava, inflate the balloon at the tip (with air or carbon dioxide) and advance the catheter through the right atrium and ventricle into the pulmonary artery. *Observe for dysrhythmias,* especially when the catheter passes through the right ventricle.

5. Advance the catheter smoothly to retard venospasm.

6. When the catheter ceases to advance, deflate the balloon and advance the catheter slightly.

7. Position the catheter tip so that the PA pressure reading is obtained with the inflated balloon.

8. Secure the catheter with a suture and close the incision. Apply a sterile dressing to the site. Tape the site securely to protect the catheter and dressing.

PROCEDURE FOR ESTABLISHING INTRAARTERIAL LINES. Intraarterial lines may be used to accom-

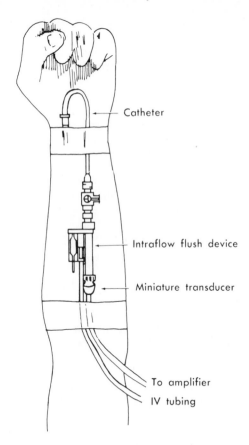

Fig. 12-8. Miniature strain gauge transducer connected to arterial catheter with Intraflow device. LuerLok stopcock is placed between catheter and Intraflow device for sampling and room air reference. A similar setup is used for venous pressure monitoring. (From Schroeder, J. S., and Dailey, E. K.: Techniques in bedside hemodynamic monitoring, St. Louis, 1976, The C. V. Mosby Co.)

plish hemodynamic monitoring. They may be established through a percutaneous puncture or cutdown.

Before installing the line in a forearm, collateral circulation should be checked by the Allen test (see p. 384).

The skin should be shaved and cleansed with an antiseptic agent such as povidone iodine. A local anesthetic may also be used.

After the arterial catheter has been installed, it is connected to a flush system (Fig. 12-8).

The emergency nurse should know the details of managing the arterial line, the flush system, and the transducer. Safety in regard to its use in an emergency setting should be understood. For example, to protect the patient and the equipment, electrical connections must be kept dry at all times. During defibrillation, the transducer should be electrically isolated or disconnected to avoid irreparable damage to the device. Of course, extreme care should always be exercised to prevent accidental disconnection of the system's parts, because exsanguination can result if the loss of integrity is not promptly recognized.

Specifics on intraarterial monitoring procedures are beyond the scope of this text.

SHOCK-RELATED COMPLICATIONS
Disseminating intravascular coagulation (DIC)

Disseminating intravascular coagulation (DIC) is a condition manifested by diffuse hemorrhage and thrombosis; it often complicates a critical illness. It is associated with gram-positive septicemia, renal allograft rejection, and liver failure. Other causes that are thought to predispose to DIC are more commonly seen by emergency personnel. These include prolonged hypotension, acidosis, hypoxemia, obstetrical complications, viremia, heat stroke, gram-negative endotoxemia (especially meningococcemia), and mismatched plasma or blood transfusions.

The emergency nurse should suspect DIC when there is acute bleeding or purpuric diathesis associated with hypotension, chemotherapy of neoplasia, sepsis, or massive blood transfusions. An abnormal baseline coagulation test may be the first clue to the problem.

Signs and symptoms. Signs and symptoms include petechiae, purpura, hemorrhagic bullae, gangrene, acral cyanosis (earlobes, fingertips, elbows, toes, and kneecaps), subcutaneous hematoma formation, and unusual bleeding following venipuncture. Maintaining a high suspicion of DIC will alert the nurse to suspect the phenomenon when encountering blood oozing from puncture sites or catheters, a sudden gastric hemorrhage associated with purpura or hematomas, or a combination of acral cyanosis and septicemia.

Emergency management. Baseline bloods should be drawn for arterial blood gases, prothrombin time, liver function studies, platelet count, and fibrinogen level. Blood cultures and a chest x-ray film (anteroposterior) should also be obtained.

In the meantime, minimize vessel catheterization and perform further studies. The physician will do careful neurological, fundoscopic, and spinal fluid assessments and plan for the patient's admission to the intensive care unit for treatment of the underlying condition. Adjunctive therapy includes heparin, EACA (epsilon aminocaproic acid), vitamin K, folic acid, vitamin B_{12}, protamine, blood products, platelets, and fibrinogen.

Shock lung

This complication of the shock state is also known as congestive atelectasis, posttraumatic pulmonary insufficiency, Da Nang lung, and adult respiratory distress syndrome (see also pp. 381-382).

Following trauma and resultant low-volume states, the lungs have decreased compliance and eventually are difficult to ventilate effectively. The steps in development are as follows:

1. Massive vascular congestion (damage to capillary beds)
2. Pulmonary edema (microaggregates form and a hydrolytic enzyme is released—"capillary leak syndrome")
3. Pulmonary hemorrhage
4. Hyaline membrane formation (capillaries covered with type I pneumocyte)
5. Bronchopneumonia (albumin enters interstitial spaces)
6. Pulmonary fibrosis (degenerative result)

The primary modes of combating this complication of shock are positive end expiratory pressure (PEEP), constant positive airway pressure (CPAP), or constant positive pressure breathing (CPPB). These special modes of ventilation decrease dead space, increase functional residual capacity, increase arterial oxygen tension by increasing compliance, and decrease arteriovenous shunting.

Micropore filters are also thought to reduce microaggregates and microemboli, which contribute to shock lung. Steroids are thought to be valuable in preventing the degenerative phenomena of the classical shock lung syndrome.

BIBLIOGRAPHY

Andreoli, K. G., and others: Comprehensive cardiac care, ed. 4, St. Louis, 1979, The C. V. Mosby Co.

Baue, A. E.: Blood volume and oligemic shock. In Hardy, J. D.: Testbook of surgery, ed. 5, Philadelphia, 1977, J. B. Lippincott Co.

Hardy, J. D.: Textbook of surgery, ed. 5, Philadelphia, 1977, J. B. Lippincott Co.

Hathaway, R. G.: Hemodynamic monitoring in shock, J.E.N. **3**(5):37-42 September-October 1977.

Hathaway, R. G.: The Swan-Ganz catheter: a review, Nurs. Clin. N. Am. **13**(3):389-407, 1978.

Mela, L. M.: Oxygen's role in health and shock. In Oxygen and cellular energy metabolism in shock, Kalamazoo, Mich., 1977, Upjohn Co.

Shubin, H., and Weil, M. H.: Bacterial shock, J.A.M.A. **235**(4):1.421, 1976.

Thal, A. P.: Septic shock. In Hardy, J. D.: Textbook of surgery, ed. 5, Philadelphia, 1977, J. B. Lippincott Co.

Thompson, W. L.: The patient in shock. From A clinical discussion from the proceedings of a symposium on recent research developments and current clinical practice in shock, Kalamazoo, Mich., 1977, Upjohn Co.

Wilson, R. F.: Shock. In A manual of practice and techniques in critical care medicine, Kalamazoo, Mich., 1976, Upjohn Co.

PART TWO

PRACTICE OF EMERGENCY NURSING

Unit III ☐ Medical and surgical emergencies

Unit IV ☐ Environmental emergencies

CHAPTER 13

Multiple trauma

One of the most challenging and critical patient care problems comes with the patient who has sustained multiple injuries. In this chapter, we will attempt to establish a plan for setting priorities when the patient is multiply traumatized.

Trauma is the third leading cause of death in the United States, following coronary artery disease and cancer. It is the number one cause of death in those under 40 years old. There are over 50 million accidental injuries each year, with over 100 thousand of these resulting in death from trauma. An additional 28,000 die from gunshot wounds. It is estimated that 10% to 50% of trauma deaths may be prevented with adequate rescue response time and proper evaluation and care.

Usually 80% of the victims of automobile accidents sustain head injuries, with 45% to 70% of these being fatal. In addition, 40% sustain leg injuries, 25% sustain chest injuries, and 15% have abdominal injuries. It has been reported that 60% of all injuries caused by automobile accidents occur as multiple systems injuries.

Multiple trauma presents a major health problem in the United States. There is a need for a system that will allow for a patient's early entrance into a medical system, prehospital care that is monitored by medical personnel, and facilities that can accommodate the critically injured patient and provide follow-up intensive care. The first step in this system is an adequate communication system. The sec-

ond step is a well-educated public, who has an understanding of how to contact the appropriate agency, how to enter the system, and how to provide basic lifesaving maneuvers.

The third step in this plan is to provide adequately educated and skilled prehospital care personnel (see Chapter 2). These people must be trained to perform an accurate initial assessment, possess good technical and communication skills, and be able to perform good, thorough, continuous assessments en route to a hospital facility.

Probably the most logical of plans for care of the multiple trauma victim is the concept of centralized trauma centers, in which trauma teams have been well trained, and medical and surgical specialists and specialized equipment are readily available. This centralized approach provides for the best care without delay, wasted manpower, or wasted time, and can offer the most modern equipment an approaches to multiple trauma care.

EVALUATION OF PRIORITIES
Assessment in the prehospital setting

Airway. When evaluating a victim of multiple trauma, one should always assume that the injuries are severe until proven otherwise. Begin with a rapid evaluation to determine priorities. Do not focus solely on chief complaint. A rapid evaluation should begin with a 5-second survey of the airway; check it for patency. If the airway is not clear, check first for proper head position. If there is suspicion of cervical spine trauma, the jaw thrust maneuver should be employed.

If you have positioned the head properly and assured that the tongue is clear of the posterior pharyngeal area, and the airway is still not clear, check for foreign bodies and other obstructions such as blood or aspiration materials, and apply appropriate therapeutic interventions (see Chapter 8).

If an airway adjunct is indicated, this is the appropriate time to use it. Consider use of the oropharyngeal airway, the nasopharyngeal airway, the esophageal obturator airway, the endotracheal tube, or cricothyrotomy, as the situation indicates.

Breathing. Next, assess the patient's breathing. If the patient is apneic, one must breathe for the patient. If the patient is breathing spontaneously, one should consider supplemental oxygen by nasal cannula, mask, or bag-valve-mask device. *All multiple trauma victims should receive supplemental oxygen.*

Assessment of breathing should include assessment for adequate ventilation. A skilled clinician should be able to place hands on the patient's chest and estimate tidal volume. If tidal volume is not adequate, ventilation must be assisted. Auscultate the lungs for bilateral breath sounds, obstructions, wheezes, rales, and rhonchi. Once again, all trauma patients should receive some sort of ventilatory assistance, whether supplemental oxygen via nasal cannula or mask or endotracheal intubation and a volume-cycled ventilator. If a volume-cycled ventilator is selected, be sure that it is set at greater than 21% oxygen and a high tidal volume (10 cc/kg) and that the inflation pressure is less than 40 mm Hg.

Circulation. Check for central circulation by palpating carotid and/or femoral pulses or auscultating for heart sounds. If central pulses are absent, chest compression must begin immediately.

At this point in the evaluation, if the victim is found to be pulseless and nonbreathing, the situation indicates a "scoop and run." This means that transportation to an adequate facility from the prehospital care setting should not be delayed, with all other definitive care adminis-

tered en route. Remember that a trauma patient who suffers a cardiopulmonary arrest is a critically ill patient and that there may be very little else that can be done for this person in the field without sacrificing precious seconds. One may, however, elect to initiate two large-bore IV lines, inflate the medical antishock trousers (MAST), and perform other lifesaving procedures such as needle thoracotomy en route to the hospital.

Cervical spine. Following assurance of the basic ABCs (airway, breathing, and circulation), one must pay particular attention to the cervical spine. Protect the cervical spine by applying a cervical collar, backboard, and sand bags, and assume that it is injured until proven otherwise. If the patient is thrashing about, one must manually apply traction to the head and cervical spine area during transport. Once the cervical spine is protected, begin a brief neurological evaluation (see Chapter 14), which should include level of consciousness and pupil reaction to light.

Chest assessment. Check the chest for obvious wounds and injuries. Be especially attuned to signs and symptoms of sucking chest wound, flail segment, pneumothorax and tension pneumothorax, and cardiac tamponade; and be prepared to apply appropriate therapeutic intervention (see Chapter 16).

Hypovolemia. Assess the victim for blood volume, and correct hypovolemic states. Check postural vital signs by first laying the patient down. Then sit the patient up with legs dependent. If the pulse rate increases by 15 beats and the blood pressure drops by 15 mm Hg, it is estimated that there is a 15% blood loss. Control any external bleeding by applying direct pressure, placing pressure on pressure points, or applying a tourniquet in life-threatening situations. If bleeding is external, estimate blood loss. Two large-bore (16-gauge or larger) intravenous lifelines should be initiated, whether or not the victim is demonstrating signs and symptoms of hypovolemia. The drip rate should be regulated according to the systolic blood pressure. The solution of choice should be crystalloid solution of either Ringers lactate or normal saline. The MAST should be placed under the victim and inflated according to protocol

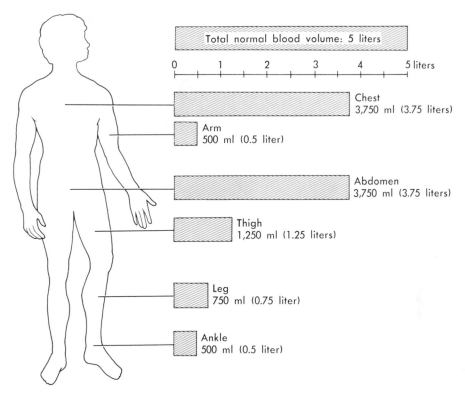

Fig. 13-1. Amount of blood that may be lost into an injured body part.

(see Chapter 18). If a MAST is not available, use the shock (Trendelenburg) position.

Remember to check vital signs and auscultate the lungs frequently of any patient who is receiving large amounts of intravenous fluids.

Hypovolemic shock usually occurs secondary to trauma (Fig. 13-1). It is a pathophysiological state in which there is poor tissue perfusion usually manifested by a systolic blood pressure of less than 80 mm Hg, a urinary output of less than 25 ml/hour, metabolic acidosis, and a rapid pulse rate. Signs and symptoms include a decreasing blood pressure with concurrent rise in pulse rate, increasing respirations, skin pallor, a decreased central venous pressure, cool extremities, clammy skin, oliguria, and vascular depression.

THERAPY. Therapeutic intervention should include close monitoring of the electrocardiogram, pulmonary artery pressure using a pressure gauge (Fig. 13-2) or transducer (pulmonary artery wedge pressure whenever possible), and frequent monitoring of vital signs. Intravenous fluids should be administered at a rate to maintain the pulmonary artery wedge pressure between 10 and 20 mm. Pulmonary artery wedge pressure less than 10 mm is indicative of hypovolemia; pulmonary artery wedge pressure greater than 20 mm indicates fluid overload. If it is not possible to monitor pulmonary artery wedge pressure, one must attempt to maintain the systolic blood pressure at greater than 90 mm Hg.

Although there is much controversy in the literature, we recommend that initial fluids be 2000 ml of a balanced electrolyte solution, such as Ringers lactate or normal saline followed by D/5/normal saline. If the patient is acidotic, one ampule (44.8 mEq) of sodium bicarbonate should be added to the IV solution. This should be followed by 25% to 50% of the continued solution as colloid or blood. One should administer one unit of fresh frozen plasma for every four to five units of whole

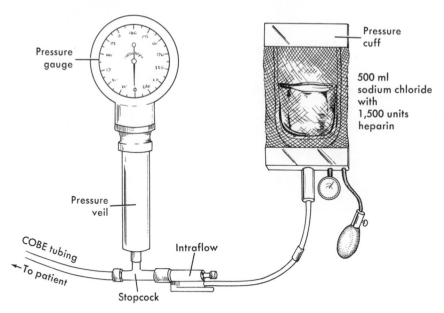

Fig. 13-2. Pressure veil method for measurement of arterial pressure.

blood cells to assure normal coagulation. One ampule (10 ml of 5% solution) of calcium chloride should be administered following every four units of whole blood cells. This is to give supplemental calcium, because free calcium is bound by the citrate added to banked whole blood cells.

Dextran (low or high molecular weight) is not advisable at this point, as it has an extremely high incidence of induced allergic reactions, causes bleeding from raw surfaces, and may sometimes make typing and cross-matching confusing.

If, following fluid administration, application of the MAST, and placement in the Trendelenburg position, hypotension continues to be a life-threatening problem, one may elect to initiate vasopressor therapy. The vasopressor of choice is dopamine (Intropin). (See Appendix F for dopamine dosage schedule.)

Fracture assessment. All fractures should be evaluated for neurological status (movement and sensation) and checked for pulses distal to the fracture site. Fractures should be splinted as they are found unless there is circulatory deficit distal to the fracture site. If there is a circulatory deficit, an attempt should be made to apply traction distal to the fracture site followed by reevaluation of circulatory status. If a neurological deficit is present, every attempt to expedite transport to a hospital facility should be made. Open wounds should be irrigated with normal saline and dressed with a wet-to-dry sterile dressing. If a femur fracture is suspected and signs and symptoms of the same are present without evidence of other fractures to that same limb, it is appropriate to apply the Hare traction splint (see pp. 439-441).

At this point in the initial assessment and therapeutic intervention, if the patient is in the prehospital care setting, it is appropriate to transport to a hospital facility, with frequent monitoring of vital signs en route. Upon arrival at the emergency department, one must immediately reassess airway, breathing, and circulation.

Assessment in emergency department

Before undressing the patient, obtain a cross-table lateral cervical spine x-ray film, which adequately views *all seven* cervical vertebrae.

The film must be read by a physician experienced in reading x-ray film. The patient should then be undressed completely, provided findings on the cervical spine film were negative. Once the patient is undressed, quickly evaluate both the front *and the back* for injuries that may have been overlooked.

History. If possible, obtain a history, both immediate and past. Ascertain facts about the accident:

EXAMPLE:

Where did it happen?	On the freeway.
How did it happen?	The car was hit broadside on the driver's side at 65 mph.
Why did it happen?	The person driving this car had a syncopal episode.
What happened?	This patient was the driver of the car that was hit broadside. He was thrown across the car and out of the passenger side, landing 30 feet from the impact. He was found lying face down on the side of the road.

Ask the patient if he has a history of past or current illness or if he is taking any medications or has any allergies.

Physical examination. Next, evaluate the patient in a thorough, head-to-toe assessment:

Check the head for lacerations, deformities, and fractures.

Check the face for lacerations, foreign bodies, and fractures.

Check the eyes for pupil responsiveness and trauma, including foreign bodies.

Check the ears, nose and throat for cerebrospinal fluid leak, trauma, and foreign bodies. Pay particular attention to examination of the larynx for fracture, as this is a diagnosis usually made by ''thinking about it'' and checking for it.

Check the neck for wounds, deformities, swelling, and appearance of neck veins.

Check the chest for symmetry, wounds, and fractures, and reassess for flail segment and tension pneumothorax or hemothorax. At this point, if obvious tension pneumothorax exists, insert chest tube(s) before obtaining chest x-ray film. Obtain arterial blood gases for analysis.

Check the abdomen for pain, rigidity, tenderness, wounds, hematomas, and girth expansion.

Check the hips and pelvic areas for dislocation, fractures, and deformities.

Check the perineum and genitalia for bleeding, fractures, and urine extravasation.

Check the vertebrae for trauma, hematomas, obvious fractures. Do a more in-depth evaluation of neurological status. (See Chapter 14.)

Check the buttocks for wounds.

Check the back for wounds and hematomas.

Radiological and laboratory evaluation. The ideal situation is to have x-ray capabilities within the emergency department, and preferably in the trauma room where the patient is being evaluated so that radiological evaluation could be going on throughout the assessment and intervention process.

Routine laboratory evaluations on the multiple trauma patient should include typing and cross-matching for at least four units of whole blood cells (more if indicated). Blood specimens should be obtained for hematocrit and hemoglobin (immediately and 1 and 2 hours after arrival at the emergency department), complete blood count (CBC), prothrombin time (PT), and partial thromboplastin time (PTT). Urine should also be sent for analysis. (See Appendix B.)

Assessment and intervention. Insert a nasogastric tube to prevent aspiration, to decompress the stomach, and to obtain gastric analysis if indicated.

Insert a Foley catheter, and monitor hourly urine output. If one has difficulty inserting the Foley catheter into a male victim, this may be indicative of a penis fracture, and one should elect to do a retrograde urethrogram to rule out fracture (see Chapter 20).

At this time it may be appropriate to perform other diagnostic studies as indicated, such as computerized axial tomography (CAT or EMI scan) peritoneal lavage (see Chapter 18), or intravenous pyelogram (IVP).

Evaluate tetanus immunization status and administer tetanus prophylaxis if indicated (see Chapter 11). Antibiotics (usually penicillin or gentamicin) are administered at this time, as well as steroids (usually dexamethasone and hydrocortisone) if indicated.

Notify consultants to medical and surgical specialties, the operating room team, and anesthesia specialists if indicated. This is also an appropriate time to notify clergy if indicated or requested.

Do not administer narcotics if blood pressure is low, if there is a decreasing level of consciousness, or if the exact extent of the injury is not known. It is not wise to administer narcotics to any trauma victim unless the injury is isolated and will not interfere with adequate patient assessment.

It is essential to remember that many of these assessments and interventions can be performed concurrently by various members of the trauma team. If, during evaluation, any of the following conditions is discovered, immediate therapeutic intervention should take place:

Airway obstruction, both upper and lower
Laryngeal fracture
Flail chest
Bilateral pneumothorax
Tension pneumothorax
Cardiac tamponade
Severe neurological trauma with decreasing level of consciousness, elevating blood pressure, and decreasing pulse with unilateral or bilateral dilated pupil
Ruptured great vessel
Respiratory or cardiac arrest

One must at all times keep a keen eye and an open mind. Be prepared to alter therapeutic intervention or respond to an unexpected happening in seconds.

OPEN CHEST MASSAGE

Open chest massage is experiencing renewed popularity with the coming of emergency medicine as a specialty. It is often indicated in the chest trauma patient and/or the multiply traumatized patient who experiences cardiopulmo-
nary arrest secondary to penetrating wounds of the heart, cardiac tamponade (following unsuccessful pericardiocentesis), severe chest trauma, tension pneumothorax with mediastinal shift (following unsuccessful needle thoracotomy or chest tube insertion), or in certain chest wall deformities (such as barrel chest), and certain spinal deformities.

This lifesaving procedure should be performed only by a physician who possesses the proper technical skills, proper equipment and a facility close by that can care for the patient following successful resuscitation. All emergency department nursing personnel should know the procedure in order to be able to prepare proper equipment and assist throughout the procedure.

Procedure
Equipment
Sterile towels
Sterile gloves
Scalpel handle and blade
Forceps
Rib spreader
Scissors
Suture
Large needle and holder
Vascular clamps
Technique
Place the patient in a supine position.
Assure that an esophageal obturator airway or endotracheal tube is in place.
Assure that two IV lines are in place. (Peripheral placement is acceptable.)
Perform simple skin cleansing.
Perform simple draping.
Make an anterolateral thoracotomy incision in the fourth or fifth intercostal space.
Spread the ribs, and retract the lungs.
Introduce a gloved hand into the chest cavity.
Open the pericardial sac if necessary.
Massage the heart, gently compressing the ventricles.
Determine if there is an injury, and repair it if possible.
Once the procedure has been accomplished, transport the patient to the operating room for irrigation, closure, chest tube placement, and so on.

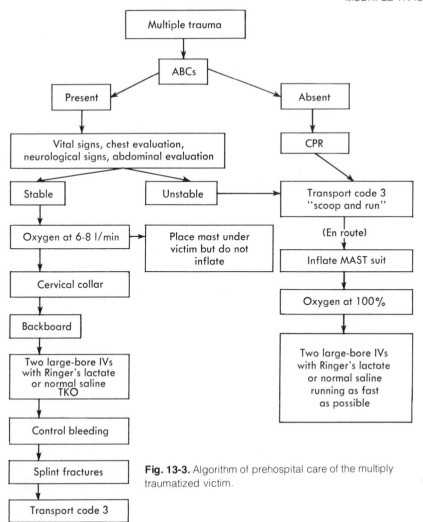

Fig. 13-3. Algorithm of prehospital care of the multiply traumatized victim.

The patient should then be transferred to the recovery room or the intensive care unit.

• • •

The key to successful resuscitation of the multiple trauma victim is a well-drilled, well-trained, and well-prepared trauma team with a strong team leader who can lead the team and make rapid, competent decisions (Fig. 13-3). Much emphasis should be placed on the team approach to preserve life and function.

BIBLIOGRAPHY

MacDonald, J. R.: Multiple trauma; field priorities and interventions, Lecture given at UCLA Postgraduate Institute on Emergency Medicine, Jan. 24, 1979, Beverly Hills, Calif.

Olivei, C. T.: Open chest massage, Crit. Care Q. **I:**1, 1978.

SUGGESTED READINGS

American Academy of Orthopedic Surgeons: Emergency care and transportation of the sick and injured, ed. 2, George Bonta Co., 1977.

American College of Surgeons, Committee on trauma: Early care of the injured patient, ed. 2, Philadelphia, 1976, W. B. Saunders Co.

Barber, J. M. and Budassi, S. A.: Mosby's manual of emergency care, St. Louis, 1979, The C. V. Mosby Co.

Houchens, B. A.: Major trauma in the rural mountain west, J.A.C.E.P. **6:**343-358, 1977.

Lanros, N. E.: Emergency nursing, Bowie, Md., 1978, R. J. Brady Co.

CHAPTER 14

Neurological emergencies

Emergency nurses frequently encounter patients with injuries of the brain and spinal cord; therefore, we must have a thorough knowledge of how to manage these problems. It involves a series of refined assessment skills, as well as basic modes to protect the patient during the acute phase of injury. This chapter deals with the mechanisms of central nervous system injury, prehospital and emergency department management of specific types of injuries, and physiological aberrations associated with disease and trauma states.

CENTRAL NERVOUS SYSTEM ANATOMY

The central nervous system comprises the brain and spinal cord. The brain is divided into several major divisions.

The cerebrum is the largest part of the brain (representing seven eighths of the total weight), and its cortex is the most sophisticated part of the brain. The white matter that lies below the cortex consists of several tracts of nervous tissue. The cerebrum is hemispheric, separated by the falx cerebri, which is actually an extension of the dura. The corpus callosum links the two hemispheres, which are largely responsible for motor activity of the contralateral half of the body. Most individuals possess a dominant hemisphere, which is largely determined by trained association processes. Each cerebral hemisphere is divided into four lobes, named according to their anatomical location under skull bones, frontal, parietal, temporal, and occipital (Fig. 14-1).

The *diencephalon* (thalamus and hypothalamus) is located in the forebrain with the cerebrum. The *thalamus* is essentially a sensory relay center (except for olfaction), and it integrates sensory impulses. Because of its anatomical location, it can facilitate or inhibit motor impulses from the cerebral cortex. It also has a role in integrating emotional behavior. The thalamus contains the pineal gland in its dorsomedial portion. Malfunction of the thalamus affects the interface of sensory cord pathways and the brainstem with the cerebral cortex.

The *hypothalamus* is responsible for regulation of renal water flow, temperature, and several endocrine-metabolic functions. It has an important role in the state of arousal along with the reticular activating systems of the brainstem and thalamus, and certainly relates to certain expressions of emotion.

The *midbrain* lies between the forebrain and the hindbrain and relates primarily to motor coordination and postural reflex patterns. The superior portion controls conjugate eye movements and the upward gaze.

The *hindbrain* contains the cerebellum, the pons, the medulla oblongata and reticular formations. The *cerebellum* is responsible for equilibrium, voluntary movement integration, position sense, and posture. The *pons* is actually a structural link and a relay station from the medulla to higher centers, as well as serving as a base for cranial nerve nuclei. The *medulla oblongata* is continuous with the spinal cord and pons. It contains a representation of all afferent and efferent spinal cord tracts. It not

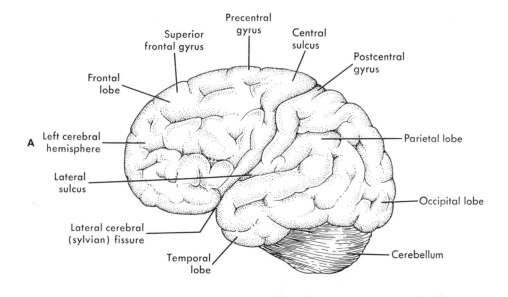

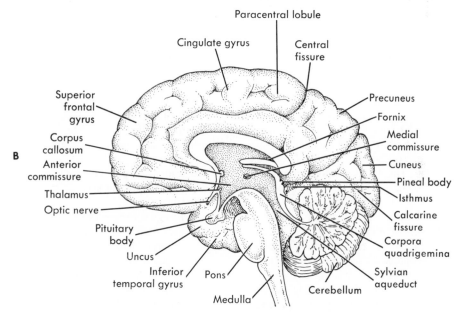

Fig. 14-1. Cerebral cortex. **A,** Lateral view; **B,** medial view.

only controls certain reflex activities but, more important, is the center for cardiac, respiratory, and vasomotor mechanisms.

The *reticular formations* are actually neurons that are interrelated and modify, in part, the reflex activity of spinal neurons. The system is sometimes thought to be responsible for wakefulness and thus called the "reticular activating system" or RAS. Injury to this brain area is likely to result in unconsciousness.

Important physiological concepts

Pressure or blood supply impairment to any cerebral area may affect the functional activity of the said brain area. Other disturbances of consequence result from anoxia or a metabolic disturbance such as hypoglycemia.

The brain tissue requires a vast amount of energy production, which is usually supplied by glucose metabolism. Since there are only minute capabilities of storing glucose, it requires a dynamic supply of circulating blood to deliver oxygen and glucose. If there is an alteration in blood supply, for even 4 to 6 minutes, brain cells are promptly affected.

Blood supply to the brain represents 20% of the oxygen and 65% of the glucose consumed by the body. In order for the brain to function normally, it requires 15% to 20% of the total circulation at all times. When any factor interferes with oxygenation or delivery of glucose, neurons fail, and seizures, unconsciousness, or other evidence of dysfunction are manifest promptly.

It is important to recall that cerebral blood flow is not affected by the same factors that cause changes in vessel size in the rest of the body, for example, catecholamines. Rather, they dilate and constrict in response to alterations in pH, $PaCO_2$ and PaO_2. For example, a hypoxic state of the blood accompanied by acidosis causes vasodilation; alkalosis causes vasoconstriction. This latter phenomenon is the basis for hyperventilation therapy as a mode to reduce intracranial hypertension (see p. 289).

Both the brain and spinal cord are bathed in about 120 ml cerebrospinal fluid (CSF), which is constantly produced, circulated, and reabsorbed. The maintenance of intracranial pressure is largely controlled by these dynamic changes in volume. If the brain is traumatized and begins to swell, for example, CSF production is slowed.

The blood-brain barrier prevents certain substances from passing between the blood and CSF. For example, certain steroids, catecholamines, and antibiotics do not transverse, and thus treatment of pathological conditions of the CNS requires a careful selection of drugs that are known for their capability of crossing this anatomic barrier. Water, glucose, and blood gases move freely back and forth to maintain a homeodynamic balance of vital elements that the brain requires to survive.

NEUROLOGICAL ASSESSMENT

The initial care of an emergency patient should not be delayed to accomplish a detailed neurological assessment, but as soon as basic life support needs have been met, a succinct physical examination should be performed to answer three major questions.

1. Is there evidence of systemic disease? Do vital signs, skin color, funduscopic findings, chest and abdominal findings, breath odor, or presence of nuchal rigidity suggest that the central nervous system (CNS) depression is secondary to systemic disease?

2. Is there evidence of a lateralizing *focal* neurological abnormality? Cranial nerves should be examined and steps taken to rule out metabolic causes of coma. Determine if a *lateral* or a *central* syndrome is present.

   Lateral syndrome — A progressive *unilateral* mass in the supratentorial region causes the medial section of the ipsilateral temporal lobe (that is, uncus) to herniate through the dural tentorium and consequently to compress the third cranial (oculomotor) nerve and the midbrain, producing an ipsilateral dilated pupil and contralateral hemiparesis.

   Central syndrome — Supratentorial masses, if diffuse or affecting both hemispheres, can compress the brainstem bilaterally to produce progressive rostral-caudal dysfunction without evidence of lateralized phenomena.

3. If rostral-caudal dysfunction is evident, what is the level and how fast is it progressing? There are five major stages (Table 14-1).

Pupillary signs

The pupils are excellent indices of rostral-caudal dysfunction. When the pupils are at rest, they should be 2 to 3 mm in diameter and symmetric. A unilateral dilated pupil may signal

Table 14-1. Rostral-caudal dysfunction signs in the comatose patient*

CNS level affected	Respiratory pattern	Level of consciousness	Pupils	Posture	Oculo-cephalic reflex†
Thalamus	Eupnea or Cheynes-Stokes respirations	Stupor, semi-coma‡	Small reactive (2 mm)	Decorticate	—
				Paratonia, gegenhalten	
Midbrain	Neurogenic hyperventilation	Coma	Midposition nonreactive (4 mm)	Decerebrate	+
Pons (Cerebellum)	Biot respirations	Coma	Midposition nonreactive (4 mm)	Flaccid	+
Medulla	Apneustic respirations§	Coma	Midposition nonreactive (4 mm)	Flaccid	+
Spinal cord					

*From Barber, J. M., and Budassi, S. A.: Mosby's manual of emergency care, St. Louis, 1979, The C. V. Mosby Co.
†Indicated by doll's eye test and caloric test.
‡There is also a decreased response to pain and decreased corneal reflexes.
§Eupnea and apnea may also characterize this stage. Some neurologists state that apneustic breathing does not occur in progressive rostral-caudal brainstem dysfunction.

ipsilateral oculomotor (third cranial) nerve compression and impending uncal herniation. Pinpoint pupils may suggest localized pons involvement or effects of opiate drugs. A midposition fixed pupil 4 to 6 mm in diameter strongly indicates progressive rostral-caudal dysfunction to the level of the midbrain. A fully dilated fixed pupil is the end result of the third cranial nerve compression.

In patients in metabolic coma, the pupils ordinarily react to strong light, except in the terminal stages. Other exceptions are:

1. Atropine and scopolamine toxicity produces fully dilated fixed pupils.
2. Anoxia or ischemia may produce dilated fixed pupils, for example, in cardiac arrest.
3. Glutethimide (Doriden) overdose produces unequal, midposition fixed pupils.

Ocular movements

Eye movements are also important in evaluating neurological phenomena. Ordinarily the eyes at rest look straight ahead or diverge slightly. (Roving eyes, either conjugate or disconjugate, occur in comatose patients with intact brainstems, but are not of particular diagnostic significance.) It is important to note, however, that this roving cannot be duplicated voluntarily and is a good detection of an individual feigning unconsciousness. An additional way to identify faking is lifting and releasing the eyelids: the eyelids in the truly comatose close gradually. This also cannot be duplicated voluntarily.

Tonic gaze is important to note. For example, in irritative cerebral lesions (such as epileptic lesions), the eyes deviate away from the side of the lesion. The eyes gaze toward the unaffected (normal) arm and leg in the event that a destructive cerebral lesion exists and allows the remaining innervated side to deviate the eyes temporarily to the side of the lesion. In contrast to cerebral lesions, those below the decussation of supranuclear oculomotor pathways in the pons cause the eyes to deviate away from the lesion since they cannot be brought past the midline toward the lesion.

Oculocephalic reflexes (doll's eye or proprioreceptive head-turning reflex) are not present in normal awake persons but become active when there is diffuse hemispheral and basal ganglion disease *if* the brainstem is intact. However, as rostral-caudal involvement progresses, they become sluggish and disappear at the level of the midbrain (Fig. 14-2).

Oculovestibular reflexes (caloric stimulation responses) are tested when a doll's eye response is absent in a comatose patient and there is no evidence of tympanic membrane damage. The fast component of nystagmus disappears as consciousness is lost, so the slow component carries the eyes tonically toward the irrigated ear for 2 to 3 minutes if the brainstem between the vestibular nuclei and extraocular muscles is intact. This reflex is rarely absent in metabolic coma.

Procedure for caloric stimulation test

1. Check the ear canals for intact tympanic membranes.
2. Elevate the patient's head 30° above the horizontal plane. The head of the bed may be elevated or the neck flexed 30° if cervical spine injury has been ruled out (see p. 306). If the neck is flexed, be certain that the airway is not compromised. The 30° elevation vertically orients the ampulla of the lateral semicircular canal.
3. Using a large-volume irrigating syringe and catheter, irrigate the ear canal with 100 ml ice water using moderate pressure. After 20 seconds, to allow for the process of heat transfer, the following eye movements are evident:

   When consciousness is lost, the fast component of nystagmus is lost, so the slow component carries the eyes tonically toward the irrigated ear for a few minutes *if* the brainstem is intact between the vestibular nuclei and extraocular muscles.

   If the patient is feigning unconsciousness or is unconscious from psychogenic causes, there will be violent nystagmus, nausea, and probably vomiting, indicating intact vestibular functioning.

   NOTE: The caloric stimulation response is rarely absent in metabolic coma.

4. Wait 5 minutes before irrigating the opposite ear.

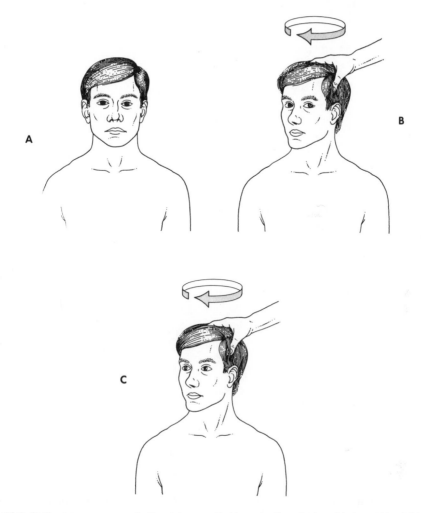

Fig. 14-2. Doll's eye maneuver. **A,** Normal gaze. **B,** Normal reflex. As head is turned to right, eyes rotate to left. **C,** Abnormal or absent reflex. As head is turned to right, eyes stay in midline position.

Motor tone and posture

Paratonia. Paratonia (gegenhalten, counterholding, or motor negativism) is a constant semivoluntary but plasticlike increase in muscle resistance throughout passive movement of the extremities, trunk, or head. It indicates a diffuse forebrain dysfunction and is the first motor indication of progressive rostral-caudal deterioration.

Decorticate and decerebrate posturing

Decorticate rigidity (Fig. 14-3, *A*) is a postural attitude that indicates injury of the brain's cortex. There is marked flexion of the wrists, arms, and digits. The upper extremities are adducted and flexed at the shoulder, and the hands are rotated internally. The legs are extended and internally rotated with plantar flexion of the foot. Symptoms may be unilateral or bilateral. Unilateral involvement is particularly characteristic of spastic hemiplegia. Decorticate rigidity indicates a large destructive lesion of the internal capsule and the rostral cerebral peduncle.

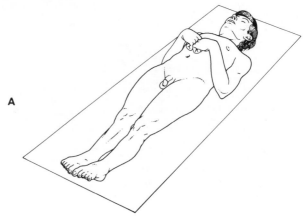

A

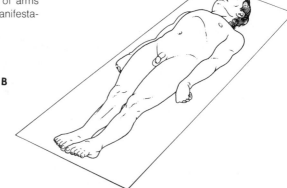

B

Fig. 14-3. A, Position assumed by patient with decorticate rigidity. Note again position in which extremities, especially upper extremities, are held. **B,** Position held by patient with decerebrate rigidity. Note position of arms and legs. Decerebrate rigidity includes other manifestations not seen here.

It is seen more often in children than adults.

Decerebrate rigidity (Fig. 14-3, *B*) is a postural attitude that characterizes midbrain or upper brainstem damage. It can occur with metabolic coma but is not considered ominous in these cases. The response occurs initially with noxious stimuli only and later may become spontaneous. There is a rigidity and contraction of all extensor muscles. The legs are extended and the feet plantar flexed. The arms are markedly extended and hyperpronated. Opisthotonus may also be evident, along with a clenched jaw and an erect head.

Decerebrate posturing is often associated with abnormal respiratory patterns and a grave prognosis.

Flaccidity. Flaccidity (or absent tone or weak flexor response) indicates rostral-caudal brainstem depression to or across the pons at the level of the trigeminal nerve.

Reflex activity

Check for corneal and gag reflexes, since reflexes are the last activity to disappear in neurological deterioration. Deep tendon reflexes may also be checked and noted (Fig. 14-4).

Hypoactivity or absence of deep tendon reflexes may indicate peripheral nerve or anterior horn cell disease and possibly certain cerebellar lesions. Hyperactive deep tendon reflexes are characteristic of pyramidal tract lesions and some psychogenic disorders. Deep reflexes may

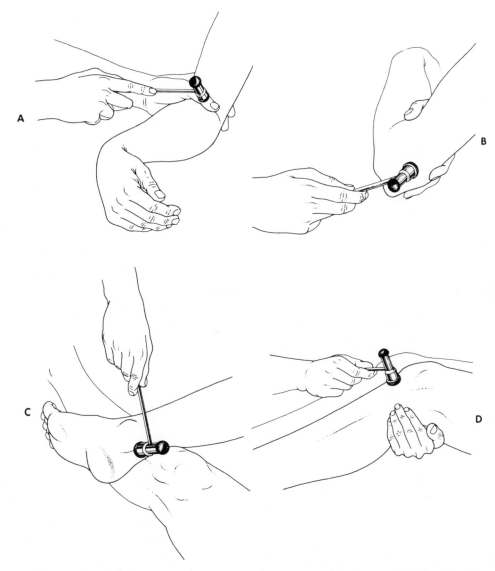

Fig. 14-4. Positions for testing the tendon reflexes. **A,** Biceps tendon. **B,** Triceps tendon. **C,** Achilles tendon. **D,** Patellar tendon.

be increased in early stages of coma and early spinal shock.

THE UNCONSCIOUS PATIENT

Assessment and management of an unconscious patient are important responsibilities of all emergency care personnel and require a thorough understanding of the following:

1. The nature and causes of altered states of consciousness
2. Techniques of evaluating the comatose patient

3. Principles of protecting the patient in coma

The level of consciousness is the most reliable indicator of cerebral injury *except* in penetrating brain injuries (caused by sharp objects *or* depressed skull fracture).

Consciousness implies an effective integration of the cerebral hemisphere and the reticular activating systems of the upper brainstem, which are responsible for mental functioning *(content)* and degree of wakefulness *(state of arousal),* respectively. Therefore, when there is a disturbance in the level of consciousness, it should be described in terms of these two components. A practical way to assess and categorize patients is to evaluate how they respond to verbal or painful stimuli, that is, determine how aware they are of *self* and *environment*.

States of consciousness can be viewed as a continuum from an *alert* and *oriented* state to *unconsciousness,* in which one fails to react to verbal or physical stimuli. Although there are several elaborate schemes for classifying various levels of consciousness, it is more useful to describe behavior rather than labeling it, since much confusion exists about terms such as "lethargy," "stuporous," "semiconscious," and "comatose."

If consciousness is normal, there is no immediate crisis. If consciousness is disturbed, pursue additional neurological assessments at once.

The patient who is unconscious may be experiencing brain dysfunction because of a wide variety of causes, including: (1) circulatory failure (hypotension, hypovolemia, low cardiac output because of pump failure, dysrhythmias, or infarction); (2) metabolic disturbances (acidosis, uremia, electrolyte disturbances, infection, drug overdose, chemical toxicity, and so on); (3) mechanical disturbances (trauma, tumors, increased intracranial pressure, cerebral edema); (4) postictal state; and (5) a large variety of unknown causes (Table 14-2).

It is important for the emergency nurse to assist in obtaining a thorough history of the present illness including the timing and nature of onset. The illnesses, complaints, or problems experienced before the period of uncon-

sciousness should be elicited. The past medical history, the taking of prescribed medications, and history of alcohol or drug consumption should be obtained from a friend or family member when possible. Any historical data that could relate to the unconscious episode must be carefully evaluated in terms of the presenting signs and symptoms other than the coma state.

The nursing care of the unconscious patient is largely devoted to maintaining an airway and to continuing to monitor the vital signs and neurological status.

Neurological status should be evaluated using a standardized and quantifiable mechanism such as the Glasgow Coma Scale, p. 280, specifically designed to objectively measure the extent and progression of neurological injury.

Initial approach to the unconscious patient

1. *Ensure that airway, breathing, and circulation are adequate.* Cardiac arrest should be suspected in all seemingly unconscious individuals. If the airway is patent, breathing is apparent, and a carotid pulse is palpable, monitor the ECG and ascertain the level of consciousness.
2. *Check the patient's response to verbal stimuli.* Call his name. This simple step may tell you that the individual is (1) alert and oriented, (2) confused (memory faulty), or (3) drowsy (arouses when stimulated but falls back to sleep when not stimulated). In emergency situations it may be necessary to use loud and repeated verbal stimulation to evoke a response. It is wise to combine such attempts at arousal with "shaking" or other similar provocation to guard against an improper conclusion when dealing with a hard of hearing patient or "heavy sleeper," who can surely appear to be unconscious. Note the characteristics of speech elicited for signs of dysphasia, dysarthria, or confusion.
3. If verbal stimuli fail to evoke a response, *employ painful* stimulating techniques. Do not use any "cruel or unusual punishment" such as pubic hair pulling, testicular pressure, or slapping, even though you suspect the patient to be feigning an unconscious

Table 14-2. Appearance of patient

Appearance	Possible diagnoses
Vital signs	
Temperature	
High	Infection (pulmonary or CNS)
Low	Carbon monoxide poisoning, overdose, shock, hypoglycemia
Pulse	
Fast	Infection (pulmonary or CNS), hypoxia
Slow	Overdose, Stokes-Adams syndrome
Irregular	Cardiac dysrhythmias
Respirations	
Kussmaul	Ketoacidosis, uremia, salicylate poisoning
Tachypneic	Shock, increased intracranial pressure
Blood pressure	
High	Increased intracranial pressure, CVA, uremia, eclampsia
Low	Shock, overdose, syncope
Skin color	
Jaundice	Hepatitis, cirrhosis
Cyanosis	Shock, COPD, hypoxia
Red or blue-red	Carbon monoxide poisoning, alcoholism
Pallor	Hypovolemia, anemia
Condition of mouth	
Wounds and scars on tongue	Epilepsy
Breath odor	
Alcohol	Alcohol
Acetone	Ketoacidosis, starvation
Chest findings	
Rales	Pulmonary edema
Consolidation	Pneumonia
Gastrointestinal and abdominal findings	
Vomiting	Elevated intracranial pressure, poisoning
Distended abdomen	Ruptured viscus
Mass	Eclampsia
Reflexes and musculoskeletal responses	
Muscular twitching	Uremia
Signs of local injury	Trauma, epilepsy
Nuchal rigidity	Meningitis, subarachnoid hemorrhage
Hemiplegia	CVA
Seizure manifestations	CVA, alcoholism, epilepsy
Head and skull	
Bulging fontanels	CNS, infection, cerebral edema, trauma

state. The recommended method of checking a response to pain is to exert pressure on nerves that are anatomically vulnerable to such exposure. Acceptable maneuvers include (1) sternal compression, (2) supraorbital compression, (3) calf pressure, (4) nipple pressure, and (5) the trapezius pinch.

a. Describe the response to painful stimuli, rather than merely stating that there is a response; for example, "the patient responds to calf pressure by withdrawing the limb."

Glasgow coma scale*

The Glasgow coma scale has been designed to quantitatively relate consciousness to motor responses, verbal responses, and eye opening. Coma is defined as no response and no eye opening. Scores of 7 or less on the Glasgow scale qualify as ''coma''; all scores of 9 or more do not qualify as ''coma.'' The examiner determines the *best* response the patient can make to a set of standardized stimuli. Higher points are assigned to responses that indicate increasing degrees of arousal.

   1. Best motor response. (Examiner determines the *best* response with *either* arm.)
   a. *6 points.* Obeys simple commands. Raises arm on request or holds up specified number of fingers. Releasing a grip (not grasping, which can be reflexive) is also an appropriate test.
   b. *5 points.* Localizes noxious stimuli. Fails to obey commands but can move either arm toward a noxious cutaneous stimulus and eventually contacts it with the hand. The stimulus should be maximal and applied in various locations, i.e., sternum pressure, or trapezius pinch.
   c. *4 points.* Flexion withdrawal. Responds to noxious stimulus with arm flexion but does not localize it with the hand.
   d. *3 points.* Abnormal flexion. Adducts shoulder, flexes and pronates arm, flexes wrist, and makes a fist in response to a noxious stimulus (decorticate rigidity).
   e. *2 points.* Abnormal extension. Adducts and internally rotates shoulder, extends forearm, flexes wrist, and makes a fist in response to a noxious stimulus (decerebrate rigidity).
   f. *1 point.* No motor response. Exclude reasons for no response; for example, insufficient stimulus or spinal cord injury.

   2. Best verbal response. (Examiner determines the *best* response after arousal. Noxious stimuli are employed if necessary.) Omit this test if the patient is dysphasic, has oral injuries, or is intubated. Place a check mark after other two test category scores after totaling to indicate omission of the verbal response section.
   a. *5 points.* Oriented patient. Can converse and relate who he is, where he is, and the year and month.
   b. *4 points.* Confused patient. Is not fully oriented or demonstrates confusion.
   c. *3 points.* Verbalizes. Does not engage in sustained conversation, but uses intelligible words in an exclamation (curse) or in a disorganized manner which is nonsensical.
   d. *2 points.* Vocalizes. Makes moaning or groaning sounds that are not recognizable words.
   e. *1 point.* No vocalization. Does not make any sound even in response to noxious stimulus.

   3. Eye opening. (Examiner determines the minimum stimulus that evokes opening of one or both eyes.) If the patient cannot realistically open the eyes because of bandages or lid edema, write ''E'' after the total test score to indicate omission of this component.
   a. *4 points.* Eyes open spontaneously.
   b. *3 points.* Eyes open to speech. Patient opens eyes in response to command or on being called by name.
   c. *2 points.* Eyes open to noxious stimuli.
   d. *1 point.* No eye opening in response to noxious stimuli.

---

*From Teasdale, G., and Jennett, B.: Assessment of coma and impaired consciousness: a practical scale, Lancet **2:**81-84, 1974.

b. Observe for unilateral responses and equality or symmetry in bilateral responses. When you are assessing response to painful stimuli, it may be possible to obtain other useful data that reflect the neurological status. For instance, in hemiparesis, pain responses will not be bilaterally equal in extremities or the resultant gestures may demonstrate unilateral motor deficits in withdrawal of the provoked part, such as striking out with one arm only, regardless of the type of stimuli. In normal subjects the trapezius pinch will cause ipsilateral pupillary dilatation (ciliospinal reflex). The absence of this phenomenon may indicate spinal cord or brainstem dysfunction.

4. If the patient is unconscious, proceed with management of the unconscious patient.

Management of the unconscious patient

For the unconscious patient who has a patent airway, is breathing, and has a pulse, typical factors in management and the rationale for each are shown in Table 14-3. Cervical injury should be ruled out before any definitive care is begun.

Table 14-3. Management of unconscious patient*

Procedure	Rationale
Give oxygen by nasal cannula at 6 to 8 liters/minute. (If the gag reflex is absent, intubation and assisted ventilation may be required; see pp. 143-148).	Nasal cannula oxygen permits suctioning while delivering a sufficient oxygen concentration.
Draw blood samples† and then establish an IV line D/5/W TKO.	D/5/W will alter blood sugar levels and interfere with baseline laboratory values in assessment of hypoglycemic states.
Give 1 ampule D/50/W unless the patient is a known alcoholic with liver disease or vitamin deficiency. For alcoholism give 100 mg thiamine IV push before the D/50/W.	Preserves neuron life. May reverse hypoglycemic cause for unconsciousness.
Give 0.4 to 0.8 mg naloxone.	Will reverse effects of selected depressant drugs and combat respiratory depression.
Assess for signs and symptoms of meningeal irritation (p. 293).	Positive findings suggest that the meninges are irritated by pus or blood (that is, meningitis or subarachnoid hemorrhage, respectively).
Insert a nasogastric tube and attach to low-power suction.	Prevents vomiting and aspiration; decompressed epigastrium facilitates physical examination.
Examine the eyes: size, equality, reaction to light, and ecchymosis.	See p. 272. Increase or decrease in pupil size could be related to drug ingestion as well as neurological pathology. Increase in size and decrease in response of pupil may be a result of nerve compression (cranial nerve III).
Search for contact lenses. If the corneal reflex is absent, protect the eyes. Consider an eye prosthesis.	Prevent misinterpretation of findings.

*From Barber, J. M., and Budassi, S. A.: Mosby's manual of emergency care, St. Louis, 1979, The C. V. Mosby Co.
†Toxicology screening and blood sugar, BUN, serum electolyte and other tests as indicated. Phenobarbital and phenytoin levels should be tested for selected patients with a history of seizure disorders. The blood alcohol level may be valuable but must exceed 350 mg/100 ml to be the sole cause of coma.

Continued.

Table 14-3. Management of unconscious patient—cont'd

Procedure	Rationale
Look for eye trauma.	See pp. 321-325.
Lift the lid and release it.	Lid closes gradually in coma. If it does not close normally, consider facial nerve involvement.
Examine fundus.	Reveals acute and chronic vascular conditions caused by hypertension, metabolic problems, or increases in intracranial pressure. Remember that papilledema is *not* an acute posttraumatic process.
Examine ears: presence of otorrhea, bleeding, or Battle's sign.	Indicates basilar skull fracture.
Repeat vital signs and initiate ECG monitoring. Obtain baseline 12-lead ECG.*	To ascertain trend in clinical symptoms. Note changes in blood pressure pattern or breathing characteristic of intracranial pathology. Monitor for dysrhythmias.
Assess body surface, front and back, for trauma. Note color (cyanosis, jaundice, cherry red color, or uremic frost), moisture, bruises, edema, surgical scars, signs of previous trauma, and sweat level at T2-C4 interface.	To rule out traumatic injury or chronic illness states that could lead to unconsciousness.
Listen for bruits over carotids and skull.	To detect vascular injury.
Check for peculiar breath odors. Note fruity acetone, almond-like, fetid, or alcoholic odors.	May indicate chemical toxicity, metabolic problems, or drug- or alcohol-related state.
Note involuntary movements and the evidence of decerebrate or decorticate posturing. Check muscle tone and movement in all extremities in response to stimulation.	Paralysis may be masked by coma. Spinal cord or peripheral nerve injury or cerebral compression from depressed skull fracture may contribute to abnormal movements. Consider effects of concurrent fractures, dislocations, and paresis, which could alter findings.
Perform modified cranial nerve check (Table 14-4).	
If not accomplished previously, draw venous blood for studies and obtain arterial specimen for blood gas testing.	As baseline and to assist in establishing cause of coma.
Anchor Foley catheter and collect urine for testing specific gravity, glucose, and ketones.	To monitor output and to assess possible causes of unconscious state.
Perform special diagnostic tests (for example, doll's eye test, caloric responses, chest and skull films, echoencephalography, EEG, CAT scan, and cerebral angiography) as indicated by clinical findings and response to therapy. (See Table 14-5 for diagnostic studies.)	

*With severe neurological injury, the autonomic stimulation and ventricular recovery time are altered. Elevated P waves, large T waves (possibly notched), prominent U waves, prolonged QT or QU intervals, and sinus dysrhythmias as well as ventricular tachycardia may occur.

Table 14-4. Modified cranial nerve testing for the comatose patient*

Nerve	Procedure
I. Olfactory	Not tested
II. Optic	Pupillary reflex: direct and consensual
III. Oculomotor	Pupillary reflex: direct and consensual *and* spontaneous or induced medial, superior, or downward eye movements
VI. Trochlear	Eye movements: spontaneous or oculocephalic reflexes, such as "doll's eyes"
IV. Abducens	
V. Trigeminal	Corneal reflex; supraorbital compression, jaw reflex
VII. Facial	Facial movement or grimace during supraorbital compression or while testing corneal reflex
VIII. Acoustic	Oculocephalic reflex and caloric stimulation
X. Glossopharyngeal	Gag, cough, carotid sinus reflexes
IX. Vagus	
XI. Spinal accessory	Spontaneous or induced shoulder elevation
XII. Hypoglossal	Tongue movement against examiner's finger

*From Barber, J., Stokes, L., and Billings, D.: Adult and child care, ed. 2, St. Louis, 1977, The C. V. Mosby Co.

Table 14-5. Special diagnostic tests*

Procedure	Value in clinical assessment and treatment
Skull films	Demonstrates shift of midline (e.g., calcified pineal body), sella erosion from chronic increase in intracranial pressure, fractures, or foreign bodies; identifies fractures of special concern, i.e., across middle meningeal groove, depressed sites, and basilar fractures; evidence of sinus or mastoid inflammation may suggest central vein thrombosis.
Cervical spine films	Detect C1 through T1 fractures or dislocations and evidence of cord compression in unresponsive patients.
Echoencephalography†	Reveals lateral shift of normally midline structures from developing mass lesions.
EEG (electroencephalography)	Reveals focal CNS lesion; a normal EEG pattern generally rules out metabolic coma.
Cerebral angiography	Pinpoints aneurysm of subarachnoid hemorrhage; assists in detecting etiology of CVA when used in conjunction with CAT scan.
Computerized axial tomography (CAT) scan (also called EMI or ACTA scan)	Demonstrates focal space-occupying lesions such as hemorrhage (increased x-ray absorption, neoplasm (increased x-ray absorption), nonhemorrhagic infarction (decreased x-ray absorption 24 hours after stroke), and ventricles (decreased x-ray absorption outlines ventricles and suggests their size and configuration); useful in detecting hydrocephalus.

*From Barber, J. M., and Budassi, S. A.: Mosby's manual of emergency care, St. Louis, 1979, The C. V. Mosby Co.
†Echoencephalograms do not rule out expanding lesions since hematomas do not consistently shift midline structures. However, if an echoencephalogram is positive, there is a need for arteriography.

PATHOPHYSIOLOGY OF HEAD INJURY AND NURSING IMPLICATIONS

The relationship of the brain to metabolic activities and other organ systems must be appreciated and understood in order to plan effectively for nursing care. The primary goal of clinical management is to establish and support optimal conditions under which the brain can recover. It is imperative, therefore, to understand the physiological consequences of head injury in relation to several hemodynamic mechanisms.

Metabolic factors

After head injury, like most other body trauma, there is a marked tendency to retain sodium and water and to lose a considerable amount of nitrogen.

Trauma evokes release of ADH, which contributes to water retention. Urinary output tends to be low and is characterized by a high specific gravity and elevated electrolyte concentrations. Sodium is retained because of stimulation of the hypothalamus, resulting in the release of ACTH and the consequent secretion of aldosterone. Renal hemodynamics also plays an important role in sodium retention. It is interesting to note, however, that there seems to be a lack of correlation between serum sodium levels and the occurrence of sodium retention. Post-trauma hyponatremia is not indicative, necessarily, of body sodium depletion and thus is not managed by therapeutic sodium administration.

Increased nitrogen loss is another significant metabolic response to trauma. Inactivity, low nutritional intake, and general physical factors such as age, sex, and state of health seem to influence this phenomenon. Skeletal muscle protein is felt to be the chief source of the nitrogen that is lost. The degree of loss seems to be proportional to the amount of trauma incurred.

Cortisol secretion, growth hormone activity, and the production of catecholamines and prolactin are accelerated, probably because of a response mediated by the hypothalamus. Glucose intolerance is present in most brain-injured persons, at least to some degree, for 3 to 5 days after the trauma. Several other intermediary metabolic responses to brain injury are also currently under clinical investigation.

Serotonin levels are generally elevated after the trauma. It is thought that serotonin in the free state produces neurological deficits and contributes to edema formation.

Excessive accumulation of acetylcholine also has been noted following brain injury. Its elevation seems to be significant, since it is capable of influencing synaptic transmission.

Most individuals with brain injury have a slightly acidotic arterial pH. Usually respiratory alkalosis develops within the first 24 hours. Urinary excretion of hydrogen ions is elevated soon after injury but decreases progressively. Early after trauma there is essentially a respiratory alkalosis and a metabolic acidosis; however, the former problem may remain obscure until fluids and oxygen are used to combat hypoxia responsible for the metabolic acidosis.

The degree of CSF metabolic acidosis shares a positive correlation with the severity of the head injury. It does not depend on the production of lactate by the traumatized, hypoxic brain. Researchers believe that CSF lactate levels are perhaps the most reliable method of determining gross brain damage. Head injury victims who have a CSF lactate concentration exceeding 27 mg/100 ml usually do not survive. CSF lactate levels, however, correlate poorly with arterial lactate levels; thus the latter is seldom used to assess brain damage. In metabolic acidosis and alkalosis, the concentration of hydrogen ions may change in opposite directions in the blood and the brain because of the slowness with which fixed acids and bases cross the blood-brain barrier and because of the ease with which molecular carbon dioxide traverses such membranes. "This means that the acid-base environment of the central nerve cells critical in respiratory control may not be altered to the same degree or even in the same direction, as is indicated by measurements made only on circulating blood" (Mountcastle, 1980, pp. 1787-1788). Arterial blood sampling is of limited use; therefore, when metabolic activity of the brain is assessed, CSF sampling is preferred.

Respiratory factors

Respiratory complications constitute the most common cause of death in victims of brain injury after 48 hours of survival (Table 14-6). Ventilatory failure may be a primary factor in producing death, or it may compound cerebral damage due to hypoxia, or it may contribute to vasodilation, which raises intracranial pressure, further compromising cerebral circulation.

Brain injury, like all trauma, tends to produce hyperventilation in the initial period after injury. High tidal volumes, some increase in respiratory rate, and actual alveolar hyperventilation characterize the clinical picture. The resultant hypocarbia is not altered even by exposure to 100% oxygen, demonstrating that hypoxemia is not the cause of this hyperventilation. Hypoxemia, however, is nearly always present, resulting from impaired ventilation-perfusion relationships associated with increased physiological dead space in the lungs and an acceleration of physiological shunting, that is, alveolar-arterial oxygen tension gradient difference. This increased ventilation-perfusion ratio accounts for hypoxemia despite hyperventilation.

Hyperventilation after head injury seems to result from intense sympathetic stimuli to the lungs, causing pulmonary vasoconstriction, pulmonary hypertension, and edema. The consequent reduction of lung compliance and the

Table 14-6. Patterns of respiration in neurological dysfunction*

Term	Description	Selected neurologic causes
Eupnea	Normal breathing	
Cheyne-Stokes respirations	Breathing characterized by regular, alternating periods of hyperpnea and apnea; breathing builds from respiration to respiration in a smooth crescendo and, as peak is reached, declines in an equally smooth decrescendo; ordinarily, hyperpneic phase endures longer than apneic phase	Deep bilateral diencephalic lesions, hypertensive encephalopathy, uremia, anoxia, or imminent transtentorial herniation
Central neurogenic hyperventilation	Sustained regular, rapid hypocapnic hyperpnea	Brain dysfunction
Biot respirations	Regular periods of hyperventilation and irregular periods of apnea	
Apneustic respirations	Ataxic, gasping, shallow breathing	Infarction at mid- or caudal pontine level, usually as a result of basilar artery occlusion; *not* characteristically observed with progressive rostral-caudal brainstem dysfunction
Posthyperventilation apnea	Respirations interrupted for up to 30 seconds after five voluntary breaths in wakeful patients	Diffuse metabolic or structural forebrain disease
Cluster breathing	Breaths follow each other in disorderly sequence with irregular pauses between them	Low pons or high medulla lesion; may be result of expanding lesion in posterior fossa (cerebellar hemorrhage)
Ataxic breathing	Completely chaotic pattern with deep and shallow breaths occurring randomly; progressively leads to apnea	Dorsomedial medulla dysfunction; may appear in relation to meningitis or acute parainfectious demyelination

*From Barber, J. M., Stokes, L. G., Billings, D. M.: Adult and child care: a client approach to nursing, ed. 2, St. Louis, 1977, The C. V. Mosby Co.

pulmonary edema trigger irritant receptors, which reflexively cause hyperpnea and bronchoconstriction.

Cheyne-Stokes respirations, characterized by regular alternating periods of hyperpnea and apnea, occur because of an increased sensitivity of the respiratory mechanism to carbon dioxide and to the occasional episodes of posthyperventilation apnea. Breathing builds from respiration to respiration in a smooth crescendo and then, when a peak is reached, declines in an equally smooth decrescendo. In most instances the hyperpneic phase endures longer than the apneic phase.

Another respiratory pattern that can be evident is "ataxic" respiratory effort, characterized by irregular rate, rhythm, and volume. The cause is thought to be damage to the medulla. It is accompanied by hypoxemia and is an ominous prognostic indicator. Finally, Biot respirations (totally irregular respiratory activity, both in frequency and volume) may occur in relation to brain injury, especially in conjunction with elevations in intracranial pressure.

Without vigorous respiratory support, hyperventilation, hypocarbia, and alkalosis create progressive pulmonary insufficiency, especially if the person remains unconscious. Alveolar-arterial gradients rise, and oxygen concentrations must be increased. Hypocarbia usually persists, despite assisted ventilation, but metabolic acid-base imbalances replace the mild respiratory alkalosis.

The nurse should appreciate limitations of mechanical ventilation and its effects on the body's own regulatory systems. Mechanical ventilation contributes to water retention, since there is a reduction in pulmonary blood volume and left atrial pressure caused by positive pressure breathing. A decrease of afferent impulses from the stretch receptors of these structures leads to additional ADH output and thus promotes water retention. This may contribute to body fluid hypotonicity and thus to cerebral edema. Excess water, in turn, creates the tendency for pulmonary failure by the addition of extravascular pulmonary water and an increased alveolar-arterial oxygen gradient.

The importance of preventing and correcting hypoxemia is apparent, since it contributes to further brain damage. Provision of a patent airway, delivery of adequate oxygen concentrations, controlling hypocarbia and its resultant vasospasms, and correcting acid-base imbalances are crucial considerations in the clinical management of a patient with head injury.

A cuffed endotracheal tube or tracheostomy may be necessary in an unconscious patient if secretions are copious, if there is an accompanying cervical spine injury that contraindicates hyperextension of the head, or in the event of soft tissue neck injuries that might compress the trachea.

Suctioning must be immediately available. Oral suctioning is preferred until the nature of injury is fully determined, because of the proximity of the cerebrum to the nasopharynx.

Cardiovascular factors

Head injury seems to result in a series of consequences that affect cardiovascular functioning, including atypical myocardial activity, pulmonary edema, and vascular pressure alterations.

Cardiac changes include ECG abnormalities such as large T waves (with normal or abnormal polarity), prominent U waves, and prolonged QT or QU intervals (see Table 14-3). These changes are the result of altered autonomic tone on functional variations of ventricular recovery time. Notched T waves, elevated P waves, and sinus dysrhythmias with wandering pacemaker, atrial fibrillation, and ventricular tachycardia also occur.

Myocardial activity changes include increased heart rate and stroke index, reduced stroke work, and a subnormal CVP reading. Intracranial pressure correlates positively with cardiac output and inversely with total peripheral resistance. A transient functional insufficiency of the ventricles seems to be present immediately after head injury. An absence of endogenous sympathetic neural stimuli may be largely responsible for the reduced ventricular contractility.

Head injury sets off a series of hemodynamic consequences that often lead to pulmonary edema. At first there is general systemic vasoconstriction, causing blood to be shunted to the pulmonary vascular bed. Ventricular compliance is lessened, and as intracranial pressure rises, there is an acceleration of venous return and cardiac output, which leads ultimately to rises in systemic and pulmonary vascular pressures. Peripheral resistance may fall, however. With continued physiological stress, there is a rise in peripheral resistance so that the diastolic pressure is great enough to ensure adequate brain perfusion. Left atrial pressure is elevated with a consequent decrease in cardiac output, and eventually pulmonary edema ensues.

Another factor that may add to the production of pulmonary edema is increased arteriovenous shunting in the lung and in the periphery. There is a rise in the volume of acidotic blood returning to the heart. Persistent autonomic stimulation does not permit the heart to relax in diastole, further encouraging failure. Since pulmonary edema and pulmonary shunting relate to intracranial pressure elevations, clinical management should incorporate attention to these phenomena. Cardiac monitoring, central venous or arterial pressures, capillary wedge pressures (see p. 257), and CSF sampling must be considered essential assessment techniques.

CEREBROVASCULAR ACCIDENT (CVA) (STROKE)

A cerebrovascular accident (CVA) is an interruption of blood supply to the brain caused by an impediment to flow, for example, clot, vasospasm, or hemorrhage. The cells supplied by the involved blood supply become anoxic and begin to die in less than 4 minutes. Furthermore, all body functions controlled or influenced by the anoxic cellular area are impaired or lost.

The usual causes of CVA are infarctions, hemorrhage, mechanical pressure (clot or tumor), and embolus (blood clot, air, or fat.) Underlying causes include hypertension, atherosclerotic processes, arteriovenous malformations, trauma, carcinoma, invasive diagnostic studies using air as contrast, aneurysms, and heart valvular or rhythm disorders.

The signs and symptoms of a CVA depend essentially on the area of the brain involved.

Sensory and motor dysfunction can include dysarthria, aphasia, hemiparesis, hemiplegia, pupillary changes in equality and reaction, incontinence, seizures, confusion, and changes in vital signs. Signs of meningeal irritation such as nuchal rigidity and vomiting may also be evident, particularly in the event of subarachnoid hemorrhage.

Emergency management is directed toward relieving the signs and symptoms. Airway maintenance is highest priority, as usual, and may require a broad range of interventions (see p. 132). Dentures should be removed, and suctioning must be employed to keep the upper airway free of secretions. If the gag reflex is absent, airway adjuncts such as an oropharyngeal airway, or endotracheal intubation must be carried out promptly. Oxygen should be given by an appropriate mechanism (see p. 151).

The physician and nurse must often rely on the family to obtain an accurate history of the problem, because the patient may be unable to provide meaningful input or to cooperate with certain parts of the examination. The medical history, current medications, recent or present illnesses, and any trauma such as falls should be fully explored to link them to the presenting phenomena.

Patients who have incurred a CVA require constant vigil because rapid deterioration is not uncommon, and because precipitant events such as seizures may occur.

HEAD INJURY
Assessment of head injuries

After ensuring that basic airway, breathing, and circulation functions are intact, the emergency nurse should carefully assess the level of consciousness of the patient with a head injury. It is important to ascertain if it is stable, improving, or deteriorating. In addition any abnormal neurological findings should be validated in terms of lateralization and symmetry. Subsequent checks should be made in regard to signs and symptoms of increasing intracranial pressure (Table 14-7), carefully noting concomitant findings such as alcohol ingestion, drug overdose, or other injuries that could influence the neurological assessment. As always with any traumatic injury involving poten-

Table 14-7. Signs of increased intracranial pressure*

Compensation ←			→ Decompensation
Early	Variable	Progressive	Late
Increased normal blind spot	Headache	Decreased level of consciousness—orientation × 3	Stupor, coma
Visual field cuts (heminanopsias)	Nausea	Eye changes	Pupils dilated and fixed
Papilledema	Projectile vomiting with position change	Deviation from midline	Decreased systolic blood pressure
Decreased visual acuity	Increased temperature	CNS damage	Increased pulse rate
	Focal signs	Side to side	Decreased respirations—arrest
	Seizures	Up and down	Bilateral decerebrate posturing progressing to flaccidity
	Eyes deviate to side of lesion	Pupillary size and reaction to light (third cranial nerve)	
	Aphasias	Doll's eyes	
	Changes in motor tone and strength	Increased systolic blood pressure	
	Focal signs are always variable.	Decreased pulse rate	
		Labored respirations (becoming alkalotic)	
		Cheyne-Stokes	
		Central neurogenic hyperventilation; forced, deep and regular; oxygen makes no difference (upper level brain stem damage)	
		Ataxic (drug overdose)	
		No regularity at all	
		Apneustic (brain stem surgery); inspire—hold; expire—hold	
		Cluster—3 respirations and apnea, 5 respirations and apnea, etc.	
		Rigidity	

*From Barber, J. M., and Budassi, S. A.: Mosby's manual of emergency care, St. Louis, 1979, The C. V. Mosby Co.

tial nervous sytem damage, assume that a cervical spine injury is present until ruled out by a cross-table lateral cervical spine film.

Never leave the patient during this period of initial assessment! Respiratory arrest, seizures, and vomiting are precipitant problems that could adversely affect the patient's chance for survival. Search for scalp wounds and skull fractures (see pp. 294 and 295, respectively). Manage any acute bleeding. Observe for rhinorrhea, otorrhea, or other clues of cerebrospinal fluid (CSF) leakage. Patients complaining of a "salty" taste in their mouth may have CSF leaks into the back of the oral cavity. Test for it by using Dextrostix or Uristix, which will be positive for glucose. CSF also separates from other bloody drainage and outlines itself with a blue halo ring on the moisture (called

the target sign). *Never* attempt to restrict the free flow of CSF, to avoid dangerous increases in intracranial pressure and meningitis via meningeal communication with a contaminated surface environment. Do not suction nasally if there is a question of CSF leaking into the throat. (Suctioning also tends to raise intracranial pressure.) Be alert to decerebrate or decorticate posturing, too.

Continue to check the airway and ventilatory pattern, since correcting an obstructed airway can improve the level of consciousness in certain cases. It is helpful to monitor blood gases at 30-minute intervals, and if the pCO_2 is above 40 mm Hg, respiratory assistance is in order. All labored respiratory patterns tend to contribute to a rise in intracranial pressure, and respiratory distress may be the result of a rise in intracranial pressure as a manifestation of a brainstem injury. Determine the causes of dyspnea, for example, position of tongue, nasopharyngeal secretions, and rhinorrhea. Correct if possible by the jaw thrust or head tilt airway maneuvers, placement of an oropharyngeal airway, endotracheal intubation, suctioning, oxygen administration, and in rare circumstances, surgical approaches.

Cyanosis and high venous pressure are associated with carbon dioxide retention and vascular dilation in the cerebral vascular system, thus altering levels of consciousness. In cervical spine injuries there may be vasomotor collapse as well as respiratory compromise, of which contribute to a shock state.

Management of cerebral edema

The emergency care team can contribute to management of cerebral edema merely by taking early steps to limit its progression. The prehospital care team has a significant responsibility in this regard.

Airway maintenance and oxygenation. There is an important interface between adequate oxygenation of the brain tissue and the development of cerebral edema. The physiological basis may be related to cerebral vasomotor paresis after concussion. Initially when the brain is concussed, increased blood flow to the brain occurs because of vascular dilation, and the consequent congestion produces edema, via activation of the medullary vasopressor mechanisms to enhance intracranial blood flow. This creates hypertension.

Plasma is then permitted to escape into tissue, and this phenomenon coupled with an eventual loss of vasomotor tone contributes to even more edema formation. Finally, cerebral blood flow is further restricted, thus aggravating the condition even more. It has been noted that early attention to airway, including intubation and ventilatory assistance, can ultimately help correct the problem, since a declining P_2CO_2 can retard cerebral blood flow, and thus edema. Simple measures such as elevating the head of the bed can also be beneficial.

Ventilation support is aimed at maintaining the pO_2 above 100 and the pCO_2 below 25 to

30. Positive end expiratory pressure (PEEP) may be useful under the direct guidance of a qualified respiratory therapist with frequent ABG analyses. A conscious patient should receive humidified high-flow oxygen (10 to 12 liters/minute) by mask.

Early nasogastric intubation to decompress the stomach and thus prevent vomiting not only protects the airway from emesis, but prevents elevations in intracranial pressure (ICP) that accompany vomiting.

Dehydration and fluid therapy. It is useful to dehydrate the brain by restricting fluid and the use of osmotic diuretics. This type of therapy, however, may require tempering if there is inherent danger from hypovolemia from concurrent traumatic injuries. The choice of IV fluid is crucial. The ideal isotonic solution having the least influence on ICP is 2.5% dextrose in half-normal saline. The rate should be TKO with no more than 500 ml used in initial resuscitation efforts, since overhydration merely increases the edema. A microdrip infusion set should be used. Isotonic agents of other varieties may be also employed as long as the rate is slow and there is concurrent monitoring of the CVP and ICP to ensure their maintenance near normal values.

Diuresis may be promoted by osmolar agents such as mannitol or by certain diuretics, such as furosemide (Lasix). Mannitol's effect peaks at 20 minutes, but furosemide does not exert a maximum effect for up to 1 hour. Some clinicians use a combination of the agents to ensure a desired result. Urea is also occasionally used to achieve dehydration of the brain. Caution should be exercised in dehydration therapy to ensure that bleeding is not the cause of increased ICP. Dehydration would, in such cases, simply create more space for the expanding hematoma.

Steroids are controversial in the management of ICP, but research has shown them to be of specific value in preventing the devastating consequences of cerebral edema. Dexamethasone (Decadron) is the agent of choice of most clinicians, since it has the least sodium-retention effects of the steroids. Since fluid and electrolyte balance are more difficult to maintain during steroid therapy, judicious laboratory monitoring is essential.

Barbiturate coma is a new technique aimed at lowering ICP and brain metabolism, thus exerting a "protecting" effect. It is induced with pentobarbital (Nembutal) in doses of 5 to 15 mg/kg IV push over 5 to 30 minutes. Maintenance doses of 1 to 3 mg/kg given every 2 hours are typical. Constant monitoring is an important nursing responsibility.* Barbiturate-induced coma has been prolonged for over 2 weeks in selected patients.

Intracranial shifts. When the brain enlarges in size because of edema or an expanding hematoma, various functions are compromised when the brain tissue becomes impinged upon by the skull bones. In the infant and young child the cranial vault is not fixed, and the suture lines and fontanels permit some intracranial expansion. However, in the adult, the rise in intracranial pressure displaces the brain, and various types of herniation can occur. A *cingulate* herniation refers to the displacement of the central hemisphere and cingulate gyrus to the opposite side beneath the falx. A *tentorial* herniation involves the displacement of the medial portion of the temporal lobe (uncus) through the tentorial incisura. Uncal herniation is characterized early by an ipsilateral dilating pupil due to cranial nerve III compression. If the cerebral peduncles are compressed, there may be a contralateral spastic weakness of the extremities. The progressive uncal herniation forces the midbrain against the opposite tentorial edge producing bilateral fixed and dilated pupils, bilateral spasticity and weakness, and finally flaccid paralysis. A common cause of temporal lobe herniation is an epidural hematoma. A third type of brain herniation is the inferior displacement of the cerebellar tonsils through the foramen magnum, leading to cardiovascular collapse and apnea. Finally, the fourth type of herniation involves the leakage of brain tissue through a skull fracture or sur-

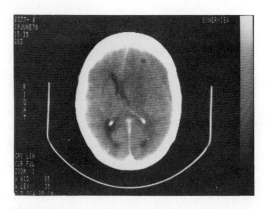

Fig. 14-5. This CT scan, performed with contrast, demonstrates a deformity of the ventricular system with a left to right midline shift secondary to deep cerebral edema.

gical opening in the brain, such as a burr hole or bone flap. Emergency nurses must be acutely aware of the consequences of herniation and be prepared to detect progressive signs of deterioration, because clinical management must be prompt and aggressive. Computerized axial tomography (Fig. 14-5) and echoencephalography (Fig. 14-6) are primary diagnostic modes.

Intracranial monitoring

The measurement of ICP is an important parameter in monitoring the clinical course of the patient with head injury. There are three basic methods: (1) intraventricular, (2) epidural, and (3) subarachnoid.

The intraventricular method employs a standard blood pressure transducer that is attached to a cannula in the ventricles. Although this method allows for withdrawing CSF samples for analysis as well as for control of ICP, it has hazards relating to infection and the need for flushing the system routinely to maintain patency. The subarachnoid method is similar in principle, but insertion of the monitoring apparatus is into the subarachnoid space. The newer epidural probe is unlikely to cause infections, and the transducer does not require calibration. Although an expensive device, it has several distinct advantages.

Nursing responsibilities in relation to ICP

---

*Parameters to be monitored during the course of coma include blood pressure, CVP, ICP, urinary output, temperature, electrolytes, CBC, coagulation studies, and brain-stem-evoked responses (see Table 14-3).

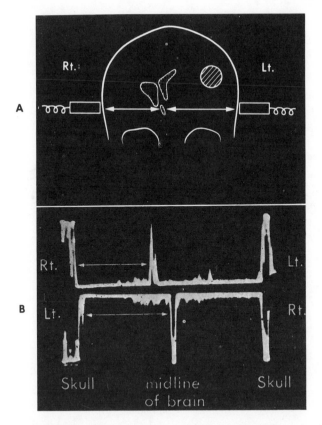

Fig. 14-6. Echoencephalography. **A,** Probe is applied in turn to temporal scalp on back side in case of left-sided mass, causing shift to right. **B,** Polaroid print of oscilloscope trace, indicating midline closer to right side of skull. (From Jennett, W. B.: Operative surgery, 3rd edition, edited by Charles Rob, Rodney Smith, and Hugh Dudley, Neurosurgery, 1979. By kind permission of Butterworths.)

monitoring vary considerably with the type of equipment and will not be considered in detail here.

The normal ICP is 4 to 14 mm Hg (50 to 200 mm H_2O). It is possible however, to exceed this range, through normal activities such as coughing, suctioning, vomiting, or defecating. Rapid increases in intracranial pressure (in less than 30 minutes) to high levels of 50 mm Hg or more signal a grave prognosis (Fig. 14-7).

Shock accompanying head injury

Shock in a patient with head injury suggests an *extracranial* cause. It can create a confusing picture when it occurs in relation to certain brain syndromes, since signs and symptoms may be similar: for example, restlessness, weakness, confusion, bilaterally dilated pupils, and syncope.

If there is hypotension in head-injured patients, it should be treated with infusion of D/5/W in Ringer's lactate and possibly the application of antishock trousers. Meanwhile, a search must be made for spinal cord trauma, which causes shock from sympathetic denervation, or intraabdominal, chest, pelvic, or long bone injuries. Intracranial bleeding in adults cannot be sufficient to cause hypovolemia. However, infants and small children with expandable cranial vaults can lose large quantities of blood and thus may be hypovolemic from head injury. Scalp wounds may bleed pro-

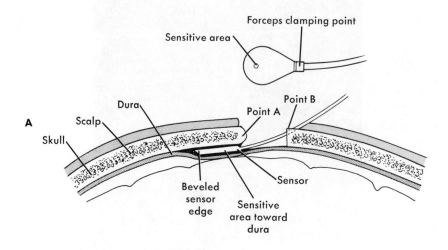

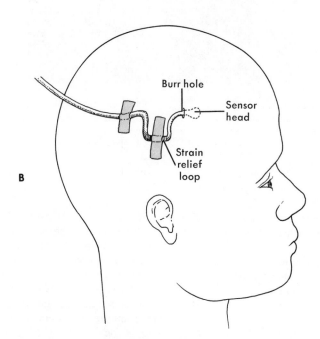

Fig. 14-7. Intracranial monitoring. **A,** Placement of epidural sensor between skull and dura to monitor intracranial pressure. **B,** External view of epidural sensor.

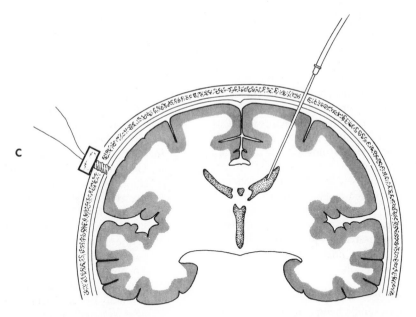

Fig. 14-7, cont'd. C, Subarachnoid *(left)* and intraventricualr *(right)* devices for measuring intracranial pressure; both require attachment to transducer using a stopcock and/or pressure tubing.

fusely, and prolonged, uncontrolled hemorrhage from this source can create shock.

Since shock contributes to hypoxia and altered cellular metabolism, it obviously leads to cerebral edema. Therefore, emergency nurses should act promptly to reverse the devastating results. Continuous monitoring of vital signs, urinary output, CVP, and other clues to cardiovascular collapse should be a high priority.

Seizures after head injury

Ordinarily no treatment is required for a single posttraumatic seizure if the patient is conscious and neurologically stable after the episode. However, there are several types of situations in which emergency nurses should be prepared to participate in anticonvulsant therapy. Among these are patients who have penetrating cranial injuries or depressed skull fractures near the motor cortex, or who exhibit patterns of neurological deterioration postictally.

Phenytoin (Dilantin) is used for acute seizures related to head injuries. A loading dose of 10 mg/kg is administered IV to obtain a rapid therapeutic blood level. Monitoring of vital signs and the ECG is crucial. If there is evidence of bradycardia, hypotension, as a prolonged QRS or PR interval, the infusion should be discontinued until cardiovascular stabilization returns. Diazepam (Valium) is the drug of choice for status epilepticus (see p. 719). Nursing care for seizures is discussed on pp. 303-305).

Signs of meningeal irritation

The irritation of the meninges, whether from trauma, intracranial bleeding, or an inflammatory process creates characteristic signs and symptoms.

Headache is the primary symptom and is usually the earliest to appear. It is caused by an increase in CSF and the stretching of edematous nerve tissue. It if often localized or it may extend down the back of the neck. Usually it increases in severity with any sudden movement such as forceful coughing or vomiting.

Nuchal rigidity, especially to flexion, is

caused by inflammation at the base of the brain. With progressive meningeal irritation, the rigidity becomes decidedly more pronounced.

Brudzinski's sign is a positive index of meningeal irritation and is elicited by passive flexion of the head on the chest, which induces flexion of the lower limbs.

Kernig's sign consists of pain and resistance on extending the leg at the knee after flexing the thigh on the body. It indicates irritation of the lumbosacral roots.

Fever is present when there is an inflammatory condition such as meningitis.

Opisthotonus is an arched body position caused by tetanic spasm. It is usually accompanied by exaggerated deep tendon reflexes, spasm, muscular twitching, and other evidence of spinal cord irritation.

Scalp lacerations

Scalp wounds should be managed quickly because they (1) bleed profusely, (2) may contribute to meningitis or brain abscess, and (3) may contribute to shock.

Scalp wounds must be cared for as a secondary consideration in relation to other neurological injuries of the skull, brain, and spinal cord. However, it is important to remember that the profuse bleeding can cause shock. Monitor vital signs and establish an IV line if shock is impending.

The patient with scalp bleeding should not be permitted to sit unattended in the waiting room or to walk, because orthostatic changes in blood pressure and syncope may contribute to accidents, especially falls.

Assessment. Detection of all scalp lacerations may not always be easy, especially in the event of multiple or profusely bleeding lacerations. Use care to part the hair and inspect all areas. Determine if the galea has been permeated, since these full-thickness scalp lacerations are prone to subgaleal abscess, particularly if there is a related skull fracture and a dural tear.

Emergency management. The nurse should control hemorrhage by compression of bleeding edges: temporal and occipital arteries may require ties; however, do not tie small arteries.

Recommendations for repair: (sample)
1. Shave a wide area after cleansing with an antiseptic soap such as Betadine.
2. Irrigate generously.
3. Remove any foreign bodies and debride as necessary. Continue to compress bleeding edges to control hemorrhage.
4. Close in one layer; even the galea can be closed in this manner. (Two-layer closure increases the risk of infection.)
   a. Use interrupted monofilament sutures, 35-gauge steel wire, or 4-0 nylon placed through all scalp layers. These may be left for 3 or 4 weeks without problems. *Do not* choose braided suture material or silk, which may cause a reaction in 6 to 8 days.
   b. To obtain a better cosmetic affect in nonhairy scalp regions, use a deep layer of 3-0 catgut in the galeal aponeurosis and a superficial layer of monofilament in the skin. Remove the superficial suture in 3 days to decrease scar formation.
5. Dress the wound.
6. Give tetanus prophylaxis.
7. Occasionally, scalp hematomas may form under contusions, but they seldom require aspiration. Large lacerations, multiple lacerations, or occlusions may require repair in the surgical suite. The nurse should ensure that scalp wounds are closed with a temporary means in open or depressed skull fractures *before* transportation to another facility.

Skull fractures

A skull fracture is a break in the continuity of the skull bones, which may or may not be accompanied by displacement of fragments (Fig. 14-8). It may be a linear break (without alteration of parts) or comminuted (several linear, fragmented interruptions of continuity). It is easy to miss some skull fractures on preliminary examinations because the bone is layered (tabled) and the surface may not be indicative of what is present immediately under the area.

The type and extent of the fracture varies

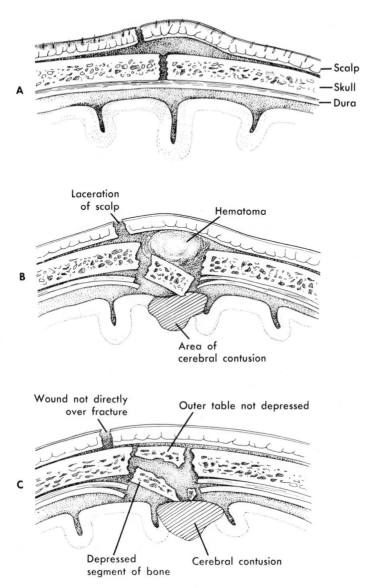

Fig. 14-8. Types of skull fractures. **A,** Simple. **B,** Depressed. **C,** Hidden. (From Barber, J., Stokes, L., and Billings, D.: Adult and child care, ed. 2, St. Louis, 1977, The C. V. Mosby Co.)

with the age of the patient and the nature of the injury, and with the mechanical agent and the amount of force behind it. In neonates, the skull may be indented without interrupting the continuity of the bone, and in young children trauma may cause separation of the sutures. Because of the absence of buttresses and immaturity of the skulls, fractures in infants do not conform to any pattern.

Skull fractures seldom require emergency treatment unless they are severely depressed, thus impinging on vital brain tissue, or are basilar, potentially irritating the meninges.

Assessment. A history of the head injury

should be obtained including the type of force and the impacting object's characteristics, (for example, sharp, blunt, heavy). Palpation of the skull is done carefully to detect changes in the continuity of the cranium. Although Battle's sign (ecchymosis of the mastoid) may not appear early after the injury, it should be considered in the inspection. Orbital ecchymoses should also be noted. Otorrhea and rhinorrhea may indicate a dural tear, so exploration should be made regarding the ear canals and the nose, respectively (see p. 288).

Usually the physician will obtain an anteroposterior and cross-table lateral films to visualize the upper cervical region as well as angulated views. Careful attention is given to any fracture that crosses the meningeal vessels of the temporal fossa, because it often contributes to severe intracranial bleeding.

Emergency management. No specific treatment is required for skull fractures *unless* they are (1) open, (2) communicating with the paranasal or mastoid sinuses, or (3) depressed.

Fractures that are open or communicating with sinuses are usually followed by meningitis. Prophylactic antibiotic therapy and observations for changes in level of consciousness are crucial factors in the hospital regimen of care.

Depressed fractures usually require elevation. (If the bone fragment is depressed sufficiently that the acute table of that bone fragment lies beneath the inner table of the adjacent bone, it requires elevation.) If the depression overlies the sagittal or lateral sinuses, anticipate profuse bleeding. There may be local effects of contusions, or the fracture may tear or obstruct dural or venous sinuses. Be prepared to treat shock. Treatment may be delayed if there is shock.

The following steps usually are involved in surgical intervention:
1. Removal of loose fragments of bone or necrotic brain, which could serve as a means of infection
2. Repair of dural lacerations
3. Bleeding control
4. Removal of in-driven bone fragments, which could cause posttraumatic epilepsy.

Basilar skull fractures. Basilar skull fractures are usually not detected on x-ray films since they occur at the very base of the skull. Clinical signs and symptoms are crucial to diagnosis, and there are four classical indices:
1. Battle's sign (ecchymosis of mastoid)
2. Hemotympanum (bleeding from the ear or visualization of blood behind the eardrum)
3. Periorbital ecchymosis (without direct eye injury) ("raccoon sign")
4. Rhinorrhea or otorrhea

The basilar skull fracture usually does not involve brain damage or coma, and other neurological deterioration is not a concern. Meningeal irritation and the threat of meningitis from spinal fluid leakage constitute the greatest hazards. Hospitalization or close outpatient observation is essential along with antibiotic therapy. The CSF leakage usually ceases in 2 to 4 weeks.

BRAIN INJURIES

Injury of the brain is obviously the most serious result of head injury. As the brain is set in motion by head injury (for example, blows), the brainstem temporarily malfunctions (because of interruption of neural transmissions) during the twisting motion, and there is an interruption of function of the reticular activating system (the center of consciousness). Unconsciousness results for a moment or two. Immediate traumatic unconscious states are always results of brainstem insult and never hematoma, because blood could not collect rapidly enough to cause compression damage. Cerebral contusions are caused by the brain raking over the bony irregularities of the calvarium. There is no immediate loss of consciousness. In fact, unconsciousness is rare with unilateral cerebral hemisphere damage.

Concussion

A concussion is a transient episode of unconsciousness (for example, "being knocked out") or brief focal neurological deficit (for example, blindness) following brain injury. A concussion has little or no residua after seconds or an hour of unconsciousness. However, the severity depends usually on the period of amnesia.

There is no specific technique for diagnosing concussion except by history, and no abnormalities can be found on neurological examination. A cerebral concussion is a diagnosis appropriate only if the patient has fully recovered from unconsciousness and no deterioration in level of consciousness is observed.

A *postconcussion syndrome,* however, has been identified; it consists of headache, dizziness, vertigo, anxiety, and fatigue. It may persist for several weeks and is usually managed by administration of aspirin.

Contusion

A contusion is local brain injury with bruising, hemorrhage, and edema (Fig. 14-9). Hemorrhage may be epidural, subdural, or subarachnoid. It may be local with or without changes

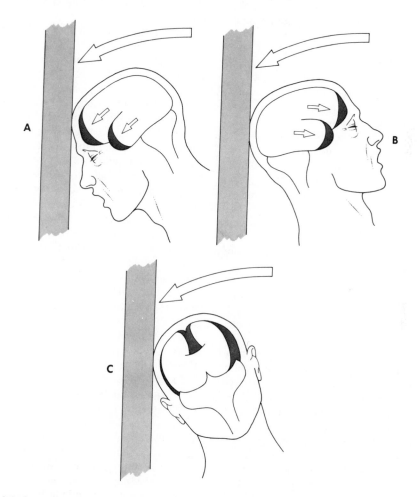

Fig. 14-9. Cortical contusion with relation to direction of head movement. **A,** Head moving forward and striking stationary surface—major injury found at tips of frontal and temporal poles. **B,** Head moving backward and striking stationary surface—major injury found in frontal and temporal lobes (contrecoup). **C,** Head moving laterally and striking stationary surface—major injury found on side opposite that which strikes surface (contrecoup). Medial surfaces of hemispheres are also injured by impingement on relativley rigid falx.

in level of consciousness. There may be resultant and prolonged coma. Coma of sudden onset with neurogenic shock may be the result of a cerebrovascular accident, ruptured aneurysm, or closed head trauma. Many patients with this severe injury do not survive, and the disability in survivors is great.

Signs and symptoms may vary from minimal weakness to complete loss of function. Seizures are likely, along with other neurological dysfunction.

All patients with contusions require hospitalization.

Dural lacerations

The dura is the final significant anatomic protection of the brain after scalp or skull injury. Laceration of the dura may or may not mean that brain injury has occurred. However, if the dura is lacerated, meningitis, brain abscess, and subdural infections can occur.

If CSF is leaking or if the brain is herniating through the dural tear, antibiotic prophylaxis and a search for other brain injury are imperative.

Hemorrhage and hematoma

In either concussion or cerebral contusion, the patient is stable or improves. Signs and symptoms depend on the area of brain that is injured. Lateralization may be apparent with hematoma formation. The life-threatening posttraumatic condition is cerebral hemorrhage, with actual rupture of blood vessels. The resultant hematoma causes an increase in intracranial pressure. Consequences of this phenomenon are important for emergency personnel to understand.

Subarachnoid hemorrhage. Subarachnoid hemorrhage occurs when vessels lying between the arachnoid and pia mater are torn and they hemorrhage into the subarachnoid space. It may result from severe head trauma and the rupture of cerebral aneurysms.

Signs and symptoms include a severe headache extending over several days, usually with marked nuchal rigidity and often photophobia. Projectile vomiting may be evident.

Management of subarachnoid hemorrhage includes surgical clamping of the bleeding source and supportive medical care for 2 to 4 weeks.

Intracerebral hemorrhage. Intracerebral hemorrhage is the most dangerous neurological bleeding, because the brain itself suffers the insult. It frequently results from blunt trauma in which the brain is severely jolted within the calvarium. Consequently, electrical activity in the brain is interrupted and there is a loss of consciousness. Aphonia and facial or extremity paralysis are not uncommon signs and symptoms.

Intracerebral hemorrhage is treated by surgical removal of the clot.

Brainstem contusion and hemorrhage. Brainstem hemorrhage can be primary (the result of a direct blow) or secondary (the result of increasing intracranial pressure). When the brainstem is injured, the reticular activating system dysfunctions and the individual is rendered comatose, or stuporous at best. It is common that respirations are abnormal and that there are bilateral pathological reflexes and posturing (for example, decerebrate posturing on painful stimulation). Occasionally there is lateralization, but this is somewhat rare and related to hematoma formation.

Cerebral hemorrhage. Cerebral hemorrhage results in signs and symptoms of increased intracranial pressure. Shock is not a related problem and, if it coexists, the clinician should search for causes other than head injury, because the calvarium cannot contain a volume of free blood sufficient to induce shock in adults. (Shock could result from intracranial hemorrhage in neonates, however.)

Extradural or epidural hematoma. Epidural hemorrhage may be severe, and death can result if the situation is not managed promptly. Ordinarily an epidural hematoma is associated with skull fracture and is commonly caused by a tear through the middle meningeal artery as a result of temporal lobe skull fracture. An epidural hematoma may be *contrecoup,* or present on the opposite side of the head from the apparent injury.

This injury should be suspected if there is a momentary loss of consciousness followed by a lucid interval and then a decreased level of con-

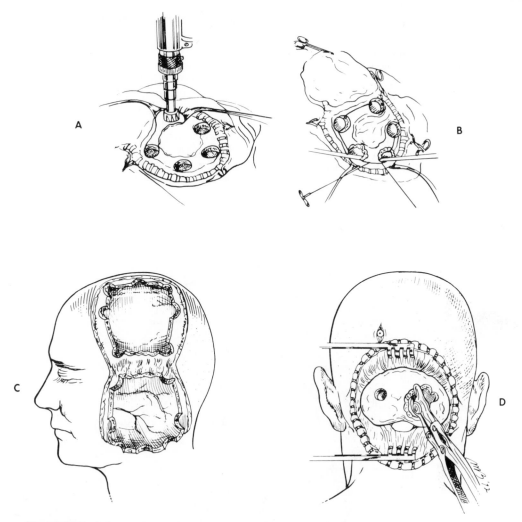

Fig. 14-10. Techniques of cranial surgery. **A,** Drilling burr holes. **B,** Using the Gigli saw. **C,** Bone flap turned down. **D,** Modification for cerebellar craniotomy. (From Barber, J., Stokes, L., and Billings, D.: Adult and child care, ed. 2, St. Louis, 1977, The C. V. Mosby Co.)

sciousness. The lucid interval may be 4 to 12 hours or even a day or two.

Extradural hemorrhages are generally arterial (middle meningeal) and can be rapidly fatal. *Do not waste time* watching for signs and symptoms of localization. Act quickly if the following appear:

1. Dilating pupil
2. Decreasing pulse
3. Increase in blood pressure
4. Decreasing respirations

Emergency intervention must include rapid surgery (burr holes) to expose the clot, to facilitate its aspiration, and to control any significant bleeding at the site (Fig. 14-10).

Subdural hematoma. A subdural hematoma is caused by active bleeding beneath the dura, and thus there is an accumulation of blood between the dural and arachnoid membranes. It occurs frequently in patients with blood dyscrasias or those taking anticoagulants. Ruptured aneurysms and arteriovenous malformations can also result in subdural hematomas.

ACUTE SUBDURAL HEMATOMA. Symptoms occur shortly after trauma, at least in the first 24 hours. It commonly occurs from massive bilateral bleeding from torn dural sinuses. The patient's condition deteriorates rapidly, and the mortality is almost 90%. It is obviously a high priority for surgery (Fig. 14-11).

CHRONIC SUBDURAL HEMATOMA. A chronic subdural hematoma may occur days, weeks, or even months after injury, and in at least half of all cases there is no history of trauma. Headache is by far the most common symptom. There is often an accompanying confusion and a decreased level of consciousness.

A chronic subdural hematoma should be suspected when there is a mild fever and leukocytosis, largely from dehydration or pneumonitis. Occasionally the subdural hematoma develops slowly and in about 12 days begins to

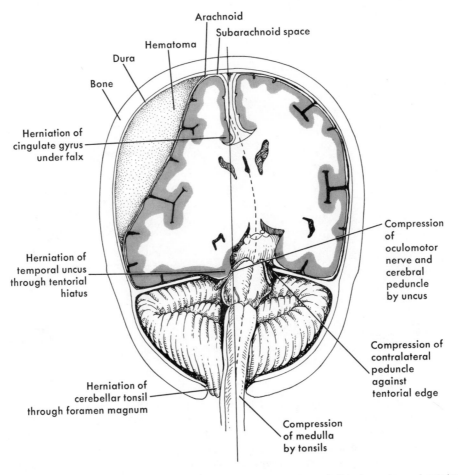

Fig. 14-11. Subdural hematoma. Although hematoma displaces and distorts surface of cerebral hemisphere, more serious and life-threatening changes are occurring in deeper structures at some distance from hematoma itself. These changes result in displacement and compression of vital centers within brainstem.

be encapsulated. In about 3 weeks the enveloped mass becomes an osmotically active "tumor" as the blood clot retracts, and a space-occupying lesion is created. The protein-rich encapsulated clot attracts fluid and expands, creating signs and symptoms of increased intracranial pressure.

There is a developing papilledema and the level of consciousness may fluctuate. CSF pressure may be normal or elevated. (Less elevation is seen in elderly patients, who have a larger subdural space.)

When an individual comes to the emergency department with headache, confusion, and a history of trauma, chronic subdural hematoma should be suspected. Chronic alcoholics who frequently fall and become disoriented are difficult to assess because of the similarity of symptoms between a head injury and an alcoholic state (see Chapter 24).

EMERGENCY DEPARTMENT ASSESSMENT. The nurse should determine the history of symptoms, noting any recent or past traumatic injuries. Particular note should be made regarding a change in sleeping habits, especially the desire to sleep later in the morning. It is significant if there are any differences in the ability to remember or if there has been an evident change in orientation or the ability to function normally. It is important to assess the body for ecchymosis that would indicate injury or a tendency to bleed with ease. Vital signs must be carefully

noted with attention to any slowed respirations and bradycardia.

X-ray films are scrutinized for linear skull fractures or a shifted calcified pineal gland. A brain scan or CAT scan may be done before angiography or other invasive diagnostic tests. If the patient is deteriorating rapidly, time should not be wasted with x-ray films.

SURGICAL TREATMENT. Large clots may not lend themselves to extraction via burr holes (see p. 299). Later, however, as the clot liquefies, this may be accomplished in some cases.

Three burr holes are usually made so that the flap can be turned if the clot is solid. If no clot is found at first, burr holes are made on the other side of the head. (False lateralizing can occur with indirect compression of central nervous system structures by impingement of the tentorial edge against the cerebral peduncle.) If there is third nerve paresis (a fixed dilated pupil) and a hemiparesis on the same side, consider the side of the abnormal pupil as the side of the expanding mass.

Disposition of the patient with head injury

The individual who is seen in the emergency department for an acute head injury may be discharged, admitted for observation, or transferred to a regional head injury center. Criteria for disposition are illustrated in Table 14-9 and in boxed material on p. 302.

Table 14-8. Summary of brain injuries

Injury	Neurological findings
Concussion	Immediate interruption of level of consciousness with gradual recovery of alertness and orientation; no abnormal neurological findings
Brainstem contusion	Immediate unconsciousness with no improvement for several hours, symmetrical neurological findings or variable lateralization
Cerebral contusion	Level of consciousness may range from alertness to coma; findings depend on area of brain that is bruised
Intracranial hematoma	Deteriorating level of consciousness with no improvement of neurological status: lateralization of pupillary dilation and paresis

*From Barber, J., Stokes, L., and Billings, D.: Adult and child care: a client approach to nursing, ed. 2, St. Louis, 1977, The C. V. Mosby Co.

Table 14-9. Criteria for disposition of patient with head injury

Category A (discharged)	Category B (admitted for observation)	Category C (transport to regional head injury center)
Concussed patients who were essentially asymptomatic on arrival. Preaccident memory is returning but immediate post-accident memory is impaired. Requires careful instructions before discharge regarding signs of neurological deterioration Scalp wound victims without any evidence of brain injury *if* head injury is only presenting complaint. (A few unusually large scalp wounds may require admission for satisfactory management, however)	Patients with concussions who are not fully oriented and who have limitations regarding immediate recall and recent memory. (Headache, if present *and* diminishing is *not* a contraindication for care in the home.) Usually may be discharged in 24 hours Preschool children. Since many erratic signs and symptoms may be inconclusive early post-trauma in this age group, at least 24 hours of observation are appropriate Basal or convex skull fracture patients should be admitted for 24 to 28 hours of observation Stuporous patients without focal or lateralizing signs who are improving neurologically, especially those with ethanol intoxication	Patients who have deteriorating level of consciousness Patients with depressed skull fractures or penetrating injury Preschool children with skull fracture Individuals with CSF otorrhea or rhinorrhea Patients with posttraumatic seizures Severely obtunded patients Patients with focal or lateralizing syndrome Multiple trauma victims requiring narcotic analgesia who have head injuries

---

Checklist for transfer of the neurologically injured

Airway	Is airway patent and secured with efficient spontaneous or supported ventilation? Is equipment available for bag-valve-mask assistance? Is oxygen supply adequate for transfer distance? Has nasogastric tube been placed to decompress the stomach? Is suctioning equipment available and functioning efficiently? Is the neck immobilized properly in a neutral position if cervical spine injury is known or suspected?
Circulation	Has blood pressure been stabilized in satisfactory range? Is at least one IV in place with an 18-gauge or larger catheter for fluid resuscitation? Is Foley catheter in place if indicated?
Other	Has receiving center been notified? Are all records and x-ray films available and ready for transfer? Is at least one transfer team member capable of giving emergency drugs if indicated during transfer? Has family been instructed regarding the details of the transfer?

SEIZURES
Classification and manifestations

Grand mal seizures. Grand mal seizures consist of sudden unconsciousness and involuntary alternating tonic and clonic movements of extremities. Respirations cease as intercostal muscles and the diaphragm become paralyzed; cyanosis may be marked. Muscles of the head and face jerk. There may be frothing from the mouth and some dyspnea when breathing is resumed. Bladder control may be lost during the attack. The entire episode lasts only a few minutes.

Status epilepticus. Status epilepticus is a series of successive grand mal seizures occurring without an interim period of consciousness. The condition is extremely serious because of the effect of hypoxia on the vital brain tissue. Prolonged seizures may result in respiratory arrest, hypertension, increased intracranial pressure, papilledema, and hyperthermia.

Petit mal seizures. In petit mal seizures there is only a momentary loss of consciousness in which the individual stares blankly for a few seconds or stops talking in the middle of a sentence. There is often no self-recognition of the episode.

Jacksonian seizures. Jacksonian seizures are focal and begin in one muscle group and spread to adjacent ones on the same side of the body. Ultimately they can become generalized, or grand mal.

Psychomotor seizures. Psychomotor seizures are manifest by the experiencing of psychic phenomena without recollection. There may be unusual motor behavior (for example, wringing of the hands, picking at objects, or undressing). Acts seem to be related to emotions such as frustrations, fear, or rage. Speech may be affected, and thoughts seem to be rambling and nonsensical.

Febrile seizures. See p. 511.

Neonatal seizures. Neonatal seizures reflect the immaturity of the central nervous system and do not manifest themselves in the usual (adult) manner. Congential anomalies, metabolic derangements, infection, and anoxia are possible causes. Signs and symptoms include transient abnormal posturing or rigidity, apneic episodes, repetitive flexion movements of the trunk, opisthotonic posturing, tremors, sudden loss of muscle tone, spasmodic crying, facial twitching or chewing movements, paroxysmal blinking or nystagmus, and hyperactivity unusual for the gestational age. Morbidity and mortality from neonatal seizures are high.

Epilepsy. Epilepsy is a form of idiopathic seizure that is recurrent and may be primary (no known cause) or secondary (from infections, trauma, congenital illness, brain tumors, and other disorders that affect the brain). The term "epilepsy" is usually employed for seizures without a known cause that begin in early childhood or young adulthood.

Emergency management of status epilepticus

The majority of seizures are self-limiting. Seizures become a life-threatening emergency in the event of status epilepticus, because of resultant hypoxia and metabolic abberations.

The airway should be enhanced and oxygen administered at a high-flow rate. An artificial airway can be used if necessary and bag-valve-mask assistance should be provided between seizure bouts. If possible, the patient should be placed in a side-lying position with suction at hand, because vomiting is a frequent occurrence as a result of air in the stomach swallowed during gasping breathing.

An IV of D/5/W should be promptly initiated as a route for anticonvulsant drugs. Drugs important in seizure management for adults include:

Diazepam (Valium) is the drug of choice for interrupting status epilepticus. It is short acting, with a half-life of only 7 minutes; thus, recurrent seizures should be anticipated. Diazepam should be given by slow IV push (not to exceed 5 mg/minute) with a total dose of 2.5 to 35 mg. Stop bolus administration just as soon as the seizure has been terminated. (Diazepam may be repeated in 15 minutes.) Dosage is based on the patient's age and weight, the duration of seizure activity, and the observed response to the drug. Expect side effects

"AEIOU TIPS" for assessing seizure disorders

A	Alcoholism	In alcoholics who are in withdrawal, seizures are quite common. As well, many alcoholics are on anticonvulsant medications and often forget or neglect to take them, particularly during drinking bouts.
E	Epilepsy	About 90% of grand mal seizures are idopathy epilepsy.
	Electrolytes	An imbalance in serum chemicals (sodium, calcium) may lead to seizures.
I	Insulin	Hypoglycemia may present with seizures. D/50/W should be given to most patients.
O	Overdose	Use of drugs such as barbiturates may lead to seizure activity when the drugs are suddenly stopped.
U	Underdose	The patient fails to take his or her medication for seizures. This is a common cause of seizures.
T	Trauma	Watch for trauma in a patient. Old trauma may lead to chronic seizure disorders.
	Tumors	Seizures may be the presenting sign of brain tumor in adults.
I	Infection	Meningitis or brain abscess may cause seizures.
P	Psychiatric	"Fake seizures"; remember that the essential thing about grand mal seizures is the unconscious state. If the patient is taking purposeful swings at you, it is not a grand mal seizure.
S	Stroke (cerebro-vascular accident)	Remember cerebrovascular causes of seizures; also ventricular fibrillation may present as a seizure, so remember to check the pulse. A transient hemiparesis may appear following a seizure. Such a temporary neurological deficit is called Todd's paralysis.

including respiratory arrest, hypotension, and cardiac arrest.

Phenytoin (Dilantin) should be begun as soon as diazepam has interrupted seizure activity. Administer an IV bolus (50 mg/minute) over 20 to 30 minutes to a total dose of 1,000 mg to achieve a 24-hour therapeutic plasma level. Monitor the blood pressure and ECG during administration (see p. 734).

Phenobarbital (½ to 2 gr) given by slow push over 5 to 10 minutes may be used with caution and repeated in 15 minutes. Since phenobarbital is a sedative, it may interfere with serial neurological testing (see p. 733).

Lidocaine (Xylocaine) may be indicated for uremic seizures.

Paraldehyde is useful for seizures related to certain alcohol withdrawal syndromes, especially those with concurrent liver disease. *Use a glass syringe,* because paral-dehyde dissolves polyethylene. Use metal connectors and rubber tubing. Shake 2 to 4 ml in 10 ml normal saline. Give by IV push at 0.5 ml/minute. The blood will turn jet black on the contact with the drug. Expect an inspiratory cramp 12 to 14 seconds after IV administration. Paraldehyde may also be given via an oil retention enema (0.2 to 0.7 ml/kg) or IM (5 ml).

As soon as feasible insert a nasogastric tube to decompress the stomach, because vomiting and aspiration are major complications of status epilepticus.

Vital signs, including temperature, should be monitored every 30 minutes, because hyperthermia results form the prolonged seizures.

Venous blood samples should be sent to the laboratory for:

Phenobarbital and phenytoin levels if appropriate

Alcohol level

Calcium and phosphate levels

Blood sugar

Toxicity screening in selected cases

BUN

Electrolytes

Magnesium

An IV bolus of D/50/W should be pushed as soon as bloods are obtained to rule out hypoglycemia-induced seizures. A baseline arterial blood gas is also recommended, with serial determinations made at least every hour to guide respiratory and drug therapy.

If there is a history of trauma, a set of skull films should be obtained. Of course, hospitalization is mandatory in status epilepticus with a thorough search for a treatable cause. CAT scans, EEGs, screening for heavy metal poisoning and for infectious and metabolic disorders are in order.

MIGRAINE

A migraine headache is presumably caused by vasospasm that produces local anoxia of the brain. After intense spasm, the affected vessels relax and become congested with blood for an extended period of time, even up to 48 hours. As dilatation progresses, there are excessive pulsations, especially of temporal arteries. As the attack continues, edema fluid containing proteolytic enzymes and pain-provoking polypeptides collects in the extracranial perivascular tissue. The pain mechanisms of dilation and pulsation are thus augmented by chemical substances produced as byproducts of the vascular phenomena. EEG changes may occur but are generally nonspecific.

The emergency management includes a reduction of environmental stimuli (such as noise and bright lights), bed rest, and vasoconstricting drugs. Ergotamine tartrate alone (Gynergen) or with caffeine added (Cafergot) is the agent of choice. Some clinicians use symptomatic treatment adjuncts including 100% oxygen, ice bags, massage, and warm baths.

HYPERTENSIVE EMERGENCIES

Emergency management of hypertension is mandatory when the diastolic blood pressure reaches 140 to 150 mm Hg or if pulmonary edema, encephalopathy, or cerebral hemorrhage occurs in relation to hypertension.

Signs and symptoms

- Diastolic blood pressure is *usually* over 140 mm Hg.
- Fundi exhibit hemorrhage, exudate, and arteriolar spasm; papilledema may be present.
- Headache, nausea, vomiting, irritability, seizures, visual disturbances, confusion, paralysis, transient focal deficits, and even coma characterize the related encephalopathy.
- Left ventricular hypertrophy and failure occur.
- Renal phenomena may include oliguria, azotemia, proteinuria, casts, and hematuria.
- Hyperreflexia is present.

Table 14-10. Guide for drug selection in hypertensive crisis*

Hypertensive emergency	Drugs of choice†	Contraindicated or use with extreme risk†
Malignant hypertension	1, 2, 3, 4, 5, 6	
Eclampsia	1, 2, 4	1, 3
Pheochromocytoma-like emergencies including those with MAO inhibitors	2, 9	All others
Intracerebral or subarachnoid hemorrhage	1, 2, 3	5, 6
Acute dissecting aortic aneurysm	2, 10	1, 4
Hypertensive heart disease with left ventricular failure	2, 3, 7, 8	1, 4
Acute encephalopathy of hypertension	1, 2, 3	5, 6
Hypertension with accompanying acute or chronic glomerulonephritis	1, 2, 4, 6, 7	3

*From Barber, J. M., and Budassi, S. A.: Mosby's manual of emergency care, St. Louis, 1979, The C. V. Mosby Co.

†*1*, Diazoxide; *2*, sodium nitroprusside; *3*, trimethaphan; *4*, hydralazine; *5*, reserpine; *6*, methyldopa; *7*, furosemide; *8*, morphine sulfate; *9*, phentolamine; *10*, propranolol.

Table 14-11. Antihypertensive drugs*

Drug	Dosage and administration precautions	Comments
Rapid-acting		
Diazoxide (Hyperstat) (See also p. 719)	300 mg or 5 mg/kg by IV *push* as rapidly as possible (30 sec)	Administer with potent diuretic
Sodium nitroprusside (Nipride) (See also p. 738)	50 mg in 500 ml D/5/W by infusion with *drop by drop* regulation via microdrip or infusion pump; administer at 0.5 to 8µg/kg/min, monitoring effect and titrating accordingly	Light-sensitive; use with diuretic; may be used with dissecting aneurysm
Trimethaphan (Arfonad) (See also p. 738)	1-2 gm/liter via infusion with *drop by drop* regulation via microdrip or infusion pump; administer at initial rate of 3-4 mg/min, monitoring effect and titrating accordingly	Use with diuretic
Less rapid-acting		
Hydralazine (Apresoline)	10 mg IV or IM every 10-15 min as needed up to 50 mg	Onset of action 10-20 min, maximum action 20-40 min; use with diuretic; consider giving propranolol *before* administering drug
Reserpine	0.5-1.0 mg initially followed by 2-4 mg q3h prn; if 4 mg is ineffective, consider other drugs	Onset of action 1½-3 hours, maximum action 3-4 hours
Methyldopa	250-1,000 mg IV given over 30 min (dilute in 100-200 ml D/5/W)	Onset of action 2-3 hours, maximum action 3-5 hours

*From Barber, J. M., and Budassi, S. A.: Mosby's manual of emergency care, St. Louis, 1979, The C. V. Mosby Co.

Emergency management

The emergency management calls for rapid establishment of an IV line of D/5/W for administration of an antihypertensive drug (Tables 14-10 and 14-11).

Blood should be drawn for electrolytes, BUN, creatinine, complete blood count with peripheral smear, and calcium.

The neurological status, the ECG, and vital signs should be monitored on a minute-to-minute basis during therapy. A Foley catheter should be considered for monitoring urinary output.

All patients with hypertensive crises are admitted for stabilization, usually to an intensive care unit setting.

SYNCOPE

Syncope is a transient loss of consciousness caused by cerebral hypoxia. Causes may include hypoglycemia, cardiac dysrhythmias (heart block, bradycardia), postural hypotension, anemia, pain, and psychogenic causes such as fear or anxiety.

Ordinarily the patient who faints is in a horizontal position, which stimulates the early return of consciousness. Placing the legs and feet in an elevated position also helps control syncope. A side-lying position is employed to prevent aspiration.

SPINAL CORD INJURIES

Emergency personnel must be well versed in handling any traumatized person who may have sustained spinal injury. Situations likely to result in such an injury include automobile and motorcycle accidents, diving accidents, falls from significant heights, and cave-ins. Prehospital care EMTs and paramedics are carefully taught the importance of extrication safety and are skilled in restoring the airway and controlling vital processes of breathing and circulation while protecting the spine from motion that could cause cord damage. It is a rule of emergency care to always suspect that spinal injury exists and manage the individual as if there were, using specific splinting and immobilization techniques. If the history of injury is unknown, emergency personnel must be alert to head and neck bruises, deformities of the spine, otorrhea, rhinorrhea, cranial nerve impairment, and depressed skull fractures (Fig. 14-12).

Cervical immobilization is usually accomplished by the use of a cervical collar. Until the collar is applied, manual head traction (by steadily pulling upward) helps open the airway and protects the cord from damage by bone fragments if a fracture has been incurred (Fig. 14-13, *A*).

The patient's body must be stabilized on a backboard for both extrication and transportation. A short backboard is often used to remove a passenger from a motor vehicular crash since it not only stabilizes the spine but also permits securing of cervical traction. Since diving accidents are classic causative forces for cervical spine injury, victims of diving accidents should be placed on a backboard before removal from the water. Of course, manual traction or a cervical collar should be employed as well, to maintain stability of the cervical region. Cravats or sandbags may also be used for immobilization during the early period after the injury (Fig. 14-13, *B*). All transfers should be done by a team of three using logrolling.

The major complications of spinal cord injury are respiratory depression (even arrest) and neurogenic (distributive) shock.

Interferences with respiration are due primarily to paralysis of intercostal muscles as a result of cervical fracture and cord damage. Because the diaphragm is responsible for the muscular activity associated with breathing, respirations are characterized by abdominal rather than chest excursions, and paradoxical respirations may be evident. Since abdominal breathing is less efficient than chest breathing, supplemental oxygen should be provided.

Fortunately, only rarely does high spinal cord injury functionally obliterate all muscles of breathing, including the phrenic nerve, which innervates the diaphragm. The consequences of phrenic nerve failure are obvious; apnea is precipitated. This must be managed promptly with artificial respirations, intubation, and administration of oxygen. Meanwhile, the carotid pulse should be palpated and if absent, chest compressions initiated (see pp. 136-137).

Shock from neurogenic causes is due to precipitant vasodilation of peripheral blood vessels that induces hypotension. It is important to differentiate this type of mechanism from hemorrhagic shock. The pulse rate and blood pressure are usually decreased in neurogenic shock; in hemorrhagic shock, the blood pressure may be also decreased, but the pulse is accelerated. The skin remains warm and dry in neurogenic shock because of dilation of cutaneous vascular beds and denervations of sweat glands. Of course if hypovolemia coexists, the shock is compounded because of the loss of reflexive vasoconstriction. Abdominal trauma should always be suspected in shock of unknown cause, because visceral as well as cutaneous sensations may not provide the essential input to detect a ruptured viscus. Peritoneal lavage is thus indicated (see p. 402). After appropriate immobilization of the spine, neurogenic shock can be treated using the shock position, intravenous fluids (D/5/Ringer's lactate at a rate to maintain the blood pressure above 100 mm Hg,* pressor agents,† and antishock trousers (see p. 247).

The patient should be carefully transported, giving attention to basic life support, neurological monitoring, and protection of the airway from aspiration. When the patient arrives at the emergency department, it is imperative that the nurse take charge of care to ensure that only personnel familiar with caring for the individual with an unstable spine be permitted

---

*The IV is chiefly established for a medication route, but some fluids may be helpful in controlling even neurogenic shock.
†Pressor agents are only judiciously used when the CVP indicates a satisfactory intravascular volume.

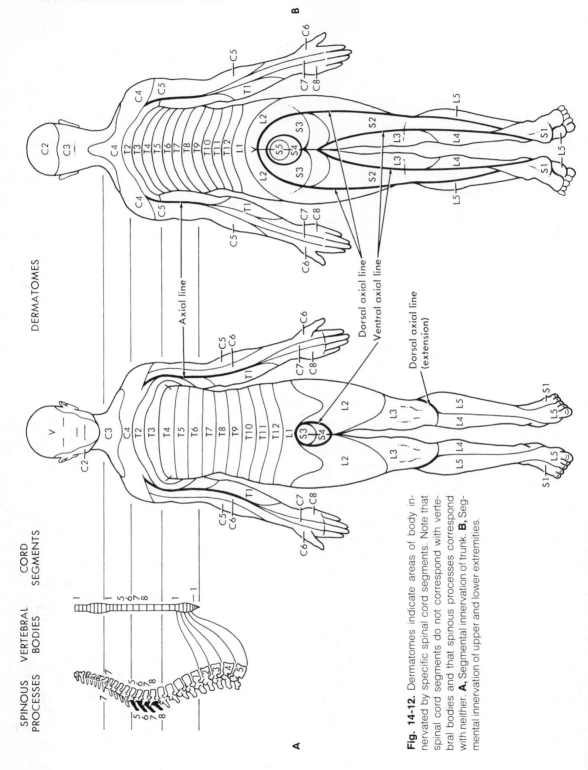

Fig. 14-12. Dermatomes indicate areas of body innervated by specific spinal cord segments. Note that spinal cord segments do not correspond with vertebral bodies and that spinous processes correspond with neither. **A,** Segmental innervation of trunk. **B,** Segmental innervation of upper and lower extremities.

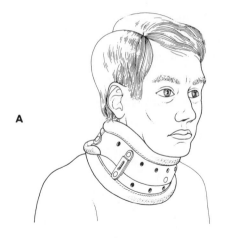

A

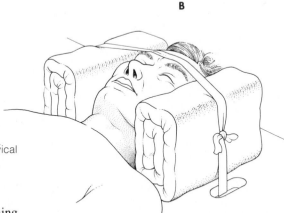

B

Fig. 14-13. Techniques for immobilization of cervical spine. **A,** Cervical collar; **B,** cravats or sandbags.

to participate in initial care activities. Clothing should be cut away along seams if necessary, and under no circumstances should tee shirts or sweaters be pulled over the head, since such movement could stress the unstable spine. Cervical spine stabilization can be assured by a cervical collar, sandbags, or wide tape across the forehead securing the head to the stretcher, preventing flexion of the neck. If emesis threatens in the patient attached to a backboard, the board can be turned sideways to protect the airway. Otherwise, in the event of vomiting, the patient must be logrolled sideways to prevent aspiration. Ideally, three people are required. One supports the hips, one the chest and shoulders, and the third stabilizes the head and neck. If lifting is required, a fourth person should be present to support the legs.

Airway management (including foreign body removal, suctioning, or intubation) should be accomplished without flexion or extension of the neck. The atonic tongue may fall backward if the patient is unconscious. Correction of this problem can be accomplished by the chin lift maneuver and employment of an oropharyngeal airway. Methods of choice for airway management when cervical spine injury is suspected are blind nasotracheal intubation or the

use of an esophageal obturator airway. Rarely, in the event of facial or mandibular complications of trauma, cricothyrotomy or tracheostomy may be required.

Baseline bloods should be drawn including a CBC, SMA-6, SMA-12, coagulation studies, a type and cross-match, and arterial blood gases.* A toxicology screen, including ETOH, may also be indicated.

A Foley catheter should be placed for decompressing the bladder and for monitoring intake and output. It is also a useful tool in detecting urinary tract trauma in relation to abdominal injuries.

Steroid therapy is characteristically initiated if spinal cord injury is present using loading doses of methylprednisolone sodium succinate (Solu-Medrol) or dexamethasone (Decadron). A careful medical history must be obtained

---

*Oxygen tension of the injured spinal cord tends to fall quickly below minimal tissue requirements; if systemic hypoxia coexists, compromise may be great. The pO_2 should therefore be maintained at or above 80 mm Hg. Intubation and the delivery of supplemental oxygen may be required.

from the patient or significant others before embarking on steroid therapy or planning for surgical intervention.

Emergency personnel should position the patient on his side to prevent aspiration of vomitus until a nasogastric tube has been placed. The side-lying position may also assist in airway maintenance by permitting secretions to drain away from the hypopharynx.

Vital signs including the ECG and CVP should be monitored carefully. It is imperative to obtain a 12-lead ECG as a baseline and to rule out myocardial infarction. Sinus bradycardia that occurs in relation to cervical spine injury does not require therapy unless nodal or ventricular escape rhythms occur. In these events, the emergency nurse should be prepared to administer atropine (0.5 to 1.0 mg).

An IV route should be established promptly with D/5/W upon the patient's arrival to ensure ready access to the blood stream for emergency medications. In addition to routine baseline blood studies, arterial blood gases, coagulation studies, and cardiac enzymes should be obtained.

While the patient is being attended in the emergency department, it is important for the nurse to be aware of the need to calm and reassure the often bewildered patient who is suddenly aphasic or possibly paralyzed. Special attention should be given to protecting paralyzed limbs or nonsensitive skin areas. Movement for any reason should be accomplished slowly and cautiously, since involved desensitized body parts are easily injured. Be certain to watch for potential sources of skin injury including pressure from lying on tubes, wrinkled sheets, or monitoring leads. Early placement of a Foley catheter will ensure that the bladder is decompressed, because a distended bladder can contribute to shock, restlessness, and even damage to the organ itself. The bladder is usually hypotonic, and the sensation of fullness is lost because of lost visceral afferent fibers.

Since the patient with spinal cord injury has difficulty maintaining body temperature because sweating and vasomotor mechanisms are disturbed, he should be protected from unusual environmental temperature stresses; ordinarily, this means keeping him lightly covered.

Motor and sensory examination

Individuals who potentially have spinal cord injuries should have motor functions evaluated. Initially, if the patient is conscious, one can ask him to "wiggle your fingers and toes" to grossly determine if motor function is possible. However, this type of test does not reflect certain central cord lesions or root deficits. In order to do a complete assessment, the motor functions must be systematically checked by major muscle groups. Muscle strength may be graded 0 to 5: 0, absent; 1, trace; 2, movement with no gravity; 3, movement against gravity only; 4, movement with resistance; and 5, normal movement and strength.

The physical examination should involve a careful check for subtle signs of spinal cord injury, including painful or limited active neck movement, tilting the head to one side, and pain upon application of pressure to spinous processes. Other clues include unusual limb responses to painful stimuli, areflexia and flaccidity of limbs, and atonic anal sphincter, priapism, and bilateral external rotation of the legs at the hips.

Reflexes should also be tested (such as, deep tendons, the Babinski, cremasteric, and bulbocavernous). "Spinal shock" is the temporary suppression of reflexes mediated by segments below the level of an acute spinal cord injury. Reflexes return over hours or days, usually beginning with perianal muscle contraction. This is elicited by the bulbocavernous reflex, stimulated by pinching the base or glans of the penis or by pulling on the Foley catheter. The rectal examination is an important way to test for a complete lesion. If the patient can feel an examining finger and can contract perianal muscles, the lesion is incomplete and the prognosis is certainly more favorable for functional return.

The sensory examination should include major dermatomes and ought to include response to pinprick and light touch. In the distal extremities, position sense should also be noted. The sensory assessment helps detect lesions of the thoracic spine that would not be identified on the motor examination alone.

Emergency nurses are often asked to assist with such examinations or may perform them independently in certain settings. In addition, they should be prepared to explain to the patient and his family or friends the purpose of the examination. It is also important to gather evidence that validates whether or not the patient is improving, deteriorating, or is stabilized after the injury. Transfer to a regional spinal cord center is advisable after stabilization if the initial receiving hospital does not have a comprehensive neurosurgical service. All stabilization procedures, including those related to the spinal cord, the airway, and cardiovascular integrity, should be accomplished before transfer.

Radiological studies

The cross-table lateral x-ray films of the cervical spine should be taken in the emergency department and interpreted before undertaking any further radiological studies. The nurse or other emergency personnel may be requested to help pull the shoulders down by wrapping elasticlike gauze (Kling or Kerlix) around the wrists, and while standing at the foot of the stretcher, pulling down toward the patient's feet forcefully while the x-ray film is being taken. All seven cervical vertebrae must be visualized for a satisfactory study.

The patient may be transported to the radiology department for thoracic and lumbar films, since adequate penetration of these regions may not be possible with portable equipment. However, under no circumstances should the emergency nurse leave the patient alone in the radiology department because unsuspecting personnel could inadvertently cause further injury to the patient, or sudden respiratory depression or arrest could occur as a complication of spinal cord injury. It is imperative that sudden vomiting be anticipated, especially until the stomach is decompressed by a nasogastric tube.

Anteroposterior films are useful for ruling out lateral and rotatory spinal dislocation.

An ''open mouth'' odontoid view is valuable in demonstrating lateral atlantoaxial articulation but can only be obtained in the conscious, cooperative patient.

Damage to the spinal cord can occur without radiographic evidence of bony abnormality, especially in the elderly.

Level of injury and types of lesions

The level of bony spinal injury may not correspond with the level of cord injury, since the structures grow at different rates. The bone increases in length during growth and development at a much faster rate than the spinal cord. For example, cervical segments of the cord may be approximately one level above the corresponding bony level, and in the thoracic region, the difference may be two levels.

Traumatic injury of the spine can be categorized as flexion, flexion-rotation, or hyperextension (Fig. 14-15). Trauma may create a disturbance in blood flow at one level that will insult adjacent cord areas.

Spinal cord lesions may be of the anterior syndrome type, producing paralysis and loss of sensation to pain and temperature. The cause is likely to be fracture-dislocations, burst fractures, and consequences of acute herniation of disc material. Posterior cord syndromes are characterized by a decrease in touch and proprioception. Central cord syndromes affect function more in upper extremities than lower extremities, but sensory losses may be quite variable. The reason for the phenomenon probably is that central fibers of the corticospinal tract supply the upper extremities, and lower extremities are served by lateral fibers. If the anterior spinal artery is obstructed or damaged, or if there is an expanding mass in the central cords, the central fibers are most noticably affected.

A lateral lesion (Brown-Sequard syndrome) affects one half of the cord, producing ipsilateral paralysis and contralateral loss of pain and temperature (Fig. 14-16). Such an injury is usually caused by a penetrating injury. Root syndromes occur often as a result of vertebral subluxation or acute herniated discs. Lost motor or sensory functions can return, since spinal roots and nerves are part of the peripheral nervous system, thus capable of regeneration if ana-

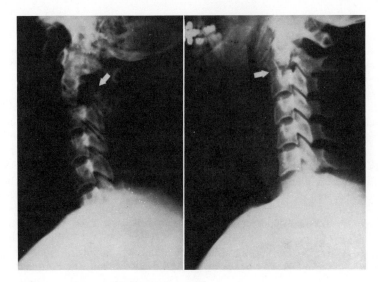

Fig. 14-14. Fracture dislocation of C2 anteriorly on C3. The body of C2 is displaced anteriorly, and pedicles are fractured *(arrow)*. In right half of photograph, dislocation has been reduced by traction, and anterior interbody fusion is performed with insertion of bone dowel *(arrow)*. (From Nishioka, H.: in Leichty, R. D., and Soper, R. T.: Synopsis of surgery, ed. 4, St. Louis. 1980, The C. V. Mosby Co.)

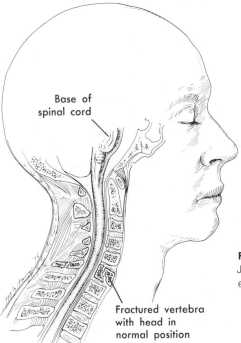

Base of
spinal cord

Fractured vertebra
with head in
normal position

Fig. 14-15. Types of spinal cord injury. (From Barber, J., Stokes, L., and Billings, D.: Adult and child care, ed. 2, St. Louis, 1977, The C. V. Mosby Co.)

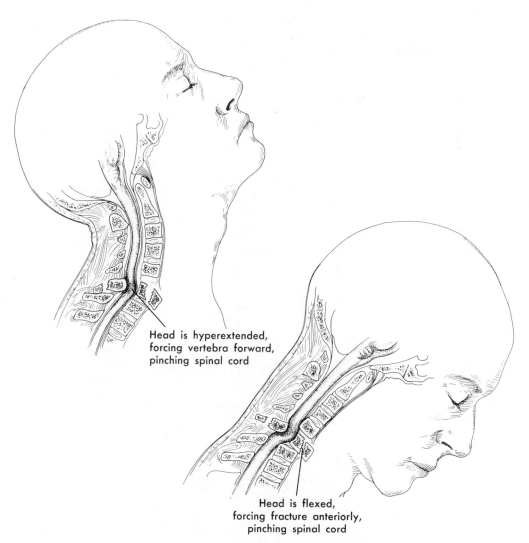

Head is hyperextended,
forcing vertebra forward,
pinching spinal cord

Head is flexed,
forcing fracture anteriorly,
pinching spinal cord

Fig. 14-15, cont'd. Types of spinal cord injury.

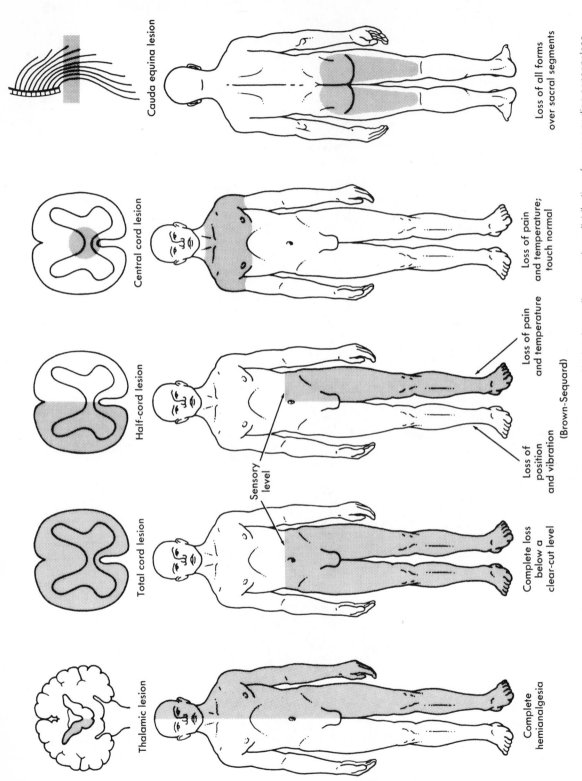

Thalamic lesion

Complete hemianalgesia

Total cord lesion

Sensory level

Complete loss below a clear-cut level

Half-cord lesion

Loss of position and vibration

Loss of pain and temperature

(Brown-Sequard)

Central cord lesion

Loss of pain and temperature; touch normal

Cauda equina lesion

Loss of all forms over sacral segments

Fig. 14-16. Common patterns of sensory abnormality. Upper diagrams show site of lesion; lower diagrams show distribution of corresponding sensory loss.

tomical continuity has not been lost. Traction and operative decompression often enhance return by eliminating impingements.

Medical management of spinal cord injury

There are several methods of treating the individual with spinal cord injury, but all are directed toward cord decompression, nurturing surviving neural tissue, and pain relief. The exact mode, of course, depends on the nature and extent of injury. Minor injuries that do not pose a serious threat to the spinal cord may require only a neck brace or plastic cervical collar. Skull tongs or a halo-ring device may be employed for lesions requiring traction (Fig. 14-17). If these devices are employed in the emergency department, the nurse should be prepared to assist with the procedures, which require scrupulous sterile technique if devices are inserted into the skull. Additional neurological

examinations and x-ray films are required to evaluate the reduction. Muscle relaxants may be administered to reduce muscle spasm, thus making reduction easier. For certain injuries, open reduction in the surgical suite will be mandatory within the first 12 to 24 hours if other factors in the patient's condition make surgical interventions feasible. The Harrington rod is one preferred method of realignment. This rod splints the spine internally. Other modes are also available and their selection is based on the preferences of the orthopedic and neurological surgeons. Satisfactory evidence of reduction may require myelography for confirmation.

Ruptured disk (herniated nucleus pulposus)

A ruptured disk is usually the result of lifting a heavy object or a fall on the back. The disk capsule tears, allowing the softer fibrocartilag-

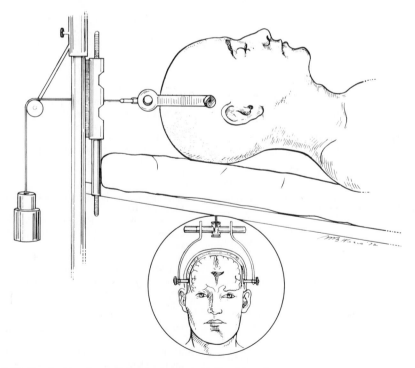

Fig. 14-17. Cervical traction with tongs. Inset shows position of tongs on skull bone structure. (From Barber, J., Stokes, L., and Billings, D.: Adult and child care, ed. 2, St. Louis, 1977, The C. V. Mosby Co.)

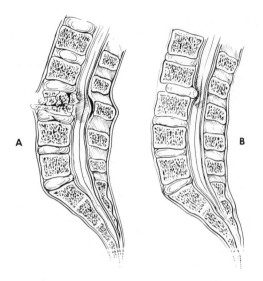

Fig. 14-18. Two causes for spinal cord compression. **A,** Compression fracture of vertebrae. **B,** Herniated nucleus pulposus. (From Barber, J., Stokes, L., and Billings, D.: Adult and child care, ed. 2, St. Louis, 1977, The C. V. Mosby Co.)

inous material to squeeze out and compress adjacent nerve roots against the vertebrae (Fig. 14-18). Lumbar injury is most common and is largely a result of improper body mechanics.

Signs and symptoms include back pain radiating down the posterior portion of the leg, difficulty walking, muscle spasm, and disorders of sensation. If the disk injury occurs near the thoracic or cervical region, there may be nuchal rigidity and pain radiating down the arm to the fingers.

Surgery, braces, casts, traction, bed rest, and physiotherapy are employed to relieve symptoms.

Whiplash injury

A whiplash injury is caused by violent hyperextension and flexion of the neck, usually as a result of a rear-end automobile accident. It produces damage to muscles, disks, ligaments, and nervous tissue in the region of the cervical spine. If the injury is linked to head rotation,

concussion and intracranial hemorrhage may be associated and deserve attention in early assessment.

Signs and symptoms include pallor and a feeling of being dazed, but no loss of conciousness. Weakness, gait disturbances, dizziness, and vomiting may also occur. An occipital headache may be severe and spread to temporal regions; it may be accompanied by nuchal ridigity and pain that radiates down the arms.

Management is symptomatic and includes bed rest, hot packs applied to the neck, analgesia, and a plastic cervical collar to minimize aggravation of the inflamed or bruised neck structures.

Whiplash injuries are frequently the source of long litigations in insurance claims.

BIBLIOGRAPHY

Ansbaugh, P.: Emergency management of intoxicated patients with head injuries, J.E.N. **3:**9-12, May/June 1977.

Barber, J. M., and Budassi, S. A.: Mosby's manual of emergency care, St. Louis, 1979, The C. V. Mosby Co.

Barber, J. M., Stokes, L. G., and Billings, D. M.: Adult and child care: a client approach to nursing, ed. 2, St. Louis, 1977, The C. V. Mosby Co.

Bhatia, S. K., and Frohlich, E. D.: Hemodynamic comparison of agents useful in hypertensive emergencies, Am. Heart. J. **85:**367, 1973.

Bickerstaff, E. R.: Neurology for nurses, ed. 2, London, 1975, English Universities Press, Ltd.

Bouzarth, W. F.: Trauma at the top, Emerg. Med. **7:**71-84, 1975.

Brock, S.: Injuries of brain and spinal cord and their coverings, ed. 5, New York, 1974, Springer Publishing Co., Inc.

Budassi, S. A.: Trauma notebook 18. Intracranial pressure: intracranial pressure monitoring, J.E.N. **5:**45-46, May-June 1979.

Cave, E. F., Burke, J. F., and Boyd, R. J.: Trauma management, Chicago, 1974, Year Book Medical Publishers Inc.

Celesia, G.: Modern concepts of status epilepticus J.A.M.A. **235:**1571-1574, 1976.

DeJong, R. N.: The neurological examination, ed. 3, New York, 1967, Hoeber Medical Division, Harper & Row, Publishers.

Dranov, J., and others: Malignant hypertension: current modes of therapy, Arch. Intern. Med. **133:**791-801, 1974.

Erikson, R.: Cranial check: a basic neurological assessment, Nursing '74 **4:**67-72, 1974.

Evening the odds in epilepsy, Emerg. Med. **6:**106-112, January 6, 1974.

Finnerty, F. A.: Hypertensive encephalopathy, Am. J. Med. **52:**672, May 1972.

Finnerty, F. A.: Hypertensive crisis, J.A.M.A. **229:**1479-1480, 1974.

Fishman, R. A.: Brain edema, N. Engl. J. Med. **293:**706-711, 1975.

Galbraith, S., and Smith, J.: Acute traumatic intracranial hematoma without skull fracture, Lancet **1:**501-503, 1976.

Galbreath, S., and others: The relationship between alcohol and head injury and its effect on the conscious level, Br. J. Surg. **63:**128-130, 1976.

Guyton, A. C.: Textbook of medical physiology, ed. 5, Philadelphia, 1976, W. B. Saunders Co.

Hekmatpanah, J.: The management of head trauma, Surg. Clin. North Am. **53:**47-57. February 1973.

Hinkhouse, A.: Craniocerebral trauma, Am. J. Nurs. **73:**1719-1722, 1973.

Hooper, R.: Patterns of acute head injury, Baltimore, 1969, The Williams & Wilkins Co.

Kaplan, G.: The psychogenic etiology of headache post-lumbar puncture. Psychosom. Med. **29:**376-379, 1967.

Keesey, J.: Neurological emergencies, Unpublished paper, Los Angeles, January 1977, U.C.L.A. Emergency Medical Institute.

Kocen, R. S.: The neuromuscular system, Edinburgh, 1976, Churchill Livingstone.

Koch-Weser, J.: Hypertensive emergencies, N. Engl. J. Med. **290:**211-214, 1974.

Liechty, R. D., and Soper, R. T.: Synopsis of surgery ed. 4, St. Louis, 1980, The C. V. Mosby Co.

Maddox, M.: Subarachnoid hemorrhage, Am. J. Nurs. **74:**2199-2201, 1974.

McDonald, E. J., Winestock, D. P., and Hoff, J. T.: The value of repeat cerebral arteriography in the evaluation of trauma, Am. J. Roentgenol. **126:**792-797, 1976.

McLaurin, M. D., Robert, L., and Scott, T.: ECG changes after experimental head trauma, J. Trauma **15:**447-450, 1975.

Meyer, J. S.: New concepts of cerebrovascular disease, Med. Clin. North Am. **54:**349-360, 1970.

Mountcastle, V. B., ed.: Medical physiology, ed. 14, St. Louis, 1980, The C. V. Mosby Co., vol. 1.

Nichol, C. E., and others: Parenteral diazepam in status epilepticus, Neurology **19:**332-343, April 1969.

Palmer, R. F., and Lasseter, K. C.: Sodium nitroprusside, N. Engl. J. Med. **292:**294-297, 1975.

Plum, F., editor: Recent advances in neurology, Contemporary neurology series, Philadelphia, 1969, F. A. Davis Co.

Plum, F., and Posner, J. B.: Diagnosis of stupor and coma, ed. 2, Contemporary neurology series, Philadelphia, 1972, F. A. Davis Co.

Pohutsky, L. C., and Pohutsky, K. R.: Computerized axial tomography of the brain: a new diagnostic tool, Am. J. Nurs. **75:**1341-1342, 1975.

Ransohoff, J., and Fleischer, A.: Insult and injury—head injuries, Emerg. Med. **8:**147-150, April 1976.

Redelman, K.: The management of acutely ill patients with ruptured intracranial aneurysm, J. Neurosurg. Nurs. **8:**69-77, December 1973.

Swift, N.: Head injury essentials of excellent care, Nursing '74 **4:**27-33, 1974.

Thorn, G. W., et al.: Harrison's principles of internal medicine, ed. 8, New York, 1977, McGraw-Hill Book Co.

Tyler, R. H.: Answers to questions on stroke, Hosp. Med. **13:**26-43, June 1977.

Warner, C. G., editor: Emergency care: assessment and intervention, ed. 2, St. Louis, 1978, The C. V. Mosby Co.

Weiss, M. H.: Head trauma and spinal cord injuries: diagnostic and therapeutic criteria. Crit. Care Med. **2:**311-316, 1974.

Yates, P. O.: The pathological basis for cerebral ischaemia. In Modern trends in neurology. Series 4, New York, 1967, Appleton-Century-Crofts.

Young, J. F.: How the brain recognizes and responds to shock, J. Neurosurg. Nurs. **8:**37-44, July 1976.

CHAPTER 15

Eye, ear, nose, throat, maxillofacial, and dental emergencies

Susan A. Budassi, Robert Kotler, and Nancy Smith

THE EYE

The eye is the main organ of one of the most precious senses the human body possesses. Many times, loss of vision can be prevented by rapid careful care in the prehospital care area and the emergency department.

To be able to deal with eye emergencies effectively and efficiently, one must have a good basic understanding of the anatomy and physiology of the eye (Fig. 15-1).

Basic anatomical descriptions

bony rim—bony process that protects the eyeball
eyelid—closes to protect the eyeball, distribute tears, and regulate amount of light
eyelashes—minimize the amount of dirt particles that enter the eye area
sclera—tough, protective coating of the eyeball
cornea—front section of the eyeball that bulges; light passes through it to the lens
retina—inner lining of the posterior eyeball; collects light
choroid—middle layer of the eyeball; supplies the retina with blood, oxygen, and other nutrients
macula—area of the retina most sensitive to light and color
lens—disc where light passes through to the posterior chamber from the cornea and the anterior chamber; light passes through the cornea, the anterior chamber, the lens, and the vitreous humor to the retina

iris—controls the amount of light entering the posterior chamber by means of expanding and contracting the opening (the pupil)
oculomotor muscles—six muscles that control eyeball movement
lacrimal glands (Fig. 15-2)—secrete fluid (tears) to soothe the eyeball and decrease friction
tears—cover the eyeball; they are distributed by the eyelids (blinking) and exit through the lacrimal puncta into the lacrimal ducts and the nasolacrimal duct
meibomian glands—secrete oil that lines the eyelid margins and prevents tears from running out of the conjunctival sacs
visual acuity—central vision; stimuli on macula
peripheral vision—vision in which stimuli are on area of the retina other than macula

When a patient with a complaint of trauma to the eye or problem with the eye is being triaged, these complaints are given priority treatment.

1. Loss of sight without pain (may be caused by central artery or vein occlusion, intraocular hemorrhage, or retinal detachment)
2. Chemical burns
3. Foreign bodies
4. Painful eyes (may be conjunctivitis, iritis, or keratitis)

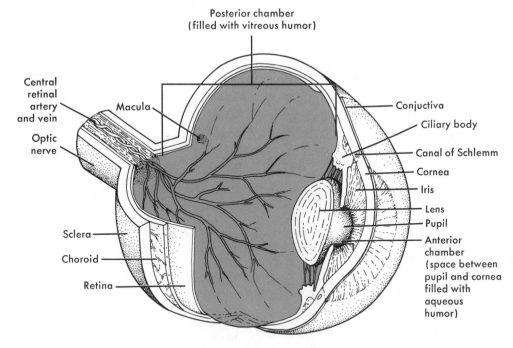

Fig. 15-1. Anatomy of the eye.

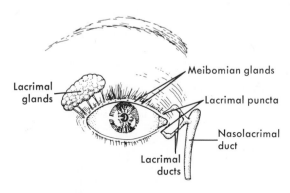

Fig. 15-2. The lacrimal glands.

Eye examination

Good lighting is essential for eye examinations. Topical local anesthetics may aid in examining an eye. It is important to remember to be gentle and to explain what is happening and what you are about to do to the patient. It is essential to recognize an eye condition or trauma early so that further complications can be avoided whenever possible.

When examining an eye, if possible, perform a visual acuity examination before the actual eye examination.

Visual acuity examination

- Do the examination with the patient wearing his glasses and then without his glasses. If the patient's glasses are not available, have the patient read the visual acuity chart through a pinhole poked in a piece of cardboard.
- Check each eye separately, then both eyes together.
- Follow specific instructions on how to conduct the examination according to the method chosen:

  The Snellen chart (Fig. 15-3) is read at 20 feet.

  The Rosenbaum Pocket Vision Screener

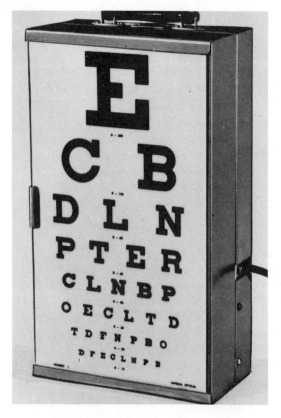

Fig. 15-3. Snellen visual acuity chart. (From Stein, H. A., and Slatt, B. J.: The ophthalmic assistant, ed. 3, St. Louis, 1976. The C. V. Mosby Co.)

(used for patients who cannot stand) is read 14 inches from the nose.

If a Snellen chart or other vision chart is not available, have the patient read newsprint, and record the distance the paper must be held in order for the patient to be able to read it.

If the patient cannot see newsprint, hold up a specific number of fingers and record the distance at which the patient can see your fingers and tell you how many you are holding up.

If the patient cannot see fingers, record the distance at which he can perceive hand motion.

If the patient cannot see hand motion, record at what distance the patient is able to perceive light.

If the patient is unable to perceive light, this finding must also be recorded on the chart.

Examples of visual acuity examination

20/20	When the patient stands at 20 feet, he can read what the normal eye can read at 20 feet.
20/40 − 2	When the patient stands at 20 feet, he can read what the normal eye can read at 40 feet (but he has missed two letters).
20/200	When the patient stands at 20 feet, he can read what the normal eye can read at 200 feet. This result is considered legally blind if the reading is obtained while the patient is wearing glasses or contact lenses.
10/200	If the patient cannot read the letters on the Snellen chart, have him stand half the distance to the chart, and record the findings as the distance he is standing from the chart over the smallest line he can read.
CF/3 feet	The patient can count fingers at 3 feet, maximum.
HM/4 feet	The patient can see hand motion at 4 feet, maximum.
LP/position	The patient can perceive light and determine from which direction it is coming.
LP/no position	The patient can perceive light but is unable to tell from which direction it is coming.
NLP	The patient is unable to perceive light.

Ophthalmoscope (Fig. 15-4). The ophthalmoscope is the basic tool in the examination of the eye. It is used to observe the posterior chamber of the eye through the pupil using a beam of light. Ophthalmoscopes have different shaped light beams and different colored light beams that are used to detect various conditions.

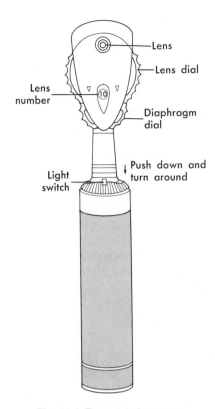

Fig. 15-4. The ophthalmoscope.

When recording information on a chart regarding the eye, use the following abbreviations:

OD	ocula dexter	right eye
OS	ocula sinister	left eye
OU	oculus uterque	both eyes
gtt	guttae	drops

Trauma to the eye

When there is trauma to the eye, always assess the patient for associated trauma, which may be more life-threatening. When there is head or facial trauma, always search for associated eye injury.

One should never put eye drops into the eye of a victim with eye trauma before examination and evaluation by a physician of the extent of injuries. If the pain from trauma is severe, it may be minimized without medication by patching both eyes and decreasing the amount of movement of the eyeball. If a patient is unconscious, be sure to check for contact lenses, and be sure to protect the cornea from drying by either instilling ophthalmic ointment and taping the eyelids shut or instilling artificial tears frequently.

Industrial accidents account for more than half of all blindness to one eye and a fifth of all blindness to both eyes. Trauma to the eye accounts for a large number of industrial accidents where safety glasses are not worn. Trauma is the number two cause of blindness in children, second only to amblyopia.

It is important to ascertain a good history from a patient with eye trauma. Questions that assist in obtaining this history follow.

What happened?

Were chemicals involved? Which ones?

Are there foreign bodies in the eye? What are they?

How did it happen?

Where did it happen?

Why did it happen?

Who witnessed it?

Was care given before arrival at the hospital? What? By whom?

Were safety glasses being worn at the time of the accident?

Is there any medical history, particularly glaucoma, diabetes, or hormone therapy?

Eyelid injuries. The eyelid serves three purposes: to protect the eye, to distribute tears, and to regulate the amount of light entering the eyeball. The eyelashes offer extra protection to the eye by minimizing dirt particles that enter the eye area.

Because the eyelid has a good blood supply, trauma to the eyelid has a very low incidence of infection, and antibiotic treatment is rarely required.

Therapeutic intervention for eyelid injuries includes irrigation of the wound with normal saline and careful approximation of the wound edges in the early postinjury period, before swelling sets in. It is important to make efforts *not* to excise any tissue, as this may cause a deformity in the eyelid and disrupt its function. If a large section of tissue is missing, one should request the services of a plastic surgeon to perform plastic reconstruction to replace lid tissue so that the cornea will be protected.

Be sure to check for a lacerated lacrimal duct when lid trauma is present. If there is lacrimal duct laceration, it should be repaired.

Orbital rim injuries. Orbital rim injury may occur as a result of a blunt or penetrating trauma to that area of the face. Periorbital ecchymosis ("black eye") may result, causing discoloration in and around the orbital rim area. Therapeutic intervention for periorbital ecchymosis includes an ice pack and examination of the orbital rim for fractures and eyeball damage. Examination should include a visual acuity examination.

If there is a fracture of the prominent supraorbital rim and the frontal sinus, be sure to check for cerebrospinal fluid rhinorrhea. If there is a visual disturbance, there may be a fracture of the orbital roof resulting in entrapment of the optic nerve.

Nonpenetrating blunt trauma to the eyeball. A blunt trauma to the eyeball may cause aqueous humor to depress the diaphragm of the iris or the ciliary bodies. When this occurs, the result is a hyphema, a hemorrhage into the anterior chamber of the eye. Any patient experiencing a hyphema *must* be referred to an ophthalmologist immediately.

If there is a partial hyphema, therapeutic intervention includes strict bedrest, heavy sedation, and bilateral eye patches for a minimum of 5 days. Some ophthalmologists choose to administer acetazolamide (Diamox), urea, or mannitol to decrease intraocular pressure. They may also administer steroids and miotics and/ or mydriatics.

Massive hyphema may occur at any time from the time of injury up to 2 weeks after the injury. This injury may cause corneal blood staining, secondary glaucoma, loss of vision, or even loss of the eye.

An eight-ball hemorrhage is a condition in which old clotted blood is found in the anterior chamber. Therapeutic intervention is to remove the clots surgically.

Retrobulbar hemorrhage may occur as a result of ruptured intraorbital vessels. It is evidenced by an eyeball that protrudes (exophthalmos) and diplopia (double vision).

A subconjunctival hemorrhage is common following trauma to the eye. It is usually left untreated and will resolve itself in about 2 weeks.

Blow-out fracture. A blowout fracture results from direct blunt trauma to the eyeball, causing an increase in intraocular pressure that fractures the orbit floor. It is diagnosed by obtaining a history of the incident and by observation of periorbital hematoma, subconjunctival hemorrhage, periorbital edema, enophthalmos, an upward gaze, and a complaint of diplopia, caused by trapping of the inferior rectus muscle and the inferior oblique muscle in the fracture. Radiological diagnosis can be made on standard facial films.

When this fracture is present, apply a cold pack. If there is bony displacement, reduce the fracture and pack the maxillary sinus. Surgery may be required to free the trapped orbital muscle. Be sure to check for associated intraocular injuries, perform a visual acuity examination, and obtain an ophthalmology consultation.

Foreign bodies. The most common foreign body in the eye is usually something small, causing the patient to complain that "there is something in my eye." Foreign bodies and corneal abrasions feel almost alike to the patient. It is important to locate the foreign body, if there is one. Often, local anesthesia will be required to adequately examine the eye. General anesthesia is usually required to adequately examine the eye of a child *and to remove a foreign body*. Always ensure that there is good lighting and a magnification source when removing a foreign body from the eye. Avoid using sharp needles and eyespuds.

FOREIGN BODIES TO THE CONJUNCTIVA. The most common foreign body is the eyelash, and it usually can be found under the upper eyelid in the tarsal conjunctiva. Therapeutic intervention includes everting the upper eyelid and irrigating with normal saline or gently removing the foreign body with a moist cotton swab or *very* carefully removing the foreign body with a 25-gauge needle at a tangential angle, and applying local antibiotics four times a day for 5 days.

An eye patch may be applied, depending on the nature of the foreign body as well as the amount of damage to the eyeball. It is also advisable to have the patient see an ophthalmologist in 1 day for a follow-up visit.

The main complication of a conjunctival foreign body is a scratched cornea. The cornea should be stained with fluorescein and, if a scratch is present, treat the injury as you would a corneal abrasion.

FOREIGN BODY TO THE CORNEA. Foreign body to the cornea is very painful to the patient. The patient will usually complain of "something under my eyelid," because the moving lid rubs up and down on the foreign body. Therapeutic intervention includes irrigation of the eye with normal saline and removal of the foreign body with a moistened cotton swab or 25-gauge needle (very carefully at a tangential angle to the eyeball). Always be sure to check for more than one foreign body. If the foreign body is metal, a rust ring will form in 12 hours. This rust ring must be removed by an ophthalmologist.

EVERTING THE EYELID (Fig. 15-5)

Have the patient look down.

Grab the lashes of the upper eyelid and gently pull down.

Apply gentle pressure on the upper lid with a cotton-tipped swab or other smooth instrument.

Evert the eyelid over the swab or instrument.

INTRAOCULAR FOREIGN BODY. Intraocular foreign bodies are easy to overlook, as they are usually caused by a high-speed, small, foreign body that penetrates the eyeball and comes to rest somewhere within the posterior chamber. Pain may be minimal. The actual opening to the posterior chamber may be small and difficult to find. One must suspect it to be able to find it.

An intraocular foreign body is *an extreme emergency*, and therapeutic intervention must occur in the very early moments of the injury. If an external eye injury is present, one must obtain a thorough history from the patient in order to suspect an intraocular foreign body.

The amount of damage to the eyeball will depend upon the size, shape, and composition of the foreign body. If surgery is required,

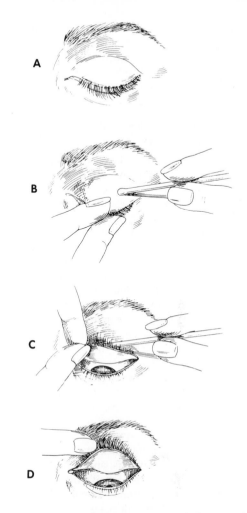

Fig. 15-5. Steps in everting the eyelid. **A,** Patient looks downward. **B,** Examiner pulls lid down with fingers. **C,** Eyelid is pulled over rod by examiner. **D,** Lid is everted. (From Barber, J., Stokes, L., and Billings, D.: Adult and child care, ed. 2, St. Louis, 1977, The C. V. Mosby Co.)

fragments that are magnetic will be easier to remove. Surgical removal prevents further damage to the eyeball, such as hemorrhage, infection, detached retina, or loss of vision.

All foreign bodies should be considered contaminated, and patients should be treated with antibiotics and checked for current tetanus prophylaxis. Many intraocular foreign bodies may be seen only on x-ray film. It is, therefore, mandatory that all suspected foreign bodies in the intraocular area be x-rayed.

Complications of intraocular foreign bodies may include infection, intraocular hemorrhage, detached retina, loss of vision, traumatic cataract, and loss of the eye.

Perforating and penetrating injuries to the eyeball

Penetrating injuries to the eyeball are usually a result of perforation by a sharp object such as a knife or a dart. In this type of injury, it is important to apply therapeutic intervention in the early stages of the injury to decrease the likelihood of further complications.

Emergency therapeutic intervention is to secure the impaled object if it is still penetrating the eyeball, and cover both eyes to decrease eye movement and reduce the possibility of further damage. Do not do a detailed examination at this time, as this should be reserved for an ophthalmologist. General anesthesia may be required in order to perform an adequate examination.

If eye tissue has not eviscerated, an ophthalmologist will most likely remove the object in surgery and suture the eye. If there is loss of vitreous humor and damage to the lens and ciliary body, enucleation may be required.

Other therapeutic intervention includes antibiotics, tetanus prophylaxis, and steroids.

Corneal lacerations. Small corneal lacerations are usually not sutured but rather left alone under a light pressure dressing. If the laceration is large, an ophthalmologist should be consulted. The ophthalmologist will most likely place sutures of either 8-0 silk or 7-0 chromic with a very fine needle.

Corneal abrasions. Corneal abrasions are common injuries. They occur when a foreign body (such as a contact lens) denudes the epithelium. It is important to obtain a history as to what caused the abrasion.

These patients will have a tearing eye, eyelid spasm, and be complaining of pain on the surface of the eye. It is diagnosed by staining the surface of the eye with fluorescein stain and observing the eyeball with a cobalt light and magnification. Use sterile, individually packaged fluorescein strips, because fluorescein solution is easily contaminated by *Pseudomonas*.

Therapeutic intervention includes local anesthesia while a visual acuity examination is being performed, local antibiotics, and patching of the injured eye for about 24 hours to prevent eyelid movement and decrease the amount of light that enters the eye. These patients should be followed up by an ophthalmologist in 1 day. The patient should be instructed *not* to use local anesthetic agents at home.

USING FLUORESCEIN STRIPS TO STAIN THE CORNEA (Fig. 15-6)

- Explain the procedure to the patient.
- Moisten the end of a sterile fluorescein strip with normal saline.
- Pull down on the lower eyelid.
- Touch the strip to the inner lower eyelid.
- Ask the patient to blink to distribute the staining solution (tears will spread it over the cornea).
- Examine the cornea using a cobalt lamp.

Conjunctival lacerations. The most common cause of a conjunctival laceration is a fingernail. Signs and symptoms include swelling and bleeding from the conjunctiva. If the laceration is small (less than 5 cm), therapeutic intervention includes local antibiotics, patching, and observation of the eye. If the laceration is large (greater than 5 cm), an ophthalmologist should be called to suture the conjunctiva.

Corneal ulcers. Corneal ulcers are common in the unconscious patient or in patients who have left their contact lenses in for an inordinate period of time. The ulcer will appear as a whitish spot on the cornea. It is painful, and the

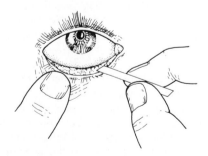

Fig. 15-6. Fluorescein staining. Touch moistened fluorescein strip to the inner canthus of the lower lid.

patient will have photophobia, profuse tearing, and vascular congestion. It will appear as a blue green cast with fluorescein staining. If *Pseudomonas aeruginosa* invades, the patient may lose his eye in a period of 48 hours. Therapeutic intervention includes antibiotics, warm compresses, and an eye patch.

Optic nerve avulsion. This type of injury does not occur very frequently. It usually results from severe trauma where the optic nerve enters the eyeball. A partial tear will result in partial blindness, whereas a total tear will result in total (permanent) blindness.

Iris injury. Traumatic iridocyclitis is an inflammation of the iris and ciliary body following contusion to the eye. It is evidenced by the presence of uveal pigment and lens tissue in the anterior chamber. Therapeutic intervention includes topical cycloplegics and topical and systemic steroids. Complications include enophthalmitis and loss of the eye.

Another type of iris injury is iris sphincter rupture. It is usually caused by trauma to the eyeball, causing the pupil to dilate and the iris to notch at the edges.

Lens injury. Lens injuries can include partial dislocations (subluxations), total dislocations (luxations) and opacifications (cataracts).

Retina and choroid injury. Trauma to the retina and choroid may produce a white elipse where the sclera is visible through the rupture. If the macula is injured, there will be a resultant decrease in visual acuity.

Problems with contact lenses

The most common problem experienced by the contact lens wearer is either chemicals or dirt particles under the lens, causing irritation of the cornea. The second most common problem is wearing the lenses too long, causing swollen, painful eyes. This usually occurs 6 to 8 hours after lens removal.

Therapeutic intervention for foreign bodies under the lens is lens removal and cleansing of the lens *and* eye before returning the lens to the eye.

If contact lenses are worn too long, a patient should refrain from wearing them for 24 to 48 hours.

Sometimes a contact lens is lost in the cul de sac, most commonly the upper one. Therapeutic intervention is to evert the eyelid and remove the lens.

There are two types of contact lenses: corneal lenses, the most common, and scleral lenses, which fit over the entire cornea and part of the scleral conjunctiva. All contact lenses float on tears and adhere to the eyeball by means of capillary attraction. Lenses come in two forms: hard or soft (also known as hydrophylic lenses).

To determine if the patient is wearing contact lenses, first ask the patient. If the patient cannot respond to your questions, check for a contact lens identification card, check for a contact lens Medic Alert bracelet, or look at the eye tangentially with a flashlight.

Removing a contact lens

Corneal

Use a suction tip designed especially for removing contact lenses; or

Use the two-hand method described in Fig. 15-7.

Soft lenses

Locate the lens and grasp it between the thumb and index finger and lift it off the cornea (Fig. 15-8).

Scleral

Retract the lower lid down and back until you can visualize the edge of the lens.

Pull the lower lid toward the ear; the lens should then slip over the eyelid.

Grasp the lens with the thumb and forefinger, and remove it (Fig. 15-9).

Burns of the eye

Chemical burns. Chemical burns are a common type of eye injury that occurs in the home and in the industrial setting. Chemical burns of the eye are (1) nonprogressive, superficial burns, usually caused by acids; (2) progressive burns caused by alkaline substances, and (3) irritants, caused by gases, such as tear gas and mace.

In any type of chemical burn, the immediate therapeutic intervention is copious irrigation with normal saline or tap water. Before examination of the eye, local anesthesia may be required.

Acid burns are usually self-limiting, because

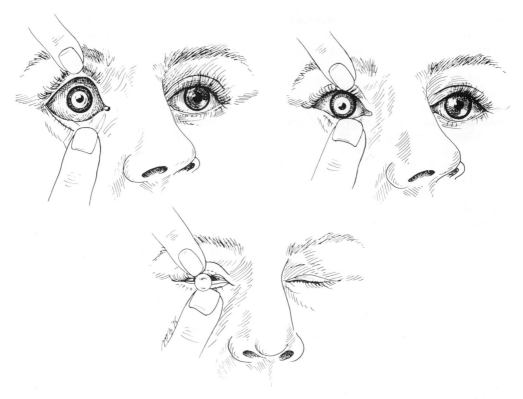

Fig. 15-7. Techniques for removing hard corneal contact lenses from an individual's eye. (From Barber, J., Stokes, L., and Billings, D.: Adult and child care, ed. 2, St. Louis, 1977, The C. V. Mosby Co.)

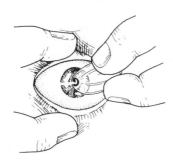

Fig. 15-8. Soft lens removal. Lift soft lens off the cornea.

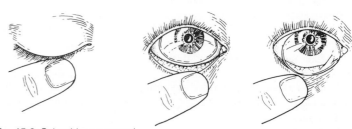

Fig. 15-9. Scleral lens removal.

as tissue denatures from the acid, the denatured tissue neutralizes the acid. Therapeutic intervention includes copious irrigation with normal saline, topical antibiotics, and cycloplegics.

Alkali burns, such as those caused by lime or ammonia, present a *very emergent* situation, because alkali causes much tissue destruction. Initially the burn may appear as white spots, and severe damage will not be evident until 3 to 4 days following the incident. Therapeutic intervention includes copious irrigation with normal saline, antibiotics, cycloplegics, and steroids.

When irrigating an eye, irrigate for 30 minutes and then check the pH of the conjunctiva, which normally is 7.0. If the pH is not normal after 30 minutes of irrigation, continue to irrigate the eye, and periodically check the pH until it returns to normal.

Specific antidotes for chemical burns

Acid burns	Sodium bicarbonate 2%
Alkali burns	Citric or boric acid
Lime burns	Ammonium tartrate 5%

Complications of acid or alkali burns of the eye include adhesions of the globe to the eyelid, corneal ulcerations, entropion (eyelashes that turn in toward the eyeball), iridocyclitis, and glaucoma.

Thermal burns. When facial burns are present, it is quite common to find associated eyelid burns. It is not common, however, to see eyeball burns, unless the burn was produced by hot metal, steam, or gasoline. Burns to the eyelids may cause lid contractures. Therapeutic intervention should include analgesia, sedation, eye irrigation, antibiotics, cycloplegics, and bilateral eye patches.

Delayed or latent action injury from direct contact with liquids and solids.* The following is a list of substances that bind chemically with tissue and have delayed onsets of toxic action.

Cardiac glycosides
Colchicine
Digitalis glycosides

Dimethyl sulfate
Dyes (cationic)
Emetine
Erythrophleine
Euphorbias
Formaldehyde
Ipecac
Manchineel
Methyl bromide
Methyl chloracrylate
Methyl dichlorpropionate
Mustard gas
Osmic acid
Podophyllium
Poison ivy
Rare earth salts
Squill
Sulfar dioxide
Surfactants
Triacetoxyanthracene

Radiation burns. There are two types of radiation burns—ultraviolet and infrared. The severity of the burn depends on the wave length and the degree of exposure.

Ultraviolet radiation burns may be seen in welders (welder's arc flash), snow skiers, and ice climbers, people who read on the beach, and people who use a sunlamp. The burn is caused when ultraviolet radiation is absorbed by the cornea, producing keratitis or conjunctivitis, or both. It is usually 3 to 6 hours after the exposure before the patient demonstrates signs and symptoms of the burn, which include feeling as though there is a foreign body in the eye, tearing, and excessive blinking. This patient may also have associated facial and eyelid burns.

Therapeutic intervention includes topical antibiotics, analgesics (systemic), cycloplegics, and bilateral eye patches. All signs and symptoms of the injury should disappear, and the condition should improve within 24 hours.

Infrared radiation burn is a much more severe type of burn than ultraviolet radiation burn. Infrared radiation burns may cause permanent loss of vision, because the infrared rays are absorbed by the iris, which results in an increase of the temperature of the lens, causing cataracts.

---

*From Grant, W. M.: Toxicology of the eye, ed. 2, 1974, p. 9. (Courtesy Charles C Thomas, Publisher, Springfield, illinois.)

COMMON TYPES OF INFRARED BURNS

- "Glass-blower's cataracts," resulting from prolonged exposure to intense heat
- Focal retinitis, caused by "elipse blindness" or exposure to an atomic bomb, where the lens condenses heat, causing a retinal scar and blindness
- X-ray burns, which are proportional to the penetration of the rays: grenz rays are soft rays that produce superficial keratoconjunctivitis and dermatitis; gamma rays are hard rays, and overexposure produces retinal damage and cataracts

When the lens is damaged, the repair process is very slow. It is, therefore, important to note that the lens remains much more vulnerable to repeated injury during the healing process.

Irrigating the eye (Fig. 15-10, *A*)

- Cleanse the external area around the eye and eyelid.
- Prepare irrigation basin or portable hairwashing tray, irrigation solution, and administration set.
- Have the patient lie down, or adjust the ENT chair to a reclining position.
- Have the patient turn his head toward the affected side.
- Pull down on the eyelid of the affected eye.
- Run irrigation fluid directly over the eyeball and lower lid cul-de-sac from the inner to the outer canthus.
- Have the patient blink occasionally to distribute the irrigation solution over the eyeball.
- Irrigate for a minimum of 30 minutes (more if indicated by the level of the pH).

CONTINUOUS EYE IRRIGATION USING THE MORGAN THERAPEUTIC LENS (Fig. 15-10, *B*). A Morgan Therapeutic Lens is a specially designed lens that is placed on the eye and used to provide continuous ocular lavage or continuous ocular medication. The lens, which is a scleral lens, is made of a hard (polymethylmethacrylate) plastic, and the tubing is made of a soft silicone plastic, with a female adapter at the distal end.

PROCEDURE (Fig. 15-10, *C*)

1. Explain the procedure to the patient.
2. Instill anesthetic ocular drops into the eye to be treated.

3. Ask the patient to "look down."
4. Retract the upper lid.
5. Grasping the lens by the tubing and the small finlike projections, slip the superior border of the lens up under the upper eyelid.
6. Then, have the patient "look up."
7. Retract the lower eyelid, and place the lower border of the lens.
8. Have the patient turn his head toward the affected side, and place a folded towel under his head to collect irrigation solution.
9. Attach the female adapter at the end of the lens tubing to
   a. a syringe filled with the solution of choice, and instill the solution at the desired rate, or
   b. intravenous tubing that is connected to solution of choice and instilled at a selected drip rate.
10. To remove the lens, follow steps 5 through 7 in reverse order.
11. Dry the patient's face and eye area with a dry towel.
12. Dispose of lens.
13. Follow any additional orders for medication instillation and eye dressing.

Medical problems involving the eye

Blepharitis. Blepharitis is an inflammation of the lid margin, usually caused by *Staphylococcus aureus*. Therapeutic intervention includes cool, moist compresses and antibiotic ophthalmic ointment.

Hordeolum. Hordeolum, or sty, is an infection of the upper or lower eyelid at the accessory gland caused by *Staphylococcus aureus*. It is evidenced by a small, external abcess, pain, redness, and swelling. Therapeutic intervention includes warm compresses four times a day until the abscess "points." Antibiotic ophthalmic ointment should also be employed. The patient should be instructed *not* to squeeze the abcess, but rather have it incised and drained by a physician when it comes to a point.

Chalazion. Chalazion is a sebaceous cyst that forms on the inside surface of the eyelid resulting from congestion of the meibomian

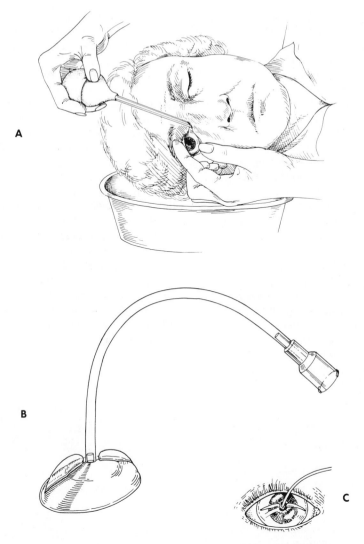

Fig. 15-10. A, Position for eye irrigation. **B,** Morgan therapeutic lens. **C,** Lens in place. (**A** from Barber, J., Stokes, L., and Billings, D.: Adult and child care, ed. 2, St. Louis, 1977, The C. V. Mosby Co.)

gland. It is evidenced by a small mass beneath the conjunctiva of the lid that is red, swollen, and quite painful. Therapeutic intervention includes antibiotic ophthalmic ointment and incision and drainage by a physician.

Keratitis. Keratitis is an inflammation of the cornea that is light-sensitive, red, and painful and causes profuse tearing. Therapeutic inter- vention includes a culture and sensitivity speci- men, warm compresses, antibiotic ophthalmic ointment, and topical steroids *(except not for Herpes type)*.

Keratoconjunctivitis. Keratoconjunctivitis is an inflammation of the outer coat of the eye. It can result from an allergic reaction, which presents with itching, redness, discharge, and tearing. Therapeutic intervention is usually the use of topical steroids. Another cause of keratoconjunctivitis may be herpes simplex, in which case *steroids should not be used!!* Herpes keratoconjunctivitis is generally treated with idoxuridine (Stoxil) or vidarabine (Vira A).

Uveitis. Uveitis is a uveal tract inflammation that usually includes the iris, ciliary body, and choroid. Signs and symptoms of this condition are unilateral and include photophobia, tearing, pain, and blurred vision. Therapeutic intervention includes warm compresses, analgesia (systemic), antibiotic ophthalmic ointment, steroids (topical), and mydriatics (to dilate the pupil and prevent adhesions of the iris and the lens).

Acute conjunctivitis. Acute conjunctivitis is a bacterial infection of the conjunctiva characterized by the eyelids ''sticking together'' when the patient wakes up in the mornings. It may be caused by staphylococcal, gonococcal, pneumococcal, *Hemophilus* or *Pseudomonas* organisms. Therapeutic intervention is antibiotic ophthalmic ointment. Before antibiotic therapy, obtain a specimen for culture and sensitivity.

Acute conjunctivitis is contagious. It is therefore essential that detailed after-care instructions be given to the patient on how to prevent disease spread.

One specific type of acute conjunctivitis is *Neisseria gonococcus,* in which there is a copious amount of purulent discharge and the conjunctiva is extremely red and swollen. Therapeutic intervention for this type of conjunctivitis is penicillin ophthalmic ointment.

Acute iritis. Acute iritis is an inflammatory condition of the iris characterized by photophobia and tenderness of the eyeball. It is *not* an infectious process. Therapeutic intervention includes cold compresses, steroids (topical), eye patch, and dark glasses.

Central retinal artery occlusion. Central retinal artery occlusion produces sudden blindness with a very poor prognosis. Therapeutic intervention includes amyl nitrate inhalation, sublingual nitroglycerine, and/or inhalation of alternating carbon dioxide and oxygen to attempt to dilate the artery and return blood supply to the retina.

Cavernous sinus thrombosis (orbital cellulitis). Cavernous sinus thrombosis is an infection (pneumococcal, staphylococcal, or streptococcal) that has spread from an infected sinus to the orbit area. Signs and symptoms of this condition include facial and eyeball edema, vascular congestion in eyelids, aching pain, pain in eyeball, conjunctival chemosis, fever, decreased visual acuity, decreased pupillary reflexes, papilledema, and paralysis of the extraocular muscles. Therapeutic intervention is antibiotic ophthalmic ointment, warm compresses, and bedrest.

Other medical problems. Some of the conditions previously discussed plus ptosis, eyelid edema, entropion, ectropion, dacryocystitis, exophthalmos, pterygium, and convergent and divergent strabismus are represented in Figs. 15-11 to 15-24.

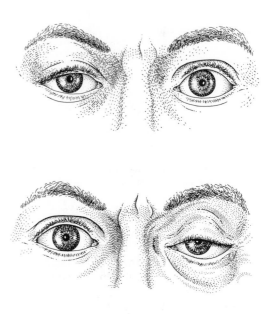

Fig. 15-11. Ptosis.

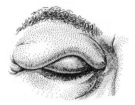

Fig. 15-12. Edema of eyelid.

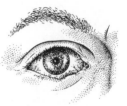

Fig. 15-13. Entropion.

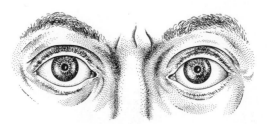

Fig. 15-14. Ectropion.

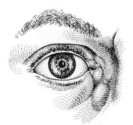

Fig. 15-15. Dacryocystitis.

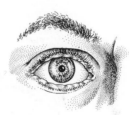

Fig. 15-16. Marginal blepharitis.

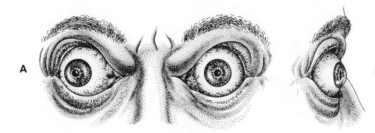

Fig. 15-17. Exophthalmos.

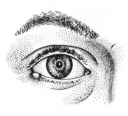

Fig. 15-18. Hordeolum.

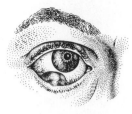

Fig. 15-19. Chalazion.

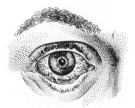

Fig. 15-20. Conjunctivitis.

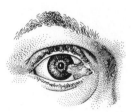

Fig. 15-21. Pterygium.

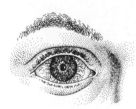

Fig. 15-22. Iritis.

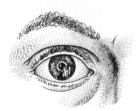

Fig. 15-23. Corneal abrasion.

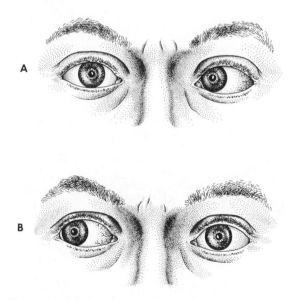

Fig. 15-24. A, Strabismus, convergent. **B,** Strabismus, divergent.

Retinal detachment

The normal function of the retina is to perceive light and send an impulse to the optic nerve. When the retina is torn, vitreous humor seeps between the retina and the choroid, resulting in the retina separating from the choroid, which decreases blood and oxygen supply to the retina. This loss of blood and oxygen supply renders the retina unable to perceive light.

Signs and symptoms of retinal detachment are flashes of light, a "veil" or "curtain" effect in the visual field, and a dark spot or particles in the vision. Therapeutic intervention is immediate strict bedrest, bilateral eye patches, tranquilizers, and possible surgery following ophthalmology consultation.

Glaucoma (Fig. 15-25)

It is estimated that approximately 1 million Americans have undiagnosed glaucoma. Glaucoma causes one out of every ten blindnesses in the United States. Acute glaucoma is a condition in which aqueous humor, secreted by the ciliary process epithelium in the posterior chamber of the eye and transported to the anterior chamber through the pupil, cannot escape from the anterior chamber, which causes a rise in the anterior chamber pressure.

Normally, aqueous humor leaves the anterior chamber and enters the vascular system via the canal of Schlemm at the junction of the iris and the cornea. This increase in anterior chamber pressure causes a decrease in circulation

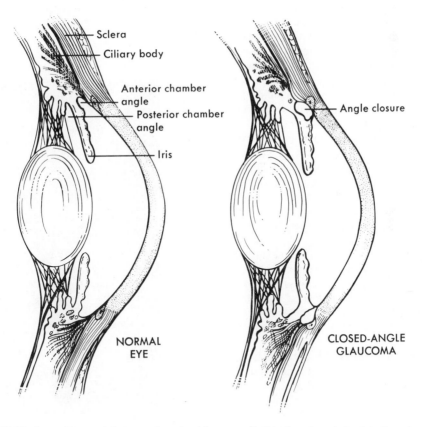

Fig. 15-25. Comparisons of the normal angle of the eye with the closed angle in closed-angle glaucoma. (From Barber, J., Stokes, L., and Billings, D.: Adult and child care, ed. 2, St. Louis, 1977, The C. V. Mosby Co.)

to the retina and an increased pressure on the optic nerve and may eventually cause blindness. *Acute glaucoma is an emergency situation,* because it may cause blindness in just a few hours.

Acute glaucoma. Acute (closed-angle) glaucoma results when there is a blockage in the anterior chamber angle near the root of the iris. Signs and symptoms of this condition include severe eye pain, a fixed and slightly dilated pupil, a hard eyeball, a foggy-appearing cornea, severe headache, halos around lights, decreased peripheral vision, and, occasionally, nausea and vomiting. Therapeutic intervention is aimed at decreasing the pupil size to allow for aqueous humor drainage. This is accomplished by frequently instilling (every 15 minutes) miotic eye drops—usually 1% or 4% pilocarpine. The strength of the solution is not so important as the frequency of instillation. Other therapeutic intervention includes sytemic analgesia (morphine sulfate is usually the drug of choice) and drugs such as acetazolamide (Diamox) to attempt to decrease intraocular pressure. Surgery may be indicated if the above therapeutic intervention is unsuccessful.

Open-angle glaucoma. Open-angle (chronic or wide-angle) glaucoma comes on gradually and is an obstruction of the canal of Schlemm. Because this condition is chronic and progresses very slowly, the patient may be unaware of its presence. Therapeutic intervention for this type of glaucoma includes instillation of miotic eye drops and surgery.

Congenital glaucoma. Congenital (infantile or juvenile) glaucoma is a failure of the anterior chamber angle to develop normally. Early signs and symptoms are copious tearing and photophobia—a baby will have the tendency to keep his eyelids shut more than usual. Therapeutic intervention is surgery.

Secondary glaucoma. Secondary glaucoma is an increase in intraocular pressure resulting from surgery, trauma, hemorrhage, inflammation, tumors, and various other conditions that may interfere with aqueous humor drainage. Therapeutic intervention varies, depending on the cause of the glaucoma.

Measuring ocular pressure with a tonometer. Tonometric examination is used to measure intraocular pressure. The Schiøtz tonometer, the most commonly used type of tonometer, has a plunger that measures the amount of indentation pressure of the cornea when the tonometer is placed on it (Fig. 15-26).

In order to properly use the tonometer, the eyeballs should be anesthetized with one to two drops of anesthetic ophthalmic drops, the patient should have the procedure thoroughly explained to him, and he should be placed in a lying position. A sterile tonometer, previously calibrated, is placed directly on the eyeball, and intraocular pressure is measured. With a Schiøtz indentation tonometer, if intraocular pressure is high, the tonometer scale will read low, because the plunger cannot indent the eyeball very much. If intraocular pressure is low, the tonometer scale will read high, because the plunger will indent the eyeball more than normal.

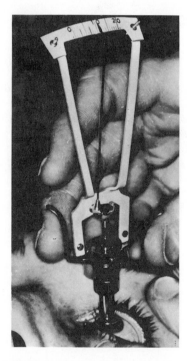

Fig. 15-26. Measurement of intracular pressure with Schiøtz tonometer. (From Stein, H. A., and Slatt, B. J.: The ophthalmic assistant, ed. 3, St. Louis, 1976, The C. V. Mosby Co.)

Table 15-1. Ophthalmological medications

Generic name	Brand name	Action
Miotics: constrict pupils; primary use to treat glaucoma		
Pilocarpine	Pilocar	Acts on myoneural junction
	Isopto Carpine	
	P.V. Carpine Liquifilm	
Carbachol	Carcholin	Acts on myoneural junction
	Carbamycholine	
	Isopto Carbachol	
	Doryl	
	P.V. Carbachol	
Echothiophate iodide	Phospholine	Cholinesterase inhibitor
	Iodide	
Isoflurophate	DFP	Cholinesterase inhibitor
	Floropryl	
Acetazolamide	Diamox	Carbonic anhydrase inhibitor; decreases aqueous humor production
Mydriatics: dilate pupils		
Sympathomimetics		
Epinephrine	Adrenalin	Mydriasis and vasoconstriction
	Epitrate	
Phenylephrine	Neo-Synephrine Hydrochloride	Mydriasis and vasoconstriction
Ephedrine	Ephedrine	Adrenergic vasoconstrictor and antiallergic
Hydroxyamphetamine	Paredrine Hydrobromide	Mydriasis
Parasympathomimetics: paralyze ciliary muscles and accommodation as well as dilate pupils		
Atropine sulfate	Isopto Atropine	Mydriasis and cycloplegia
Cyclopentolate	Cyclogyl	Mydriasis and cycloplegia
Homatropine hydrobro-	Homatrocel	Mydriasis and cycloplegia
mide	Isopto Homatropine	Anticholinergic and sedative
Scopolamine	Hyoscine	Mydriasis and cycloplegia
Tropicamide	Mydriacyl	
	Mydriaticum	
Physostigmine salicylate	Eserine	Mydriasis and cycloplegia
	Neostigmine	
	Physostol	
Cycloplegics: paralyze ciliary muscles and accommodation		
Cyclopentalate hydro-	Cyclogyl	Mydriasis and cycloplegia
chloride		
Anesthetics: for surface anesthesia		
Procaracaine hydrochlo-	Ophthaine	Local anesthesia
ride		
Tetracaine	Pontocaine	Local anesthesia
Antibiotics		
Tetracycline hydrochlo-	Achromycin	Antimicrobial
ride		
Chloramphenicol	Chloromycetin	Broad-spectrum antibiotic
Polymyxin B with neomy-	Cortisporin	For nonpurulent, bacterial infections
cin	Neo-Polycin	
Gentamicin sulfate	Garamycin	For gram-positive bacteria
Erythromycin	Ilotycin	For superficial topical infections
	Dista	
Sulfisoxazole	Gantrisin	Bacteriostatic
Sulfacetamide sodium	Sulamyd	Gram-negative and gram-positive bacterio-static

Continued.

Table 15-1. Ophthalmological medications—cont'd

Generic name	Brand name	Action
Steroids: decrease inflammatory response		
Dexamethasone	Decadron	Decreases inflammatory response
Combination steroid-antibiotics		
Prednisolone acetate	Metimyd	Antiinflammatory/antibacterial
Prednisolone sodium phosphate with sodium sulfacetomide	Optimyd	Antiinflammatory/antibacterial
Neomycin sulfate and hydrocortisone acetate	Neo-Cortef	Antiinflammatory/antibacterial
Terramycin/oxytetracycline/hydrocortisone acetate	Terra-Cortril Cortril	Antiinflammatory/antibacterial
Neomycin sulfate with methylprednisolone	Neo-Delta-Cortef Neo-Medrol	Antiinflammatory/antibacterial
Herpes simplex inhibitors		
Idoxuridine	Stoxil	Inhibits herpes simplex virus
Vidarabine	Vira-A	Inhibits herpes simplex virus when nonresponsive to Stoxil or if there is an allergic reaction to Stoxil
Combination eye drops		
Various combinations of phenylephrine hydrochloride, methyl cellulose, boric acid, sodium borate, sodium chloride, ethylene diamine tetraacetate, and benzalkonium chloride	Ocusol Murine Visine Prefrin	To "soothe tired eyes" and decrease redness

A normal indentation tonometer reading is 11 to 22 mm Hg. A lower reading indicates increased intraocular pressure and a higher reading indicates decreased intraocular pressure.

Eye drops and ophthalmic ointments

Eyedrops are instilled into the eye to decrease pain, administer antibiotic therapy, increase the size of the pupil, decrease the size of the pupil, decrease allergic reactions of the eye, or cleanse the eye.

Procedure for instilling eye drops
- Explain the procedure to the patient.
- Pull the lower eyelid downward.

- Instill one to two drops of the intended solution into the cul-de-sac (the center of the inner lower lid).
- Have the patient blink to distribute the solution.
- Instruct the patient *not* to squeeze his eyelids tightly shut, because this will cause the medication to leak out.

Procedure for instilling ophthalmic ointment
- Explain the procedure to the patient.
- Pull the lower eyelid downward.
- Have the patient look up.
- Apply ointment in a thin line into the inner

aspect of the lower lid from the inner to the outer canthus.

- Have the patient blink to distribute the ointment.
- Instruct the patient *not* to squeeze his eyelids tightly shut, as this will expel the ointment.

NOSE AND THROAT EMERGENCIES
Foreign bodies of the throat

If a patient comes to the emergency department complaining of a foreign body in the throat, the history should not be ignored. Despite the spontaneous passage of some foreign bodies, one must assume presence of the foreign body until proven otherwise.

Common foreign bodies include coins, peanuts, straight and safety pins in children; large boluses of meat and fish bones in adults. Foreign bodies may be multiple.

Signs and symptoms of foreign bodies in the throat include:

Pain
Drooling
Sight of foreign body
Dysphasia
Stridor
Hematemesis
Hemoptysis
Cyanosis (which calls for immediate resuscitative efforts)

The physical examination should include complete head and neck examination, including indirect laryngoscopy. X-ray examinations, including "end inspiratory" and "end expiratory" chest films in anteroposterior and lateral projections, may be diagnostic.

Frequent sites of foreign body lodging area:

Base of tongue
Tonsilar fossae
Pyriform sinuses (of hypopharynx)
Cricopharyngeus muscle
Aortic indentation of esophagus
Left mainstem bronchus

The use of emetic agents is condemned; so is the practice of ingesting a large piece of bread or even using a piece of cotton soaked in a radiopaque medium as a marker to detect blockage by a foreign body of the esophagus. This practice is considered inadvisable because it merely may add a second and obscuring foreign body to further compound the problem.

Removal should be performed by a trained specialist, preferably in an operating room, where adequate and varied instrumentation is available.

Foreign bodies of the nose and ear canals

Foreign bodies in the nose and ear canals are frequent in children and patients with emotional problems. Foreign bodies in any of these passages will eventually cause bleeding and foul discharge. Adequate examination requires the following.

Proper lighting
Suction
Topical anesthesia
Specific instrumentation

If the patient is not cooperative, then examination and removal should be performed under general anesthesia.

Caustic ingestion

Household cleaning products (lye, ammonia, sulphuric acid, and liquid drain cleaners) are the most frequently ingested caustic agents. On examination, there may be signs of injury to the upper ear and food passages, including erythema, ulceration, and denuded areas. However, the presence or absence of such within the visible areas of oral cavity, pharynx, and larynx does not preclude or necessarily indicate similar injury to distal areas. Therefore, endoscopic examination (usually under general anesthesia) may be required.

Specific antidotes may be given if the patient is seen within 30 minutes of ingestion. Emesis should be avoided; so should the passage of a Levin tube or other indwelling tubes. The patients are generally admitted to the hospital for observation and treatment.

Epistaxis

Nosebleeds are the most common ENT problem seen in the emergency department. The most common site is from the anterior septal mucosa, Kiesselbach's or Little's area. In older patients, more bleeding sites are found in the posterior nose or along the roof of the nose.

The first priority is to determine the source of the bleeding. Because most patients are anxious and frightened by the bleeding, they should be sedated before the examination. Intravenous morphine is excellent for its analgesic and sedative qualities. The following equipment should be available for proper intranasal examination.

Electric headlight

Suction apparatus with Frazier metal suction tips, sizes 9 through 12

Waterproof aprons for patients and examiners

A large basin for expectoration

Topical nasal decongestant/anesthetic, such as 5% cocaine, 0.5% phenylephrine or 1% tetracaine

Large cotton pledgets

Tongue blades

Electrocautery equipment, suction apparatus, or silver nitrate or chromic acid sticks

Nasal balloon or nasostat

After the patient has been reassured and sedated, the nasal cavities are suctioned of blood clots, and decongestant anesthetic solution is sprayed into the nose. Alternatively, long (3-inch) cotton pledgets are saturated with the solution and placed deeply into the nasal fossa. The patient then pinches both nostrils for 5 or 10 minutes while awaiting vasoconstriction and anesthesia. The nose is then resuctioned after the pledgets of cotton are removed. The nose is reexamined. If the mucosal shrinkage is not adequate and topical anesthesia is not satisfactory, the process of spraying and/or packing is repeated and another waiting period endured. Thereafter, the bleeding source should be identifiable as a fresh trickle of blood from this specific site. If the source is the anterior septum, the area is cauterized by method of the operator's choice. If the bleeding is posterior or from the vault of the nose and nonaccessible to "spot" cautery, then an inflatable nasal balloon, nasostat, or posterior pack is inserted that will exert pressure within the entire nasal chamber; these patients must be admitted to the hospital (Fig. 15-27).

The assurance of control of the nosebleed is made by observing no fresh blood from the nostrils or into the oropharynx from the nasopharynx.

Patients in whom spot cautery has been successful are advised to refrain from exertional activities for 1 week and given a prescription for a mild sedative and a nasal decongestant spray to be used for approximately 1 week.

Airway obstruction

Patients with acute airway obstruction are among the most critical seen in the emergency department. Causes may range from foreign body enlargement to acute epiglottitis to facial or laryngeal fracture.

Complete resuscitative equipment must be immediately brought to the bedside.

Laryngoscope

Suction apparatus

Variety of endotracheal tubes

Topical anesthetics

Equipment for "stab tracheostomy" or cricothyrotomy

Formal tracheostomy is not recommended as an emergency department procedure.

The most critical decision made in the emergency department is whether to immediately reestablish the airway in a patient with airway obstruction, presuming that the site of obstruction has been determined. This decision is based upon a clinical evaluation of the patient's condition. Young children, because of their inherently small airways, and older patients, because of their weaker constitutions, are the groups in whom time delay can be catastrophic.

In *most* clinical conditions of upper airway obstruction seen in the emergency department, suctioning of the pharynx, repositioning, or endotracheal intubation will obviate the need for tracheostomy. It is recommended that the intubator be skillful and experienced, lest precious time be lost by a series of inexpert attempts at intubation. An anesthetist, anesthesiologist, or otolaryngologist should be summoned to give whatever aid may be necessary.

Neck trauma

Auto accidents and assaults generate most neck injuries in the emergency department.

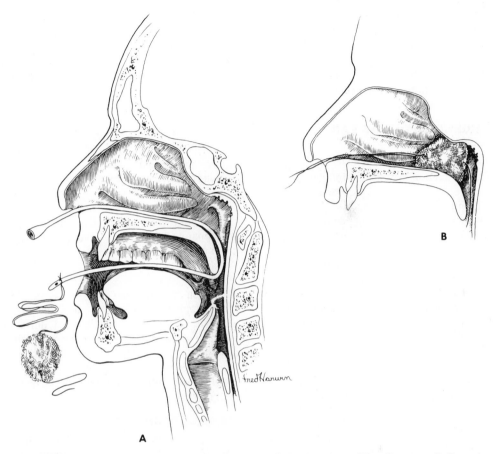

Fig. 15-27. A, Steps used in passing a postnasal pack. **B,** Pack in place. (From Deweese, D. D., and Saunders, W. H.: Textbook of otolaryngology, ed. 4, St. Louis, 1973, The C. V. Mosby Co.)

Neck trauma's most serious sequelae are cervical spine fracture and laryngeal injury. The former is suspected by cervical muscle tenderness and spasm with or without neurological deficit. Cross-table, lateral cervical spine x-ray films can be obtained in the emergency department without moving the patient, thus reducing the risk of further injury.

Penetrating neck wounds (stab or gunshot wounds) are generally not lethal. The most critical of these injuries are the vascular wounds, since they may carry a mortality as high as 40%. When such serious injuries occur, they are recognized by:

Persistent bleeding from the wound

Expanding hematoma of the neck

Airway compression

Absence of extremity pulses

Bruits

Central nervous system defects

The signs and symptoms of a severe laryngeal injury include:

Hoarseness

Dysphonia

Aphonia

Stridor

Hemoptysis

Neck tenderness

Crepitus

Flattening of the laryngeal prominence

Indirect or direct laryngoscopy may reveal the following vocal cord abnormalities.

Lacerations

Hematoma

Edema

Vocal cord immobility

In such circumstances, the examiner may consider intubation or stab tracheostomy if the airway is threatened.

EMERGENCIES OF THE EAR
Otitis externa

Otitis externa (swimmer's ear) is a bacterial or fungal infection that has the following symptoms.

Ear pain

Narrowing of the canal by edema

Tenderness of the cartilaginous ear canal

Drainage

Hearing loss due to accumulation of debris in the ear canal

It is differentiated from acute otitis media by the tenderness of the outer ear and canal, which is absent in a middle ear infection. Otitis externa occurs most often during outdoor swimming seasons.

The treatment consists of suctioning debris from the ear canal and placing a wick of cotton saturated with a topical ear drop preparation, with or without a steroid ingredient. The wick is left in place from 48 to 72 hours while the otological topical solution is instilled on the indwelling wick three to four times a day. After the wick is removed, the drops are continued for a total treatment of 10 days. Narcotic analgesics are necessary to relieve pain for the first 24 to 48 hours.

Acute otitis media

Generally preceded by an upper respiratory tract infection, this middle ear inflammation is heralded by

Hearing loss

Otalgia

"Fullness" in the affected ear

Examination findings may include:

Redness of the tympanic membrane

Either withdrawal or bulging of the tympanic membrane

White or yellow discoloration

Blebs on the eardrum surface (bullous myringitis)

In the event of imminent perforation or bullae on the eardrum that are producing severe pain, an otolaryngologist should be summoned to perform a myringotomy. Otherwise the patients are treated with analgesics or antibiotics and decongestants.

Vertigo

Most, but not all, causes of vertigo are otological. Common causes of vertigo in emergency room patients include:

Head trauma with concussion

Temporal bone fracture

Acute labyrinthitis

The following additional symptoms may accompany the vertigo, making the patient quite miserable.

Tinnitus

Hearing loss

Nausea and vomiting

Spontaneous nystagmus, accentuated with head movement, can be detected during the physical examination. When the syndrome is disabling, hospitalization may be required; otherwise otolaryngological consultation is sought, and outpatient treatment is begun in the emergency room.

MAXILLOFACIAL TRAUMA

When a person comes to the prehospital care arena or the emergency department with maxillofacial trauma, it is often easy to overlook the fact that there may be other, more serious, life-threatening problems occurring. Most injuries to the face either bleed profusely externally or produce a large amount of swelling and ecchymosis because of the vascularity in the facial area.

One of the most serious life-threatening problems is an obstructed airway, either by the tongue, blood or other debris. Always assure, first, that the airway is clear and patent, that breathing is present (or being done artificially), and that there is an acceptable circulatory situation. In the initial ABC assessment of the facial trauma victim, one should also include assessment of the cervical spine. All facial trauma victims should be considered to have head and neck trauma until proved otherwise.

Initial therapeutic intervention includes

A Airway: If the patient is unable to maintain an open airway, employ the jaw thrust maneuver (avoid the head tilt maneuver whenever possible) in conjunction with the oropharyngeal airway or nasopharyngeal airway, or employ nasotracheal intubation or the esophageal obturator airway (see Chapter 8).

B Breathing: Assess ventilatory status. Administer supplemental oxygen by nasal cannula or face mask.

C Circulation: Assure that adequate perfusion is occurring.

C Cervical spine: Protect the cervical spine by first avoiding hyperextension of the neck. Observe the neck for any obvious injury (bleeding, bruising, or swelling) or fractures. Whenever possible, use a cervical collar and immobilize the neck. If in the emergency department, obtain a cross-table lateral cervical spine x-ray film, if indicated.

Control bleeding using the direct pressure technique. If there is a suspected skull or facial fracture, apply pressure at the wound edges.

Because facial trauma should be considered to be head and cervical spine trauma as well, a baseline neurological evaluation should include level of consciousness, neurological signs, visual signs, an ear examination (to check for hematotympanum) and a check for Battle's sign.

Before soft tissue repair, the eyes should be examined. Check for ocular damage, check visual acuity (see pp. 319-320), check for loss of vision and diplopia, and do a funduscopic examination to check specifically for hyphema and detached retina.

Next, check the facial nerve, parotid gland, and Stensen's duct (which drains the parotid gland). If any of these are severed, primary repair is essential. If unfamiliar with this type of repair, one may choose to consult an otolaryngologist or a plastic surgeon.

One should check for patency of the four cranial nerves the run through the face: the third (oculomotor), fourth (trochlear), fifth (trigeminal), and seventh (facial).

To check for damage to the facial nerve, four of the five branches should be tested. The temporal branch may be tested by having the patient raise his eyebrows and wrinkle his forehead. The zygomatic branch is tested by having the patient manipulate the orbicularis oris muscle and squeeze his eyes tightly shut. To test the buccal branch, have the patient elevate his upper lip and wrinkle his nose. And, to test the marginal mandibular branch, observe the patient for a depression and loosening of the lower lip. Table 15-2 shows how to assess the other three cranial nerves that ennervate the face.

If saliva is leaking out of the parotid gland, it is essential to do an early primary repair by inserting a catheter into the proximal end of the gland and suturing the gland over the catheter. Once the repair is completed, the catheter should be left in place for 10 days.

On initial assessment, also check for symmetry of the infraorbital rim, the zygomatic arch, the anterior wall of the antrum, the an-

Table 15-2. Cranial nerves involved in facial trauma*

Nerve	Name	Activity	Elicits	Test by
Third	Oculomotor	Motor	Eyeball movement; supplies 5 of 7 ocular muscles	Pupil response; ocular movement to four quadrants
Fourth	Trochlear	Motor	Eyeball movement (superior oblique)	Same as above
Fifth	Trigeminal	Motor and sensory	Facial sensation; jaw movement	Assessing pain, touch, hot and cold sensations, bite, opening mouth against resistance

*From Barber, J. M., and Budassi, S. A.: Mosby's manual of emergency care, St. Louis, 1979, The C. V. Mosby Co.

gles of the jaw, and the lower borders of the mandible. Look for malocclusion of the teeth, point tenderness, and cerebrospinal fluid leak from the ears and nose.

Facial injuries may be skeletal, soft tissue, or both. Simple soft tissue injuries may be managed in the emergency department, but the following circumstances suggest that the repair be performed by a facial specialist, ideally in the operating room.

Wounds requiring multiple layer closure
Wound requiring extensive debridement
Wound requiring repair of fascia, nerve, or muscle

Bony injuries require the following additional information before definitive diagnosis.

Historical review, including past history of facial bone fracture
Loss of consciousness
Sensory deficit
Loss of smell
Loss of taste
Hearing deficit
Inability to speak
Disequilibrium

Motor deficit such as muscle weakness due to motor nerve injury must be determined in all facial injuries.

Facial lacerations

Immediate repair of facial lacerations is important in order to allow for good scar formation and to reduce the incidence of infection. Facial lacerations should be sutured within the first 8 hours of the accident. A laceration that is 8 to 24 hours old may be sutured, but systemic antibiotics should also be initiated. A facial laceration that is more than 24 hours old must be soaked with a saline preparation; then the wound should be cleansed, debrided, and then sutured. The patient should be placed on systemic antibiotics. Once the wound is cleansed, irrigated debrided, and sutured, a topical antibiotic ointment is usually a sufficient dressing.

Facial lacerations should be sutured without tension.

In order to properly cleanse a wound, the wound should be injected wtih local anesthesia (usually 1% lidocaine with epinephrine). Epinephrine causes vasoconstriction, decreases bleeding, and increases the absorption time of lidocaine. When using lidocaine with epinephrine, bleeding will decrease in 7 minutes, and anesthesia will effectively begin to work in another 7 minutes. Without epinephrine, it may take as long as 20 minutes to receive an anesthesia effect.

If the wound is small, it may be sutured under local anesthesia. If the wound is large, one may elect to do a nerve block.

Some areas of the face require special consideration. For example, edema progresses rapidly in the eyelids; therefore, they should be sutured as soon as possible following the injury. When lips are sutured, it is important to assure that the vermillion border is intact. Eyebrows should be approximated when suturing and should never be shaved, because they may not grow back. When a laceration of the cheek occurs, be sure to check for an intact parotid gland and Stensen's duct. Lacerations of the tongue may sometimes be left without suturing. When suturing the tongue of a small child, sedate the child at least ½ hour before the procedure. If a laceration is a through-and-through laceration of the cheek, usually the mucosal layer is left open to drain.

Any patient with a soft tissue injury or an open fracture should have current tetanus prophylaxis.

When the patient is discharged from the emergency department, he should be instructed to keep the wound clean and dry, cleanse around the wound area with hydrogen peroxide solution three times a day, and apply a topical antibiotic ointment after each cleansing. He should also observe the wound for signs of possible infection (heat, redness, swelling), and return for suture removal in 4 days. These patients should also be given a list of warning signs for those who have suffered head trauma (see Chapter 14 and Appendix D).

Facial fractures

Because automobile and motorcycle accidents are the major cause of facial trauma in the United States, many of the patients who come to the emergency department with facial trauma have other concurrent injuries. Although a facial fracture may be the most obvious injury, care must be taken not to overlook the not-so-obvious, but perhaps, much more life-threatening injuries that may also be present. A facial fracture, unlike a laceration, may have its repair delayed for more than 7 days, usually without serious consequences.

Signs and symptoms of facial fractures include:

Pain
Swelling
Discoloration
Deformity
Malfunction
CSF otorrhea
CSF rhinorrhea
Facial bone fracture is detected clinically by:
Inspection
Palpation
Radiographic study

Fractures of the nasal bones, zygoma, and mandible are the frequently seen in the emergency department. Underlying sinus fracture is not unusual and requires immediate antibiotic coverage. Other bodily injuries that are life-threatening, such as chest, cranial, or abdominal injuries should not be overlooked, since facial injuries themselves do not cause death, but other system injuries do. The life-threatening potential of facial injuries lies in the bleeding and airway obstruction that are features of some severe maxillofacial injuries.

Nasal fracture. The most common of facial fractures is a nasal fracture, which usually occurs as a result of blunt trauma to the front or side of the nose. An x-ray film is not usually required to make a diagnosis. Diagnosis is made by obtaining a good history of the incident and observing for depression, swelling, deformity, and crepitus. One may be able to actually feel the fracture. A blunt blow to one side of the nose may cause depression on the injured side. A heavier blow may cause both sides to be broken with or without septal dislocation. A very great force may cause a flattened bridge and a comminuted fracture.

Nasal fractures may bleed internally into the throat, as well as externally. Pay particular attention to maintenance of the airway.

Once swelling has occurred, reduction of the fracture should be delayed until the swelling subsides. Always check for septal hematoma, which should be excised and packed. The patient should be checked for current tetanus status. Any fracture of the nose should be treated as an open fracture, and the patient should be given antibiotics.

Therapeutic intervention for nasal fractures includes a cold pack to the bridge of the nose and face, a protective splint over the fracture, and control of bleeding. Once this is accomplished, initiate regional anesthesia by injecting 1% lidocaine with epinephrine into the infraorbital area, the anterior nasal spine, and the dorsum of the nose. Anesthetize the nasal mucosa by packing it with cotton pledgets soaked in 5% cocaine solution.

Once regional anesthesia has taken effect, manipulate and mold the impacted bone and cartilage with fingers and forceps. Pack the inside of the nose to decrease bleeding. If the septum is fractured, be sure to pack both sides. A protective splint should be applied and left in place at least 2 weeks.

Nasal septal hematoma is one complication of a facial fracture that is worthy of explaining for one of its sequellae: permanent nasal deformity. Following severe trauma to the nose, the septal cartilage may be fractured. Bleeding between intact mucosal coverings on either side of the septal cartilage may dissect these nourishing coverings from the cartilage, causing avascular necrosis and "saddling" or depression of the nasal dorsum. This complication may be prevented by thorough examination of the nasal interior. Should bulging of the septum with red violet discoloration be visible, particularly with complete bilateral nasal airway obstruction, then surgical drainage and packing of the septum by an otolaryngologist is indicated.

Zygomatic arch fracture. Zygomatic arch fractures are usually caused by blunt trauma to the side of the face and upper cheek. The most common type of zygomatic arch fracture is known as the tripod fracture, in which there is not only a fracture of the zygomatic arch, but also a fracture of the infraorbital rim and the frontal zygomatic suture line.

The diagnosis of zygomatic arch fracture is made by visual appearance (look down at the face from above and behind; the fracture side will appear flat), by palpating the infraorbital rim fracture itself, by the patient demonstrating limited eye movement in the upward gaze, and by noting swelling in the area of the injury. One can also use the mnemonic TIDES:

T   Trismus (tonic contractions of the muscles of mastication)
I   Infraorbital hypesthesia or anesthesia
D   Diplopia (double vision)
E   Epistaxis
S   Symmetry (appearance of depressed cheek; look down over the forehead to observe)

Diagnostic radiology includes a Caldwell and Waters view, lateral and submentovertex views, or a basilar view.

Therapeutic intervention includes local cold pack, regional anesthesia, and closer or open reduction. Remember to be particularly aware of a cerebrospinal fluid leak caused by a fractured cribriform plate.

Orbital blow-out fracture. See p. 322.

Maxillary fracture. Automobile accidents, fist fights, and direct blows to the face with blunt instruments often cause maxillary fractures. The French pathologist LeFort struck corpses in the face with clubs and classified the resultant fractures.

LeFort I (Fig. 15-28, *A*). A fracture of the transverse alveolar process that involves the front teeth in a bilateral fracture up to the nose. It is diagnosed by malocclusion of the teeth. Therapeutic intervention should include cold packs to the area of injury and internal fixation.

LeFort II (Fig. 15-28, *B*). A fracture of the pyramidal area, including the central part of the maxilla to the nasal area. It is diagnosed by grasping the front teeth and observing the nose moving with the dental arch. Therapeutic intervention includes a cold pack to the area of injury and an ex-

tensive reduction, including internal stabilization and fixation. Note that very special attention should be paid to the airway, because these victims bleed profusely from the nose and pharynx.

LeFort III (Fig. 15-28, *C*). This is a total craniofacial separation that includes a tripod fracture and craniofacial detachment. Diagnosis is made by grasping the front teeth and noting that the nose and dental arch move without frontal bone movement. Therapeutic intervention includes a cold pack to the area of injury, bedrest with the head of the bed elevated, antibiotics, and open reduction with internal fixation. It is important to check for cerebrospinal fluid leaks, because it is common to see an associated fracture of the cribriform plate.

Mandibular fracture. Mandibular fractures are the second most common type of facial fractures and may be associated with other fractures (such as the condyles). Many of these fractures are open. This is a common football or baseball injury, as it is caused by a severe force to the jaw.

It is diagnosed by noting malocclusion of the teeth, pain, bone or fragment displacement, palpation of fractures, and bleeding between the teeth. One can also place two tongue blades together and have the patient bite down on them in the molar area. A fracture will produce pain. If there is no pain, there is usually no fracture.

Therapeutic intervention includes a cold pack to the area of injury, immobilization of the fracture area (usually by wiring), antibiotics, and current tetanus immunization.

Fractures that require no therapeutic intervention. There are several facial fractures that do not require treatment. These are a nondisplaced facial fracture, a fracture of the anterior wall of the maxillary antrum, a fracture of the coronoid process of the mandible, and a fracture of the condyle in children.

Once again, remember that all facial trauma victims should be considered to have head and cervical spine injuries until proved otherwise. These persons should be observed, either in the

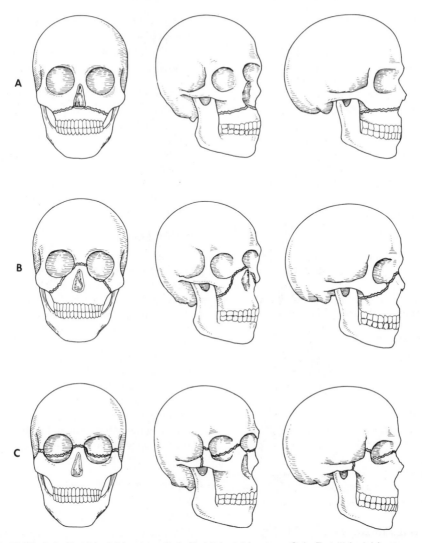

Fig. 15-28. A, LeFort I facial fracture. **B,** LeFort II facial fracture. **C,** LeFort III facial fracture.

emergency department or by a responsible individual at home for signs and symptoms of head trauma.

DENTAL EMERGENCIES

Patients with dental emergencies usually come to the emergency department complaining of pain or trauma or both. There are, generally speaking, two types of dental pain that bring a patient into the emergency department, es-

pecially in the middle of the night or on a holiday when a dentist is not readily available. These two types of pain are maxillofacial pain and dental pain. Maxillofacial pain can be characterized into major and minor neuralgias.

Major neuralgias

Trigeminal neuralgia (tic douloureaux). Trigeminal neuralgia is a degenerative process or pressure on the trigeminal nerve; it usually occurs in persons over 40 years old. The pain is described as excruciating and paroxysmal and usually radiates (1) along the eye and up into the forehead, (2) from the upper lip, through the nose and cheek, up into the eye, and (3) into the lower lip and on the outside of the tongue. An acute onset of unknown etiology is known as Bell's palsy.

The signs and symptoms are a droopy corner of mouth, inability to close the eye, difficulty eating, and difficulty swallowing.

Therapeutic intervention is a trigeminal nerve block.

Glossopharyngeal neuralgia. Glossopharyngeal neuralgia resembles trigeminal neuralgia but is characterized by severe pain in the middle ear, the back of the throat, and the tonsils, leading to dysfunction or protruding of the tongue.

Therapeutic intervention consists of phenytoin (Dilantin) or carbamazepine (Tegretol).

Minor neuralgias

Minor neuralgias include sphenopalatine neuralgia, occipital neuralgia, and geniculate neuralgia.

Dental pain

The most common cause of dental pain is tooth decay or pulpal disease. Pulpal disease has three phases:

1. Hyperemic. The vascular system responds to an external stimulus, such as dental caries (cavity) or dental trauma; this is a reversible condition.
2. Pulpitis. The pulp becomes infected.
3. Pulpal necrosis. The pulp dies; fluid and pressure build, causing pain.

Therapeutic intervention consists of analgesia and referral to a dentist.

Other causes of dental pain

Fractured teeth
Periodontal disease (in the gums)
Foreign bodies (such as a toothbrush bristle)
Dry socket
Pressure from a prosthetic device
Mandibular fractures
Vincent's angina, or "trench mouth" (ulcers of the tonsils and pharynx)

Pericoronitis (pain of wisdom teeth erupting)
Causalgia (severe burning pain 2 to 3 weeks following tooth extraction; usually stress related)
Sinusitis
Glossodynia (a burning pain in the tongue usually caused by fungal infection following antibiotic administration)
Fractured styloid process
Hematomas (usually resulting from injections of anesthetic)
Coronary artery disease (referred pain to jaw)
Carcinoma
Unerupted teeth (especially in children)

Toothaches

The most common cause of toothaches is pulpal disease or dental caries. The tooth becomes extremely sensitive to heat and cold. The pain may be reversible if the decay can be removed and the tooth restored. This type of pain is paroxysmal and usually begins with a heat or cold stimulus. Irreversible pain indicates that the tooth will require either a root canal (endodontics) or extraction. This pain usually occurs spontaneously and continues to worsen, especially at night when intracranial pressure increases.

Therapeutic intervention for both consists of topical eugenol (oil of clove) or other analgesia and referral to a dentist.

Chipped (broken) teeth

Chipped or broken teeth are the most frequently seen dental emergencies in the emergency department. It is a common injury in children and in participants in contact sports. The four center upper teeth are the teeth most frequently injured.

Check for bleeding from gums and from pulp. Bleeding from pulp requires an emergency dental consultation. As these injuries are frequently associated with head injuries, be sure to check the mouth and pharynx area for pieces of teeth and debris that may obstruct the airway.

Avulsed teeth

Avulsed teeth are teeth that have been torn from the mouth by trauma. If found, these teeth may be reimplanted. It is important to place the tooth in a saline solution, irrigate the wound, anesthetize the wound area, and reimplant the tooth as soon as possible following the accident. Once the tooth is reimplanted it should be wired or splinted in place and a referral should be made to a dentist or oral surgeon. The blood supply to the tooth comes through the pulp, so the viability of the tooth depends upon the patency of the pulp.

Teeth that have been driven into the gums, especially in children, should be left alone. No attempt should be made to pull the teeth out of the gums. These teeth will usually return to their normal position within 1 month if left alone.

Remember, again, to look for teeth and foreign bodies, such as prostheses and bridges, in the mouths of trauma patients and remove these objects to avoid airway obstruction. If a head injury is suspected in a patient with dental trauma, the patient should be admitted to the hospital for 24-hour observation.

Dental abscess

Abscesses in the periapical areas usually result from pulpal necrosis, which results from caries or trauma. Periodontal abscesses usually result from bony destruction at the peridontal membrane, which forms a pocket and an abscess.

Therapeutic intervention consists of drainage of the abscess, antibiotics, analgesics, hot packs on the area, warm saline rinses every 2 hours, aspirin or other antipyretic for fever above 38.3° C (101° F), and referral to a dentist.

Periodontal emergencies

gingivitis — inflammation of the gums characterized by redness, swelling, pain, and bleeding
periodontal disease — loss of periodontal bone; appears similar to gingivitis; definitive diagnosis is made on x-ray films
necrotizing ulcerative gingivitis — painful bleeding, foul-smelling breath, lymphadenopathy, chills, fever, and malaise; therapeutic intervention consists of debridement, antibiotics, warm hydrogen peroxide rinses every 2 hours, soft toothbrush, and a dental consultation

pericoronitis — painful eruption of wisdom teeth accompanied by swelling, lymphadenopathy, and trismus; therapeutic intervention is by removal of tissue over the tooth, warm saline rinses, antibiotics, and dental referral for possible tooth extraction

Postoperative bleeding

Often a patient comes to the emergency department bleeding from the mouth with a history of recent tooth extraction or recent oral surgery. Usually all that is needed is to apply a pressure pack over the area of hemorrhage. If the bleeding persists, a hemostatic dressing such as Gelfoam, Surgicel, or thrombin should be packed into the socket. A home remedy that may also be effective is to place a teabag over the socket. (The tannic acid produces hemostasis.) If the packing is unsuccessful, sutures may be placed or the bleeding vessels may be cauterized. The patient should be cautioned to avoid mouth rinses until the bleeding has completely stopped, to eat a soft diet, and to use intermittent ice packs.

Dry socket (alveolalgia)

Dry socket usually occurs 3 to 5 days after surgery, when a blood clot is lost and bone is exposed. Therapeutic intervention consists of eugenol (oil of clove) packed into the socket, analgesia, and dental referral.

Note about local anesthesia

Both infiltration and regional block techniques may be used when applying dental anesthesia. Strict attention to detail must be paid when injecting the anesthesia. Complications of anesthesia injection include facial paralysis (from injecting into the parotid gland), blurred vision (from injecting into the optic nerve), trismus, and hematoma. Therapeutic intervention is simply to observe the patient until the effects of the anesthesia wear off.

BIBLIOGRAPHY

Anderson, R. D., Jr.: Ocular emergencies. In Warner, C. G., editor: Emergency care: assessment and intervention, ed. 2, St. Louis, 1978, The C. V. Mosby Co.

Barber, J. M., and Budassi, S. A.: Mosby's manual of emergency care: procedures and practice, St. Louis, 1979, The C. V. Mosby Co.

Barber, J. M., Stokes, L. G., and Billings, D. M.: Adult and child care: a client approach to nursing, ed. 2, St. Louis, 1977, The C. V. Mosby Co.

Boles, R., Crumley, R. L., Schindler, R. A., and others: The face inside and out, Emerg. Med. **10:**27, February 1978.

Brunner, L. S., and Suddarth, D. S.: Eye problems. In The Lippincott manual of nursing practice, Philadelphia, 1974, J. B. Lippincott Co.

Chee, H. Y.: Emergency ocular care. In Barry, J., editor: Emergency nursing, New York, 1978, McGraw-Hill Book Co.

Coe, R. O., Jr.: Emergency eye care. In Stephenson, H. E., Jr., editor: Immediate care of the acutely ill and injured, St. Louis, 1974, The C. V. Mosby Co.

Duke-Elder, S., and Mac Faul, P. A.: System of ophthalmology: mechanical injuries, Vol. 14, Part 1 and 2, St. Louis, 1972, The C. V. Mosby Co.

Dupont, J.: Eye, ear, nose and throat emergencies. In Giving emergency care competently, Nursing Skillbooks, Nursing '78, Horsham, Pa., 1978, Intermed Communications.

Grant, W. M.: Toxicology of the eye, ed. 2, Springfield, Ill., 1974, Charles C Thomas Co.

Kirchner, F. R.: Management of neck and face injuries. In McSwain, N. E.: Traumatic surgery, Flushing, N.Y., 1976, Medical Examination Publishing Co., Inc.

Kruger, G.: Fractures of the jaw. In Kruger, G., editor: Textbook of oral surgery, ed. 4, St. Louis, 1974, The C. V. Mosby Co.

Lanros, N. E.: Assessment and intervention in emergency nursing, Bowie, Md., 1978, Brady Co.

Leake, D., Doykos, J., Habal, M. B., and Murray, J. Z.: Longterm follow-up of fractures of the mandibular condyle in children, Plast. Reconstr. Surg. **47:**127, 1971.

Mechner, F., and Saffiotti, L. J.: Patient assessment: examination of the eye, Part I and Part II, Am. J. Nurs. **74:** P.I. 1-24, 1974; and **75:**P.I. 1-24, 1975.

Moore, L. T.: Emergency management of facial injuries. In Warner, C. G., editor: Emergency care: assessment and intervention, ed. 2, St. Louis, 1978, The C. V. Mosby Co.

Schaefer, A. J.: Care of the patient with ocular injuries. In Cosgriff, J. H., and Anderson, D. L., editors: The practice of emergency nursing, Philadelphia, 1975, J. B. Lippincott Co.

Seelenfreund, M. H., and Freilich, D. B.: Rushing the net and retinal detachment, J.A.M.A. **235:**25, 1976.

Shira, R.: Emergency treatment of patients with facial trauma. In Douglas, B., editor: Introduction to hospital dentistry, ed. 2, St. Louis, 1970, The C. V. Mosby Co.

Stein, H. A., and Slatt, B. J.: The ophthalmic assistant: Fundamentals of clinical practice, ed. 3, St. Louis, 1976, The C. V. Mosby Co.

Vaughan, D., Cook, R., and Asbury, T.: General ophthalmology, Los Altos, Calif., 1975, Lange Medical Publications.

Wilson, R. F., and Zamick, P.: Trauma to the face. In Walt, A. J., and Wilson, R. F.: Management of trauma: pitfalls and practice, Philadelphia, 1975, Lea & Febiger.

CHAPTER 16

Chest trauma

A patient with chest trauma may have one of the most life-threatening emergencies encountered in the emergency department. There has been an increase in the number of chest traumas as a result of the increased number of traffic accidents and the increase of social violence. Twenty-five percent of all trauma deaths in the United States are due to chest trauma, and 25% to 50% of all chest traumas result in death. Trauma deaths account for the number one loss of lifetime working years (3,800,000 working years/year), with head trauma being the number one cause of death and chest trauma number two. It is interesting to note that heart disease accounts for a yearly loss of 2,000,000 lifetime working years and cancer for 1,800,000 lifetime working years.

The major causes of blunt trauma to the chest are an automobile steering wheel and bicycle handlebars. Gunshot wounds and stabbings account for the majority of penetrating injuries.

Many of these injuries are emergent, and one must diagnose and apply therapeutic intervention almost concurrently.

ANATOMY AND PHYSIOLOGY

The thoracic cavity extends from the first rib and adjacent structures above, to the diaphragm, and includes the 12 pairs of ribs. It contains the lower airway, intrathoracic structures such as the heart and pericardium, the lungs, the inferior and superior vena cavae, and aorta, and the esophagus.

The lungs are elastic structures that have a natural tendency to collapse. They are prevented from collapsing by negative pressure

found between the lungs and the chest wall in the pleural space. When the chest wall expands, negative pressure increases, and the lungs, concurrently, fill with air from the upper airways and expand (Fig. 16-1). If negative pressure is lost, the lungs will collapse (Fig. 16-2).

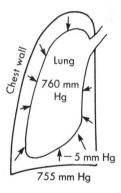

Fig. 16-1. Negative pressure in the chest cavity.

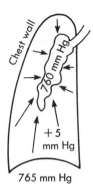

Fig. 16-2. Loss of negative pressure in the chest cavity.

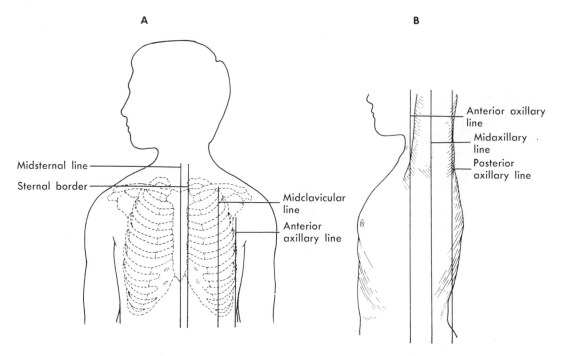

Fig. 16-3. Anatomical references lines. **A,** Anterior. **B,** Lateral. **C,** Posterior. **D,** Anterior intercostal spaces. **E,** Posterior aspect.

The chest wall expands with the assistance of the muscles of respiration. These are grouped into two categories: the main muscles and the accessory muscles. The main muscles of respiration are the diaphragm and the intercostal muscles. The diaphragm separates the thoracic cavity from the abdominal cavity. It contains the phrenic nerve, which originates at the fourth cervical vertebra. On expiration the diaphragm is located at about the sixth intercostal space. On deep inspiration, it is located at about the fourth lumbar spine.

The accessory muscles used in respiration are the pectoralis major, which is a chest wall muscle that pulls on the anterior chest, the sternocleidomastoid muscle, which has its main body in the neck and pulls on the upper chest, and the abdominal wall muscles.

When the intercostal muscles elevate the chest wall and the diaphragm drops down, negative pressure increases in the pleural space, and the lungs expand with air entering the air-

ways—inspiration. When the intercostal muscles drop, the chest wall and the diaphragm raises up, negative pressure decreases in the pleural space, and the lungs contract, with air exiting through the airways—expiration.

In order to adequately and accurately describe an injury, one must be familiar with surface anatomy as described in Fig. 16-3. Any wound below the nipples should also be considered an abdominal injury as well.

EVALUATION OF CHEST INJURIES

Any patient with chest trauma should be considered to have a serious injury until proved otherwise. Airway, breathing, circulation, and cervical spine should always be of primary concern. Chest injuries that may produce problems with any of these are flail chest, sucking chest wounds, pneumothorax, tension pneumothorax, hemothorax, and cardiac tamponade. Other injuries, such as esophageal rupture, tracheobronchial tree rupture, diaphragmatic rupture,

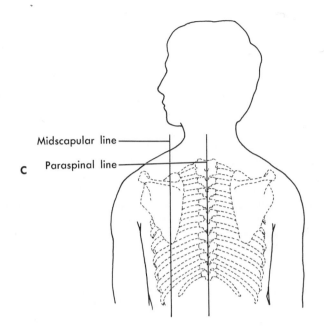

Midscapular line
Paraspinal line

C

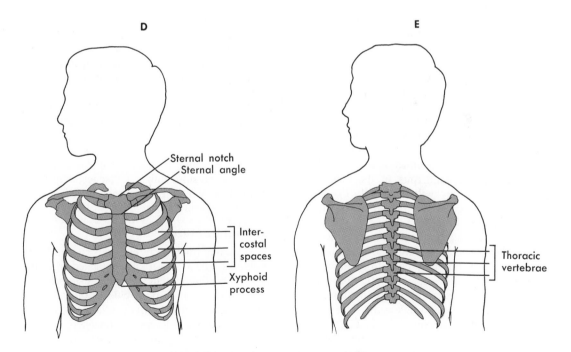

D

E

Sternal notch
Sternal angle

Inter-
costal
spaces

Xyphoid
process

Thoracic
vertebrae

Fig. 16-3, cont'd. For legend see opposite page.

aortic rupture, pulmonary contusion, and myocardial contusion, may not demonstrate immediate airway, breathing, or circulatory impairment, but they may be fatal.

Rib fractures

Rib fractures are common chest injuries, particularly in the athlete involved in contact sports and in the elderly. These patients will appear with a history of trauma to the chest, pain that increases with inspiration, and local pain and crepitus over the fracture site.

First rib fracture is often associated with clavicle fracture and sometimes with scapula fracture. One may also see perforation of the subclavian artery or vein or tracheobronchial injury with first rib fracture. This rib is not well exposed, and trauma is not common. If the first rib has been fractured, it has taken a great force to fracture it. With first rib fractures, consider other injuries as well.

When the lower ribs are fractured, consider concurrent injury to the kidneys, the spleen on the left, and the liver on the right. If three or more ribs are fractured, the patient should be considered a multiple trauma victim, and one must search for other injuries.

Diagnosis can be made by palpating the fractures or by x-ray film. Therapeutic intervention is individual. If the fracture is simple and nondisplaced, rest, local heat, and simple analgesia are recommended. For the elderly and those with jagged fractures, displaced fractures, known pulmonary disease, or multiple trauma, hospitalization is recommended. Rib fractures are particularly dangerous in the elderly, as their vital capacity will be greatly decreased. Chest strapping for rib fractures is no longer recommended, because it decreases ventilation and may cause atelectasis and pneumonia.

If chest pain is severe and ventilation is compromised, one may elect to employ either local infiltration of an anesthetic solution directly into the fracture site or by intercostal nerve block above and below the fracture site. If an intercostal nerve block is elected, one must obtain a chest x-ray film before and after the procedure to assure that pneumothorax has not taken place.

Flail chest

When two or more adjacent ribs are fractured in two places (anteriorly and laterally) or the sternum is detached, the result is a free-floating segment of ribs and chest, or sternum, that has lost continuity with the rest of the chest. This segment does not move symmetrically and responds to intrathoracic pressure changes rather than aiding in respirations. A paradoxical chest wall motion ensues, and respiratory distress results. When negative pressure increases (inhalation), the flail segment is drawn in (Fig. 16-4, *B*). When negative pressure decreases (exhalation), the flail segment is pushed out (Fig. 16-4, *C*). This motion of the flail segment is called paradoxical motion. Diagnosis of flail chest is made by observation of the flail segment, shortness of breath, and difficulty breathing. Therapeutic intervention is aimed at stabilizing the chest wall by placing the victim with the flail side down (Fig. 16-5, *A*) in a semi-Fowler position, sandbagging the flail segment (Fig. 16-5, *B*), taping (either wide tape, or taping an object) the flail segment (Fig. 16-5, *C*), placing manual pressure over the flail segment (Fig. 16-5, *D*) or attaching the center of the flail segment to a towel clip, which is attached to a weighted line, draped over an IV pole (Fig. 16-5, *E*). One must also give oxygen at high flow under positive pressure through an endotracheal tube and start an IV of Ringer's lactate or normal saline through a large-bore cannula.

One should think about an associated myocardial contusion or possible underlying pulmonary contusion with a flail chest. Also, be aware of a developing pneumothorax that may result from positive pressure ventilation.

Sternal fracture

A sternal fracture rarely causes significant problems unless it is totally detached from the ribs and becomes a flail segment. A sternal fracture, however, may be a clue to other underlying injuries, such as myocardial contusion. It is not uncommon to find a detached sternum following use of an automatic chest compressor in CPR. Therapeutic intervention is identical to that for a flail chest.

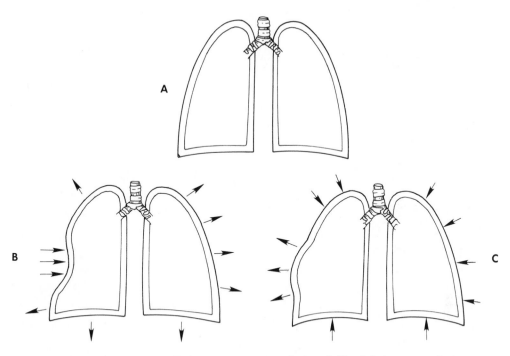

Fig. 16-4. A, Normal lungs. **B,** The flail chest on inspiration. **C,** The flail chest on expiration.

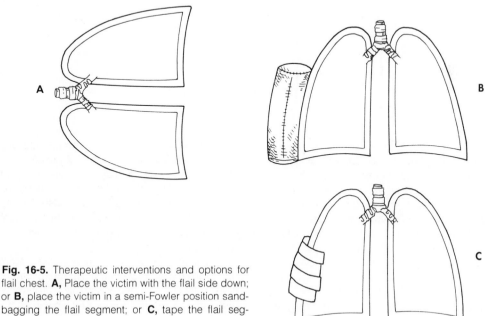

Fig. 16-5. Therapeutic interventions and options for flail chest. **A,** Place the victim with the flail side down; or **B,** place the victim in a semi-Fowler position sandbagging the flail segment; or **C,** tape the flail segment; or; *Continued.*

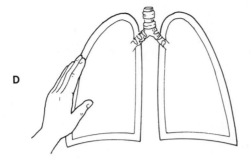

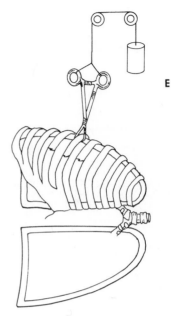

D

E

Fig. 16-5, cont'd. D, place manual pressure over the flail segment; or **E,** attach the center of the flail segment to a towel clip that is attached to a weighted line, draped over an IV pole.

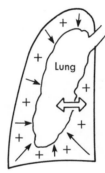

Fig. 16-6. Simple pneumothorax.

Simple pneumothorax

Air enters the pleural space and causes a loss of negative pressure. This loss of negative pressure causes a partial or total collapse of the lung on the affected side (Fig. 16-6). It may be due to a hole in the chest wall, the lungs, the bronchus, the trachea, or a ruptured aveoli. Spontaneous pneumothorax usually occurs in young men between the ages of 20 and 40, and is probably due to the rupture of subpleural blebs.

Diagnosis is made by eliciting a history of blunt trauma to the chest or sudden onset of sharp (pleuritic) chest pain, auscultating decreased breath sounds on the affected side, hyperresonance on percussion, shortness of breath and tachypnea, and positive findings on chest x-ray films. The patient may also demonstrate syncope and Hamman's sign (a ''crunching'' sound with each heartbeat due to mediastinal air accumulation).

Therapeutic intervention may range from simply observing the patient (if the pneumothorax is small), to placement of a large-bore needle in the second intercostal space in the midclavicular line, the fifth intercostal space in

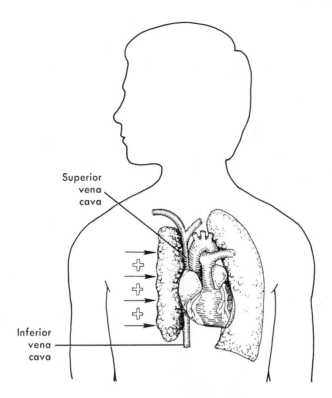

Fig. 16-7. Tension pneumothorax.

the midaxillary line on the affected side, or placement of a chest tube in the same location(s). These patients should be placed in a semi-Fowler position and be administered high-flow oxygen.

Tension pneumothorax

When air enters the pleural space on inspiration and cannot escape during expiration (similar to a one-way valve effect) a tension pneumothorax forms. As the positive pressure increases on the affected side, the lung on that same side collapses and a mediastinal shift occurs that compresses the heart and great vessels and the trachea. This shift, in turn, compresses the lung on the unaffected side and impedes venous return to the right atrium by putting pressure on the inferior and superior vena cavae (Fig. 16-7).

Consequently, one will note much neck vein enlargement. The patient's ventilation will de-crease because of increased intrathoracic pressure, and he may become severely short of breath. Shock may ensue because of the lack of oxygenated blood flow to the heart. Other signs and symptoms of tension pneumothorax are a history of chest trauma, severe shortness of breath, paradoxical movement of the chest, a deviated trachea (toward the unaffected side), cyanosis, distant heart sounds, and hyperresonance on percussion. Definitive diagnosis may be made on x-ray film.

If the patient is severly symptomatic, do *not* delay therapeutic intervention until an x-ray film is taken—act immediately.

Therapeutic intervention includes maintenance of airway, breathing, and circulation, oxygen at high flow under positive pressure, needle thoracotomy in the second intercostal space in the midclavicular line or the fifth intercostal space in the midaxillary line, placement of a chest tube, and IV therapy with Ringer's

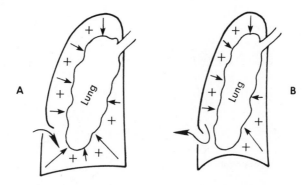

Fig. 16-8. Sucking chest wound. **A,** Inspiration. **B,** Expiration.

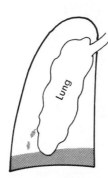

Fig. 16-9. Hemothorax.

lactate or normal saline through a large-bore cannula.

If tension pneumothorax is not corrected, cardiac output will continue to fall and the patient will die.

Sucking chest wound

A sucking chest wound is an open pneumothorax with a chest wall defect. Air passes from the atmosphere through the chest wall into the pleural space and out again (Fig. 16-8). When an opening is made in the chest wall, there is a resultant loss of intrathoracic pressure. If a flap forms and air can be sucked into the pleural cavity but cannot be released, positive pressure will begin to increase and a tension pneumothorax will result.

Diagnosis is made by obtaining a history of penetrating trauma to the chest and by hearing a sucking sound on inspiration as the chest wall rises, the diaphragm drops, and air is sucked into the chest cavity through the opening in the chest wall.

The goal of therapeutic intervention is to stop the wound from sucking by covering the wound with an occlusive dressing such as petrolatum-impregnated gauze. One must pay particular attention to airway, breathing, and circulation. The patient should also receive high-flow oxygen. The integrity of the pleural space may be restored with a chest tube.

If, following placement of the occlusive dressing, a tension pneumothorax begins to form, remove the occlusive dressing to convert the tension pneumothorax to a simple pneumothorax.

Hemothorax

A hemothorax is a collection of blood in the pleural cavity (Fig. 16-9). Blood accumulation may be mild (up to 300 ml), moderate (300 to 1400 ml), or severe (1400 to 2500 ml). Se-

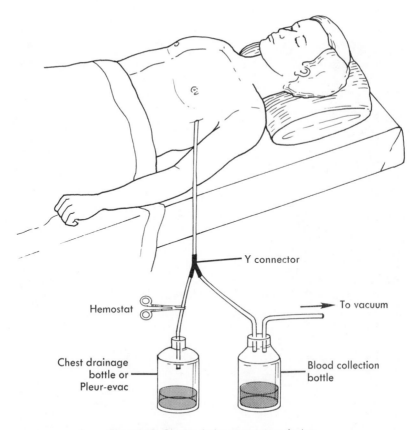

Fig. 16-10. Gravity drainage autotransfusion.

vere blood loss may be life threatening because of resultant hypvolemia and the tension that is forming.

Signs and symptoms of hemothorax are similar to those in pneumothorax and tension pneumothorax with the addition of tachycardia, hypotension, dullness on chest percussion, and other associated signs of shock, such as cold, clammy skin, and tremors.

Therapeutic intervention is aimed at treating the shock condition (MAST, IVs, oxygen, Trendelenburg position) as well as relieving the pressure from the pleural cavity by inserting a chest tube (or tubes) into the fifth intercostal space in the midaxillary line. Chest drainage should be measured and recorded. Surgery may be indicated if drainage is greater than 200 ml/hour over 24 hours.

If trauma volume is high or if there is a shortage of whole blood, one may elect to employ autotransfusion, in which blood draining from the patient's chest tube is filtered and transfused back into that same patient (see p. 249) (Fig. 16-10).

Chest tubes and chest drainage

If air or blood is accumulating in the pleural cavity, there will be a reduction of negative pressure. Both air and blood must be removed, and negative pressure must be restored. A method to remove both air and blood is insertion of a chest tube. The chest tube is normally placed in either the second intercostal space in the midclavicular line (for air) or in the fifth intercostal space in the midaxillary line (for fluid). It is attached to a water seal suc-

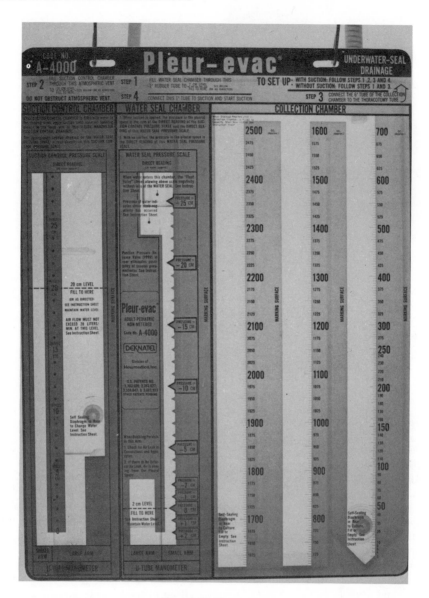

Fig. 16-11. Pleur-evac.

tion that acts as a one-way valve, allowing blood or air to escape but not allowing backflow.

There are various types of chest drainage systems available, either improvised or commercial. Regardless of the system chosen, the goal is the same: to remove blood or air from the pleural cavity and allow for lung reexpansion.

The most common system used today is the Pleur-evac (Fig. 16-11), a plastic disposable system equivalent to the three-bottle drainage system in which the first bottle is the collection bottle, which collects drainage from the patient's chest, the second bottle is the water seal, and the third bottle is the pressure regulating bottle (Fig. 16-12).

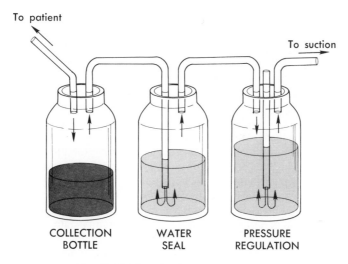

Fig. 16-12. Three-bottle drainage system.

Ensure that the system is kept sterile and air-tight. Secure all connections with adhesive tape. The chest tube and connecting tubing should be "milked" periodically to evacuate any clots that may have formed. Be sure to measure the amount of drainage and record it, both in nurse's notes and on the collection chamber.

LUNG INJURIES
Pulmonary contusion

A pulmonary contusion may be localized or generalized ("wet lung") and is usually associated with other severe injuries. In pulmonary contusion, blood extravasates into the parenchyma, causing tissue anoxia and change in tissue permeability. It may also cause tracheal obstruction.

Diagnosis is made by suspecting it, and by observing increasing hyperpnea, dyspnea, and the development of an ineffective cough.

Therapeutic intervention includes oxygen at high flow, limiting fluids during the resuscitation and early ICU period, and using whole blood, plasma, or salt-poor albumin to replace blood loss. One should also employ diuretics and steroids. If the contusion is severe, it is advisable to give the patient positive pressure using an endotracheal tube.

LACERATION OF THE PARENCHYMA

Lacerations of the parenchyma are usually caused by penetrating trauma or fractured ribs. They are usually self-limiting and rarely require therapeutic intervention.

TRACHEOBRONCHIAL TREE INJURIES

Injuries to the tracheobronchial tree are usually due to blunt trauma or penetrating trauma, such as gunshot wounds or stab wounds and usually involve the trachea and mainstem bronchus.

Signs and symptoms vary greatly, but may include airway obstruction, atelectasis, hemoptysis (usually massive), mediastinal and subcutaneous emphysema, and tension pneumothorax.

Diagnosis is usually made on observation of progressive mediastinal and subcutaneous emphysema or on direct bronchoscopic examination, and by observing other signs and symptoms.

Therapeutic intervention includes maintaining an open airway, placing a chest tube, administering high-flow oxygen, placing the patient in a semi-Fowler position, and immediate surgical repairing of the tear.

DIAPHRAGMATIC INJURIES

Injuries to the diaphragm may be caused by either blunt or penetrating trauma. With any injury at or below the level of the nipples, diphragmatic injury must be considered. If there is injury to the diaphragm, this is indicative of other severe trauma.

Diagnosis can be made by observing pain that is referred to the shoulder. Depending on the size of the injury, some herniation of the bowel may be present and visible on x-ray film.

Therapeutic intervention includes stomach decompression by placement of a nasogastric tube, evacuation of any hematoma that may have formed, and surgical repair of the rupture.

CARDIAC INJURIES
Contusions

Cardiac contusions occur more frequently than are diagnosed and are frequently associated with other injuries. One should always suspect contusion in any patient giving a history of blunt trauma to the chest, particularly by a steering wheel or a bicycle handlebars. One should also suspect cardiac contusion in any patient following cardiopulmonary resuscitation.

Diagnosing is made primarily by suspecting it. There may be ST and T wave changes on ECG, although these may not be evident for 12 to 24 hours. One should draw serum enzymes (SGOT, SGPT, and LDH) for baseline levels. Often these patients will complain of shortness of breath, dyspnea, and chest pain, and one will observe tachycardia, hypotension, and possible arrhythmias (usually supraventricular). If trauma is significant, cardiac output may drop and cardiogenic shock may ensue.

Therapeutic intervention is similar to that for acute myocardial infarction and includes oxygen therapy, semi-Fowler position, analgesia, treatment of dysrhythmias, and admission to the coronary care unit. These patients should be closely monitored for dysrhythmias and cardiogenic shock.

Penetrating injuries

Most patients with penetrating injury to the heart die rapidly—very few reach the hospital.

If penetrating injury is identified, it is imperative to aggressively treat the shock and transport to a capable medical facility as soon as possible.

If the patient survives the trip to the emergency department, immediate thoracotomy is the treatment of choice. Some emergency department physicians may even elect to place the patient on a cardiopulmonary bypass machine during the procedure.

If there is myocardial rupture, the patient will demonstrate hypotension, an elevated CVP, and distended neck veins, decreased ECG voltage, and decreased heart sounds. The mortality rate in myocardial rupture is high. The right ventricle is more frequently ruptured than the left because of the superficial position of the right ventricle. Therapeutic intervention is pulmonary toilet, digoxin, diuretics, immediate thoracotomy, and repair of the rupture.

When the aortic valve ruptures, there is sudden onset of severe chest pain, severe shortness of breath, dyspnea, hemoptysis, a "roaring" load murmur, and signs of congestive heart failure and pulmonary edema. Therapeutic intervention is immediate surgery for valve replacement.

Many penetrating injuries of the heart may produce cardiac tamponade. Tamponade may be treated with pericardiocentesis is early recognition is made.

Cardiac tamponade

The heart is surrounded by a fibrinous sac known as the pericardial sac. Tamponade occurs when a relatively minor wound of the heart bleeds into the pericardial space (Fig. 16-13). Blood begins to build up in the pericardial sac because either it cannot escape or it cannot escape as fast as the bleeding occurs. Blood accumulation interferes with the filling of the ventricles and the pumping action of the heart, and cardiac output falls. The heart will begin to compensate by becoming tachycardic, but then it deteriorates.

As the heart rate increases, venous pressure increases, blood pressure falls, and heart sounds diminish (Beck's triad). Neck veins

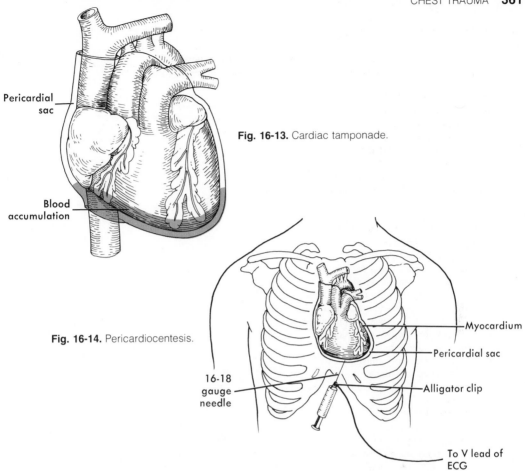

Fig. 16-13. Cardiac tamponade.

Fig. 16-14. Pericardiocentesis.

distend, the patient becomes dyspneic and demonstrates Kussmal respirations. One will also note a paradoxical pulse and cyanosis.

Therapeutic intervention includes fluid administration to elevate CVP, oxygen at high flow, high Fowler position, and pericardiocentesis.

Pericardiocentesis. Pericardiocentesis is a procedure whereby a 16- to 18-gauge intracardiac needle is introduced into the pericardial sac for withdrawal of blood or fluid that is compressing the myocardium. The needle is attached to a large syringe (usually 30 to 50 ml). The hub of the needle is connected to the lead of an ECG machine by means of an alligator clip (Fig. 16-14). The needle is inserted about 3 cm to the left of the xiphoid

process (the subxiphoid approach) and directed toward the left shoulder. The ECG machine should be running and recording continuously on the V-lead selector. The needle is advanced slowly until it penetrates the pericardial sac and reaches the myocardium. When the needle touches the myocardium, a current of injury pattern will appear on the V-rhythm strip. When this occurs, the needle is withdrawn a few centimeters, negative pressure is placed on the plunger, and the pericardial sac is aspirated. Withdrawal of as little as 15 ml of blood or fluid may be lifesaving. Following pericardiocentesis, the patient should be observed closely for the possibility of further bleeding. If bleeding reoccurs, one may choose to repeat the pericardiocentesis or one may

Assessment and therapeutic
intervention of the chest trauma victim

Maintain airway, breathing, and circulation
Obtain a quick history
- What happened?
- Was there a weapon involved? An automobile?
- How long ago did it happen?
- Where does it hurt?
- Is there any medical history?

Perform a quick (1-minute) evaluation
- Check for shortness of breath and cyanosis.
- Chest vital signs.
- Check skin color and temperature.
- Check wound size and location.
- Check for paradoxical chest movement.
- Check for distended neck veins.
- Listen for respiratory stridor.
- Listen for bilateral breath sounds.
- Look for epigastric and supraclavicular indrawing.
- Give rough estimate of tidal volume.
- Check for tracheal deviation.
- Assess intercostal muscle use.
- Assess accessory muscle use.
- Check for subcutaneous emphysema.
- Look and listen for sucking chest wounds.
- Listen to heart sounds.

Therapeutic intervention
- Maintain airway.
- Assure adequate air movement.
- Cover any open chest wound.
- Control flail segment.
- Insert needles or chest tube into anterior chest wall if tension pneumothorax is present.
- Initiate an IV line (two or more lines if possible—but do *not* delay transport to do this.)
- Do pericardiocentesis, if indicated.
- Get chest x-ray film if more than three ribs are fractured, because victim is considered multi-traumatized and one must search for other associated injuries. It is essential at this time to obtain cross-table lateral cervical spine x-ray film for detection of cervical spine injury before initiating any other diagnostic tests or moving the victim.
- Frequently recheck vital signs.
- Monitor for dysrhythmias.

elect to recommend thoracotomy for surgical repair.

Complications of pericardiocentesis include laceration of a coronary artery, laceration of a lung, laceration of a ventricle, dysrhythmias, and further increasing the cardiac tamponade.

GREAT VESSEL INJURIES

The great vessels, the superior and inferior vena cavae and the aorta, are subject to both penetrating and blunt injuries. A penetrating injury to a great vessel is one of the most lethal injuries to the human body. It the victim reaches the hospital alive, immediate thoracotomy is indicated, as well as high-flow oxygen, two to three large-bore IVs, and the MAST.

Ten to twenty percent of victims of blunt trauma resulting in tears of the great vessels survive the initial accident and reach the hospital alive. It is believed that his percentage survives because blood is contained by the adventitia, forming a false aneurism.

The most common cause of sudden death following an automobile accident is a ruptured aorta. The usual mechanism of injury is a rapid acceleration-deceleration force that causes a tortion and shearing force at the point of fixation of the aorta (ligamentum arteriosum), resulting in a transverse tear and exsanguination or massive tamponade. This patient is rarely salvageable.

Diagnosis can be made by observing signs and symptoms of cardiac tamponade or exsanguinating hemorrhage and mediastinal widening, by auscultating a murmur in the left parascapular region, and by a marked difference in blood pressure from right to left arm.

Therapeutic intervention is limited to large-bore IVs with IV solution running as rapidly as possible, high-flow oxygen, the MAST, and immediate surgical intervention, which is usually the patient's only hope for survival.

RUPTURED BRONCHUS

A ruptured bronchus, most commonly near the carina and the right mainstem, may be lethal if not diagnosed and treated immediately. Diagnosis is made by identifying the resultant tension pneumothorax and looking specifically for the rupture.

Therapeutic intervention is high-flow oxygen, chest tube placement, and immediate surgical repair of the rupture.

ESOPHAGEAL RUPTURE

The esophagus is subject to both blunt and penetrating trauma; foreign bodies and esophagoscopy are often the cause of penetrating trauma. With penetrating trauma, rupture is often at the pharyngoesophageal junction. In blunt trauma, rupture often occurs just above the diaphragm.

Esophageal rupture is a rare event, but when it occurs, it is very often fatal. One should consider esophageal rupture whenever there is a first or second rib fracture.

Diagnosis is made by observation of sudden onset of severe chest pain or severe upper abdominal pain, pneumothorax, pain on swallowing, mediastinitis and subcutaneous emphysema, mediastinal crunch (Hamman's sign), increased respirations, pleural effusion, and gastric contents or bile in the chest tube.

Therapeutic intervention includes large-bore IVs, high-flow oxygen, and immediate surgery.

SUMMARY

The primary focus in any patient with chest trauma should be maintenance of airway, breathing, and circulation. Assure an adequate airway, and administer oxygen at high flow. Initiate two large-bore IVs with Ringer's lactate or normal saline if possible. Seal any open chest wounds and splint fractures. Rapid transport, diagnosis, and treatment are essential. These patients should be considered critical until proved otherwise.

BIBLIOGRAPHY

Anyanwu, C. H.: Mitral incompetence and VSD's following nonpenetrating injury, Thorax **31:**113-117, 1976.

Applebaum, A., Karp, R. B., and Kirklin, J. W.: Surgical treatment for closed thoracic aortic injury, J. Thor. Cardiovasc. Surg. **77:**458-460, 1976.

Barber, J. M., and Budassi, S. A.: Mosby's manual of emergency care, St. Louis, 1979, The C. V. Mosby Co.

Bryant, L. R., Mobin-Uddin, K., Dillon, M. L., Hinshaw, M. A., and Utley, J. R.: Cardiac valve injury with major chest trauma, Arch. Surg. **107:**279-283, 1979.

Budassi, S. A.: Chest trauma, Nurs. Clin. No. Amer. **13:** 533-541, 1978.

Chambers, A. A.: Traumatic aortic rupture, J.A.M.A. **229:**463, 1974.

Cordell, R. A.: Evaluation of major cardiac and vascular injury to the chest, Emerg. Med. Serv. July/August 1977, pp. 11-16.

Crawford, W. O.: Pulmonary injury in thoracic and nonthoracic trauma, Rad. Clin. No. Amer. **11:**527, 1973.

Defore, W. W., Mattox, K. L., Hansel, H. A., and others: Surgical management of penetrating injury of the esophagus, Am. J. Surg. **134:**734-738, 1977.

Doty, D. B., Anderson, A. E., Rose, E. C., and others: Cardiac trauma, Ann. Surg. **180:**452-60, 1974.

Flint, L. N., Jr.: Injuries to major vessels: an overview of current concepts, Heart and Lung **5:**301-306, 1976.

Haddon, W. J., and Baker, S. P.: Injury control, Washington, D.C., 1978, Insurance Institute for Highway Safety.

Hardy, J. D., Tompkins, W. C., Ching, E. C., and Chaves, C. M.: Esophageal perforations and fistulas, Ann. Surg. **177:**788-796, 1973.

Jackson, D. H., and Murphy, G. W.: Nonpenetrating cardiac trauma, Mod. concepts Cardiovasc. Dis. **45:**123-128, 1976.

Kish, G., Kozloff, L., Joseph, W. L., and Adkins, P. C.: Indications for early thoracotomy in the management of chest trauma, Ann. Thor. Surg. **27:**23-28, 1976.

Lance, E., and Sweetwood, H.: Chest trauma: what to do in the first critical minutes, In Robinson, J., editor: Giving emergency care competently, Harsham, Pa., 1978, Nursing '78 Books, Intermed. Communications, pp. 71-79.

Kiedtke, A. S., and deMuth W. E., Jr.: Nonpenetrating cardiac injury, Am. Heart J. **86:**687, 1973.

Maloney, J. V., Jr., Schmutzer, K. J., and Raschke, E.: Paradoxical respiration and pendelluft, J. Thorac. Cardiovasc. Surg. **41:**291, 1961.

Marsh, D. G., Sturm, J. T.: Traumatic aortic rupture: roentgenographic indications for angiography, Ann. Thor. Surg. **21:**337-340, 1976.

Mattox, K. L.: Management of penetrating chest trauma, Hosp. Med. **13:**8-13, 1977.

Moraes, C. R., Victor, E., Arruda, M., Cavalcanti, I., and others: Ventricular septal defect following nonpenetrating trauma: case report and review of the surgical literature, Angiology **24:**222-229, 1973.

Naclerio, E.: Chest injuries, New York, 1971, Grune & Stratton, Inc.

Naclerio, E.: CIBA symposium on chest trauma, **22:**3, Summit, N.J., 1970, The CIBA Corp.

Oliver, C.: Open thoracotomy, Crit. Care Q. **1:**67-70, 1978.

Payne, D. D., DeWeese, J. A., Mahoney, E. B., and Murphy, G. W.: Surgical treatment of traumatic rupture of the normal aortic valve, Ann. Thor. Surg. **17:**223-229, 1974.

Pories, W. J., and Gaudiani, V. A.: Cardiac tamponade, Surg. Clin. No. Am. **55:**573, 1975.

Rea, W. J., Gallivan, G. J., Ecker, R. R., and Snugg, W. L.: Traumatic esophageal perforation, Ann. Thor. Surg. **14:**671-677, 1972.

Reul, G. J., Jr., Beall, A. C., Jr., Jordan, G. L., and Mattox, K. L.: The early operative management of injuries to the greater vessels, Surgery **74:**862, 1973.

Rutherford, R. B.: Thoracic injuries. In the management of trauma, Philadelphia, 1973, W. B. Saunders Co.

Rutherford, R. B., Hunt, H. H., Jr., Brickman, R. D., and Tubb, J. M.: The pathophysiology and treatment of progressive tension pneumothorax, J. Trauma **8:**212, 1968.

Sawyers, J. L., Lane, C. E., Foster, J. H., and Daniel, R. A.: Esophageal perforation: an increasing challenge, Ann. Thor. Surg. **19:**233-238, 1975.

Sinclair, M. C., and Moore, T. C.: Major surgery for abdominal and thoracic trauma in childhood and adolescence, J. Ped. Surg. **9:**155, 1974.

Smith, J. M. III, Grover, F. L., Marcos, J. J., Arom, K. V., and Trimble, J. K.: Blunt traumatic rupture of the atria, J. Thorac. Cardiovasc. Surg. **71:**617-620, 1976.

Stallone, R. J., Ecker, R. R., and Sampson, P. C.: Management of major acute thoracic vascular injuries, Am. J. Surg. **128:**249, 1974.

Symbas, P. N.: Traumatic injuries of the heart and great vessels, Springfield, Ill., 1972, Charles C Thomas Publisher.

Symbas, P. N.: Cardiac trauma, Am. Heart J. **92:**367-396, 1976.

Symbas, P. N.: Penetrating cardiac wounds: a comparison of different therapeutic methods, Ann. Surg. **183:**377-381, 1976.

Trinkle, J. K., Richardson, J. D., Franz, J. L., Grover, E. L., and others: Management of flail chest without mechanical ventilation, Ann. Thorac. Surg. **19:**355, 1975.

Von Koch, L., DeFore, W. W., Mattox, K. L.: A practical method of autotransfusion in the emergency center, Am. J. Surg. **133:**770-772, 1977.

Webb, W. R.: Thoracic trauma, Surg. Clin. No. Am. **54:**1170, 1974.

CHAPTER 17

Chest pain and respiratory emergencies

CHEST PAIN OF CARDIAC ORIGIN

Of the total 600,000 people who die from myocardial infarction each year, 200,000 to 300,000 die in the first two hours of the infarction, before they have reached the hospital. Myocardial infarction may be medically treatable, and it has been statistically shown that the mortality rate from infarction can be reduced significantly if the patient receives proper medical care in the early phases of the infarction—thus, the advent of the mobile coronary care unit, where early care can be brought to the victim at his home or at the scene of the infarct.

Certain factors can increase the incidence of myocardial infarction. As these risk factors are compounded, the risk of myocardial infarction is also compounded. The known risk factors are cigarette smoking, hypertension, obesity, diabetes mellitus, a type A personality, lack of exercise, increasing age, poor diet, and family history of coronary artery disease. As an example, if a person smokes two packs of cigarettes a day, that person will have increased his risk of myocardial infarction by a multiple of four. Coronary artery disease is more prevalent in males than females; however, the female incidence is increasing. It has been demonstrated that, the greater number of risk factors a person has, the greater are his chances of having a myocardial infarction.

It has been conservatively estimated that more than 5.5 million people over the age of 18

have coronary artery disease. Coronary artery disease is a combination of two words: *atheroma,* which means lipid deposits, and *sclerosis,* which means smooth cell fibrosis.

Angina pectoris

When the myocardium becomes hypoxic, a retrosternal discomfort occurs known as angina pectoris. It is believed that this occurs as a result of an increased oxygen demand, an increased cardiac output, and the inability of that oxygen to reach the myocardium because of a block in the coronary arteries. The most prevalent cause of coronary artery occlusion is atherosclerosis. Other causes are emboli, coronary artery spasm, and dissecting aortic aneurysm.

Differential diagnosis of angina can be made by the history obtained from the patient. It is important to obtain answers to such questions as, What precipitated the pain? What relieved the pain? Did it come on suddenly? How long was the episode of pain? Five minutes? More? Less? What did the pain feel like? Was it stabbing? Crushing? Burning? Tearing? Where was the pain? Did it radiate to any other spot? Did you take nitroglycerine? Did it relieve the pain? The pain location of angina is different in different persons but usually stays in the same spot in that person from episode to episode.

Types of angina (Table 17-1). There are three types of angina: *Stable angina* or typical angina occurs as a predictable event following

Table 17-1. Differential diagnosis of angina*

	Stable angina	Unstable (preinfarction) angina
Location of pain	Substernal; may radiate to jaws and neck and down arms and back	Substernal; may radiate to jaws and neck and down arms and back
Duration of pain	1 to 5 minutes	5 minutes, occuring more frequently
Characteristic of pain	Ache, squeezing, choking, heavy; burning	Same as stable angina, but more intense
Other symptoms	None, usually	Diaphoresis; weakness
Pain worsened by	Exercise; activity; eating; cold weather; reclining	Exercise; activity; eating; cold weather; reclining
Pain relieved by	Rest; nitroglycerin; isordil	Nitroglycerin, isordil may only give partial relief
ECG findings	Transient ST depression; disappears with pain relief	ST segment depression; often T-wave inversion; but ECG may be normal

*From Barber, J. M., and Budassi, S. A.: Mosby's manual of emergency care: practices and procedures, St. Louis, 1979, The C. V. Mosby Co.

such activities as exercise or body strain. The typical angina attacks in *unstable angina,* or preinfarction angina, are prolonged, the attacks occur more frequently, and the episodes become more severe. *Prinzmetal angina,* or variant angina, occurs at rest. This pain usually occurs at the same time each day. During the attack, the patient may demonstrate an elevated ST segment. Prognosis in Prinzmetal angina is poor. There is a 50% mortality rate during the first year. In the early stages of the disease if coronary catheterization results are favorable, coronary artery bypass surgery is usually recommended.

Treatment of angina. The aims of treating angina are to increase coronary blood flow and to reduce myocardial oxygen demand. *Nitroglycerin* is the drug of choice in the treatment of angina pectoris. It is administered sublingually in $\frac{1}{100}$, $\frac{1}{150}$, and $\frac{1}{200}$ grain tablets. Nitroglycerin works by dilating the coronary arteries, reducing afterload (thereby decreasing blood pressure), reducing preload (venous return to the heart), and reducing left ventricular end diastolic pressure (LVEDP).

Myocardial infarction

Myocardial infarction, a localized ischemic necrosis of an area of the myocardium, is caused by a narrowing of one or more of the coronary arteries, possibly due to a spasm, hemorrhage, thrombus, or other unknown cause. The primary cause of coronary artery narrowing is believed to be atherosclerotic plaques. Other causes of myocardial infarction are hypovolemic shock as a result of hemorrhage or dehydration, embolic occlusion, or syphilitic aortitis. The size and the location of the infarct depend upon the coronary artery that is affected and the level at which the artery is blocked.

The most common myocardial infarction location is the anterior wall. This type of infarction is due to occlusion of the anterior descending branch of the left coronary artery. If the circumflex branch of the left coronary artery is blocked, an anterolateral infarction results. Posterior infarction is caused by a block in the right coronary artery. Inferior wall myocardial infarction can be caused by a block either in the left anterior descending or the right coronary arteries.

Pain (characterized as "crushing," "burning," "sharp," "heavy," and a variety of other descriptions) is described by one third of the victims of myocardial infarction. The pain has been said to last anywhere from several minutes to several weeks. It is theorized that localized hypoxia, lactate buildup, and sensory response of the hypoxic arteries contribute to pain. The location of pain varies: it may localize in the substernal area, or it may radiate into

Table 17-2. Serum enzymes in myocardial infarction*

Enzyme	Elevation (hours after infarction)	Peak	Return to normal
CPK (6-30)	2-5 hours	24-48 hours	2-3 days
SGOT (12-40)	6 hours	24-48 hours	3-4 days
LDH (150-300)	6-12 hours	48-72 hours	5-6 days
	6-12 hours	48-72 hours	10+ days
SGPT (6-53)	6-10 hours	24-48 hours	5 days

*From Barber, J. M., and Budassi, S. A.: Mosby's manual of emergency care: practices and procedures, St. Louis, 1979, The C. V. Mosby Co.

the jaw and down the left arm. The victim may experience nausea, vomiting, and hiccoughs because of phrenic nerve stimulation.

One will observe that blood pressure decreases, because poor pump action causes a decreased cardiac output. Sodium and water retention may occur as a result of decreased cardiac output and increased venous pressure. When myocardial infarction occurs, a proportional amount of ventricular failure occurs. When venticular failure is severe, the stroke volume decreases, resulting in an increase in ventricular diastolic pressure. The body's sympathetic response decreases the peripheral blood flow. A decrease in blood flow and pressure to the kidneys leads to a slow glomerular filtration rate. Because of this, the renal cells are stimulated, and renin production begins. With this increase in renin production, the angiotensin level increases. Angiotensin causes secretion of aldosterone. The combination of aldosterone increase and decreased glomerular filtration rate causes sodium and water retention and produces edema.

When auscultating the heart, one may hear a decreased first heart sound due to decreased myocardial contractility. One may also hear an increased second sound because of an increase in pulmonary artery pressure. An S_3 may be heard as a result of ventricular dilatation and increased ventricular fluid pressure. A pericardial friction rub may be heard as a result of transient pericarditis.

One may elicit pulsas alternans as a result of left heart failure. Increased pressure because of congestion causes a backflow of blood into the neck veins, which distends them when the patient is at a 45° angle. One will also see a prominent early V wave with a rapid, deep Y wave descent. The patient may also have an elevated temperature caused by inflammation and necrosis of myocardial tissue. As myocardial cells die and become necrotic, enzymes leak into the serum (Table 17-2).

The patient is diaphoretic as an autonomic nervous system response. The patient may demonstrate signs of anxiety as a result of pain and fear. The pulse rate increases because of a low output state and sympathetic nervous system response as a compensatory mechanism. The patient may also demonstrate cyanosis, caused by a decreased oxyhemoglobin and a decreased blood supply to the peripheral vascular system.

Pulmonary edema

Pulmonary edema, also known as "backward failure" or circulatory overload, is a result of backward pressure into the left atria and lungs, which causes an increased pressure in the pulmonary capillaries. This increase in pressure causes fluid to leak out of the capillaries and into the alveoli, producing what is commonly known as pulmonary edema. Pulmonary edema is a commonly seen acute medical emergency that requires prompt recognition and rapid management. When it is recognized and treated early, results of the treatment are usually dramatic and favorable. The normal fluid content in relation to the lung mass is 20%. In acute pulmonary edema, fluid content sometimes reaches greater than 1000%.

It is important to remember that pulmonary edema is a symptom of some other underlying disorder and should not be considered a diagnosis. It is most commonly of cardiac origin, although there are several other conditions that may also cause it. Some of the more frequent causes of pulmonary edema are myocardial infarction with left ventricular failure, aortic insufficiency, aortic stenosis, mitral stenosis, amyloidosis, myocarditis, hypertension, coronary artery disease, dysrhythmias (particularly tachycardia of greater than 180 beats/minute and bradycardia of less than 30 beats/minute), hyperthermia, hyperthyroidism, exercise, and severe congestive heart failure. Other causes are adult respiratory distress syndrome, heroin overdose, methadone overdose, inhalation of toxic substances, pulmonary embolism, high altitude, neurogenic causes, volume overload, anemia, uremia, disseminated intravascular coagulation, near drowning, renal impairment, lymphatic obstruction, bacteremic sepsis, beriberi, and anesthesia.

The onset of pulmonary edema is usually sudden. The initial complaint will likely be shortness of breath, even though the underlying process may have been going on for a prolonged period of time. The patient may also complain of tightness across the chest, anxiety, inability to lie down, a decreased exercise tolerance, paroxsysmal nocturnal dyspnea and orthopnea, cough, Cheyne-Stokes respirations, central and peripheral cyanosis, rales, rhonchi, and wheezes, distended neck veins, an S_3 gallop and decreased heart sounds, peripheral edema, tachycardia, and pink, frothy sputum.

The goals of therapy in pulmonary edema are to decrease hypoxia, improve ventilation, decrease pulmonary capillary wedge pressure, and improve myocardial contractility.

While obtaining a brief history from the patient or the family, assure that the ABCs are adequate. Check the patient's vital signs. He will usually be tachypneic, tachycardic, and hypertensive. It is estimated that 75% of patients experiencing pulmonary edema with congestive heart failure are hypertensive. Monitor the patient carefully for dysrhythmias. The pulmonary edema may be the result of a dysrhythmia, or dysrhythmias may be present because of hypoxia.

Lung auscultation will reveal rales and rhonchi; wheezes suggest cardiac asthma, which is caused by a reflex spasm of the airways.

When auscultating the heart, one will often hear an S_3 gallop rhythm of ventricular distension and/or muffled heart sounds.

Because there are no valves in the internal jugular vein, it can act as a manometer for the right atrium. To observe the jugular vein, the head should be turned to the left or the right and the vein should be observed at the posterior border of the sternocleidomastoid muscle. Place the patient in a semi-Fowler position. If the neck veins are distended more than 2 inches above the sternal notch, this suggests right atrial congestion. Examine the patient for peripheral edema, especially in dependent parts of the body, such as the arms, legs, feet, and sacral area.

Therapeutic intervention. It should be remembered that the following therapeutic interventions are meant to improve circulatory and ventilatory dynamics and will not alter the underlying disease process. Following initial life-threatening therapeutic intervention, one must study the cause of the pulmonary edema further.

HIGH FOWLER POSITION. The initial step in treating pulmonary edema is to place the patient in a high Fowler position. The patient should have his legs over the edge of the bed in a dependent position whenever possible. One will find that it will not be necessary to convince the patient to do this; he will insist on sitting up because he cannot tolerate lying down. This position decreases venous return to the heart, decreases the work of breathing, and increases tidal volume.

OXYGEN THERAPY. Administer oxygen to treat the hypoxic state. Therapy should begin with a nasal cannula with an oxygen flow of 6 to 8 liters/minute. When the patient is in a controlled environment, administer 100% oxygen by mask with intermittent positive pressure breathing (IPPB). This type of oxygen administration requires much reassurance and direction, because the patient will have the sensation that he is suffocating.

IV LINE. Initiate IV therapy with D/5/W at a keep open rate. This line is for the adminis-

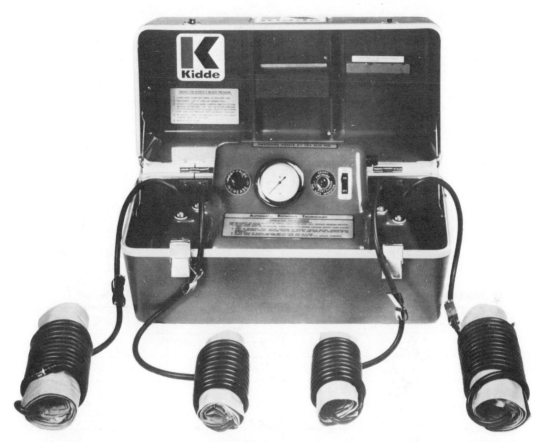

Fig. 17-1. Automatic rotating tourniquets. Cuffs are applied to four limbs and inflated and deflated periodically to rotate. (Courtesy Walter Kidde and Co., Inc., Belleville, N.J.)

tration of medications. Attach a control volume measuring device to the IV bottle.

ROTATING TOURNIQUETS. There is much controversy in the literature at present about the use of rotating tourniquets. Be sure to check with the facility at which you work regarding the policy regarding rotating tourniquets. Rotating tourniquets, also known as a "medical phlebotomy," are used to decrease venous return to the heart. They can either be individual wide-band cuffs or commercially available automatic rotating tourniquets (Fig. 17-1).

MORPHINE SULFATE. The patient should be medicated with morphine sulfate 8 to 15 mg in 2- to 3-mg increments, slow IV push every 3 minutes. Given to cause venous dilatation and venous pooling, morphine thereby causes

a decreased venous return to the heart. It also has the effect of a sedative, which allows the patient to be less anxious and slows his rate of breathing. It should be given with much caution, as it may cause respiratory depression. Attention must be paid to the rate and depth of respirations following administration, especially in patients with a history of chronic obstructive respiratory disease. Naloxone (Narcan) is a narcotic antagonist that may be administered (0.4 to 0.8 mg by IV push) if the patient develops respiratory distress as a result of morphine administration.

DIURETICS. Diuretics are given to decrease intravascular volume and produce a fluid loss. The diuretic of choice is furosemide (Lasix). The second drug of choice is ethacrynic acid.

ROTATION TOURNIQUETS TIME CHART

Right arm off	Left arm off	Left leg off	Right leg off
11:15	11:30	11:45	12:00

Furosemide will elicit a response in 5 to 15 minutes following IV administration.

DIGITALIS. To increase myocardial contractility and improve cardiovascular function, digitalis may be given.

AMINOPHYLLINE. Aminophylline may be used for its effect on the lungs, where it produces bronchodilitation and decreases bronchospasm. It also increases heart rate and myocardial contractility. The hazard of aminophylline administration is that it may produce life-threatening ventricular dysrhythmias.

PHLEBOTOMY. Although decreasing in popularity, phlebotomy is still employed in some institutions. In phlebotomy, 100 to 500 ml of venous blood are drawn from the patient's circulatory system in an attempt to reduce venous return to the heart.

ARTERIAL BLOOD GAS ANALYSIS. Arterial blood gas values should be measured; the following blood gas values are desirable: pO_2, 80 mm Hg; pCO_2, 30 to 40 mm Hg; and pH, 7.4.

REASSURANCE. Besides all the therapeutic measures, one should offer this patient as much reassurance as possible. These patients are very frightened and often have the feeling that they are suffocating and going to die. Verbal and touch reassurance is very important. Your words and touch can help them relax a bit and "breathe easier."

FOLEY CATHETER. We mention placement of a Foley catheter last because it should be used only if the patient cannot urinate by himself or if the patient is unable to control urination.

High-altitude pulmonary edema. Besides being the result of a medical illness, pulmonary edema can result from a person being exposed to a high altitude without the benefit of acclimation. High altitude pulmonary edema occurs when there is a rapid ascent to altitudes above 10,000 feet and the person is performing heavy physical activity for the first 3 days while at this altitude. Signs and symptoms of this disorder occur 6 to 36 hours after the initial exposure. It may also be seen in those who normally dwell at high altitudes, go to sea level for 2 or more weeks, and then return to the high altitude. This occurs in the absence of underlying cardiovascular disease or pulmonary disorders. It demonstrates itself as marked pulmonary hypertension and is treated with bed rest and oxygen therapy.

Congestive heart failure

Congestive heart failure occurs when the heart fails to function adequately as a pump. This results in venous congestion, a decreased stroke volume and cardiac output, and an increase in peripheral systemic pressure. Its onset may be sudden or gradual. It may be seen alone or in conjunction with pulmonary edema. The onset of congestive heart failure is a symptom of an underlying problem, which may include hypertension, fluid overload, intracranial injuries, myocardial infarction, and valvular heart disease. It may also be seen as a result of coronary artery disease, cardiomyopathy, and dysrhythmias (especially tachycardias of more than 180 beats/minute and bradycardias of under 30 beats/minute). Sometimes fever, hyperthyroidism, and adult respiratory distress syndrome may result in congestive heart failure. It may also be seen in oxygen toxicity syndromes, following pneumothorax, uremic pneumonia, intracranial tumors, and administration of certain drugs such as methotrexate, busulfan, hexamethonium, and nitrofurantoin.

Congestive heart failure is identified by the following: severe shortness of breath, dyspnea, weakness, dependent edema, distended neck veins, bilateral rales, an increased circulation time, and hepatomegaly.

While obtaining a brief history from the patient or family or friends, be sure to assess the patient for the adequacy of his airway, breathing, and circulation. Once these are established, check the vital signs, monitor the heart for dysrhythmias, auscultate the lungs and the heart, and observe the patient for the presence of distended neck veins and peripheral edema.

Therapeutic intervention includes placing the patient on bed rest and in a high Fowler position, administering oxygen therapy, digitalis, and diuretics, maintaining an intravenous line at a keep open rate, keeping track of accurate intake and output, applying rotating tourniquets if indicated, and weighing the patient.

Acute pericarditis

Acute pericarditis is an inflammation of the pericardial sac. It may occur as a result of trauma, infection, coronary artery disease, or neoplasms. Coxsackievirus, streptococci, staphylococci, tuberculosis, and *H. influenzae* are generally the causes in younger people; there are other causes in the middle-aged and elderly.

These patients will have severe chest pain, which increases with respirations and increased activity, fever, chills, and dyspnea. They will appear diaphoretic, and they may be hypotensive. Tachycardia or other dysrhythmias may be present, as well as a pericardial friction rub that increases in intensity when the patient leans forward. The patient complains of general malaise and demonstrates ST segment elevations of 1 to 3 mm in all ECG leads except a V_R and V_1.

Therapeutic intervention should include oxygen by nasal cannula at 4 to 6 liters/minute, sedation, and analgesia, bed rest, and much reassurance. This patient may also be placed on antibiotics.

Be aware that, if pericardial effusion results, there is great danger of cardiac tamponade.

Cardiac tamponade

Cardiac tamponade is a condition in which blood leaks into the pericardial sac and causes a compression of the heart. It may result from trauma, infection, or other rarer causes, such as neoplasms. The pericardial sac is nondistensible and, when filled with blood, may cause the cardiac output to drop. A positive effect of tamponade is that the tamponade places a pressure on the heart and may control hemorrhage. When the tamponade is great and a large amount of compression occurs, the patient may go into shock and die.

In cardiogenic shock, tamponade causes a decreased venous return to the heart, which elevates central venous pressure, distends the neck veins, and decreases cardiac output. This decreased cardiac output causes a compensatory vasoconstriction along with increased peripheral vascular resistance, which will initially demonstrate itself as a slightly elevated blood pressure.

As little as 150 to 200 ml of blood in the pericardial sac may cause a patient to go into profound shock. Removing 10 to 20 ml of blood from the pericardial sac may be enough to save a person's life.

Common signs and symptoms of cardiac tamponade are Beck's triad of elevated blood pressure, distended neck veins, and distant heart sounds. Other common signs are tachycardia and a central venous pressure of over 15 mm Hg. These are the cardinal signs of cardiac tamponade. If these signs are seen, immediately suspect tamponade. Other signs and symptoms include a decreased arterial pressure, a weak, thready pulse, cyanosis, increased respiratory rate, dyspnea, paradoxical pulse, restlessness, a widening cardiac silhouette, and finally, shock.

Therapeutic intervention includes an IV of D/5/W, oxygen at 6 liters/minute by nasal cannula, and pericardiocentesis (see pp. 361-362).

Paradoxical pulse. Paradoxical pulse is a finding in one third of the victims experiencing cardiac tamponade. Its cardinal sign is an abnormal fall in systolic blood pressure during inspiration. To check for a paradoxical pulse, apply a blood pressure cuff to the patient's arm, and pump the cuff up above the systolic sounds. Slowly deflate the cuff until the first systolic sound is heard. During normal inspiration the systolic sound will disappear. Deflate the cuff until all systolic sounds can be heard during both inspiration and expiration. The difference in millimeters of mercury between the pressure at which the systolic sound disappears during inspiration and the pressure at which *all* systolic sounds can be heard is called the paradox. A difference of more than 10 mm mercury indicates a paradoxical pulse.

CHEST PAIN OF AORTIC ORIGIN
Aortic dissection

One of the most commonly seen life-threatening disorders of the aorta is a dissection. It occurs primarily in men and is frequently seen in conjunction with hypertension and arteriosclerotic heart disease. It may also be seen following chest trauma and with Marfan's Syndrome.

An aortic dissection is a tear in the intimal layer of the aorta. As a result of this tear, blood leaks between the intimal layer and the medial layer. A type I dissection occurs in the ascending aorta and extends beyond the aortic arch. A type II dissection is a dissection of the ascending aorta alone. A type III dissection begins beyond the left subclavian artery.

As the aorta dissects, it may occlude the major vessels that branch off the aorta. These include the myocardial vessels, cerebral vessels, mesenteric vessels, and renal vessels.

Rupture of a dissection may cause either (1) cardiac tamponade, as a result of blood filling the pericardial sac or (2) rupture into the chest cavity, causing exsanguination.

Signs and symptoms of aortic dissection include a complaint of "excruciating" or "tearing" anteroposterior pain, dyspnea, orthopnea, diaphoresis, pallor, apprehension, syncope, tachycardia, unilateral absence of major arterial pulses, blood pressure differences between arms, hypertension, pulsation at the sternoclavicular joint, murmur of aortic insufficiency (in ascending aorta dissection), hemiplegia or paraplegia, and shock. The chest pain will most likely be confused with that of myocardial infarction, severe back strain, pericarditis, or peptic ulcer. A widening mediastinum will show up on x-ray film.

Therapeutic intervention includes a high Fowler position, high-flow oxygen using nasal cannula, an IV of D/5/W, antihypertensive agents, much support and reassurance, and possible preparation for surgery.

CHEST PAIN OF PULMONARY ORIGIN
Pulmonary embolus

The signs and symptoms of pulmonary embolus are frequently confused with those of myocardial infarction, pneumothorax, rib fractures, or other entities that present with chest pain. Because of this, pulmonary embolus is one of the most difficult conditions to diagnose in the emergency department.

Pulmonary embolus is the complication of a disease or condition whereby an embolus lodges in a branch of the pulmonary artery, causing a partial or total occlusion and, there-fore a pulmonary infarct. The embolus usually comes from the venous system of the legs, the pelvis, or the right heart. The embolus may consist of blood, fat, air, bone, amniotic fluid, or a foreign body.

Pulmonary embolus is most commonly seen following trauma, surgery, or a long bone fracture. It is also seen occasionally with obesity, a decreased peripheral circulation, congestive heart failure, and thrombophlebitis. Cardiac diseases or prolonged bed rest may cause pulmonary embolus. It may also occur in conjunction with acute infections, blood dyscrasias, childbirth (amniotic fluid emboli), SCUBA diving (air emboli), poor intravenous techniques (air emboli), oral contraceptives, or neoplasms.

When discussing pulmonary emboli, one should stress the preventive factors of this possibly devastating entity. Instruct your patients to ambulate frequently when taking a long trip by car, airplane, or other mode of transportation. Also instruct them to avoid long periods of standing where venous pooling may cause serious problems. Patients should be encouraged to ambulate early during the postoperative period. If a patient must be on bed rest, Ace wraps or elastic stockings should be employed on the lower extremities. These people should also have range-of-motion exercises performed several times daily.

When initiating an IV line, practice good IV technique; do not allow air to enter the tubing. Move severely traumatized patients carefully. It may also be wise to administer prophylactic antibiotics to those who risk developing pulmonary emboli.

Common signs of symptoms of pulmonary embolism are shortness of breath, tachypnea, tachycardia, and anginalike chest pain. They will also develop pallor and/or cyanosis, anxiety, an occasional decreased blood pressure, and possible wheezes. It may demonstrate itself on electrocardiogram as a right bundle branch block and right axis deviation with peaked P waves in the limb leads and a depressed T wave in the right precordial leads (V_1, V_2, V_3). Occasionally, however, there may be no signs and symptoms that precede the terminal event, or symptoms may be vague.

Therapeutic intervention includes maintenance of the basics of airway, breathing, and circulation, administration of oxygen at a high flow rate, an IV line of D/5/W, analgesia (usually meperidine—do not give morphine sulfate), bronchodilators, and management of dysrhythmias. Clotting times should be monitored using the Lee-White clotting time method. Heparin should be administered usually in a dosage range of 7,500 to 10,000 units initially, then 500 units every 4 hours. Posteroanterior and lateral chest x-ray films will help confirm the diagnosis. Remember that these patients require much reassurance, as they are usually quite frightened.

Spontaneous pneumothorax*

A spontaneous pneumothorax is generally caused by the rupture of a pulmonary bleb. These blebs are found in younger people (16 to 26 years) as a congenital anomaly. They are seen in older people as a process that has developed from chronic obstructive pulmonary disease (COPD). Some of the other causes of spontaneous pneumothorax may be the administration of mechanical ventilation, the rupture of a cyst, an abscess or fungal disease, cancer or tuberculosis, trauma, chest compression in cardiopulmonary resuscitation, tracheostomy, or subclavian line placement.

Signs and symptoms may be minimal if the pneumothorax is small. However, if it develops to greater than 40%, the patient will demonstrate dyspnea, tachypnea, cyanosis, and sudden, pleuritic chest pain. There will be a decrease in breath sounds, and the patient will appear agitated.

If a tension results, one will notice a decreased motion of the chest wall, a deviated trachea, distended neck veins, a mediastinal shift, tympany on percussion and eventually, shock.

The goal of therapeutic intervention is to reexpand the collapsed portion of the lung. In order to do this, one must administer oxygen at

---

*Additional information and definitive procedure guidelines for pneumothoraces that require surgical repair can be found in Chapter 16.

high liter flow, initiate an IV line of D/5/W, place the patient at rest in a high Fowler position, and either place needles in the anterior chest wall or a chest tube in the second or fifth intercostal space in the midaxillary line to decompress the chest cavity. (See also pp. 354-359.)

When therapeutic intervention is applied in tension pneumothorax, it is important to remember that an absolute diagnosis is made by chest x-ray examination. However, if the symptoms are severe, do *not* delay definitive therapy until a chest x-ray film is obtained.

Pleurisy

Pleurisy is an inflammation of the lining of the chest cavity. It results from tuberculosis, pneumonia, trauma, and tumors. Dry pleurisy (fibrinous) presents as sharp chest pain that increases with inspiration, with the patient taking short quick breaths and sometimes lying on his affected side. Therapeutic intervention includes bed rest, analgesia, sedation, and oxygen administration.

Exudative pleurisy (with effusion) usually results from an infectious process. The patient has dyspnea, an elevated temperature, and a history of dry pleurisy. Therapeutic intervention includes bed rest, analgesia, a thoracentesis to remove fluid, antipyrectics, and oxygen at moderate flow rates.

Pneumonia

Pneumonia results from an acute bacterial, viral, or fungal infection. It may be preceded by an upper respiratory tract infection, an ear infection, or an eye infection, or it may occur as the primary illness, without other medical precipitating causes. It occurs primarily in young children, elderly people, and those who are debilitated.

Pneumonia may be classified according to the causative organism (pneumococcal or streptococcal) or according to location (bronchial or lobar). People who develop pneumonia often have been bedridden or have an underlying cardiac or pulmonary disorder. Other causes include smoking, diabetes mellitus, exposure to extreme changes in environmental tempera-

Table 17-3. Antibiotics in pneumonia

Type of pneumonia	Antibiotic
Pneumococcal	Penicillin
Staphylococcal	Methicillin
Gram-negative organisms	Gentamycin
Micoplasma	Erythromycin, tetracycline, doxycycline
Aspiration	Penicillin, steroids
Viral	No known therapy

tures, steroids, or immunosuppression therapy. Pneumonia is often seen in alcohol or drug abusers, who have a tendency to aspirate. It is also seen in other conditions in which the victim has aspirated.

A patient with pneumonia has an elevated temperature of 39.4 to 40° C. He will be diaphoretic and may complain of chest pain that may be referred diaphragmatically and mistaken for gastrointestinal disorder. He will have a productive cough, be tachypneic, tachycardic, cyanotic, and apprehensive, complaining of abdominal distension, vomiting, and headache.

The aim of therapeutic intervention is to relieve respiratory distress and control infection. This can be accomplished by administering humidified oxygen and antibiotics (Table 17-3), controlling fluid and electrolyte balance, and encouraging the patient to cough, turn, and breathe deeply frequently.

Occasionally pneumonia is complicated by rupture of a pneumatocele, which produces a pneumothorax or an empyema. Therapeutic intervention for both is placement of a chest tube (see p. 357).

CHEST PAIN OF OTHER ORIGINS
Hyperventilation syndrome

Hyperventilation is one of the most commonly seen conditions in the emergency department. It may occur as a result of an anxiety disorder, or it may be a response to a disease process such as myocardial infarction, salicylate overdose, or intracerebral bleeding. So it is

of utmost importance to treat this patient with extreme caution and pay attention to other presenting signs and symptoms of an underlying disorder.

A patient who comes to the emergency department with a chief complaint of hyperventilation brings with him a difficult diagnostic problem. It is important to avoid "tunnel vision" and to keep one's mind open to all possibilities for a diagnosis. Remember that hyperventilation may be a response to an organic process—one in which the traditional treatment of breathing into the paper bag would cause severe impairment to the patient. Medical illness must be ruled out before assuming that the victim is hyperventilating as a response to hysteria.

Hyperventilation can be a sign of many illnesses, including anxiety, pregnancy, fever, liver disease, trauma and hypovolemia, pulmonary embolus, stress, ketoacidosis, high altitude reaction, thyrotoxicosis, pulmonary hypertension, and pulmonary edema, anemia, CVA or intracerebral catastrophe, a central nervous system lesion, and fibrotic lung disease.

Hyperventilation causes the arterial pCO_2 to drop (hypocapnea) and cerebral vasculature to constrict, causing a respiratory alkalosis and demonstrated as symptoms of tetany.

Signs and symptoms of hyperventilation syndrome include anxiety and panic, shortness of breath, tingling of the fingers and toes and periorbital numbness, carpopedal spasm, confusion, syncope, and occasionally, chest pain.

Therapeutic intervention includes pointing out to the patient what he is doing. Explain what is happening and why. Act in a calm and reassured manner. Have the victim talk to you—it is very difficult to hyperventilate while talking. As a last resource, have the victim rebreathe into a paper bag (carbon dioxide rebreathing).

Again, remember to look for underlying causes of the hyperventilation before treating it as a reaction to an emotional state.

• • •

Other causes of chest pain may be of abdominal origin. With such illnesses as a hiatus

Table 17-4. Differential diagnosis of chest pain*

Cause	Onset of pain	Characteristic of pain	Location of pain
Acute myocardial infarction	Sudden onset; lasts more than 30 minutes to 1 hour	Pressure, burning, aching, tightness, choking	Across chest; may radiate to jaws and neck and down arms and back
Angina	Sudden onset; lasts only a few minutes	Aches, squeezing, choking, heaviness, burning	Substernal; may radiate to jaws and neck and down arms and back
Dissecting aortic aneurysm	Sudden onset	Excruciating, tearing	Center of chest; radiates into back; may radiate to abdomen
Pericarditis	Sudden onset or may be variable	Sharp, knifelike	Restrosternal; may radiate up neck and down left arm
Pneumothorax	Sudden onset	Tearing, pleuritic	Lateral side of chest
Pulmonary embolus	Sudden onset	Crushing (but not always)	Lateral side of chest
Hiatus hernia	Sudden onset	Sharp, severe	Lower chest; upper abdomen
Gastrointestinal disturbance or cholecystitis	Sudden onset	Gripping, burning	Lower substernal area, upper abdomen
Degenerative disk (cervical or thoracic spine) disease	Sudden onset	Sharp, severe	Substernal; may radiate to neck, jaw, arms, and shoulders
Degenerative or inflammatory lesions of shoulder, ribs, scalenus anterior	Sudden onset	Sharp, severe	Substernal; radiates to shoulder
Hyperventilation	Sudden onset	Vague	Vague

*From Barber, J. M., and Budassi, S. A.: Mosby's manual of emergency care, St. Louis, 1979, The C. V. Mosby Co.

History	Pain worsened by	Pain relieved by	Other
Age 40 to 70 years; may or may not have history of angina	Movement, anxiety	Nothing; no movement, stillness, position, or breath holding; only relieved by medication (morphine sulfate)	Shortness of breath, diaphoresis, weakness, anxiety
May have history of angina; circumstances precipitating; pain characteristic; response to nitroglycerin	Lying down, eating, effort, cold weather, smoking, stress, anger, worry, hunger	Rest, nitroglycerin	Unstable angina appears even at rest
Nothing specific except that pain is usually worse at onset			Blood pressure difference between right and left arms, murmur of aortic regurgitation
Short history of upper respiratory infection or fever	Deep breathing, trunk movement, maybe swallowing	Sitting up, leaning forward	Friction rub, paradoxical pulse over 10 mm Hg.
None	Breathing		Dyspnea, increased pulse, decreased breath sounds, deviated trachea
Sometimes phlebitis	Breathing		Cyanosis, dyspnea, cough with hemoptysis
May have none	Heavy meal, bending, lying down	Bland diet, walking, antacids, semi-Fowler position	
May have none	Eating, lying down	Antacids	
May have none	Movement of neck or spine, lifting, straining	Rest, decreased movement	Pain usually on outer aspect of arm, thumb, or index finger
May have none	Movement of arm or shoulder	Elevation and arm support to shoulder, postural exercises	
Hyperventilation, anxiety, stress, emotional upset	Increased respiratory rate	Slowing of respiratory rate	Be *sure* hyperventilation is from nonmedical cause!

hernia, a gastric or peptic ulcer, pancreatitis, esophageal spasms, or other entities such as Mallory-Weiss syndrome or Borhave's syndrome, the patient may complain of chest pain. These are discussed in Chapter 18. Additional problems that could possibly cause chest pain are musculoskeletal disorders involving trauma, degenerative disc disease, xiphoidalgia, costrochondritis, Mondor's disease, or postherpetic syndrome (Table 17-4).

RESPIRATORY PROBLEMS

It is important to be familiar with the meaning of several terms that are used frequently in respiratory disorders.

ventilation—the amount of air passing into and out of the lungs
hypoventilation—not enough air going in and out of the lungs
hyperventilation—too deep and too rapid respirations
tidal volume—amount of air breathed in on each normal breath
tachypnea—a respiratory rate greater than 20/minute
dyspnea—shortness of breath (objective)
orthopnea—difficult breathing except in an upright position
stridor—crowing sound heard with upper respiratory obstruction

To assess the tidal volume without the assistance of a sophisticated piece of equipment, one should place the back of one's hand near the patient's mouth and nose to feel for air movement and place the hands on the patient's lower rib margin and feel for chest movement. With a little practice, one can become very accurate at assessing total volume this way.

One should begin assessment of any patient complaining of respiratory distress with the basic airway, breathing, and circulation. Once it is assured that these are present, listen for noises. If there is noise, there is obstruction. Check the patient's level of consciousness. Check skin vital signs of color, moisture, and temperature. Waht do the respirations sound like? What do they look like? Are they shallow? Deep? Is the patient using accessory muscles of respiration, such as the sternocleidomastoid muscles, the abdominal muscles, or is there

supraclavicular indrawing? Last, check for paradoxical movement of the chest wall.

Dyspnea

Dyspnea is the subjective finding that the victim is short of breath. It is one of the most frequently seen complaints in both the prehospital and emergency care settings and is one of the findings in many disease and trauma entities. It is essential to make a rapid and accurate assessment of the problem and intervene therapeutically as fast as possible before disaster sets in.

To be able to accurately assess the problem, one must ask questions, such as when the shortness of breath began, and what, if known, caused it to happen. It is important to know whether the episode came on gradually or suddenly. Ask the patient if the problem is in getting air into his lungs or in getting air out of his lungs. This may be a repeated episode, and he may be able to tell you what happened the last time this happened and how it was treated. He also may be able to tell you if this episode is worse or less severe than previous episodes.

Ask the patient about a history of lung disease or heart disease. Ask him if he has a history of asthma or hypertension. Be sure to use terms with which he is familiar. Ask the patient if he smokes, is taking any medications, or has difficulty walking short distances or up stairs.

Look for the objective signs of shortness of breath of obvious respiratory distress, flaring of the nostrils, cyanosis, pallor, and decreasing level of consciousness.

It a patient is indeed short of breath, be sure that the ABCs of airway, breathing, circulation are present or have been established. If the patient is still conscious, place him in a high Fowler position and administer oxygen. If the patient has a history of chronic obstructive lung disease, run the oxygen at 2 liters/minute. If there is no history of lung disease, administer oxygen at 6 to 8 liters/minute per nasal cannula or mask (if the victim will tolerate it). Initiate an IV line of D/5/W to keep the vein open. Also administer aminophylline 250 mg in 25 ml D/5/W over 5 to 10 minutes.

Asthma

Asthma is an obstruction of air flow to or from the lungs that may be caused by secretions, swelling, or spasms. This produces bronchospasm, hypoxia, and anxiety. Between attacks the lungs and the bronchial tree are normal.

It is estimated that over 8 million people in the United States have asthma. It may occur at any age and is believed to be caused by a bronchial tree that is sensitive to inhaled substances, such as pollen, molds, feather dust, animal dander, dust, gases, insecticides, and foods such as chocolate, milk, or seafood.

Besides these, asthma may be caused by excessive stress, depression, cigarette smoke, a pulmonary embolus, nasal polyps, other allergies, or cardiovascular problems.

Therapeutic intervention includes administration of epinephrine 1:1000 solution in a subcutaneous dosage of 0.1 to 0.3 ml. This dosage may be repeated at 20-minute intervals up to a total of three doses. If the epinephrine is not successful in clearing the asthma, one may elect to administer aminophylline in a pediatric dosage of 4 mg/kg or 500 mg in 50 ml D/5/W in an adult, to run intravenously over 20 minutes, followed by an IV drip of 500 mg aminophylline in 1000 ml D/5/W to run slowly (at least over 6 hours). Before placing these patients on oxygen, obtain an arterial blood gas. If arterial pH demonstrates severe acidosis, sodium bicarbonate should be administered accordingly. Monitor fluid and electrolyte balance, and replace accordingly. Treat dysrhythmias routinely, and offer the patient much reassurance.

Status asthmaticus

Although there are various definitions of status asthmaticus, generally defined it is a state of severe asthma that has not responded to subcutaneous epinephrine doses. One can make a definitive diagnosis by examining the patient's history, in which he will tell you that his dyspnea has gradually increased over the past few days, that his chest feels tight, and that his cough has been nonproductive. He will be found to have tachycardia and inspiratory-expiratory wheezes. Remember that if the asthma is so severe, there may be no air movement and there may be no wheezes. This patient will be anxious and will be sitting in an upright position and forward using his accessory muscles of respiration to breathe. He may tell you that he has used his isoproterenol (Isuprel Medihaler) several times without success. He will appear mildly cyanotic, and his neck veins will distend on expiration.

Therapeutic intervention includes determination of arterial blood gases, administration of high-flow oxygen, initiation of an IV line of D/5/W, and administration of epinephrine 0.4 ml of a 1:1,000 solution subcutaneously every ½ hour for three to five doses. This should be followed by a drip of 500 mg aminophylline in 50 ml D/5/W over 5 to 10 minutes in an adult or 3 to 4 mg/kg every 8 hours in a child, not to exceed 12 mg/kg in 24 hours. Intermittent positive pressure breathing (IPPB) should be administered, with a solution of either isoproterenol or N-acetylcysteine. If indicated, intubation through the endotracheal route should be performed. Also consider the use of sodium bicarbonate, steroids, sedation, antacids, and expectorants if indicated. Be sure to keep an accurate record of intake and output.

Bronchitis

Bronchitis is a chronic irritation of the bronchial mucosa, causing a frequent and productive reoccuring cough. It is caused by such things as cigarette and cigar smoke, air pollution, or chronic inhalation of irritating substances. It is commonly seen in the middle age group, more frequently in men than women, and may be a precursor to chronic obstructive lung disease.

The patient has dyspnea and a productive cough that increases in the evenings and in damp, rainy weather.

Therapeutic intervention includes removing the cause of the irritation and having the patient rest and drink plenty of fluids. One may also elect to employ bronchodilators, expectorants, and antibiotics if necessary. If the problem is a chronic one, the patient may choose to move to a dry, warm, dust-free climate.

Chronic obstructive lung disease

Chronic obstructive lung disease (also known as chronic obstructive pulmonary disease, COPD, COLD and emphysema) is a process in which the alveoli of the lungs enlarge and lose their elastic property and the alveolar wall begins to destruct. Because of the inelasticity of the alveoli, the patient is unable to exhale adequately, and there is much difficulty with adequate gas exchange at the alveolar level.

The exact cause of chronic obstructive lung disease is not known, but it is thought to have a positive connection to cigarette smoking, because 90% of patients who have this disease are smokers with a history of smoking more than one pack of cigarettes per day for many years. Other causative factors are thought to be pulmonary irritants such as air pollution, industrial inhalants (especially silicone), and tuberculosis.

When this patient comes to the emergency department, he will usually tell you that he has a history of emphysema and that he is experiencing dyspnea that has increased in severity over the past several days. He will appear cyanotic, especially in the lips, fingernails, and earlobes. His fingers will probably be clubbed, as this is a process which has gone on for a prolonged period of time. Assessment will show that the patient has a prolonged expiratory phase of respiration, and breath sounds are faint, with wheezes and rales present. He demonstrates a prolonged expiratory phase of respiration, and he uses his accessory muscles of respiration. One notices subclavicular and tracheal indrawing on inspiration. His cough is productive, and he offers a history of many years of smoking. He may have a barrel chest.

Therapeutic intervention in the acute phase of this disease includes placing the patient in a high Fowler position, administering oxygen at low liter flow (2 liters/minute by nasal cannula), initiating an IV line of D/5/W, and administering aminophylline 250 mg in 25 ml D/5/W to run over 5 to 10 minutes. When administering oxygen, be very careful to observe the patient for a positive response. Remember that the most serious, life-threatening event to the patient is hypoxemia. So, if the patient is not responding favorably to the initial therapy, do not hesitate to administer oxygen at a higher liter flow.

Smoke inhalation

When a person is exposed to a fire, besides being burned, he may also suffer from smoke inhalation or inhalation of a noxious gas that was created as a product of combustion. Although the burns may be minor, the inhalation of smoke may be life-threatening, because severe pulmonary damage may result in chemical pneumonitis, asphyxiation due to increased carboxyhemoglobin levels, or pulmonary edema.

When synthetic materials burn, the products of combustion usually include noxious gases (Table 17-5). These may produce additional pulmonary problems.

It is important to obtain a good history if a patient has been exposed to smoke or noxious gases. Find out how long the victim was exposed, if he was in a confined space, the type of material that was burning, and how much of the material was burning.

The primary manifestation of smoke inhalation is pulmonary edema, which may not exacerbate for 24 to 48 hours. Signs and symptoms of smoke inhalation include a mild irritation of the upper airway and a burning pain in the throat or chest. He may have singed nasal hairs, carbonaceous sputum, facial burns, and hypoxia. Pulmonary auscultation may reveal rales, rhonchi, or wheezes. He will be dyspneic and restless. He may cough, have a hoarse voice, and show other signs of pulmonary edema. If a patient has a history of being exposed to smoke of other noxious gases without other signs of pulmonary irritation, he should be observed for a period of several hours before being allowed to leave the hospital.

Therapeutic intervention for victims of smoke inhalation includes maintenance of the basic ABCs of airway, breathing, and circulation, administration of high-flow humidified oxygen, and an IV line of D/5/W TKO. Arterial blood gases should be drawn, and appropriate therapy should be administered in accordance with results. Encourage the patient to

Table 17-5. Data on toxic products of combustion*

Material	Use	Major toxic chemical products of combustion
Polyvinyl chloride	Wall and floor covering, telephone cable insulation	Hydrogen chloride (P)† Phosgene (P) Carbon Monoxide
Polyurethane foam	Upholstery	Isocyanates (P) (Toluene-2, 4-diisocyanate) Hydrogen cyanide
Lacquered wood, veneer, wallpaper	Wall covering	Acetaldehyde (P) Formaldehyde (P) Oxides of nitrogen (P) Acetic acid
Acrylic	Light diffusers	Acrolein (P)
Nylon	Carpet	Hydrogen cyanide Ammonia (P)
Acrilan	Carpet	Hydrogen cyanide Acrolein (P)
Polystyrene	Miscellaneous	Styrene Carbon monoxide

*From Genovese, M., Tashkin, D. P., Chopra, S., and McElroy, C. R.: Transient hypoxemia in firemen following smoke inhalation, Chest **71**:441, 1977.
†P = Pulmonary irritant.

cough and breathe deeply, and provide for chest physical therapy and tracheal toilet. These patients should be admitted to the hospital and should be observed for 24 to 48 hours. They may require endotracheal intubation, cricothyreotomy, or tracheostomy. Consider also bronchodilators, steroids, and a nasogastric tube.

Adult respiratory disease syndrome

Adult respiratory distress syndrome (also known as ARDS, shock lung, pulmonary contusion, Da Nang lung, congestive atelectasis, wet lung, and posttraumatic lung) is pulmonary congestion that occurs suddenly and causes atelectasis and hyaline membrane formation because of a decrease in surfactant and the buildup of mucous along the alveoli. It is acute and progressive respiratory failure that may be caused by a variety of conditions, such as a cardiopulmonary bypass, infection, pulmonary edema, and inhaled toxants. It may also be caused by hemorrhagic shock and multiple transfusions, contusions of the lung itself, fat emboli, aspiration, overdose, or eclampsia. It is also seen frequently in conjunction with diffuse intravascular coagulation (DIC).

The lungs initially appear normal, and then there is progressive atelectasis, increased interstitial and alveolar edema, and a marked ventilation-perfusion abnormality that results in progressive hypoxemia and difficulty breathing as lung compliance decreases.

Signs and symptoms of shock lung include dyspnea and tachypnea, cyanosis, hypoxemia, hypocapnea, pulmonary hemorrhage, and hypotension.

Therapeutic intervention includes maintenance of the basic ABCs of airway, breathing, circulation, endotracheal intubation or tracheostomy, ventilation with a volume-cycled ventilator with positive and expiratory pressure (PEEP) at 5 to 15 cm water pressure, diuretics, salt-poor albumin, fluid restriction, and possibly the administration of steroids and/or anticoagulants. One must also pay strict attention to providing meticulous pulmonary toilet.

PEEP prevents alveoli collapse, increases functional residual capacity, improves the V/Q relationship, combats pulmonary edema, and enhances FIO_2. PEEP is dangerous to use, however, because it increases the chance of oxygen toxicity and fluid overload, and it decreases cardiac output. It may cause a pneumothorax and infection. If one has chosen to use PEEP, and it has not proved effective, one may elect to place the patient into a hyperbaric oxygen chamber. Some practitioners choose to employ the bypass oxygenator.

Near drowning

Each year in the United States there are over 8,000 drowning deaths. Over half of these deaths occur in home swimming pools. Worldwide statistics indicate the over 140,000 drowning deaths occur in the world each year. Drowning is the second leading cause of accidental death in the United States each year and the fourth leading cause of death in children. It accounts for 10% of all accidental deaths, with 47% of these deaths are in children under the age of 4. The highest incidence of drowning occurs in those from 15 to 19 years of age. It is interesting to note that the incidence is five times higher in men than women.

Drowning or near drowning may result when a person cannot stay afloat because he is fatigued; he panics; or he experiences an acute medical/surgical emergency, such as myocardial infarction, seizure, or trauma. It may also result from hyperventilation before a long underwater swim, or it may be an attempted suicide.

Signs and symptoms of near drowning include progressive dyspnea, auscultatory wheezes, rales, and rhonchi, tachycardia, cyanosis, and a cough that produces a pink, frothy sputum. His temperature may be elevated but may initially be below normal because of a low water temperature. The patient may complain of chest pain and demonstrate mental confusion. He may have seizures and increased

muscle tone, and he may lapse into coma or cardiopulmonary arrest (Table 17-6).

Therapeutic intervention for the near-drowning victim includes maintenance of the basic ABCs of airway, breathing, and circulation. If indicated, employ advanced cardiac life support. Be sure to protect the cervical spine, as this may have caused the near drowning. Initiate an IV line, and administer plasma or a plasma substitute if possible. Administer oxygen under intermittent positive pressure breathing (IPPB), and employ PEEP. Suction the airway frequently. Correct any acid-base imbalance after obtaining a specimen for arterial blood gas values. Administer antibiotics, steroids and, isoproterenol (for bronchospasm). It would be wise at this point in the therapeutic intervention to place a nasogastric tube and a central venous pressure line or a Swan-Ganz catheter. This patient should be admitted to an intensive care unit for close observation for at least 24 hours.

Drowning is categorized into three types: dry, wet, and secondary. *Dry* drowning occurs in 10% to 20% of cases. It occurs when the victim asphyxiates because he cannot inspire oxygen as a result of laryngotracheal spasm, which prevents the entrance of water as well as air into the lungs. This results in cerebral anoxia, edema, and unconsciousness. The victims of dry, near drowning have the best chance of survival.

The second type of near-drowning is *wet* drowning. This occurs in 80% to 90% of cases. This victim usually makes a violent respiratory effort and consequently fills his lungs with water.

The third type of drowning is *secondary* drowning, which occurs with the recurrence of respiratory distress following a successful resuscitation and recovery from the initial incident. This often occurs as pulmonary edema or aspiration pneumonia, and may result anywhere from 3 minutes to 4 days after the initial incident.

Pulmonary edema that results from near drowning may occur as a result of both fresh water and salt water.

Salt water is a hypertonic solution and causes

Table 17-6. Significant differences between salt and fresh water aspiration*

Salt water	Fresh water
Hypoxia	
Greater degree of hypoxia; fluid in alveoli interferes with ventilation	Alteration of normal surface tension properties of surfactant with subsequent collapse of the alveoli; atelectasis; uneven ventilation and recurrent collapse continue until surface active material regenerates
Blood volume	
Hypertonic fluid draws water into the alveolar spaces causing a persistent hypovolemia; increase in blood osmolarity and viscosity	Hypotonic water rapidly absorbed into the circulation; transient hypervolemia; decrease in blood osmolarity and viscosity; elevated CVP
Serum electrolytes	
Changes usually insignificant; hyperkalemia may result from severe hypoxia and acidosis	
Picture may be complicated by ingestion of large amounts of salt water	
Hemoglobin	
Hemolysis occurs after aspiration of at least 11 ml of fluid/kg body weight, with a possible decrease in hemoglobin	
Hematocrit	
Technical problems make correct measurements almost impossible and interpretation difficult	
Cardiac changes	
Sufficient water to cause ventricular fibrillation is seldom aspirated	
Central venous pressure	
An increase in CVP coincides with hyperventilation; falls rapidly to normal when only small amounts of liquid have been aspirated	
Aspiration of large amounts of fluid results in initial rise in CVP, followed by a rapid drop to zero	Aspiration of large quantities of fluid results in a persistent rise in CVP
Neurological effects	
When sea water is ingested in large quantities, the magnesium ion may cause lethargy, drowsiness, and coma	
Urinary system	
Acute renal failure due to tubular necrosis resulting from hypoxia and hypotension	Acute renal failure due to hemolysis and hypotension

*From Warner, C. G., editor: Emergency care: assessment and intervention, ed. 2, St. Louis, 1978, The C. V. Mosby Co.

fluid to transverse the alveoli because of an osmotic pull across the alveolar capillary membrane, resulting in pulmonary edema. This type of near drowning also causes hemoconcentration and hypovolemia.

Fresh water is a hypotonic solution, and fluid rapidly tranverses out of the alveoli by diffusion. Fresh water contains contaminants such as chlorine, algae, and mud that cause surfactant breakdown and fluid seepage into the alveoli, also resulting in pulmonary edema. This type of near drowning causes hemodilution and hypervolemia and its resultant consequences. Pulmonary edema in both salt water and fresh water near drownings is complicated by the inflammatory response of the body.

MEASUREMENT AND MONITORING
Drawing blood for blood gas measurement*

Selection of site

Choose the radial, brachial, or femoral artery (Figs. 17-2 to 17-4).

Avoid limbs demonstrating poor circulation.

Avoid limbs where hematomas are present.

If the radial artery is selected, check for the presence of a positive Allen test.

ALLEN TEST. To assess for Allen's sign, palpate both the radial and ulnar pulses. Occlude both arteries with firm pressure and raise the arm to balance the hand. Release the ulnar ar-

---

*Modified from Budassi, S. A.: J.E.N. **3**(2):24-27, 1977.

tery and assess for return of color to the hand. If the hand *does not perfuse* (negative Allen's sign), this indicates that the ulnar artery is not capable of maintaining circulation to the hand. Therefore, do not attempt a radial artery puncture in the extremity (Figs. 17-5 and 17-6).

Suggested equipment

Container of crushed ice (plastic bag or emesis basin is fine)

Rubber or cork stopper or commercial blood gas cap

5-ml *glass* syringe

Two 22-gauge 1.5-inch needles

Two alcohol swabs

Sodium heparin, 0.5 ml (1000 units/ml)

One small dry gauze pad

Gummed label for syringe

Laboratory requisition slip with the following information: concentration of oxygen patient is receiving and by what route (FIO_2) and patient's rectal temperature at the time

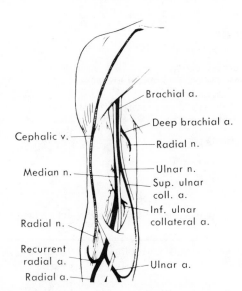

Fig. 17-2. Brachial artery, a continuation of axillary artery. *Advantages:* Easy to locate, not much arterial spasm, and easy to immobilize. *Disadvantages:* Radial and medial nerves in close proximity and venous system in close proximity making venous sampling possible. (From Budassi, S. A.: J.E.N. **3**[2]: 24-27, 1977.)

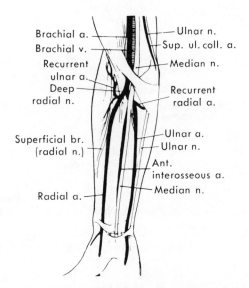

Fig. 17-3. Radial artery extends from neck of radius to median side of styloid process. *Advantages:* No close proximity to nerves and no close proximity to veins; thus venous sampling is unlikely. *Disadvantages:* Puncture may produce spasm, and artery is very small. (From Budassi, S. A.: J.E.N. **3**[2]:24-27, 1977.)

the specimen is collected (Both parameters affect calculation of values.)

Drawing the specimen

1. Explain the procedure to the patient.
2. Draw up 0.5 ml heparin into a *glass* syringe.
3. Flush the syringe with heparin (expel all air bubbles).
4. Replace the needle.
5. Select the puncture site.
6. Straighten the limb of the selected puncture site; position on a firm surface.
7. Palpate the artery: assess the pulse and position of artery.
8. Cleanse area over the puncture site with an alcohol swab (be sure to use plenty of friction and allow alcohol to dry before actual puncture).
9. Immobilize the artery between two fingers (be careful not to contaminate the puncture site).

10. Penetrate both the skin and the artery at a 45° to 90° angle, holding the syringe like a pencil (Fig. 17-7).
11. If the syringe begins to fill and the plunger begins to move spontaneously, this is usually an indication that the needle is in the artery.
12. If the syringe does not begin to fill spontaneously, withdraw the needle slightly (you may have gone all the way through the artery).
13. If systolic blood pressure is less than 100 mm Hg, the syringe may not fill spontaneously and it may be necessary to manually withdraw the plunger (for example, during CPR).
14. If the blood sample is not bright red or is bluish, this may indicate that the specimen is venous, and another attempt at an arterial specimen should be made.
15. Obtain 3 to 5 ml of arterial blood sample

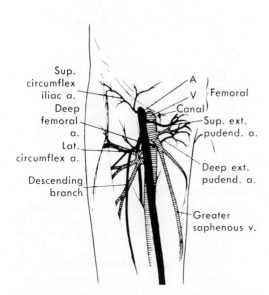

Fig. 17-4. Femoral artery branches from abdominal aorta and branches to superficial epigastric, superficial circumflex iliac, external pudendal, deep femoral, and descending genicular arteries. *Advantages:* Easily accessible. *Disadvantages:* May have large amount of interstitial bleeding before it is noticed. Close proximity to vein makes venous sampling possible. (From Budassi, S. A.: J.E.N. **3**[2]:24-27, 1977.)

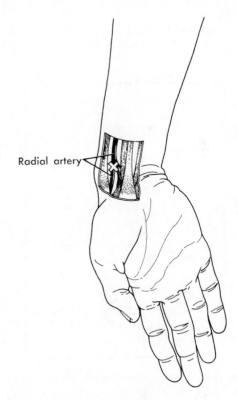

Fig. 17-5. Anatomical location of radial artery.

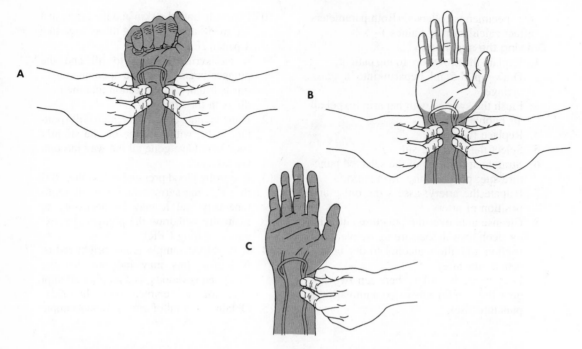

Fig. 17-6. To assess for Allen's sign, **A,** occlude both arteries with firm pressure, and **B,** raise arm to blanch hand. **C,** Release ulnar artery for return of color to hand.

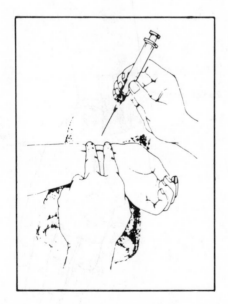

Fig. 17-7. Puncture of radial artery. (From Budassi, S. A.: J.E.N. **3**[2]:24-27, 1977.)

(some laboratories will accept less for analysis).

16. Withdraw the needle quickly.
17. Apply direct pressure with dry gauze.
18. Maintain pressure for 5 minutes (make certain to time it on your watch or the wall clock—it is difficult to estimate 5 minutes).

Care of specimen

1. Expel all air bubbles from the sample.
2. Stick the needle into a cork or rubber stopper, or remove the needle and cap the syringe.
3. Place the gummed label (containing patient's name and hospital number) on the syringe.
4. Place the syringe into the container of ice.
5. Send to laboratory immediately along with completed laboratory request form. (If you have a small laboratory, it frequently will help if you call the laboratory before obtaining the arterial speci-

	pH	CARBONIC ACID	BICARBONATE
ACIDOSIS	Low	Increase	Decrease
ALKALOSIS	High	Decrease	Increase

Acid-base balance is normally maintained by three different body systems: the respiratory system, the renal system, and the buffer system.

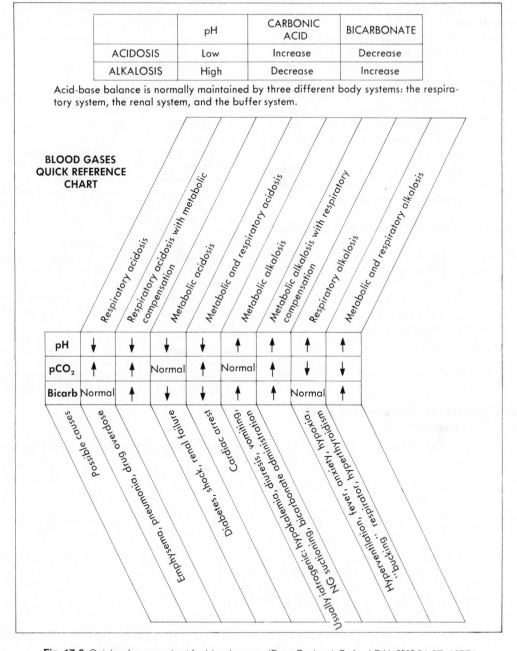

BLOOD GASES QUICK REFERENCE CHART

	Respiratory acidosis	Respiratory acidosis with metabolic compensation	Metabolic acidosis	Metabolic and respiratory acidosis	Metabolic alkalosis	Metabolic alkalosis with respiratory compensation	Respiratory alkalosis	Metabolic and respiratory alkalosis
pH	↓	↓	↓	↓	↑	↑	↑	↑
pCO₂	↑	↑	Normal	↑	Normal	↑	↓	↓
Bicarb	Normal	↑	↓	↓	↑	↑	Normal	↑

Possible causes: Possible drug overdose; Emphysema, pneumonia, drug overdose; Diabetes, shock, renal failure; Cardiac arrest; Hypokalemia, diuresis, vomiting; Usually iatrogenic: hypokalemia, bicarbonate administration; Hyperventilation, fever, anxiety, hypoxia; "bucking" respirator, hyperthyroidism

Fig. 17-8. Quick reference chart for blood gases. (From Budassi, S. A.: J.E.N. **3**[2]:24-27, 1977.)

men so that the blood gas analyzer can be calibrated before the arrival of the specimen in the lab.)

Aftercare

Assure that pressure is maintained over the puncture site for at least 5 minutes (sand bags will not do—use fingers!)

Do not use dressings or Band-aids that interfere with visualization of the puncture site. Patients with blood dyscrasias or who are anticoagulated may require a longer period of pressure to ensure that bleeding has ceased.

Observe the puncture site for at least 1 minute following removal of manual pressure for formation of a hematoma.

Reassess pulse.

Interpretation of arterial blood gas values
(Fig. 17-8)

Notice the pH value. 7.35 to 7.45 = normal; above 7.45 = alkalosis; below 7.35 = acidosis.

Note the bicarbonate level. 22 to 26 mEq = normal; metabolic alkalosis; below 22 mEq = metabolic acidosis.

Notice the pCO_2 value. 35 to 40 mm Hg = normal; above 45 mm Hg = respiratory acidosis; below 35 mm Hg = respiratory alkalosis.

Make an acid-base "diagnosis" based on the above criteria. Consider the effect on blood gas values of compensatory mechanisms. While the values are abnormal, they may not all fit the criteria. The variance is caused by the compensatory action—see the examples below.

acid —a hydrogen ion donor; carbonic acid (H_2CO_3) is an acid

base —a hydrogen ion acceptor; bicarbonate (HCO_3) is a base

acidosis —increased acid concentration and/or decreased base concentration; a pH of less than 7.4 is considered acidosis; a pH less than 7.3 is considered within the "danger range"; severe acidosis is a central nervous sytem depressant; *signs and symptoms:* judgement errors, lethargy, disorientation

alkalosis —increased base concentration and/or decreased acid concentration; a pH greater than 7.4 is considered alkalosis; a pH greater than 7.6 is considered within the "danger range"; severe alkalosis is a central nervous sytem excitant; *signs and symptoms:* tingling of fingertips, muscle spasms, seizures

pH —the hydrogen ion concentration of a solution; the relationship of carbonic acid (H_2CO_3) and bicarbonate (HCO_3) determines the pH of human serum; acid-base balance is a function of the ratio of carbonic acid (H_2CO_3) to bicarbonate (HCO_3)

ECG monitoring and plotting an axis
ECG MONITORING

Monitoring on a four-lead monitoring system (with an automatic lead switch button) is shown in Figs. 17-9 and 17-10.

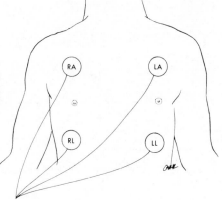

Fig. 17-9. Lead placement for four-lead monitoring system (with automatic lead switch button). (From Barber, J. M., and Budassi, S. A.: Mosby's manual of emergency care, St. Louis, 1979, The C. V. Mosby Co.)

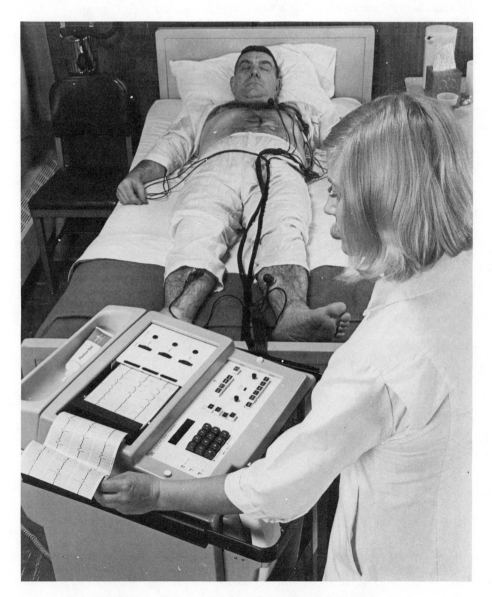

Fig. 17-10. Strip recorder. (Courtesy Hewlett-Packard, Palo Alto, Calif.)

Monitoring on a three-lead ECG monitor (without an automatic lead switch button) is shown in Fig. 17-11. Leads II and MCL₁ are the best leads to monitor for dysrhythmias.

Standard 12-lead ECG. The standard 12-lead ECG takes 12 views of the heart's electrical activity and records it on a wax-coated, standardized ECG paper.

BEFORE YOU BEGIN

1. Check to be sure that all leads are placed correctly (Figs. 17-12 and 17-13).
   a. "Green and white on the right." "Christmas trees (red and green) below the knees."
   b. Assure that there is a conduction medium between the electrodes and the patient.
   c. Avoid placing the electrodes over large muscle masses.
2. Assure that lead wires are not touching anything metal (this will cause 60-cycle interference).
3. Explain to the patient what you are doing.

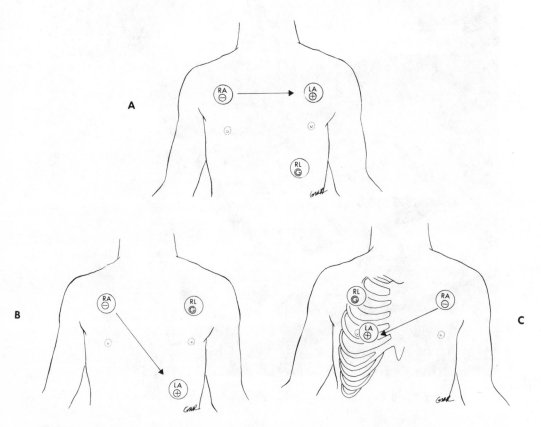

Fig. 17-11. Monitoring on a three-lead system (without automatic lead switch button). **A,** Lead I. **B,** Lead II. **C,** Lead MCL₁. Leads II and MCL₁ are best leads to monitor for dysrhythmias. (From Barber, J. M., and Budassi, S. A.: Mosby's manual of emergency care, St. Louis, 1979, The C. V. Mosby Co.)

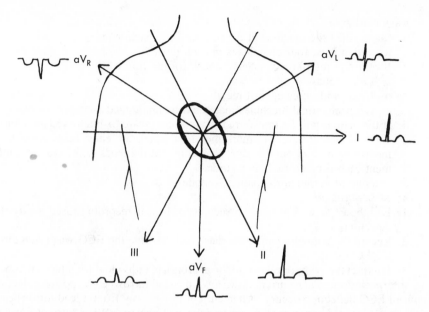

Fig. 17-12. The six limb leads. (From Barber, J. M., and Budassi, S. A.: Mosby's manual of emergency care, St. Louis, 1979, The C. V. Mosby Co.)

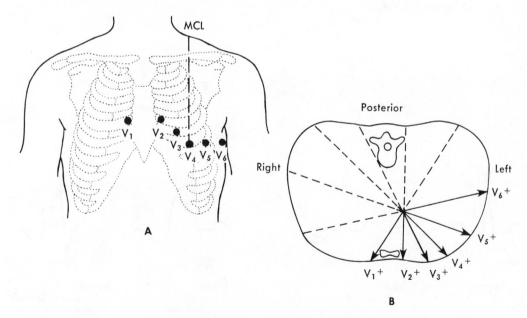

Fig. 17-13. A, Electrode positions of the precordial leads: V_1, fourth intercostal space at right sternal border; V_2, fourth intercostal space at left sternal border; V_3, halfway between V_2 and V_4; V_4, fifth intercostal space at midclavicular line; V_5, anterior axillary line directly lateral to V_4; V_6 midaxillary line directly lateral to V_5. **B,** Precordial reference figure. Leads V_1 and V_2 are called right-sided precordial leads; leads V_3 and V_4, midprecordial leads; and leads V_5 and V_6, left-sided precordial leads. (Modified from Andreoli, K., and others: Comprehensive cardiac care: a text for nurses, physicians, and other health practitioners, ed. 4, St. Louis, 1979, The C. V. Mosby Co.)

WHEN YOU BEGIN

1. Standardize the machine at the beginning of each lead.
2. Record at least four complexes in each lead.
3. If 60-cycle interference occurs, check for the following:
   a. Loose leads.
   b. Leads and wires against metal.
   c. Other electrical machines that could be unplugged.
4. If the patient will be transferred to a coronary care or intensive care unit where a daily ECG will be done, mark the chest where the chest leads are placed (with methylene blue or another dye) to ensure that the leads will have the same placement each time an ECG is recorded.
5. Attempt to maintain the patient's modesty.

AT THE CONCLUSION

1. End the ECG with at least 15 seconds of lead II recording (used for dysrhythmia detection).
2. Record the patient's name, the date, and the time the ECG was taken directly on the ECG strip.
3. Interpret the strip, or relay it to the appropriate individual for interpretation.

Interpretation. When current flows toward a lead (arrowheads, positive electrode), an upward ECG deflection occurs. When current flows away from a lead (arrowhead, positive electrode), a downward deflection of the ECG occurs. When current flows perpendicular to a lead (arrowhead, positive electrode), biphasic deflection of the ECG occurs.

When examining a 12-lead ECG, examine each of the 12 leads individually and note any of the following:

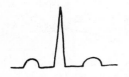 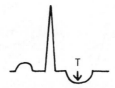 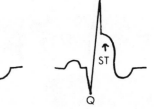

Normal

Ischemia
Decreased blood supply
T wave inversion
May indicate ischemia
without myocardial infarction

Injury
Acute or
recent; the
more elevated
the ST segment,
the more recent
the injury

Infarct
Significant Q wave
greater than 1 mm
wide and half the
height + depth of
the entire complex
Indicates myocardial
necrosis

The leads directly recording the area of infarct will demonstrate changes. An anterior wall myocardial infarction appears in leads V_1, V_2, and V_3.

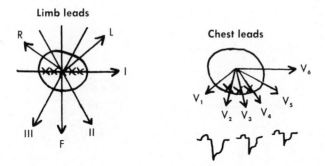

An inferior wall myocardial infarction appears in leads II, III, and aV_F.

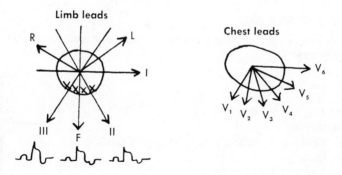

A lateral wall myocardial infarction appears in leads I, aV_L, V_5, and V_6.

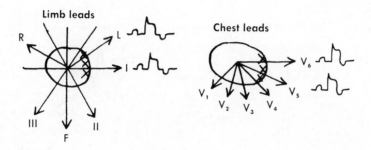

A posterior wall myocardial infarction appears in leads V_1 and V_2. The first R wave is tall, there is a depressed ST segment, and there is an elevated T wave.

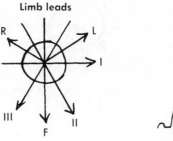

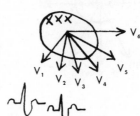

PLOTTING A SIMPLE AXIS

An axis is a graphic representation of the main vector in the heart.

EQUIPMENT
12-lead ECG
Graph paper
Ruler
Writing instrument

PROCEDURE
1. Draw leads I and aV_F lines on graph paper.

2. Examine lead I of the ECG.
   a. Determine if it is positive or negative.
   b. Determine by how much.

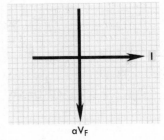

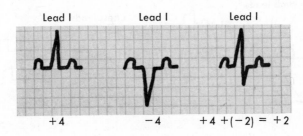

3. Plot the positive inflection or negative deflection on the graph paper by drawing a perpendicular line.
   a. Positive goes *toward* the lead.
   b. Negative goes *away from* the lead.

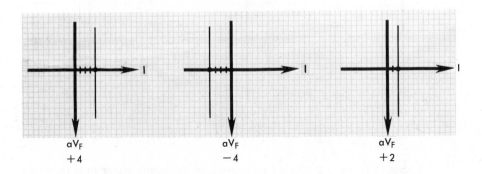

aV$_F$	aV$_F$	aV$_F$
+4	−4	+2

4. Examine lead aV$_F$ of the ECG.
   a. Determine if it is positive or negative.
   b. Determine by how much.

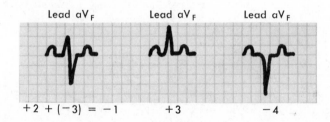

Lead aV$_F$ Lead aV$_F$ Lead aV$_F$

$+2 + (-3) = -1$ $+3$ -4

5. Plot the positive inflection or negative deflection on the graph paper by drawing a perpendicular line.
   a. Postive goes *toward* the lead.
   b. Negative goes *away from* the lead.

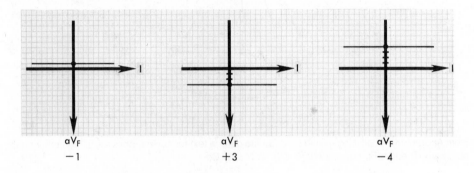

aV$_F$	aV$_F$	aV$_F$
−1	+3	−4

6. The intersection of the plots of leads I and aV_F is the axis.

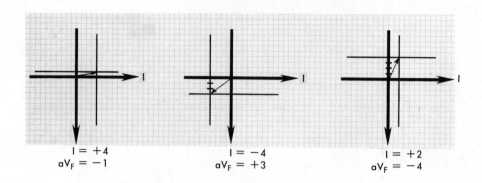

7. Superimpose a protractor compass over the graph paper to determine the exact degree of axis or estimate the degree of axis by quadrants.

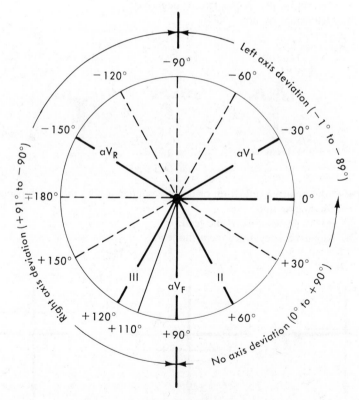

From Andreoli, K., et al.: Comprehensive cardiac care: a text for nurses, physicians, and other health practitioners, ed. 4, St. Louis, 1979, The C. V. Mosby Co.

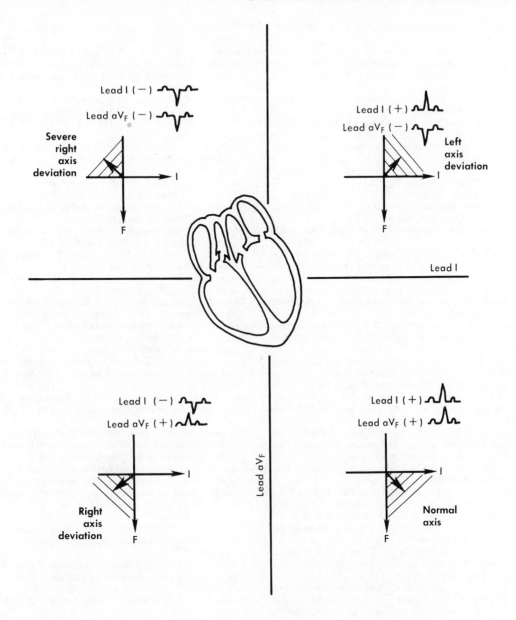

BIBLIOGRAPHY

Anagnostopoulos, C. F.: Acute aortic dissection, Baltimore, 1975, University Park Press.

Bache, R. J.: Effect of nitroglycerine and arterial hypertension on myocardial blood flow following acute coronary artery occlusion in the dog, Circulation **57**:557, 1978.

Barber, J. M., and Budassi, S. A.: Mosby's manual of emergency care, St. Louis, 1979, The C. V. Mosby Co.

Berte, J. B.: Pulmonary emergencies, Philadelphia, 1977, J. B. Lippincott Co.

Biddle, T. L.: Acute pulmonary edema, Hosp. Med. **13:** 56, December 1977.

Borer, J. S., Redwood, D. R., Levitt, B., and others: Reduction in myocardial ischemia with nitroglycerine or nitroglycerine plus phenylephrine administered during acute myocardial infarction, N. Eng. J. Med. **293:**1008, 1975.

Burch, G. E., and DePasquale, N. P.: Congestive heart failure—pulmonary edema. In Weil, M. H., and Shabin, H. editors: Critical care medicine, New York, 1976, Harper and Row.

Chatterjee, K., Swan, H. J. C., Kaushil, V. S., and others: Effects of vasodilator therapy for severe pump failure in acute myocardial infarction on short-term and late prognosis, Circulation **53:**797, 1976.

Clarke, E. B., and Higgeman, E. H.: Near-drowning, Heart Lung **4:**946, 1975.

Comroe, J.: Physiology of respiration, ed. 2, Chicago, 1974, Yearbook Medical Publishers.

Collinsworth, K. A., Kalman, S. M., and Harrison, D. C.: The clinical pharmacology of lidocaine as an antiarrhythmic drug, Circulation **50:**1217, 1974.

Dack, S.: Acute pulmonary edema, Hosp. Med. **14:**3, 1978.

Dalen, J. E., Alpert, J. S., Cohn, L. H., and others: Dissection of the thoracic aorta: medical or surgical therapy? Am. J. Cardiol. **34:**803, 1974.

Dauchot, P., and Gravenstein, J. S.: Bradycardia after myocardial ischemia and its treatment with atropine, Anesthesia **44:**501, 1976.

DeGowin, E. L., and DeGowin, R. L.: Bedside diagnostic examination, New York, 1969, MacMillan Publishing Co., Inc.

Epstein, S., Kent, K., Goldstein, R., and others: Reduction of ischemic injury by nitroglycerine during acute myocardial infarction, Physiol. Med. **292:**29, 1975.

Fowler, N. O.: Pericardial disease. In Hurst, J. W., editor: The heart, ed. 3, New York, 1974, McGraw-Hill Book Co.

Fuhs, M. F.: Respiratory crisis in nursing skillbook series: giving emergency care competently, Horsham, Pa., 1978, Intermed Communications, Chapter 6.

Fishman, A. P.: Shock lung: a destinative non-entity, Circulation **48:**921, 1973.

Galant, S. P.: Status asthmaticus. In Pascoe, D. J., and Grossman, M., editors: Quick reference to pediatric emergencies, Philadelphia, 1973, J. B. Lippincott Co.

Greenburg, M. I., and Walter, J.: Axioms in smoke inhalation, Hosp. Med. **14:**100, 1978.

Genovese, M., Tashkin, D. P., Chopra, S., and others: Transient hypoxemia in fireman following smoke inhalation, Chest **441:**71, 1977.

Gold, H. K., Leinbach, R. C., and Sanders, C. A.: Use of sublingual nitroglycerine in congestive failure following acute myocardial infarction, Circulation **46:**839, 1972.

Hancock, E. W.: Constrictive pericarditis: clinical clues to diagnosis, J.A.M.A. **232:**176, 1975.

Hopewell, P. C.: The adult respiratory distress syndrome, Ann. Rev. Med. **27:**343, 1976.

Luria, M. H., Knoke, J. D., and Margolis, R. M.: Acute myocardial infarction: prognosis after recovery, Ann. Intern. Med. **85:**561, 1976.

Madias, J. E., and Hood, W. B., Jr.: Reduction of ST-segment elevation in patients with anterior myocardial infarction by oxygen breathing (brief communication), Circulation **53:**Supplement 1, 198, 1976.

Maroko, P. R., Radvany, P., Braunwald, E., and Hale, S. L.: Reduction of infarct size by oxygen inhalation following acute coronary occlusion, Circulation **52:**360, 1976.

Mason, D. T.: Congestive heart failure: mechanisms, evaluation and treatment, New York, 1976. Dun-Donnelly Pub. Co.

Miller, R. H.: Textbook of basic emergency medicine, ed. 2, St. Louis, 1980, The C. V. Mosby Co.

Pontoppidan, H.: Acute respiratory failure in the adult, N. Engl. J. Med. **287:**690, 1972.

Raffin, R. A., and Theodore, J.: Separating cardiac from pulmonary dyspnea, J.A.M.A. **238:**2066, 1977.

Robin, E. D., Cross, C. E., and Zelis, R.: Pulmonary edema, N. Engl. J. Med. **288:**292, 1973.

Severinghaus, J. W.: Symposium on high altitude physiology, London, 1971, Churchill-Livingstone.

Shabetai, R., Fowler, N. O., and Guntheroth, W. G.: Hemodynamics of cardiac tamponade and constrictive pericarditis, Am. J. Cardiol. **26:**480, 1970.

Shibel, E. M., and Moser, K. M., editors: Respiratory emergencies, St. Louis, 1977, The C. V. Mosby Co.

Shoemaker, W. C.: Algorhythm for early recognition and management of cardiac tamponade, Crit. Care Med. **3:**39, 1975.

Stein, L., Shubin, H., Weil, M. H.: Recognition and management of pericardial tamponade, J.A.M.A. **255:**503, 1973.

Thomas, D. M.: The smoke inhalation problem: Proceedings of the Symposium on Occupational Health Hazards of the Fire Service, Notre Dame University, 1971, International Association of Fire Fighters, Washington, D.C.

VanLeeuwen, G. J.: Immediate care of common emergencies in children. In Stephenson, H. E., editor: Immediate care of the acutely ill and injured, St. Louis, 1974, The C. V. Mosby Co.

Vismara, L. A.: Identification of sudden death risk factors in acute and chronic coronary artery disease, Am. J. Cardiol. **39:**821, 1977.

Warren, J., and Lewis, R.: Beneficial effects of atropine in the prehospital phase of coronary care, Am. J. Cardiol. **37:**68, 1976.

Wilson, A. F.: Drug treatment of acute asthma, J.A.M.A. **237:**1141, 1977.

Wilson, R.: Acute high altitude illness in mountaineers and problems at rescue, Ann. Intern. Med. **78:**421, 1973.

Wyman, M. G., Lalka, D., Hammersmith, L., and others: Multiple bolus technique for lidocaine administration during the first hours of an acute myocardial infarction, Am. J. Cardiol. **41:**313, 1978.

CHAPTER 18

Abdominal emergencies

The emergency nurse must be familiar with four types of acute abdominal conditions:

1. Inflammation with or without rupture of a hollow viscus.
2. Gastrointestinal hemorrhage.
3. Obstruction of a hollow viscus.
4. Penetrating or blunt abdominal trauma.

Many of the conditions seen in the emergency department are the result of long-term disease processes, whereas others are suddenly developing conditions requiring prompt management.

THE ACUTE ABDOMEN

The term "acute abdomen" refers to any abdominal condition that requires consideration for immediate surgery. Signs and symptoms indicate an acute condition, but the underlying problems may range from long-term pathological conditions to sudden trauma. The necessity for systematic clinical decision making is obvious, since certain conditions giving rise to the acute abdomen may be life-threatening, such as ruptured aortic aneurysm, ruptured spleen, and ruptured ectopic pregnancy. There are numbers of other conditions that must be managed within hours to prevent increased chances for morbidity and mortality, such as perforated ulcer, ruptured appendix, and intestinal trauma. Finally, certain acute conditions can be managed on a delayed basis (up to 12 hours) in order to take advantage of preoperative preparation, such as acute cholecystitis, appendicitis, incarcerated hernia, and mesenteric thrombosis.

Emergency personnel may contribute meaningfully to management of the acute abdomen by careful history taking and abdominal examination. It must be remembered that there are many conditions that mimic an acute abdomen, including inferior wall myocardial infarction, narcotic withdrawal, peritonitis, lobar pneumonia, renal colic, acute sickle cell disease, diabetic ketoacidosis, lead poisoning, and black widow spider bites. The history taking must be thorough in order to avoid the pitfalls inherent in the easily confused mimickers of the acute abdomen (Table 18-1).

Guidelines for trauma-related abdominal complaints

1. Manage hypovolemic shock with aggressive fluid administration. Avoid venesections or IVs in the lower extremities, since the vena cava may be damaged. Consider antishock trousers.
2. Obtain a detailed history of trauma. Ascertain if seat belts were in place in automobile accidents. If so, determine the type.
3. Search for fractures of ribs, pelvis, or lower vertebral bodies, since they frequently account for intraabdominal injury.
4. Nausea and vomiting frequently accompany abdominal complaints. Decompress the stomach with a nasogastric tube at the earliest feasible time to prevent vomiting and aspiration. Have suction at hand.

Assessment of pain

1. Did the pain have a gradual or sudden onset? What is its duration? (Steady, unrelenting

Table 18-1. Diseases producing an acute abdominal condition*

"Hot" abdomen (pain and tenderness)	"Warm" abdomen (pain but minimal if any tenderness)	"Cold" abdomen (shock—often no pain or tenderness)
1. Appendicitis	1. Early bowel obstruction	1. GI bleeding
2. Cholecystitis	2. Viral enteritis	
3. Perforated peptic ulcer	3. Gastritis	
4. Pancreatitis	4. Peptic ulcer	
5. Pelvic inflammatory disease	5. Renal stones	
6. Diverticulitis	6. Mesenteric adenitis	
7. Ruptured ectopic pregnancy		
8. Acute renal infections	**Mimics of the "warm" abdomen (extraabdominal causes)**	
9. Regional enteritis	1. Myocardial disease	
10. Ulcerative colitis	2. Respiratory disease	
11. Dissecting or ruptured aneurysm	3. Crises (sickle cell, diabetes, syphilis, Schönlein-Henoch purpura)	
12. Mesenteric arterial occlusion	4. Spinal cord tumor	
	5. Glaucoma	

*From Liechty, R. D.: In Liechty, R. D., and Soper, R. T.: Synopsis of surgery, ed. 4, St. Louis, 1980, The C. V. Mosby Co.

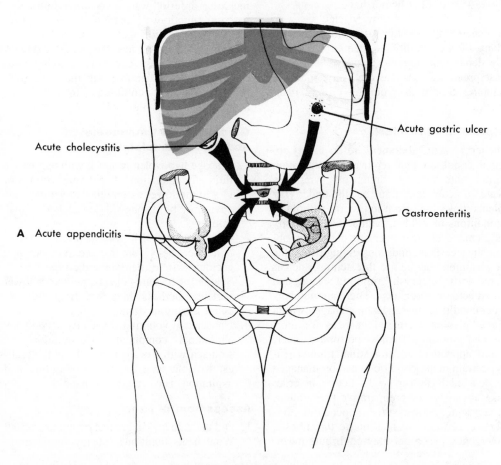

Fig. 18-1. A, Pain radiates to umbilicus in several acute abdominal conditions. **B,** Pain from acute abdominal conditions may radiate (note arrows) or may localize, such as in appendicitis. (From Barbar, J. M., and Budassi, S. A.: Mosby's manual of emergency care, St. Louis, 1979, The C. V. Mosby Co.)

pain is usually related to nonobstructive factors such as ulcerations of mucosa, ischemia, or peritonitis.)

2. Describe the pain including any radiation (Fig. 18-1). Is it colickly, suggesting obstruction of a hollow viscus?

3. Elicit the factors that make it better or worse, such as turning onto the opposite side, sitting up, taking a deep breath.

It is important for emergency personnel to obtain information about associated phenomena such as vomiting. For example, did pain precede the vomiting? If yes, this is usually characteristic of a surgical problem. Elicit whether the vomitus is undigested or digested food, and if it contains obvious bile or blood. Projectile vomiting is usually indicative of pyloric obstruction and should be noted.

Bowel functioning can also provide valuable clues to the nature of the problem. Is there evidence of obstruction? Constipation? Obstipation? Diarrhea? Tenesmus? Melena? Change in stool caliber? Is there a fecal impaction? Flatus expulsion? (Flatus can be expelled even with bowel obstruction.)

Explore menstrual status, because menstrual-related pain may mimic an acute abdomen. Of course, always consider ectopic pregnancy as a cause of abdominal crisis.

Urinary tract symptomatology can be confused with other abdominal complaints. Be certain to consider genitourinary problems when

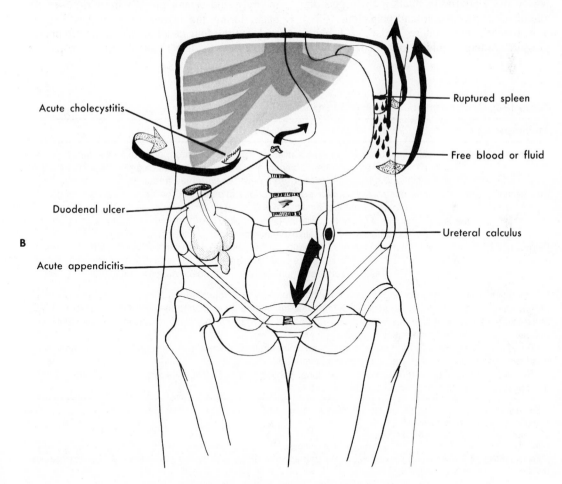

Acute cholecystitis

Duodenal ulcer

B

Acute appendicitis

Ruptured spleen

Free blood or fluid

Ureteral calculus

Fig. 18-1, cont'd. For legend see opposite page.

you are searching for an explanation of the acute abdomen (see Chapter 20).

Baseline physical and laboratory data

When the patient with abdominal complaints arrives in the emergency department, note the patient's position and his level of comfort. Characteristically, individuals with peritonitis tend to lie quietly; those with colic exhibit writhing pain. Pancreatitis symptoms become worse when the recumbent position is assumed. One can readily appreciate the need to note the patient's behavior in relation to postural changes. The abdominal examination should be accomplished early. See Table 18-2 for findings to be alert for in relation to inspection, auscultation, percussion, and palpation.

A baseline temperature, pulse, and blood pressure reading should be obtained, and laboratory work should include CBC, electrolytes, BUN, blood smear, hemoglobin and hematocrit, and amylase (Table 18-3).

The physician will probably request a supine and upright abdominal film, an upright chest film (to demonstrate free air), and possibly an IVP (Table 18-4).

There are two specialized diagnostic tests of particular importance to the emergency nurse, namely, peritoneal lavage and culdocentesis.

Peritoneal lavage. A peritoneal lavage is a safe diagnostic procedure used to demonstrate intraabdominal bleeding. It is an especially useful adjunct to diagnosis when the individual is intoxicated, comatose, or under the influence of drugs and cannot provide meaningful feedback during the examination. It has largely replaced the four-quadrant aspirating tap previously used to detect intraabdominal bleeding

Table 18-2. Components of abdominal examination*

Technique	Findings to be noted
Inspection	Ascites, distention, Grey Turner's† or Cullen's‡ sign, old scars, caput medusa,§ external hernia, visible or pulsating mass, or hematoma at level of lumbar spine (indicative of significant retroperitoneal bleeding usually resulting from pelvic or vertebrae fractures)
Auscultation	Bowel sounds, obstructive sounds, bruits (anterior and posterior), friction rub over the liver (Listen for bowel sounds for at least 5 minutes)
Percussion	Liver span, gaseous distention, ascites, shifting dullness, or fixed area of dullness in upper left quadrant (Ballance's sign) indicative of subcapsular or extracapsular spleen hematoma
Palpation	Point of maximum tenderness, rebound as well as direct tenderness and guarding, organomegaly, palpable masses, Murphy's sign,‖ subcutaneous emphysema (displacement of intrathoracic air), or result of retroperitoneal, duodenal, distal colon, or rectal injury

Abdominal pain, tenderness, and rigidity may indicate peritoneal irritation from blood or abdominal contents or may attend fractured ribs or contusions. Differentiate the finding by infiltrating the site of the rib fractures with anesthetic and then note changes in abdominal findings. If frank abdominal injury is present, the anesthetic will not affect the expressed tenderness or rigidity.

Raise the patient's head to distinguish abdominal wall pain from visceral pain. Visceral pain is lessened with head elevation, but abdominal wall injury pain is unaltered.

Rectal and pelvic examinations may also be done. (Obtain a stool guaiac measurement and check for high anterior tenderness and displacement of the prostate.)

*From Barber, J. M., and Budassi, S. A.: Mosby's manual of emergency care, St. Louis, 1979, The C. V. Mosby Co.
†Purplish discoloration on the flank.
‡Purplish discoloration around the umbilicus.
§Plexus of veins surrounding the umbilicus in periportal cirrhosis.
‖Test for cholecystitis: When a thumb is placed over the gallbladder on expiration, the patient experiences pain and catches his breath.

Table 18-3. Laboratory studies*

Test	Significance
Hemoglobin and hematocrit	Provide baseline data only. Usually do not reflect recent hemorrhage. Several hours may elapse before hemodilution will be reflected by the hematocrit.
Complete blood count	Provides baseline data. Splenic injury should be suspected if the leukocyte and platelet counts rise sharply without significant dehydration.
Type and cross-match	Preparatory to blood component therapy.
Arterial blood gas	Provides baseline data to assess ventilatory status.
Electrolytes	Provides baseline data.
SGOT	Provides baseline data.
Total bilirubin	Provides baseline data.
Coagulation studies	Hemostasis must be evaluated before extensive therapy or surgery.
BUN and serum creatinine	Provide baseline data. A rising BUN or serum creatinine level may indicate impaired renal function 24 to 48 hours after trauma, but these are usually not valuable initially.
Serum amylase	A high serum amylase level may suggest, but not confirm, pancreatic injury. Some patients have no rise in amylase levels despite injury to the pancreas, and others have elevations without visceral damage.

*From Barber, J.: Nurs. Clin. North Am. **13:**221, June, 1978.

Table 18-4. Radiological studies*

Film	Demonstrates
Flat plate of abdomen	Loops of intestine separated by fluid; fractures of lower ribs, pelvis, spine; position of organs and psoas muscle
Upright plate of abdomen	Free air under the diaphragm suggesting hollow viscus rupture†
Lateral decubitus film	Free air above flank†
Upright chest film	Injury or rupture of diaphragm
Flat plate of chest	Intestinal organ herniation into left chest, which may not be visible on upright
IVP	Renal injury
Abdominal angiography (reserved for poor surgical risks)	Intravisceral hematomas
Excretory urography	Urinary tract integrity or injury before surgically exploring or removing a kidney
Radioisotope scanning	Defects of liver, kidney or spleen of 2 cm or greater

*From Barber, J.: Nurs. Clin. North Am. **13:**221, June, 1978.
†The patient must sit upright or lie on his side for 10 minutes before the film to permit air to rise. Absence of air does not rule out hollow viscus rupture, however. Haziness or a "ground glass" appearance caused by accumulated air and fluid is a late sign.

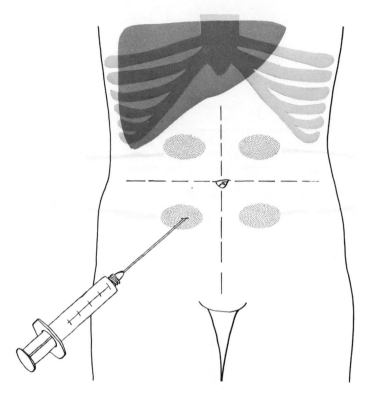

Fig. 18-2. Four sites for quadrant tap to detect free blood, bile, pus, and other materials from a ruptured viscus. (From Barber, J. M., and Budassi, S. A.: Mosby's manual of emergency care, St. Louis, 1979, The C. V. Mosby Co.)

(Fig. 18-2). Peritoneal lavage is a highly reliable diagnostic test that is simple to perform in a short time span in the emergency department. It can usually be completed in 15 to 20 minutes.

The essential equipment for peritoneal lavage consists of surgical antiseptic solution, sterile drapes and gloves, local anesthetic, scalpel, peritoneal dialysis catheter (with or without a trochar), a 5- to 10-ml syringe with a small-gauge needle, a 20-ml syringe, 1,000 ml Ringer's lactate, IV tubing, skin retractors, suture, sterile sponges, and a small dressing for covering the stab wound.

It is imperative to obtain baseline abdominal films before the procedure, because air can enter the abdomen during the tap, thus confusing later x-ray films. If the patient is conscious, the procedure should be briefly explained while preparations are in progress. The bladder must be decompressed by catheterization immediately before the lavage to avoid accidental bladder perforation as the trochar is introduced (Fig. 18-3). Nasogastric intubation may also be advisable to reduce abdominal distention.

ASSISTING WITH THE PROCEDURE. The patient is positioned recumbent, and the abdominal wall is surgically prepared and draped. An anesthetic wheal is raised 2 to 3 cm below the umbilicus (or in another adjacent site if a midline surgical scar is present). A small stab wound is made and the skin and subcutaneous tissues are retracted to accommodate introduction of the trochar. It is crucial that absolute hemostasis be accomplished at this point, because escaping blood could lead to a false indication of intraabdominal bleeding. Sterile

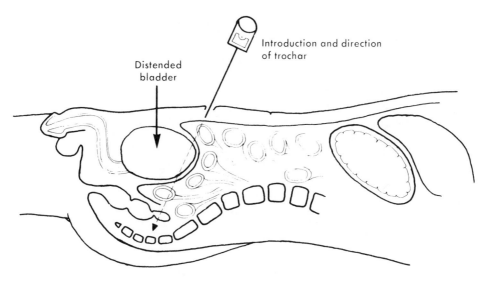

Distended
bladder

Introduction and direction
of trochar

Fig. 18-3. Distended bladder could be easily perforated during introduction of trochar for peritoneal lavage. Foley catheter should always be anchored before this procedure. (From Barber, J. M., and Budassi, S. A.: Mosby's manual of emergency care, St. Louis, 1979, The C. V. Mosby Co.)

sponges should be used as necessary. If the patient is conscious and is able to cooperate, he should be instructed to tense his abdomen as the trochar is introduced and the catheter is threaded into the cavity. A 20-ml syringe is attached to the catheter for aspirating a sample of peritoneal fluid. If the aspirate is grossly bloody, the lavage is considered ''positive'' and is terminated.

If there is slight or no evidence of blood, up to 1,000 ml Ringer's lactate is infused over 15 minutes (10 to 20 ml/kg). The patient is rolled from side to side to mix the solution with peritoneal fluids. The IV bag or bottle is then placed on the floor to permit the fluid to be siphoned from the abdominal cavity. When the return is complete, the catheter is removed and the stab wound sutured with 4-0 nylon. Antibiotic ointment and a small dressing may be applied to protect the site.

ANALYSIS OF FINDINGS. The lavage fluid is examined for opacity by the newsprint method before samples are sent to the laboratory for hematocrit, CBC, amylase, free bile determination, and culture and gram stain.

The newsprint method is designed to evaluate the amount of free blood in the fluid by an opacity examination using newsprint held behind a test tube of the lavage fluid. If the fluid looks entirely clear, the lavage is considered negative. If it is bloody but newsprint can be read through the fluid, it is indication for further diagnostic study. If newsprint can be seen but not read, it is 94% positive for blood, and surgery is usually indicated. If no newsprint can be seen looking through the test tube, there is 100% chance of significant intraabdominal injury, and surgery is indicated.

Culdocentesis. A culdocentesis (Fig. 18-4) may be indicated for female patients to detect free intraabdominal blood, which tends to migrate to the cul-de-sac, the most dependent part of the peritoneal cavity.

The nurse should explain the procedure to the patient if feasible, and assist her into lithotomy position. After the physician introduces the speculum, the posterior fornix is sponge dried and prepared with an antiseptic solution. A syringe with an 18-gauge spinal needle is inserted into the cul-de-sac, and suction is applied by using the syringe as an aspirating device over 1 minute while slowly withdrawing the needle. The aspirate is examined for blood as previously described.

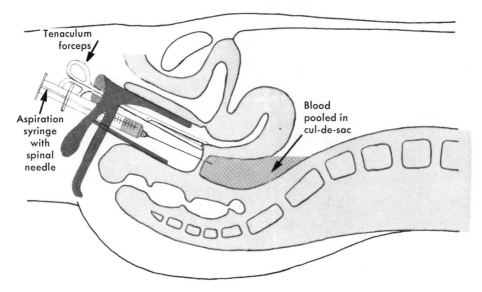

Fig. 18-4. Culdocentesis may be useful in detecting pooled blood from blunt abdominal injury in female trauma patient. (From Barber, J. M., and Budassi, S. A.: Mosby's manual of emergency care, St. Louis, 1979, The C. V. Mosby Co.)

INFLAMMATORY CONDITIONS
Pancreatitis (acute)

Acute pancreatitis is usually revealed in a painful epigastric episode after a large intake of food and alcohol. Some patients describe the pain as "boring through to the back." Abdominal pain, nausea, vomiting, and abdominal distention follow. There is usually marked epigastric and abdominal tenderness, as well as rigidity of the abdominal wall. Shock may be present in severe cases because of acute plasma volume depletion.

Emergency management consists of initiating an IV of D/5/W after drawing baseline venous bloods for CBC, hemoglobin and hematocrit, electrolytes, alkaline phosphatase, blood sugar, amylase, and bilirubin. ECG, CVP, and vital signs monitoring should be instituted, along with frequent assessments of urinary output and specific gravity. A nasogastric tube should be inserted and connected to intermittent suction, since paralytic ileus often accompanies acute pancreatitis. Some physicians prefer to initiate antibiotic therapy at once and to obtain a baseline chest film, since up to 50% of all patients with acute pancreatitis have pulmonary complications. Following admission to the hospital,

anticholinergic therapy and further medical or surgical measures are undertaken. Meperidine (Demerol) is the drug of choice for pain control, because it has a minimal effect on the sphincter mechanism of the pancreatic ducts.

Ulcerative colitis

A patient with known ulcerative colitis may come to the emergency department with complications such as perforation or sepsis. A classic history reveals bloody diarrhea with 10 to 30 stools per day along with abdominal cramping, weakness, weight loss, and in severe cases an immensely dilated colon. If perforation has occurred, the individual will be gravely ill with fever, tachycardia, and signs of generalized septicemia and peritonitis.

An IV of Ringer's lactate should be established at once to combat hypovolemia and as a route for antibiotic therapy. Baseline blood studies appropriate to the acute abdomen should be drawn and electrolyte imbalances corrected as necessary (see p. 402). The ECG, vital signs, and urinary output should be closely monitored during the stabilization period to guide clinical management of the shock state and to detect additional complications. A stool

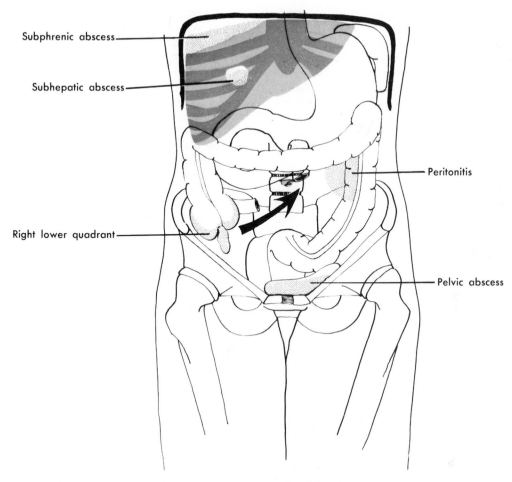

Subphrenic abscess

Subhepatic abscess

Right lower quadrant

Peritonitis

Pelvic abscess

Fig. 18-5. Perforation in acute appendicitis can lead to abscess formation in several locations within abdominal cavity. (From Barber, J. M., and Budassi, S. A.: Mosby's manual of emergency care, St. Louis, 1979, The C. V. Mosby Co.)

culture should be obtained to rule out a contagious disease as the cause of the diarrhea and other signs and symptoms of abdominal distress. Of course, specific medical therapy depends on the diagnostic findings. Surgery may be required in severe cases in which medical management fails to control the acute condition. Barium studies are not attempted, since they may precipitate a toxic megacolon. A toxic megacolon is essentially a severely dilated colon (usually transverse) accompanied by shock, fever, explosive bloody diarrhea, and often a "silent-peritonitis" abdomen.

Abdominal abscesses

The most common locations for abdominal abscesses are the iliac fossa, lower pelvis, below the diaphragm, and in and about any intra-abdominal or retroperitoneal organs. There may be a characteristic elevation of the diaphragm, gas bubbles, and obliteration and/or asymmetry of fat planes that suggest abscess formation.

Appendicitis

Inflammation of the vermiform appendix is usually caused by an obstruction of its lumen; thus, the early pain is likely to be colicky and referred to the epigastric region or periumbilical midline (Fig. 18-5). The individual may report anorexia and vomiting along with the pain and accompanying muscle spasm. As suppuration occurs in a progressive inflammatory process, the midline pain is superceded by radiating right lower quadrant pain. Other patterns, not uncommon, are low back, hip, or suprapubic radiation. Female patients should have a pelvic exam to rule out an inflammatory gynecological condition that could be responsible for pain. Male patients should undergo rectal examination to detect prostatitis and other genitourinary tract inflammation. Fever may not be evident unless there is severe dehydration or there has already been a rupture of the appendix.

X-ray films provide the best diagnostic clues to appendicitis. Free intraperitoneal air, gas patterns suggesting obstruction, and any lesions should be carefully considered. An appendiceal fecalith, although not commonly detected on x-ray film, is a valuable indicator of appendicitis. Any individual suspected of having acute appendicitis should be admitted for observation.

An IV of Ringer's lactate is initiated, and analgesics are given as necessary. A nasogastric tube is inserted and attached to suction. Blood is drawn for CBC, electrolytes, and blood sugar, and fever is managed with surface cooling and antipyretics (acetaminophen) and aspirin. If and when the diagnosis is confirmed, immediate surgery is advisable to prevent rupture and peritonitis.

GASTROINTESTINAL BLEEDING

One of the most frightening experiences that an individual can experience is a massive bleeding episode from the upper gastrointestinal tract. Even a small amount of blood in emesis can create considerable anxiety. The nurse in the emergency department should recognize this and give prompt attention and ensure close monitoring for the patient.

Acute gastrointestinal bleeding

Active upper GI bleeding (proximal to the ligament of Treitz) can be induced by peptic ulcers, esophageal varices, hemangiomas, Mallory-Weiss syndrome,* and prolapsing gastric mucosa. Although upper GI bleeding can be chronic, most emergency cases involve acute bleeding. A loss of 25% of the circulatory volume (or over 1,500 ml) within a few hours creates a characteristic clinical picture. Signs and symptoms include:

Bright red or "coffee ground emesis"

Hypovolemic shock

It is important to note that these phenomena may not both be apparent at once, so concealed bleeding should be suspected, especially if there is a history of previous bleeding or medical conditions that predispose to GI hemorrhage, such as peptic ulcers, cirrhosis, and tumors.

Emergency management. The shock room should be used for acute GI bleeding, since vigorous resuscitation may be required. Conscious patients may be permitted to sit upright during initial assessment procedures unless they are shocky. Unconscious patients should be positioned in a side-lying, head-down position to prevent aspiration if vomiting should occur. Antishock trousers may be useful to help combat shock and distend upper extremity veins for IV establishment. However, if esophageal varices are suspected, the abdominal section must not be inflated, since increased abdominal pressure aggravates bleeding.

The emergency nurse should promptly establish an IV line using a large-bore device, since whole blood is likely to be required. A second line for additional fluid and CVP monitoring is also desirable. As the IV route is tapped, blood samples should be drawn for baseline studies including typing and cross-matching, CBC, clotting studies, hemoglobin and hematocrit,† electrolytes, BUN, SGOT, creatinine, liver profile, amylase, and total bilirubin. Arterial blood gas samples for baseline studies should be drawn and oxygen administered as necessary to maintain the pO_2 at 100 mm Hg during

---

*A tear in the mucosal and submucosal tissue of the esophagus or stomach at or near the gastroesophageal junction.
†Changes in values related to acute GI hemorrhage require 12 to 36 hours.

resuscitation. The initial fluids should consist of Ringer's lactate or normal saline. The first 1,000 ml should be infused within 20 minutes. Blood products should be obtained for subsequent therapy.

Meanwhile, a large nasogastric tube (a Salem-sump) should be introduced to permit gastric decompression and to facilitate lavage with iced normal saline. This procedure is often begun promptly if shock is not profound, but may be delayed until basic life support activities are completed in the event of profound shock because the introduction of cold stimuli places an additional demand on cellular metabolism.

The purpose of the iced saline lavage is to arrest active bleeding. A 30- to 50-ml syringe is employed, and the procedure is continued until the aspirate is clear. Clear nasogastric aspirate indicates that the stomach is free of active bleeding and that prior bleeding has ceased. Coffee ground aspirate or dark blood is indicative of earlier bleeding resulting in acid hematin (hemoglobin combined with hydrochloric acid). If this coffee ground aspirate clears after lavage, active bleeding has probably ceased. Persistent pinkish or red-tinged aspirate after repeated lavage points to active hemorrhage.

A chest x-ray film and an upright film of the abdomen should be obtained as soon as circumstances permit diagnostic studies. A 12-lead ECG should be recorded, too, to search for a silent myocardial infarction. The ECG should be monitored constantly along with vital signs to support general management of the hypovolemic shock.

Additional measures for esophageal varices. The infusion of vasopressin (Pitressin) into the superior mesenteric artery may be useful to induce diffuse vasoconstriction and to lower portal pressure through constriction of the splanchnic arterial bed. Side effects of IV infusion (or intraarterial infusion into the superior mesenteric artery) include abdominal colic, bowel evacuation, systemic arterial hypertension, and coronary vasoconstriction. The drug can lead to myocardial infarction and thus is contraindicated for patients with coronary artery disease.

Esophageal balloon tamponade (Sengstaken-Blakemore tube) can be useful because it mechanically compresses varices in the esophagus and cardia of the stomach. The triple lumen tube has two balloons, one for anchoring and one for compression. The third lumen is used for gastric aspiration and lavage (Fig. 18-6).

Indications for surgery. If medical measures fail to control upper gastrointestinal bleeding, surgery may be indicated. The patient should be hospitalized, and invasive diagnostic studies (such as barium studies, endoscopy, angiography) delayed until the individual has been well stabilized by the emergency or intensive care teams.

Lower gastrointestinal bleeding

Bleeding of the large bowel and rectum is associated with carcinoma, diverticulitis, ulcerative colitis, cecal ulcers, hemorrhoids, and polyps.

Control of bleeding usually requires surgery when the site of origin is discovered. Most bleeding from diverticulitis ceases spontaneously. Emergency management consists primarily of treating hypovolemic shock (see p. 244).

Insertion of a nasogastric tube

1. Measure the tube from the tip of the earlobe to the tip of the nose and down to the xiphoid process *or* from the tip of the nose to the umbilicus. Mark this length with tape.
2. Lubricate the tube with a water-soluble lubricant.
3. Position an alert patient upright (with the head tipped slightly forward) for insertion. A weak or comatose patient should be in the left side-lying, head-down position.
4. Quickly thread the tube through the nares while the patient swallows small amounts of water, unless contraindicated. Observe respirations carefully. If severe choking or coughing occurs, withdraw the tube and reattempt placement. (Vagal stimulation caused by gagging can cause respiratory arrest. Always anticipate the need for resuscitation equipment when placing a nasogastric tube.)

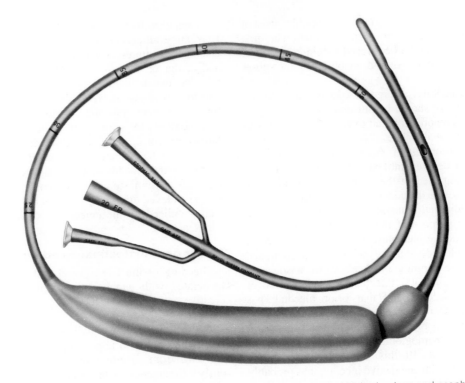

Fig. 18-6. Sengstaken-Blakemore tube. Note gastric balloon used to hold tube in place and esophageal balloon that is used to provide pressure on varices. Third lumen is used to aspirate gastric contents. (Courtesy Davol, Inc., Providence, R.I.)

Test the tube placement by:

a. Listening with a stethoscope for air (1 to 3 cc) injected into the stomach through a syringe.

b. Aspiration of stomach contents.

c. Placing the open end of the nasogastric tube under water to check for the presence of air.

5. Secure the tube with taping when the proper positioning has been assured.

6. Connect the tube to suction.

a. Double lumen tubes may be attached to low *continuous* suction.

b. A single lumen tube should be attached to low *intermittent* suction.

Procedure for anchoring a Sengstaken-Blakemore tube

1. Explain the procedure to the patient.

2. Check the balloons for patency and the ability to maintain inflation.

3. The pharynx may be anesthetized. Some physicians prefer that the gag reflex remain intact.

4. Insert the lubricated tube through the nares for approximately 50 cm. Check for stomach position.

5. Fill the gastric balloon with 200 to 250 ml Hypaque, and double clamp it. Apply gentle traction to check for placement and to pull it against the cardioesophageal junction.

6. Aspirate the stomach contents to check for continued bleeding; if it is present, inflate the esophageal balloon.

7. Inflate the esophageal balloon to a pressure of 25 to 45 mm Hg measured by a sphygmomanometer. Double clamp the tube. Provide slightly less than 1 kg continuous pressure on the tube to maintain placement.

8. Obtain an abdominal x-ray film to verify the placement.

9. A small nasogastric tube may be passed to the upper part of the esophageal balloon for esophageal aspiration, if necessary.

10. Schedule esophageal balloon deflation every 8 to 12 hours.

11. Monitor the patient closely for airway obstruction, and keep scissors at the bedside to deflate the balloons in the event of accidental dislodgement.

BOWEL OBSTRUCTION

Bowel obstruction can be caused by a wide variety of phenomena, including adhesions, strictures, carcinoma, ileus, intussusception, volvulus, regional enteritis, hernias, gallstones, fecal impactions, abscesses, and hematomas. The obstruction can be primary (mechanical) or secondary to inflammation or neurogenic disturbances. The dangers of intestinal obstruction relate to fluid depletion, strangulation of the bowel and perforation.

Obstruction of the bowel can be easily confused with several other conditions including a distended bladder, hypokalemic abdominal distention, constipation, and inflammatory conditions that create an alteration of air-fluid levels. Signs and symptoms of acute obstruction depend on the location of the obstruction and its duration and include distention, constipation, obstipation, fecal emesis, pain that is dull and cramping, changes in bowel sounds, or absence of bowel sounds. A partial obstruction is sometimes encountered in which bowel contents are expelled around the obstruction (for example, an impaction) often in the form of liquid or loose stool mixed with blood and mucous. Lesions far from orifices develop less dramatic presentations in most instances, and symptoms appear more insidious. High obstructions usually have precipitant pain and vomiting. It is evident from these varied findings that history is an extremely important adjunct to diagnosis.

Bowel sounds

Listening for bowel sounds is an essential component of the emergency nurse's assessment skills (see p. 130). Absent bowel sounds indicate a paralytic ileus, but one should remember that, to document the absence of sounds, auscultation must be continuous for 3 to 5 minutes over the small intestinal region. (Colon sounds occur only at 15- to 20-minute intervals.) If bowel sounds are present, their characteristics are valuable to diagnosis and should be carefully described in accordance to tonal quality, temporal relationship to pain, and so forth. Sounds caused by a mechanical obstruction are characteristically high-pitched, rushing, and continuous. Pain that coexists has a direct relationship to peristaltic activity and thus increases and declines with waves.

Other abdominal findings

Palpation of the abdomen may reveal mild tenderness, rebound tenderness over a general region, or localized pain. It is important to inspect the abdominal wall during palpation, because old surgical scars may suggest adhesions, a common cause of obstruction after surgery. Hernias (incarceration) should be suspected, and the femoral and inguinal regions closely examined. X-ray studies are a vital element of establishing a definitive diagnosis of the obstruction and its consequences (Table 18-5).

Emergency management

In the emergency department the nurse should establish an IV of Ringer's lactate or D/5/W and draw venous bloods for typing and cross-matching, electrolytes, amylase, CBC, hemoglobin and hematocrit, and blood sugar. A urine specimen should be collected for urinalysis. Antibiotics may be given if there are indices of frank peritonitis, impending perforation, or other high-risk phenomena. A nasogastric tube should be inserted and attached to suction to relieve distention of the GI tract.

The individual should be prepared for the various x-ray studies designed to detect the exact nature of the obstructive process (Table 18-5). Of course, if fluid and electrolyte imbalances require therapy, it is initiated in the emergency department even before the establishment of the diagnosis. Other preparatory activities for surgery are performed according to the anticipated procedure, giving attention to relief of discomfort and allaying anxiety by providing explanations of procedures be-

Table 18-5. X-ray and clinical evidence of specific bowel obstructions*

Type	X-ray findings	Clinical signs and symptoms
Bowel obstructions (general)	Air-fluid levels may appear as a "string of beads" and thus serve as important diagnostic clue to mechanical obstructions. More than two fluid-air levels present reflect mechanical obstruction and/or adynamic ileus. Fluid-filled loops form proximal to impediment and are indicative of a bowel obstruction. Routine films or contrast studies show air-fluid levels, distortion, abscess formation, narrow lumens, mucosal destruction, distention, and deformities at the site of torsion.	Pain, distention, vomiting, obstipation, and constipation.
Strangulating obstruction	"Coffee bean" sign on x-ray film (dilated bowel loop bent on itself, assuming shape of a coffee bean). Gas- and fluid-filled loops may have unchanging locations on multiple projection films. A pseudotumor (a closed loop obstruction filled with water that looks like a tumor) may be present.	Abdominal tenderness, hyperactive bowel sounds, leukocytosis, rebound tenderness, fever.
Gallstones	Air in gallbladder tree, distention of small bowel, and visualization of a stone.	
Hernia		Extraabdominal or intraabdominal hernias may be present: in men, most commonly inguinal; in women, right-sided femoral hernias.
Volvulus	See Figs. 18-7 and 18-8.	Torsion of mesenteric axis creating digestive disturbances.
Intussusception	"Coiled spring" appearance on contrast x-ray film.	

*From Barber, J. M., and Budassi, S. A.: Mosby's manual of emergency care, St. Louis, 1979, The C. V. Mosby Co.

ing performed or anticipated (Figs. 18-7 and 18-8).

Ingested foreign bodies

Emergency management of the individual who has accidentally *or* intentionally ingested a foreign body initially requires careful history taking. It is essential to determine when the foreign body was swallowed and under what circumstances. Attempt to elicit its size, shape, condition, or other characteristics that could provide clues to the potential damage that it could cause within the gastrointestinal tract. It is also valuable to know if the insertion was accidental or intentional, and if there is a history of other earlier episodes of a similar nature.

The mouth and pharyngeal area should be carefully inspected for local tissue trauma evidenced by bleeding. lacerations, or other injury. Be alert to edema that could impair normal ventilations. Observe respirations carefully to detect abnormalities in the work and effect of breathing.

The airway, as well as the gastrointestinal tract should be examined radiologically, with special attention given to the pharynx and the esophagus. If a foreign body is noted to be impacted in the esophagus, it should not be expected to advance into the stomach without additional propulsion. Esophagoscopy can be used to either extract or propel the foreign material.

An overwhelming number of foreign bodies (90%) are eliminated without incidence once they have passed through the stomach. Exceptions, although uncommon, include long, slender objects that become impacted in the

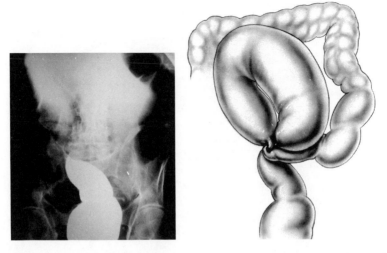

Fig. 18-7. Sigmoid volvulus. Radiograph shows large fluid-filled mass and typical bird-beak deformity outlined in barium in distal sigmoid colon. Diagram shows the twist. (From Liechty, R. D.: In Liechty, R. D., and Soper, R. T.: Synopsis of surgery, ed. 4, St. Louis, 1980, The C. V. Mosby Co.)

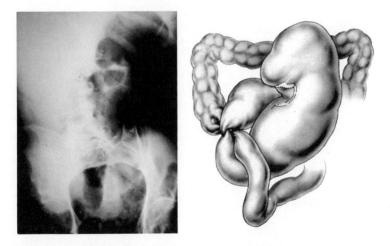

Fig. 18-8. Cecel volvulus. Note dilated gas-filled cecum in left upper quadrant on radiograph. Diagram shows the twist. (From Liechty, R. D.: In Liechty, R. D., and Soper, R. T.: Synopsis of surgery, ed. 4, St. Louis, 1980, The C. V. Mosby Co.)

pylorus, duodenum, duodenojejunal flexure, ileocecal region, or sites of congenital anomalies such as stenoses (Fig. 18-9). Fortunately, impaction and duodenal perforation are rare and are most likely to occur in children under 2 years of age.

The average time for foreign bodies to pass completely through the gastrointestinal tract is 5 days. The progress of foreign bodies should be followed by x-ray films at 48-hour intervals. Concurrently, there should be a careful examination of all stool, since x-ray films should be

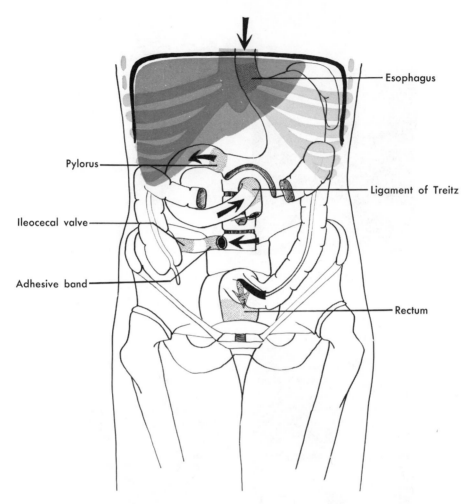

Fig. 18-9. Six common sites for foreign body obstruction or perforation of gastrointestinal tract. (From Barber, J. M., and Budassi, S. A.: Mosby's manual of emergency care, St. Louis, 1979, The C. V. Mosby Co.)

stopped as soon as the foreign body is eliminated to avoid unnecessary exposure to radiation.

Surgical intervention is indicated if there are signs and symptoms of impaction *or* if the foreign body fails to advance after 2 weeks.

Instructional points. Intestinal stimulants or cathartics should never be used to hasten elimination of an object, because the intense peristalsis that they induce could invite perforation of the gastrointestinal tract. It is important to stress this to parents, because they may be tempted to use such agents to shorten the interval of anxious waiting for the foreign body to be passed. Nurses should also explain that special foods or dietary additives will in no way protect the lining of the stomach or intestine form the trauma of a migrating object, and a normal diet should be continued.

It is helpful to suggest ways to collect and examine stool for the foreign body, that is, plan for defecation into a receptacle other than the commode to avoid retrieving stool from water, use a tongue blade or ice cream stick to search the stool before discarding, and so on. Advise parents to be certain that all of a foreign body is eliminated, not such a portion.

Individuals who have ingested foreign bodies should promptly return to the emergency department if these signs or symptoms of impaction or bowel perforation are noted: vomiting, obstipation, fever, abdominal pain and rigidity, hip pain, diarrhea, changes in characteristics of urine (secondary to kidney perforation), or blood in the stools.

ABDOMINAL TRAUMA
Penetrating abdominal injuries

Penetrating wounds of the abdomen require surgical exploration. Since 25% to 30% are associated with intrathoracic injury, careful study of the chest structures is indicated. Before surgical exploration and debridement, IV antibiotics should be initiated along with other emergency care routines.

Blunt abdominal trauma

Blunt abdominal trauma is a challenging clinical problem and may result in death from hypovolemia or peritonitis if undetected (Fig. 18-10). Occasionally the individual has a massive shock syndrome and requires vigorous anti-shock therapy. If antishock trousers have not been applied in the field, strong consideration should be given to their use. Two large-bore IVs should be established, with one line designated for central venous pressure monitoring. If a peripheral IV cannot be established, a venesection should be done. It is imperative to avoid the lower extremities, because there could be damage to the inferior vena cava, and hence the right heart volume would not be enhanced. Since nausea and vomiting often accompany acute abdominal problems, a nasogastric tube should be inserted to decompress the upper gastrointestinal tract and prevent the dangers of aspiration. A Foley catheter should be anchored to decompress the bladder and as an aid to monitoring output. However, extreme caution should be used if there is hematuria or other signs of urinary tract insult. Never force a catheter into the urethra! If any resistance is encountered, or if there is history of a straddle-type injury, a urology consultation should be obtained before proceeding with catheterization. Occasionally in urinary tract trauma, the individual will feel a sense of urgency to void, but voluntary voiding should be discouraged, since it could allow urine to extravasate into the peritoneum (see Fig. 20-2).

The indications for emergency surgery include unexplained hemorrhagic shock, peritoneal perforation, increasing abdominal tenderness or rigidity, evidence of peritonitis, visualized free air in the abdomen, positive peritoneal lavage or culdocentesis, enlarging abdominal mass in the absence of pelvic or vertebral fractures, or a progressive drop in hemoglobin and hematocrit in the absence of hypotension, especially in the second 24 hours after injury.

Ordinarily if there is a high suspicion of intraabdominal contamination, the physician will choose to start IV antibiotics at once so an adequate blood level can be attained before the additional stress of surgery is placed on the defense mechanisms.

Usually patients with a high index of suspicion of having blunt abdominal trauma will be admitted for at least 24 hours of observation; however, in some instances, the decision may be reached to discharge the individual if the studies performed yielded negative results. In this event, it is essential that the emergency nurse give adequate instructions to the patient regarding the warning signs of intraabdominal compromise. In all cases, a referral should be made for a 3- to 5-day follow up. Document instructions and the referral carefully in the emergency department record for future legal protection and reference.

Ruptured spleen

A ruptured spleen is a life-threatening injury requiring prompt identification and management by the emergency care team. Signs and symptoms can develop over several hours, or the presentation may be dramatic, with hypovolemic shock. Clues to suspecting a ruptured spleen follow.

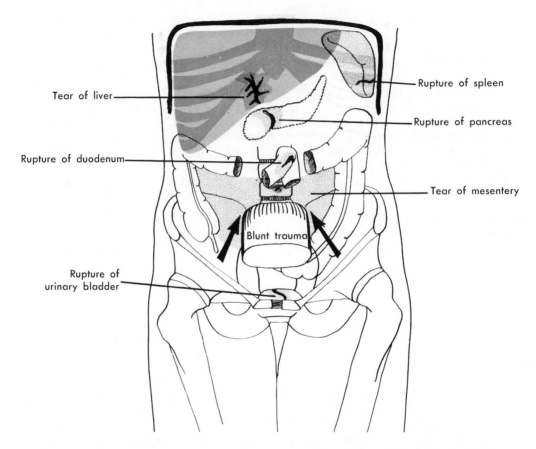

Tear of liver

Rupture of duodenum

Rupture of urinary bladder

Rupture of spleen

Rupture of pancreas

Tear of mesentery

Blunt trauma

Fig. 18-10. Some possible consequences of blunt trauma. (From Barber, J. M., and Budassi, S. A.: Mosby's manual of emergency care, St. Louis, 1979, The C. V. Mosby Co.)

1. Severe upper left quadrant pain
2. Palpable mass in the splenic region
3. Fall in hematocrit
4. Rapidly developing hypovolemic shock

The index of suspicion should be high after injuries to the upper left quadrant, lower left chest, or left flank. Lower left rib fractures and the confirmation of a hemopneumothorax should arouse suspicion of severe splenic trauma.

The emergency management should include that cited in relation to blunt abdominal trauma, and additionally, a spleen scan with selected angiography. X-ray studies charcteristically reveal a complete or partial loss of the splenic outline, displacement of the gastric fundus, slight elevation of the left portion of the diaphragm, downward displacement of the splenic flexure, fluid in the abdomen, loss of the left kidney outline and psoas margin, and fracture of one or more of the lower left ribs.

If splenic rupture is confirmed, immediate splenectomy is indicated. If confirmation is obtained, the individual should be hospitalized, since delayed rupture (up to 72 hours) can occur (Fig. 18-11).

Special considerations for the pregnant patient

If a suspected or known pregnant patient sustains abdominal trauma, an obstetrical consultant should be obtained at once. The third tri-

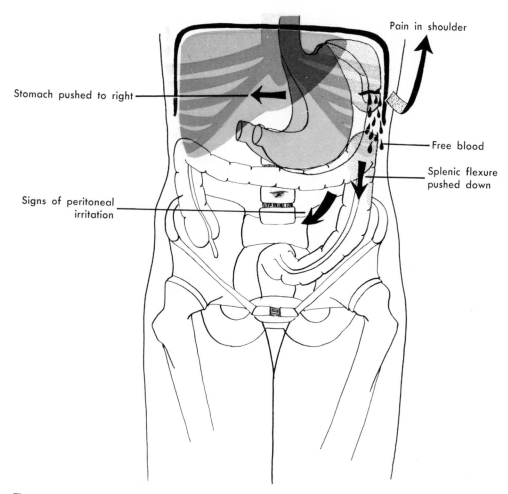

Fig. 18-11. Clinical indices of a ruptured spleen, other than shock. (From Barber, J. M., and Budassi, S. A.: Mosby's manual of emergency care, St. Louis, 1979, The C. V. Mosby Co.)

mester pregnant woman should be positioned side-lying with the legs elevated and the gravid uterus displaced to the right to relieve vena caval compression and resultant hypotension. Not only do these maneuvers help restore a normotensive state in the absence of trauma, but additionally, if there is bleeding within the pelvis or in the lower extremities, vena caval compression obstructs circulation and contributes to increased hemorrhage.

Oxytocic drugs should not be given in the event of vaginal bleeding and uterine contrac-

tions, since they could contribute to fatal uterine contractions and bleeding.

Whole blood and packed cells are recommended for fluid resuscitation because they tend to improve fetal arterial oxygenation. Crystalloids or colloids such as dextran would not provide these salient benefits. Avoid vasopressors, because they decrease uterine blood flow and thus increase fetal hypoxia.

If diagnostic x-ray films are thought to be necessary, they should be kept to a minimum, and the uterus should be shielded as much as possible. Fetal monitoring is an important adjunct to emergency care and should be employed when feasible.

SUMMARY

Acute medical and surgical abdominal conditions can result in serious consequences, including hemorrhage, sepsis, and death, if not detected early and managed aggressively. A thorough history, systemic abdominal examination, selected laboratory studies, and x-ray films are helpful in establishing a diagnosis. Peritoneal lavage is highly valuable for assessing, intra-abdominal bleeding resulting from blunt abdominal trauma.

Nurses in the emergency department should be thoroughly familiar with acute abdominal problems and aware of their role in initial stabilization and assistance with the tests and procedures that facilitate diagnosis.

BIBLIOGRAPHY

Batalder, D. J., and others: Value of G-suit in patients with severe pelvic fracture, Arch. Surg. **109:**326, 1974.

Beck, K., and others: Color atlas of endoscopy and biopsy of the intestine, Philadelphia, 1975, W. B. Saunders Co.

Bouchier, I. A. D.: Gastroenterology, Baltimore, 1973, The Williams & Wilkins Co.

Davidson, I., Miller, E., and Litwin, M. S.: Gunshot wounds of the abdomen, Arch. Surg. **111:**862, 1976.

Davis, J. J., Cohn, I., and Nance, F. C.: Diagnosis and management of blunt abdominal trauma, Ann. Surg. **183:**672, 1976.

Eldridge, W. W.: Foreign bodies in the gastrointestinal tract, J.A.M.A. **178:**665-667, 1961.

Ellis, P. D.: Portal hypertension and bleeding esophageal and gastric varices: a surgical approach to treatment, Heart Lung **6:**791-798, 1977.

Engrav, L. H., and others: Diagnostic peritoneal lavage in blunt abdominal trauma, J. Trauma **15:**854, 1975.

Gammill, S. L., and Nice, C. M.: Air fluid levels: their occurrence in normal patients and their role in the analysis of ileus, Surgery **71:**771,780, 1972.

Generelly, P., Moore, T. A., III, and LeMay, J. T.: Delayed splenic rupture: diagnosed by culdocentesis, J.A.C.E.P. **6:**369-371, 1977.

Greenberger, N., and Winship, D.: Gastrointestinal disorders: a pathophysiologic approach, Chicago, 1976, Year Book Medical Publishers, Inc.

Jergens, M. E.: Peritoneal lavage, Am. J. Surg. **133:**365-369, 1977.

Kawai, K., and Tanaka, H.: Differential diagnosis of gastric diseases, Chicago, 1974, Year Book Medical Publishers, Inc.

Kazarian, K. K., Devanesan, J. D., and Mersheimer, W. L.: Diagnostic peritoneal lavage: technique, complications and interpretations, N.Y. State Med. J. **75:**2149-2151, 1975.

Looser, K. G., and Crombie, H. D.: Pelvic fractures: an anatomic guide to severity of injury, Am. J. Surg. **132:**638, 1976.

Meads, G. E., et al.: Traumatic rupture of the right hemidiaphragm, J. Trauma **17:**797-801, 1977.

Montegut, F. J.: Tube paracentesis without lavage, J. Trauma **13:**142-144, 1973.

Nance, F. C., and others: Surgical judgment in the management of penetrating wounds of the abdomen, Ann. Surg. **179:**639, 1974.

Nelson, S. W.: Extraluminal gas collections due to diseases of the gastrointestinal tract, Am. J. Roentgenol. **115:**225-248, 1972.

Olsen, W. R., and Hildreth, D. H.: Abdominal paracentesis and peritoneal lavage in blunt abdominal trauma, J. Trauma **11:**824-829, 1971.

Pops, M. A.: Emergency management of gastrointestinal bleeding, Unpublished paper, Los Angeles, 1976, U.C.L.A. Postgraduate Institute on Emergency Medicine, pp. 1-4.

Schwartz, G. F., and Polsky, H. S.: Ingested foreign bodies of the gastrointestinal tract, Am. Surg. **42:**236-238, April 1976.

Shahinpour, N.: The adult with bleeding esophageal varices, Nurs. Clin. North Am. **12:**331-343, 1977.

Soter, C. S.: The use of barium in the diagnosis of acute appendiceal disease: a new radiological sign, Clin. Radiol. **19:**410-415, 1968.

Spitz, L.: Management of ingested foreign bodies in childhood, Br. J. Med. **4:**469-472, November 20, 1971.

Steele, M., and Lim, R. C.: Advances in management of splenic injuries, Am. J. Surg. **130:**159, 1975.

Thal, E. R., and Shires, G. T.: Peritoneal lavage in blunt abdominal trauma, Am. J. Surg. **125:**64-69, 1973.

Wein, A. J., and others: Controversial aspects of blunt renal trauma, J. Trauma **17:**662-666, 1977.

Wilson, R., and others: Shock in the emergency department, J.A.C.E.P. **5:**678-690, 1976.

X-rays in focus: radiology of the stomach and duodenum, Nurs. Times **73:**13-16, April 21, 1977.

CHAPTER 19

Limb trauma

One of the greatest sources of disability in all age groups in the United States is limb trauma. One must stress the importance of early management and correct therapeutic intervention to preserve life and limb, prevent disability, and promote good healing.

The skeleton is composed of 206 bones and provides the framework of the body. It also functions to provide support for the body, attachments for muscles, leverage, and protection to the vital organs (Fig. 19-1).

Two types of bones comprise the skeleton. Cancellous (spongy) bone is found in the skull, the vertebrae, the pelvis, and the long bone ends; cortical (dense) bone is found in the long bones. Bones have blood, nerve, and lymphatic supply that allows the injured bone to repair itself. They are covered by a layer known as the periostium, which provides an additional blood supply. Bones are labeled as long, short, flat, or irregular in accordance with their shape.

Bone is connected to bone by a fibrous connective tissue known as *ligament*. Another type of fibrous connective tissue that connects muscle to bone is known as *tendon*. The dense connective tissue found between the ribs, in the nasal septum, the ear, the larynx, the trachea, the bronchi, between the vertebrae, and on the articulating surface of the bone is known as *cartilage*. Cartilage has no neurovascular supply.

Radiographs in this chapter are courtesy Western Radiologic Medical Group, Inc., Los Angeles. Special thanks to Cindy Allen, RT, Administrative Secretary.

Joints are areas where two bones are connected to provide mobility and stability, flexion and extension, medial and lateral rotation, and abduction and adduction. Anatomically speaking, a joint consists of two bone articulating surfaces covered with cartilage, a two-layered sac containing synovial membranes for lubrication, and a capsule that becomes dense and forms a ligament. Movement is provided by muscles that overlie the joints and attach bone to bone with tendons.

When one encounters a victim with possible limb trauma, it is first essential to assess airway, breathing, and circulation before proceeding to treat the injured limb. One must also perform a rapid assessment to detect other major trauma, such as head, cervical spine, chest, or abdominal trauma. If obvious head or cervical spine trauma is present or suspected, one must provide protection and preventive therapeutic intervention to these areas.

Once one is assured that no life-threatening injury has been left unattended, immobilize the traumatized extremity by splinting it both above and below the trauma site as well as splinting the trauma site itself. Splinting is provided to prevent further damage and reduce the amount of pain in the injured limb. It is essential to evaluate the neurovascular status of the limb both before and after immobilization, by assessing for pulses distal to the trauma site, checking skin color, temperature, and capillary refill, and testing for sensation and movement distal to the trauma site. If neurological or vascular status is compromised, one must attempt to apply traction to reduce the

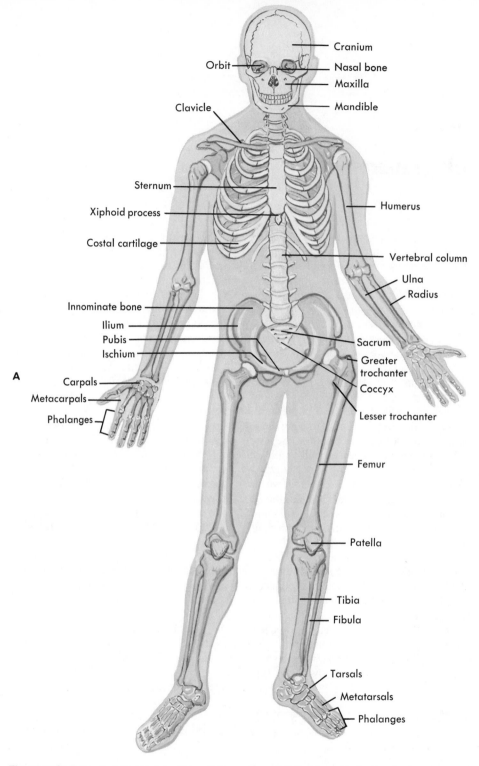

Fig. 19-1. Skeleton. **A,** Anterior view. (From Anthony, C., and Thibodeau, G.: Textbook of anatomy and physiology, ed. 10, St. Louis, 1979, The C. V. Mosby Co.)

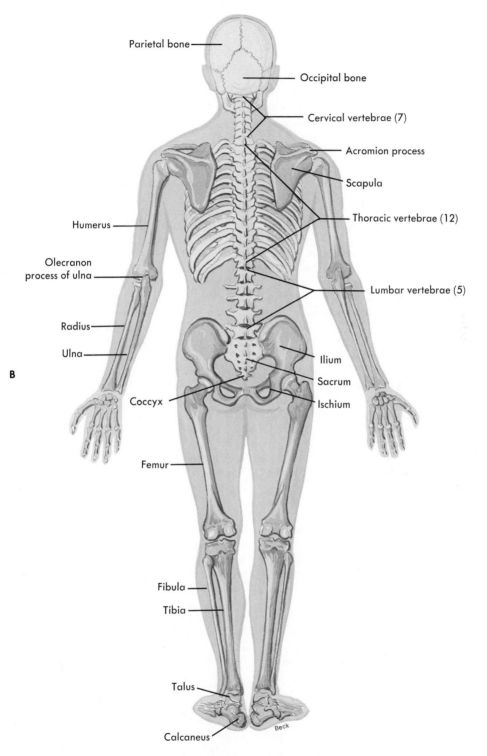

Parietal bone

Occipital bone

Cervical vertebrae (7)

Acromion process

Scapula

Humerus

Thoracic vertebrae (12)

Olecranon
process of ulna

Lumbar vertebrae (5)

Radius

Ulna

B

Ilium

Sacrum

Coccyx

Ischium

Femur

Fibula

Tibia

Talus

Calcaneus

Beck

Fig. 19-1, cont'd. Skeleton. **B,** Posterior view.

fracture and to allow for neurological and vascular function to return.

Whenever possible, the injured limb should be elevated and a cold pack applied to the injury site to keep the amount of swelling to a minimum. It may benefit the patient to obtain a brief history of the circumstances surrounding the accident, the mechanism of injury, and any past medical history and/or medications the patient is currently taking.

Careful observation must be made of any swelling, discoloration, contusions, abrasions, and obvious deformities. If an open fracture is evident or if a puncture site is present but no bone is protruding,* irrigate the wound with sterile normal saline solution, apply a dry sterile dressing over the wound, followed by a light compression dressing. The injury should then be splinted. *Never* attempt to reduce an open fracture in the prehospital care setting.

If bleeding is present, apply pressure either over the bleeding site or around the edges of the wound. A tourniquet should be used *only as a lifesaving measure* when bleeding cannot be controlled by other methods. If a tourniquet has been applied and all circulation to the limb has ceased for a prolonged period of time, the limb may have to be amputated.

At this point in therapeutic intervention, if the victim is still in the prehospital care setting, it is appropriate to transport the victim to a hospital facility.

Once the victim has reached the emergency department, providing that measures have been taken to assure that the cervical spine has been protected, the patient should be totally undressed and examined both anteriorly and posteriorly for other associated injuries that may have been overlooked in the field.

SOFT TISSUE INJURIES

Soft tissue injuries frequently involve the limbs. They may be injuries to the skin and underlying tissues, such as muscle, tendon, cartilage, ligament, veins, arteries, and nerves.

The skin may be traumatized in several ways.

---

*If a puncture site is present but there is no bone end protruding, one should assume that the puncture site was made by a jagged bone end or a missile, and one should treat it as an open fracture.

If the epithelial layer is removed, exposing the dermal layer, an *abrasion* wound is created. A *contusion* is a bruise in which vessels are damaged but the skin is not disrupted. It is usually the result of a blunt force. A *hematoma* forms when blood escapes into the subcutaneous space. When skin is disrupted through the dermal layer, a wound is formed known as a *laceration*. Disruption of the skin by a sharp pointed object is a *puncture* wound. If the puncturing object remains imbedded in the skin and tissues, this is an impaled object. It should not be removed until the wound and the impaling object's location can be thoroughly evaluated.

When applying therapeutic intervention for soft tissue injuries, one must always first consider airway, breathing, and circulation. Once these three parameters are assured, control bleeding by applying direct or indirect pressure to the wound. If there is an impaled object present, secure it so that it will not be removed accidentally. Place a dry sterile dressing over the wound, and evaluate the injured area if possible. Apply a cold pack to the wound to minimize swelling. Be sure to check with the patient regarding the currency of his tetanus prophylaxis status.

Crush injuries

Although there are many types of soft tissue injuries, several are common to the emergency department. *Wringer injuries* were seen much more frequently in the days when wringer washing machines were commonly found in the home. A patient with this type of injury may come to the emergency department following an industrial accident in which the victim's arm was caught by the wringer of a commercial washing machine, causing a crush injury. These wounds should be treated by cleansing the wound and dressing it with a sterile bulky dressing. Before dressing the wound, evaluate the limb for distal pulses and neurological status. The limb should be elevated above the level of the heart, an x-ray film should be ordered, and one should check for current tetanus prophylaxis status. At this point, if the injury is isolated to a limb, one should consider analgesia. Depending upon the extent of damage, one may elect to consult with a specialist in orthopedics, neurosurgery, or vascular or hand surgery for further therapeutic intervention.

Other types of crush injuries occur when a heavy object falls on an extremity. Therapeutic intervention is the same as that for wringer injuries.

Impaling injuries

Impaling injuries are seen frequently and are usually the result of an industrial accident in which the victim falls onto a sharp, immobile object. Whenever possible, secure the impaling object without removing it. Assess the neurovascular status of the limb distal to the impaling object. Consider analgesia if the injury is isolated. Once again, check for currency of tetanus prophylaxis status. Order x-ray films of the appropriate body parts involved, and call in appropriate surgical consultants if necessary.

Gunshot wounds

Gunshot wounds usually result from acts of violence or hunting accidents. The amount of damage resulting depends upon the type of weapon used, the caliber of ammunition used, the distance from which the weapon was fired, and what part of the body was hit. In general, a person who has been a victim of a gunshot wound, following assessment of the ABCs, should have the wound cleansed and dressed with a dry sterile dressing until it can be evaluated by a physician. Be sure to check for pulses and neurovascular status, and assess the limb if possible. One item often overlooked in the excitement of the injury and other therapeutic intervention is the status of the patient's tetanus prophylaxis.

Knee injuries

Knee injuries are a common form of soft tissue injury where rotational or extraflexion trauma results in a medial meniscus, collateral ligament, or cruciate ligament strain or tear. Signs and symptoms of this type of injury include a history of trauma to the knee, swelling, ecchymosis, effusion, pain, and tenderness. Therapeutic intervention includes a compression bandage, knee immobilizer, or cylinder cast, depending on the extent of the injury, elevation of the injured limb, a cold pack to the injured area for the first 24 hours (intermittently), and instructions to the patient as to how to use crutches for the purpose of not bearing weight. If the injury is assessed to be a ligament tear, it should be surgically repaired within 24 to 48 hours of the time of the injury.

Fingertip injuries

Fingertip injuries are common in the emergency setting. The most common type of fingertip injury is a crush injury to the distal phalanx resulting from a heavy object falling on the fingertip or the fingertip being caught in a house or car door. Therapeutic intervention is to apply a soft, bulky, protective dressing. The finger should be x-rayed to rule out fractures. If a hematoma is forming under the fingernail, nail trephination should be carried out by penetrating the fingernail over the site of the hematoma with a nail drill, a scalpel, or a superheated paper clip to relieve the blood collecting under the nail.

Another type of fingertip injury that is seeing increasing frequency is high-pressure paint/grease gun injuries. This injury occurs when the victim is cleaning the tip of a high-pressure gun and the gun releases a stream of paint or grease into the fingertip and up into the hand under very high pressure. Particular caution must be paid to the history in this case, as the injury will appear only as a small pinhole in the tip of the finger. Therapeutic intervention requires surgical debridement of the paint/grease-injected limb with the patient under general anesthesia.

Strains

Other types of soft tissue injuries include *strains* and *sprains* of the extremities. A strain is a weakening or overstretching of a muscle where it attaches to the tendon. Strains may occur as the result of almost any type of movement, from simply stepping off a step the wrong way and twisting the ankle to a wrenching force as a result of an automobile accident. Most commonly, strains are seen as a result of athletic injuries.

A patient with a *mild strain* complains of local pain, point tenderness, and slight spasm of the muscle. Therapeutic intervention includes a compression bandage, elevation of the limb above the level of the heart for 12 hours, application of a cold pack intermittently for the same period of time, and light weight bearing on the injured part.

A *moderate strain* finds the patient complaining of local pain, point tenderness, swelling and discoloration, and inability to use the limb for prolonged periods of time. Therapeutic intervention includes a compression bandage, elevation, and cold pack for 24 hours, analgesia, and light weight bearing only.

When the strain is *severe,* the patient complains of local pain, point tenderness, swelling, discoloration, and offers a history of a "snapping noise" at the time of the injury. Therapeutic intervention includes a compression bandage, elevation, and a cold pack for 24 to 48 hours, analgesia, and no weight bearing for 48 hours.

Sprains

A *sprain* is a ligament injury. The mechanism of injury may be the same as that of a strain, but in general, it is usually a much more traumatic force. A sprain occurs when a joint exceeds its normal limit. The most common sprains are seen in the ankles, knees, and shoulders. A *mild sprain* produces slight pain and slight swelling. Therapeutic intervention includes a compression bandage, elevation, a cold pack for 12 hours, and light weight bearing. A *moderate sprain* causes pain, point tenderness, swelling, and inability to use the limb for more than a short period of time. Therapeutic intervention includes a compression bandage, elevation, and cold pack for 24 hours, and light weight bearing with the use of crutches.

A severe sprain involves tearing of the ligaments, which causes pain, point tenderness, swelling, discoloration, and inability to use the limb. Therapeutic intervention includes a compression bandage or a cast, elevation, and a cold pack for 48 hours, and light to no weight bearing, using crutches.

Ruptured Achilles tendon

With the advent of tennis and racquetball as major pasttimes in the United States, one should expect to see an increasing incidence of *ruptured Achilles tendon.* This injury usually occurs in athletes over 30 years old who actively participate in start-and-stop sports in which one steps off abruptly on the forefoot with the knee forced in extension. The patient will complain of a sharp pain from the heel and up into the back of the leg. There is a sudden inability to use the foot of the injured extremity; a deformity develops, and the patient exhibits a positive Thompson's sign: when the calf muscle is squeezed, with the leg extended and the foot over the end of the table, the heel will not pull and no upward motion will be seen.

A person who has sustained a ruptured Achilles tendon should have a compression bandage applied, along with elevation of the extremity and a cold pack until surgery can be performed to repair the tendon.

PERIPHERAL NERVE INJURIES

Throughout the text, neurovascular function has been mentioned. Neurovascular function may be altered not only by mechanical, chemical, or thermal trauma to an extremity, but also by malignancies, toxins, metabolic factors, or collagen disease. The most common causes of peripheral nerve injuries are lacerations, penetrating wounds, fractures, and dislocations. One should be familiar with the distribution of nerves, the origin of motor branches, and the muscles that they supply. When testing for motor loss, one should be able to visualize the tendon or muscle body being tested (Table 19-1).

Other more sophisticated diagnostic tests, such as electromyography, electrical stimulation, and nerve conduction tests, are performed in the inpatient setting and are not appropriate for emergency department use. Likewise, peripheral nerve injury repair should take place in the operating room and not in the emergency department.

FRACTURES

A fracture is a disruption or break in the bone. Generally, there are signs and symptoms common to most fractures. These include angulation and/or deformity, pain, point tenderness and region tenderness, swelling, lack of move-

Table 19-1. Modes for assessing common peripheral nerve injuries*

Nerve	Frequently associated injuries	Assessment technique†
Radial	Fracture of humerus, especially middle and distal thirds	Inability to extend thumb in "hitchhiker's sign"
Ulnar	Fracture of medial humeral epicondyle	Loss of pain perception in tip of little finger
Median	Elbow dislocation or wrist or forearm injury	Loss of pain perception in tip of index finger
Peroneal	Tibia or fibula fracture, dislocation of knee	Inability to extend great toe or foot; may also be associated with sciatic nerve injury
Sciatic and tibial	Infrequent with fractures or dislocations	Loss of pain perception in sole of foot

*From Barber, J. M., and Budassi, S. A.: Mosby's manual of emergency care, St. Louis, 1979, The C. V. Mosby Co.
†Test is invalid if extension tendons are severed or if severe muscle damage is present.

ment, and crepitus (grating of bone ends). Other findings are obvious bony fragment protrusion, decreased neurovascular status, including decreased distal pulses, decreased skin temperature distal to the fracture site, cyanosis, decreased sensation, and occasionally, shock.

Fractures are divided into two general categories: closed or simple fractures, in which the bone is broken but the skin is not disrupted; and open or compound fractures, in which the bone is protruding, the bone has punctured the skin and returned into the limb, or a foreign object has penetrated the skin and bone, causing a fracture.

Types of fractures

A *transverse fracture* results from an angulation force or a direct trauma (Fig. 19-2).

An *oblique fracture* results from a twisting force (Fig. 19-3).

A *spiral fracture* results from a twisting force while the foot is firmly planted (Fig. 19-4).

A *comminuted fracture* results from a severe direct trauma. The fracture has more than two fragments (Fig. 19-5).

An *impacted fracture* results from a severe trauma, causing the fractured bone ends to jam together (Fig. 19-6).

A *compression fracture* results from a severe force to the top of the head or the os calcis, causing a forcing together of the vertebrae (Fig. 19-7).

A *greenstick fracture* is the result of a compression force. It usually occurs in children in

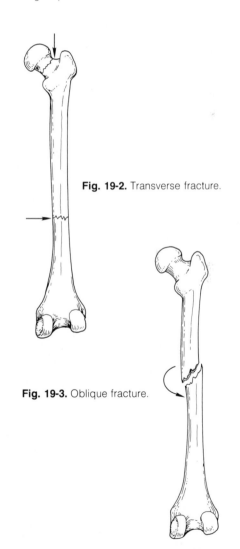

Fig. 19-2. Transverse fracture.

Fig. 19-3. Oblique fracture.

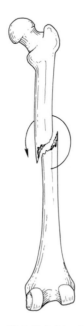

Fig. 19-4. Spiral fracture.

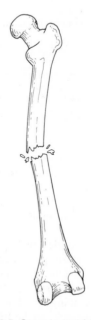

Fig. 19-5. Comminuted fracture.

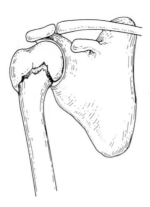

Fig. 19-6. Impacted fracture.

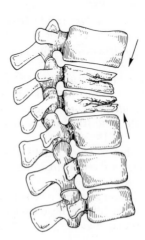

Fig. 19-7. Compression fracture.

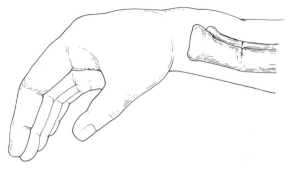

Fig. 19-8. Greenstick fracture.

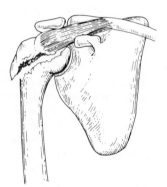

Fig. 19-9. Avulsion fracture.

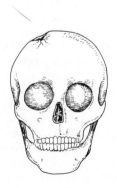

Fig. 19-10. Depression fracture.

the grammar school and junior high school age groups (Fig. 19-8).

An *avulsion fracture* is the result of a forceful contraction of a muscle mass, causing a bone fragment to break away at the insertion (Fig. 19-9).

A *depression fracture* is the result of a blunt trauma to a flat bone. This type of fracture is usually associated with a great deal of soft tissue damage (Fig. 19-10).

Assessment

General assessment of a patient with a suspected limb fracture should include checking for pain or point tenderness, pulses distal to the fracture site, pallor (skin color) distal to the fracture site, paresthesia (tingling or numbness) of the extremity, and paralysis of the extremity. These indices are known as the "five Ps." Other entities to check for are deformity, swelling, crepitus, discoloration and other associated wounds.

Therapeutic intervention

Begin with the general assessment as indicated above. Determining the mechanism of injury helps determine the fracture diagnosis. Immobilize the fracture site by splinting the extremity to include the joints above and below the fracture site whenever possible. Once splinting has been accomplished, reassess the limb for neurovascular status. If compromise is present, apply traction in an attempt to restore integrity. Elevate the limb if possible to decrease the amount of swelling and hemorrhage. Apply a cold pack to the injured area to cause vasoconstriction and decrease swelling, spasm, and pain.

When a limb is traumatized, a fracture should be suspected until it is proved otherwise by x-ray films, which are the most definitive way of confirming a fracture. If possible, the x-ray film should include the joints above and below the trauma site, as these joints are often injured and the injury is oftentimes overlooked. The x-ray film should also include both anterior and lateral views of the injured limb, because some fractures can only be visualized from one angle.

When limbs are fractured, they may cause damage to vessels that leads to hypvolemia and shock. A jagged bone may lacerate vital organs, arteries, veins, and/or nerves. Open fractures may lead to serious infections. Fractures may also lead to fat emboli, which may occur anywhere from 24 to 48 hours after the fracture. They are most commonly seen in conjunction with pelvic, tibial, or femoral fractures, but may also be associated with other types of fractures. Fat embolism has a high mortality rate and is a life-threatening situation. The patient develops a sudden onset of tachycardia accompanied by an elevated temperature, an altered level of consciousness, decreased respirations, cough, shortness of breath, cyanosis, petechiae, and pulmonary edema. Immediate therapeutic intervention includes oxygen delivery at a very high flow rate, support of airway, breathing, and circulation, and possible administration of steroids and heparin according to physician or facility policy.

Victims with multiple fractures are frequently hospitalized. Many of these victims have had an accident that has occurred as a result of alcohol abuse, where they have fallen, been struck by an automobile, or been involved in a collision of two motor vehicles. If hospitalization is prolonged, these people may begin to experience delirium tremens. It is, therefore, essential to ask questions about alcohol use when obtaining the initial history. One must give appropriate attention to the patient with a history of chronic alcoholism. Therapeutic intervention for a patient experiencing delirium

tremens is diazepam (Valium) IV, chlorpromazine (Thorazine), and IV alcohol (see also Chapter 24).

Upper torso fractures

The following upper torso fractures are commonly seen:

Clavicle

Shoulder

Scapula

Ribs (see Chapter 16)

Sternum (see Chapter 16)

Clavicular fracture. Fracture of the clavicle is a common type of fracture that can be found in all age groups (Fig. 19-11). It is particularly common in children. It usually results from a fall on the arm or the shoulder or direct lateral trauma to the shoulder such as contact injury in which athletes run into each other. The victim complains of pain in the clavicular area and point tenderness, and he will not raise his arm. Swelling, deformity, and crepitus are present. One will also notice that the victim tilts his head toward the side of the injury with his chin directed toward the opposite side. One should assess the neurovascular status of the arm, support the arm, and place the shoulders in a figure eight support (Fig. 19-12). The patient should be instructed to apply a cold pack to the injured area for 12 to 24 hours (intermittently) and to see an orthopedic specialist or be referred to the orthopedic clinic for follow-up.

Shoulder fracture. A shoulder fracture is a fracture of the glenoid, humeral head, or humeral neck (Fig. 19-13). It is common to see shoulder fractures in the elderly as a result of a fall on an outstretched arm, or as a result of direct trauma to the shoulder. When this same mechanism of injury occurs in a younger person, it usually results in a shoulder dislocation. However, a fracture occurs in an elderly person because of a weaker bone structure.

When a person has a shoulder fracture, he will complain of pain in the shoulder area and point tenderness; he will not be able to move his arm; and there will be gross swelling and discoloration. Therapeutic intervention includes

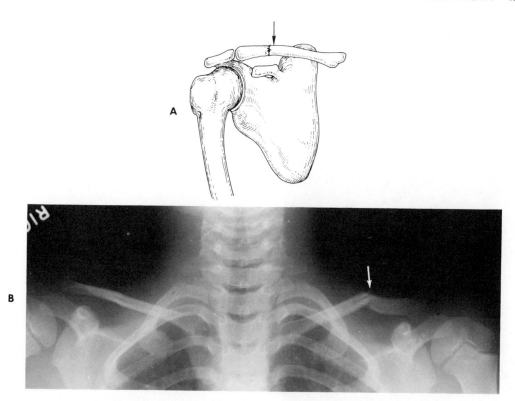

Fig. 19-11. **A,** Fracture of clavicle; **B,** arrow on radiograph shows fracture.

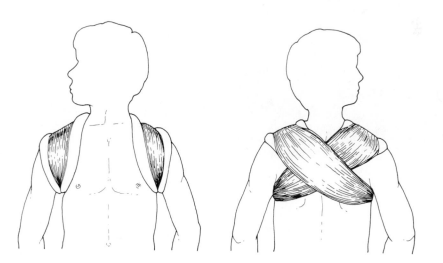

Fig. 19-12. Figure eight support.

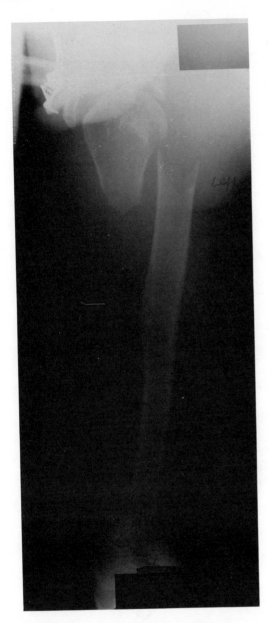

Fig. 19-13. Radiograph of shoulder fracture.

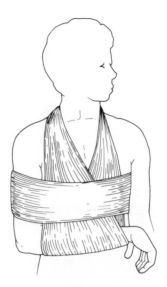

Fig. 19-14. Sling and swath.

admits the patient to the hospital where skeletal traction is applied. If the fracture has been unable to be reduced by the manipulative method, an open reduction may have to be performed. One must pay particular attention to the fact that a humeral neck fracture may cause axillary nerve damage.

Scapular fracture. A scapular fracture (Fig. 19-15) may be seen in any age group. This injury is usually the result of a violent direct trauma. It may, however, be seen as the result of a severe muscle contraction. The patient complains of pain on shoulder movement and point tenderness. There is usually bone displacement and swelling over the injured area. Therapeutic intervention includes assessment of neurovascular status, a compression bandage over the scapula if the bone is nondisplaced, a sling and swath bandage, and a cold pack for the first 24 hours. Complications include injuries to the underlying ribs or viscera.

Arm fractures

Fractures of the upper arm. Fractures of the upper arm (humeral shaft) are seen commonly

assessment of the neurovascular status, a sling and swath (Fig. 19-14), and a cold pack over the area of the injury. An orthopedic surgeon generally reduces the fracture and either immobilizes the fracture with a sling and swath or

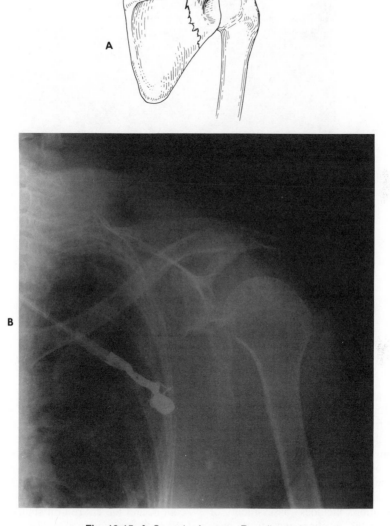

Fig. 19-15. A, Scapular fracture; **B,** radiograph.

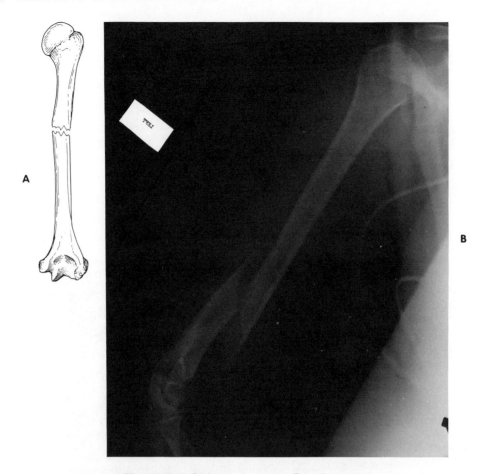

Fig. 19-16. A, Fracture of humerus; **B,** radiograph.

in children and in the elderly (Fig. 19-16). This type of fracture results from a fall on the arm, a direct trauma, or in association with a dislocation of the shoulder. It is a painful fracture; the victim complains of point tenderness, and one will note swelling, the inability or hesitance of the victim to use his arm, a severe deformity or angulation, and crepitus. Therapeutic intervention includes assessment of neurovascular status, a sling and swath bandage, a cold pack, and assessment for other injuries, because humeral shaft fractures are frequently associated with chest trauma. When the patient arrives in the emergency department, the fracture is usually reduced by closed reduc-

tion. If vascular or neurological compromise is present, one should apply mild, steady, downward traction. The arm is casted, applying a long plaster splint from the acromial process, down around the elbow, and back up to the acromial process. It is then wrapped with a compression elastic bandage (to allow for swelling). The axilla should be padded with cotton, and the entire arm should be stabilized and supported with a sling. Besides routine cast care instructions, the patient should be instructed to exercise his wrists and fingers frequently. There is a danger of radial nerve damage in a fracture of the middle or distal portion of the shaft. There is also a possibility of hem-

Fig. 19-17. A, Fracture of elbow; **B,** radiograph.

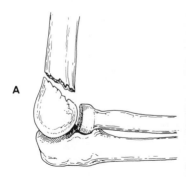

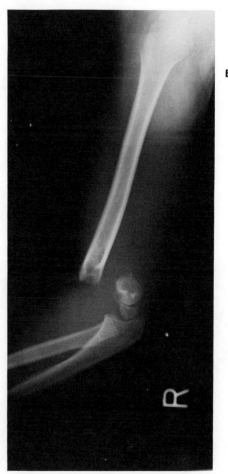

orrhage if bleeding is not controlled in the early moments of the injury.

Elbow fractures. Elbow fractures are seen most commonly in young children and young athletes. They result from a fall on an extended arm or on a flexed elbow (Fig. 19-17). This is a common result of a fall from a skateboard. The patient complains of pain and point tenderness. There is a great deal of swelling, as this injury is frequently associated with much soft tissue damage. The patient does not move his elbow, and a deformity is present. Because of the massive swelling, there may be vascular compromise, resulting in decreased circulation to the hand. Therapeutic intervention requires immediate assessment of vascular status. The arm should be splinted in the position in which it is found—not always an easy task. If possible, a sling and swath bandage should be applied, as well as a cold pack. If neurovascular compromise is evident, attempt to flex the arm at a greater angle. The fracture may be reduced manually or it may have to be reduced by placement of a pin and traction. If the fracture is reduced in a closed manual fashion, it is usually casted and placed in a sling. The complications of this type of fracture are brachial artery laceration, median or radial nerve damage, and Volkmann's ischemic contracture.

Volkmann's ischemic contracture results from ischemia to the muscles and nerves. Signs and symptoms of this condition are inability to move the fingers (manipulation of the fingers causes severe pain), severe pain in the forearm flexor muscles (even after reduction), inability to obtain a radial pulse, swelling, cold temperature of the extremity, cyanosis, and decreased sensation. Temporary therapeutic intervention includes removal of the cast and extension of the forearm with application of cold packs. It is essential to obtain immediate orthopedic consultation for further therapeutic intervention.

Forearm fractures. Forearm (radius and ulna) fractures are seen commonly in both adults and children. They usually result from a fall on an extended arm or as a result of a di-

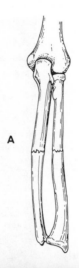

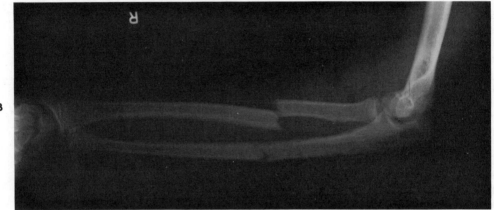

Fig. 19-18. A, Fractures of radius and ulna; **B,** radiograph.

rect blow (Fig. 19-18). The patient exhibits signs and symptoms of pain, point tenderness, swelling, deformity and angulation, and occasional shortening of the extremity. Therapeutic intervention includes assessment of neurovascular status, a splint to immobilize the fracture, a sling, and a cold pack. Many of these fractures can be manipulated with closed reduction technique. They are then casted with the elbow in 90° of flexion. The shoulder and the fingers should be free of the cast and allowed motion. Complications include rare neurovascular compromise and Volkmann's ischemic contracture.

Wrist and hand fractures

Fractures of the wrist. Fractures of the wrist are common in the elderly but may occur in any age group (Fig. 19-19). The most common mechanism of injury is a fall on an extended arm and an open hand. These patients complain of pain, swelling, and deformity. One should first assess the neurovascular status of the wrist and hand. The fractured limb should be splinted as it is found. The arm should be placed in a sling, and a cold pack should be applied. Because one can anticipate much swelling, one may elect to place a compression bandage over the fracture site. Oftentimes these

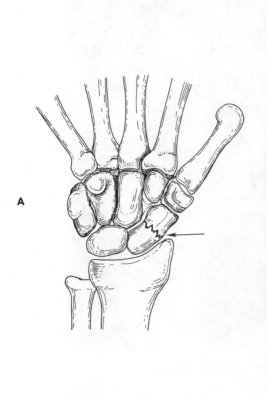

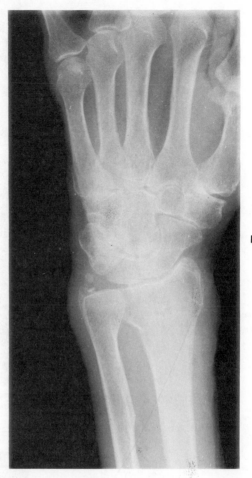

A   B

Fig. 19-19. A, Wrist fracture; **B,** radiograph.

fractures can be manipulated in a closed reduction procedure and then casted and placed
in a sling. Occasionally an open reduction is
necessary to pin the fracture segments. Aseptic
necrosis is a rare complication resulting from
fractures of the wrist.

A fracture of the distal radius and ulna is
known as a silver fork deformity and results
from a fall onto an extended hand. This type
of fracture is also known as a *Colles* fracture.
If a patient has a Colles fracture, it is wise to
check the mechanism of injury. Occasionally
these victims fall from a height and fracture
their os calcis (heel) and also sustain a compres-

sion fracture of the lumbodorsal vertebrae. The
victim may then fall forward as a result of the
pain from the lumbar fracture. As he falls forward, he extends his hands to break his fall,
and the result is an associated Colles fracture.

Carpal and metacarpal fractures. Fractures
of the carpals and the metacarpals are common
injuries in athletes, particularly those involved
in contact sports (Fig. 19-20). Some of the
more common types of fractures of the carpals
and metacarpals result from such activities as
fighting, which causes a fracture of the fifth
metacarpal, known as a ''boxer's fracture.''
Another common type of fracture is an avul-

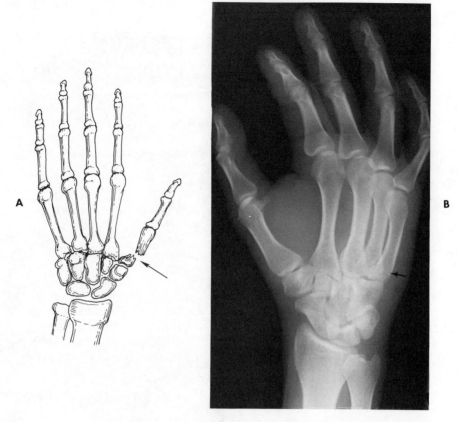

Fig. 19-20. A, Fracture of metacarpals; **B,** radiograph.

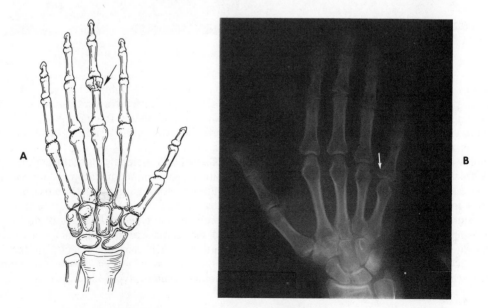

Fig. 19-21. A, Fracture of phalange; **B,** radiograph.

sion fracture, which results when someone throws a baseball and causes the distal attachment of the extensor tendon to tear loose, bringing with it a segment of bone. Other common carpal and metacarpal fractures result from industrial crush injuries.

Signs and symptoms of fractured carpals and metacarpals include pain, severe swelling, deformity, inability to use the hand, and, frequently, an open fracture. Therapeutic intervention includes assessment of neurovascular status, control of bleeding, covering the open wounds with a dry, sterile, bulky dressing, splinting the fracture in a functional position, application of a cold pack, and pressure to the wound with a compression bandage. The fracture is usually casted in the emergency department.

Phalange fractures. Fractured phalanges (fingers) are common in all age groups (Fig. 19-21). Signs and symptoms are similar to those of carpal and metacarpal fractures, and therapeutic intervention is basically the same.

Sometimes phalange fractures have an associated hematoma beneath the fingernail (a subungual hematoma), and the victim complains of a severe, throbbing pain. Therapeutic intervention in this case is nail trephination. Therapeutic intervention for phalange fractures is usually splinting the finger involved. Occasionally an operative reduction will have to be performed to realign the fractured segments.

Pelvic fractures (Fig. 19-22)

Pelvic fractures occur frequently in middle-aged and elderly adults. It is estimated that 65% of patients with pelvic fractures have other associated injuries. It is also estimated that 8% to 10% of patients with pelvic fractures die. This injury commonly occurs as a crush injury from an automobile or motorcycle accident or as a result of direct trauma, a fall from a height, or sudden contraction of a muscle against resistance. The patient exhibits signs and symptoms of tenderness over the pubis when the iliac wings are compressed, para-

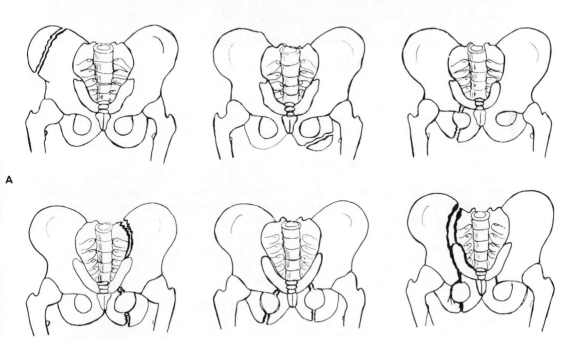

A

Fig. 19-22. A, Pelvic fractures. (**A** from Barber, J. M., and Budassi, S. A.: Mosby's manual of emergency care, St. Louis, 1979, The C. V. Mosby Co.)

Continued.

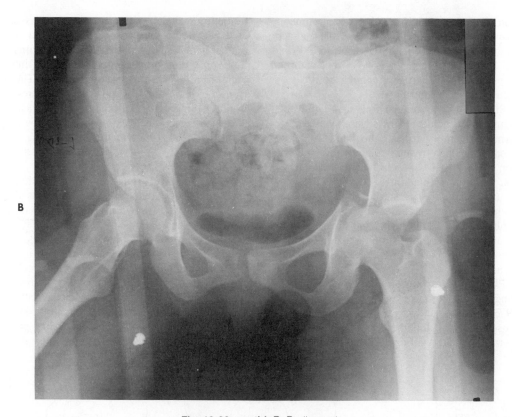

Fig. 19-22, cont'd. B, Radiograph.

spinous muscle spasm, sacroiliac joint tenderness, paresis or hemiparesis, pelvic ecchymosis, and hematuria. The patient may also demonstrate signs of blood loss as evidenced in tachycardia, hypotension, and other signs of pending shock.

Therapeutic intervention includes immobilization of the spine and the legs using a long board, flexing the knees to decrease pain, oxygen at high liter flow, monitoring vital signs every 5 minutes, initiation of two large-bore IV lines for volume replacement (run at a rate in accordance with blood pressure and pulse measurements), placing the antishock trousers under the patient and inflating as necessary (see pp. 247-249). These patients should be transported to a hospital facility rapidly, in order that early x-ray studies, peritoneal lavage, and typing and cross-matching can be accomplished

in minimal time. These patients have a tendency to bleed profusely and should be typed and cross-matched for at least five units of whole blood. The average amount of blood lost is two units.

Complications of pelvic fractures include bladder trauma, genital trauma, lumbosacral trauma, ruptured internal organs, shock, and death.

In-hospital therapeutic intervention may include bed rest, with either pinning and traction or casting, following closed or open reduction.

Hip fractures (Fig. 19-23)

Hip fractures are common in the elderly, where the fracture usually results from a fall or a minor trauma. When a hip fracture occurs in a younger person, it is usually the result of

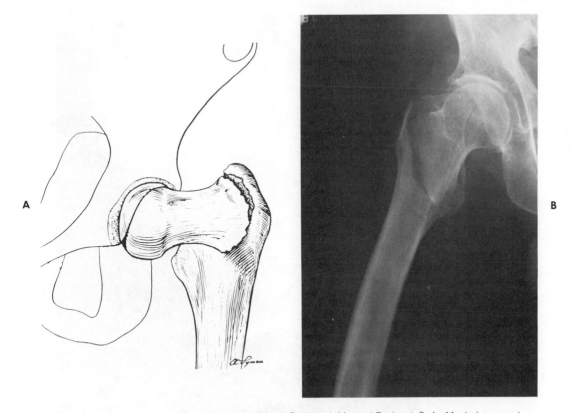

Fig. 19-23. A, Hip fracture; **B,** radiograph. (**A** from Barber, J. M., and Budassi, S. A.: Mosby's manual of emergency care, St. Louis, 1979, The C. V. Mosby Co.)

a major trauma. These patients complain of pain in the hip joint and the groin area, severe pain with movement of the leg, inability to bear weight, external rotation of the hip and leg, and minimal shortening of the limb. If the injury is extracapsular and associated with a trochanteric fracture, the patient complains of pain in the area of the lateral hip, one sees an increased shortening of the extremity, and the degree of external rotation is greater.

Immediate therapeutic intervention includes splinting the hip, either to a long board or one leg to the other, checking pulses and neurological status distal to the fracture site, and taking frequent vital signs (at least every 5 minutes). Once the patient reaches the hospital, early immobilization should be accomplished, and surgical intervention is probable.

Complications of hip fracture are the immediate complications of hypovolemia and shock and the later complications resulting from prolonged bed rest.

Leg fractures

Femoral fractures (Fig. 19-24). Femoral fractures occur in all age groups, usually the result of a major trauma. The patient complains of severe pain and an inability to bear weight on the injured leg. There is a noticeable deformity, swelling, and angulation. The limb shortens as a result of severe muscle spasm. One may also note crepitus over the fracture site.

Therapeutic intervention includes use of the Hare traction splint (Fig. 19-25) or other type of long-leg splint, such as a Thomas splint, to apply traction to the limb. One should not

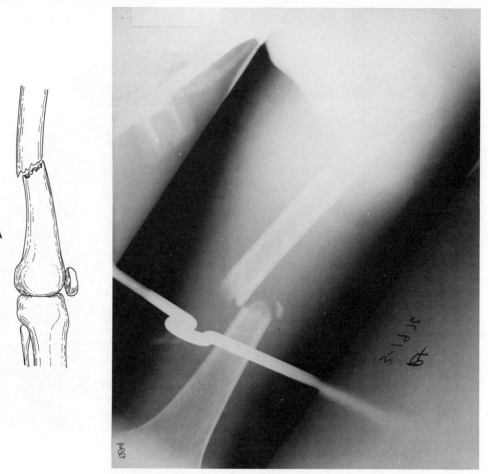

Fig. 19-24. A, Fracture of femur; **B,** radiograph.

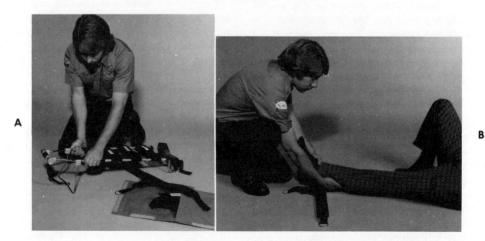

Fig. 19-25. Hare traction splint application. **A,** Remove cover. Twist collet sleeves to unlock. Place splint parallel to injured leg. Adjust splint to desired length, approximately 8 to 10 inches past foot. Twist collet sleeves to lock (excessive pressure not required). Fold down heel stand until it locks into place. Slide heel stand up splint about 5 inches. Position Velcro support straps (two above knee and two below knee) and open. **B,** Remove tri-ring ankle strap from cover and place under patient's heel with padded side against foot. Place bottom edge of heel even with lower edge of sponge.

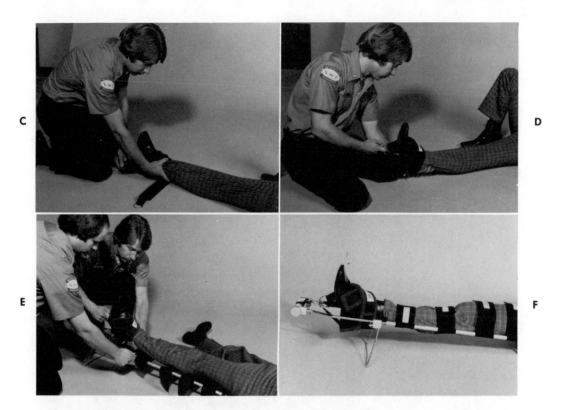

Fig. 19-25, cont'd. C, Criss-cross top straps over instep, keeping straps high up on instep. **D,** Grasp all three rings, bottom ring first, and exert manual traction to align leg using slow firm pull. Steady foot by placing one hand under heel. When establishing manual alignment, be sure to support lower portion of involved extremity just below point of fracture. **E,** While maintaining manual traction, have an assistant place splint under leg with half-ring placed just below the buttock. Secure half-ring strap. Once alignment is started, continue to maintain constant manual traction until alignment has been secured by splint. **F,** Insert the S hook into three D rings, heel ring first. Twist knurled knob to apply traction. Tighten until strap is snug. Injured leg is now in traction. Fasten the Velcro straps, which may also be used to apply pressure over an open wound. Position strap so it will close over bleeding area, apply gauze pad, and secure strap. The patient may now be moved. You should adjust location of heel stand after patient has been placed on cot so that solid contact is established with cot. (Manufactured exclusively by Dyna Med, Inc., 6200 Yarrow Drive, Carlsbad, Calif. 92008.)

use a long-leg air splint with a closed foot, as one will not be able to assess distal neurovascular status. It is also not advisable to use the other leg as a splint. Whenever possible and whenever time permits, initiate two large-bore IV lines for volume replacement. Be sure to check for distal pulses and distal neurological status. Check, also, for other associated injuries. One should obtain frequent vital signs

(at least every 5 minutes). Apply a cold pack to the injured area. If the injury is isolated, consider analgesia. Once the victim arrives at the hospital, he should be prepared for traction, pin placement, or surgery.

Complications of femoral fracture include hypovolemia. It is not infrequent to lose two units of blood into the thigh of a fractured femur. As a result of the severe muscle spasm

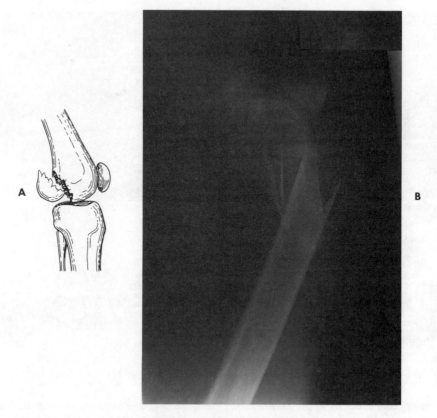

Fig. 19-26. A, Knee fracture; **B,** radiograph.

causing the bone ends to move, severe muscle damage may result. Also, often associated with femur fracture is knee trauma, which could be very easily overlooked. The greatest complication of femoral fracture is shock caused by hypovolemia. There is also a possibility of fat emboli.

Knee fractures. Knee fractures are either supracondylar fractures of the femur or intra-articular fractures of the femur or tibia (Fig. 19-26). This type of injury may occur in all age groups and is usually the result of an automobile, motorcycle, or automobile-pedestrian accident that results in a direct trauma to the knee. The patient complains of knee pain, an inability to bend the knee or straighten the knee (depending upon the position of the knee following the accident), swelling, and tenderness.

Therapeutic intervention should include a long leg splint or one leg secured to another, check of distal pulses, and distal neurological status. Depending upon the extent of the injury, the patient may have to be prepared for surgical repair and will most likely be casted. The most common complication of knee fracture is neurovascular compromise.

Patellar fractures. Patellar fractures are commonly seen in all age groups (Fig. 19-27). They usually occur as a result of a direct trauma from a fall or an impact with the dashboard of a car or from indirect trauma, such as a severe muscle pull. The patient complains of pain in the knee. The fracture can often be palpated by the examiner. Frequently there is an open fracture. Therapeutic intervention includes covering the open wound and applying

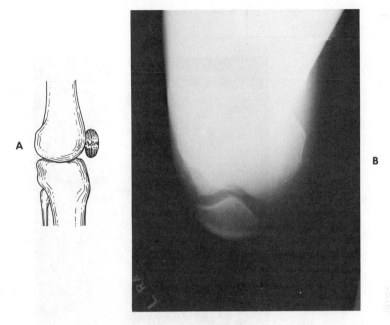

Fig. 19-27. A, Patellar fracture; **B,** radiograph.

a cold pack and a long-leg splint. When the patient arrives in the emergency department, the limb should be x-rayed to determine the extent of the fracture. If the fracture is nondisplaced, the leg is usually placed in a long-leg cylinder cast. If the fracture is displaced, there should be an attempt to realign the parts. Sometimes it is necessary to send the patient to surgery for an open reduction and perhaps even a pinning. Remember that the patella is an important part of the knee in that it aids in leverage of the knee and protects the knee joint.

Tibial and fibular fractures. Tibial and fibular fractures are seen commonly in all age groups (Fig. 19-28). They result from direct or indirect trauma or a rotational force. The patient complains of pain in his leg, point tenderness, swelling, deformity, and crepitus. Many tibial and fibular fractures are open fractures. These injuries should be splinted as they are found without attempt at realignment unless there is neurovascular compromise. Be sure to check for neurovascular status before and after splinting. Most of the time the leg can be

splinted with a long-leg splint. If there is an open fracture, it should be irrigated with sterile normal saline and covered with a dry sterile dressing. Apply a cold pack to the area of the wound. Upon arrival in the emergency department, x-ray films should be obtained, and the extent of the injury should be determined. Open or closed reduction may be necessary. The patient's leg is almost always casted. If the fibula alone is fractured (which is very unusual) a walking cast is usually applied, as the fibula is not a weight-bearing bone.

Complications of tibial and fibular fractures can include soft tissue damage, infection, neurovascular compromise, and Volkmann's ischemic contracture.

Ankle fractures. Fractures of the ankle are commonly seen in all age groups (Fig. 19-29). These types of injuries occur as a result of direct trauma, indirect trauma, or torsion. The patient complains of pain in the area of the injury, inability to bear weight on the extremity, point tenderness, swelling, and deformity. Therapeutic intervention includes a soft splint,

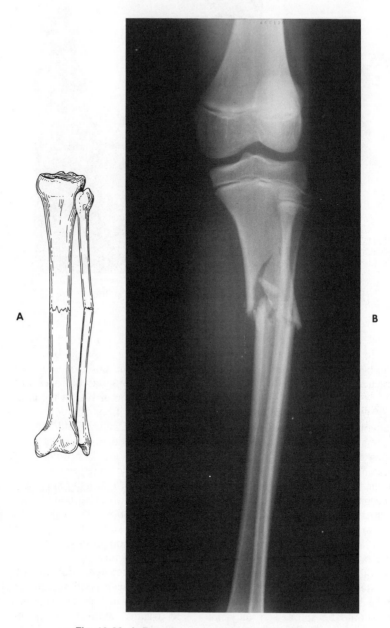

Fig. 19-28. A, Tibial/fibular fracture; **B,** radiograph.

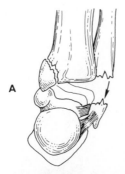

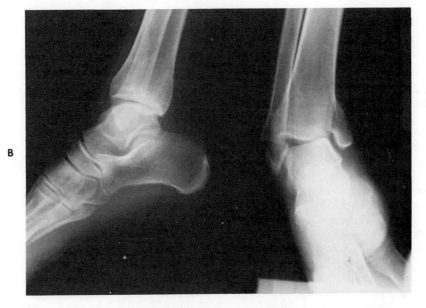

Fig. 19-29. A, Ankle fracture; **B,** radiograph.

check of neurovascular status, a cold pack, and elevation. X-ray films are obtained upon the patient's arrival in the emergency department. Depending upon the extent of damage, the patient may need a closed or open reduction, pinning, and most likely a cast. Depending on the extent and location of the injury, the patient may be placed in a walking cast. The most common complication from this type of injury is neurovascular compromise.

Foot fractures

Tarsal and metatarsal fractures. Fractures of the tarsals and metatarsals are common in all age groups (Fig. 19-30). They occur as a result of automobile accidents, athletic injuries, crush injuries, or direct trauma. The patient complains of pain in his foot. He will hesitate to bear weight on his foot. There is point tenderness, deformity, and swelling. Therapeutic intervention includes a compression dressing and a soft splint. When the patient arrives in the emergency department, an x-ray film is obtained to determine the extent of the injury. The fracture(s) should be reduced if necessary, and the patient should have his foot placed in a cast. He may be allowed to walk on crutches without weight bearing. Complications from this type of injury are rare.

Heel (os calcis) fracture. Fractures of the

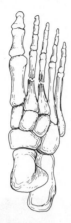

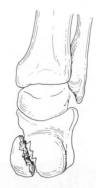

Fig. 19-30. Foot fracture.

Fig. 19-31. Heel fracture.

heel (os calcis) are usually seen in the young adult and usually result form a fall from a height in which the patient lands on his feet (Fig. 19-31). The patient complains of pain in the heel area and point tenderness, and demonstrates swelling and perhaps dislocation. Therapeutic intervention includes a compression dressing, elevation of the injured extremity, and a cold pack. Upon arrival in the emergency department, the patient should have x-ray studies performed. Management usually includes reduction of the fracture if necessary and application of a below-the-knee, weight-bearing cast. Occasionally open reduction is necessary. Complications of this type of injury are frequently, an associated lumbosacral compression fracture, and rarely, a Colles fracture.

Toe (phalangeal) fractures. Fractures of the toes (phalanges) are commonly seen in all age groups (Fig. 19-32). They are usually caused by kicking a hard object or running into an immovable object (stubbing the toe). The patient complains of pain in the toe area, and one will notice swelling and discoloration. Therapeutic intervention includes a compression dressing, a rigid splint, elevation, and a cold pack. Following x-ray studies in the emergency department, felt or cotton is placed between the fractured toe and the toe next to it. The two toes are then taped together so that the uninjured toe acts as a splint. The patient may bear weight as tolerated and is instructed to wear

shoes that do not put weight on the toes from the anterior aspect. Complications from this type of injury are rare.

Fracture healing

Fractures may heal poorly as a result of improper immobilization, poor reduction, insufficient immobility, too much traction on the injured extremity, a decreased neurological or vascular supply, and infection.

DISLOCATIONS

Dislocations occur when a joint exceeds its range of motion and the joint surfaces are no longer intact. Soft tissue injury within the joint capsule and surrounding ligaments, severe swelling, and possible vein and artery damage are commonly seen with this type of injury. One can frequently project a diagnosis before obtaining confirming x-rays by soliciting the mechanism of injury.

In general, dislocations produce severe pain, deformity at the joint, an inability to move the joint, swelling, and point tenderness. Therapeutic intervention includes careful palpation of the joint and splinting the injury as it is found. One should *not* attempt to relocate the joint in the prehospital setting unless there is severe neurovascular compromise. It is important to transport the patient early so that the emergency department physician or orthopedic surgeon can reduce the dislocation early under

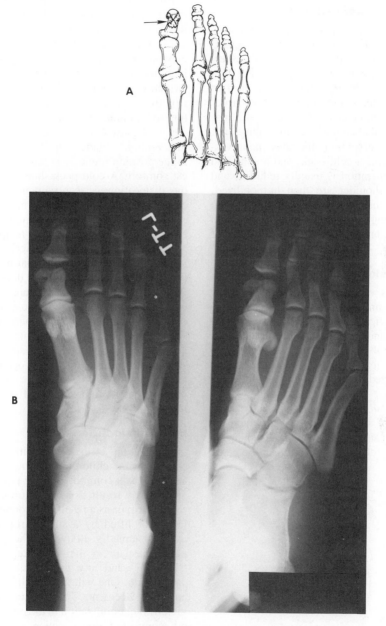

Fig. 19-32. A, Toe fracture; **B,** radiographs.

adequate anesthesia. One should be very careful to check for associated fractures.

Acromioclavicular dislocation

Acromioclavicular separations are commonly seen in athletes (Fig. 19-33). They are caused by a fall or a force on the point of the shoulder. The patient complains of great pain in the joint area. He will not be able to raise his arm or bring it across his chest. One will note a deformity and point or area tenderness, swelling, and possibly a hematoma over the injury site. Therapeutic intervention includes neurovascular assessment, a cold pack, and a sling and swath. The separation is usually reduced, and the arm and shoulder are then immobilized. Occasionally, the patient will have to be taken to the operating room for an open reduction and wiring. Complications form this type of injury are rare.

Shoulder dislocation

Dislocations of the shoulder usually occur in the young and in athletes. There are two general categories for dislocations of the shoulder: anterior and posterior dislocations. Each type has several variations but will not be discussed in this text. For more information, the reader is referred to the bibliography at the end of the chapter.

Anterior shoulder dislocations usually occur as the result of an athletic injury in which the athlete falls on an extended arm that is abducted and externally rotated. The result is a force that

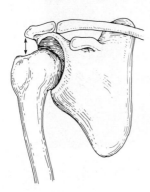

Fig. 19-33. Acromioclavicular separation.

pushes the head of the humerus anterior to the shoulder joint (Fig. 19-34).

Posterior dislocations are rare. They are usually found in patients with seizures in which the arm is abducted and internally rotated.

In all shoulder dislocations, the patient will complain of severe pain in the shoulder area, an inability to move his arm, and a deformity (which is sometimes difficult to see in a posterior dislocation). It is estimated that 55% to 60% of shoulder dislocations seen in the emergency department are recurrent. Therapeutic intervention includes support of the extremity in the position found or in the position of greatest comfort. A cold pack should be applied. If the dislocation is recurrent and relocation is easy to do, it may be performed in the field (however, this is not advisable). Be sure to check for distal pulses, skin temperature and moisture, and distal neurological status. Upon arrival in the emergency department, the patient should have x-ray films done before the joint is relocated, unless there is neurovascular compromise. Once the joint is relocated, one should immobilize the joint by placing a sling and swath bandage or other commercially available device on the injured side. The patient should be referred to an orthopedic surgeon. Complications from this type of injury are neurovascular compromise and associated fractures.

Elbow dislocation

Dislocations of the elbow joint are seen most commonly in children, teenagers, and young adults. It is a common athletic injury (Fig. 19-35). It may result from a fall on an externally rotated arm or as a result of a young child being jerked or lifted by a single arm (known also as "nursemaid's elbow"). The patient complains of pain in the joint area. It may feel "locked," and any movement may produce severe pain. One will note swelling, deformity, and displacement. Therapeutic intervention includes immobilization in the position of greatest comfort for the patient, assessment of neurovascular status, and a cold pack. When the patient arrives in the emergency department, following x-ray studies of the injured

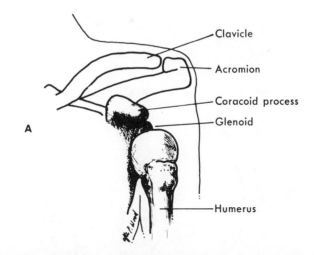

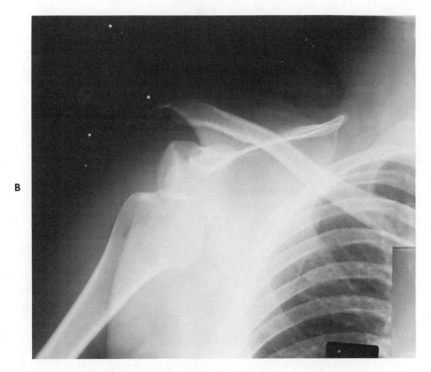

Fig. 19-34. A, Shoulder dislocation; **B,** radiograph. (**A** from Barber, J. M., and Budassi, S. A.: Mosby's manual of emergency care, St. Louis, 1979, The C. V. Mosby Co.)

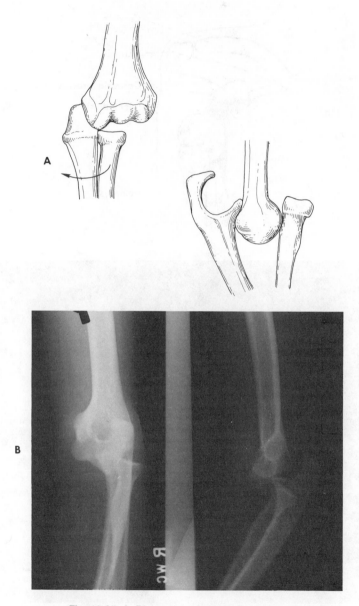

Fig. 19-35. A, Dislocation of elbow; **B,** radiograph.

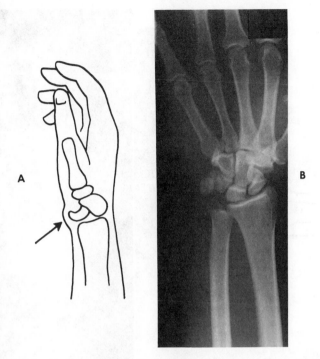

Fig. 19-36. A, Dislocation of wrist; **B,** radiograph. (**A** from Barber, J. M., and Budassi, S. A.: Mosby's manual of emergency care, St. Louis, 1979, The C. V. Mosby Co.)

extremity, the joint should be relocated. Once the joint is relocated, it is immobilized. The position of immobilization depends on the type of dislocation. The most common complication of this type of injury is neurovascular compromise.

Wrist dislocation

Dislocation of the wrist is an injury seen most frequently in the athlete, although it may be seen in all age groups. It usually results from a fall on an outstretched hand (Fig. 19-36). The patient complains of severe pain in the wrist area. Swelling, deformity, and point tenderness are evident. Therapeutic intervention includes a splint, a sling and swath bandage, and a cold pack. Upon arrival in the emergency department, the patient should have x-ray films of the injured extremity, followed by relocation of the joint. It is then followed by casting to immobilize the joint. Complicatons of this

type of injury are neurovascular compromise, especially median nerve damage.

Hand or finger dislocation

Hand or finger dislocations are most commonly seen in athletes. This injury usually results from a fall on an outstretched hand or finger. It may also result from direct trauma to the tip of the finger (Fig. 19-37). The patient complains of pain in the area of the injury and inability to move the joint. One will note deformity and swelling. One should splint the injury in the position of comfort and apply a cold pack until x-ray films are obtained and interpreted and relocation of the joint is attempted. The injured area is then usually splinted to immobilize the joint.

Hip dislocation

Hip dislocations are common to all age groups. This injury usually results from a major

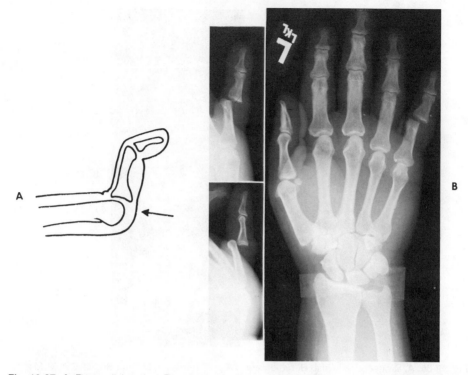

Fig. 19-37. A, Finger dislocation; **B,** radiograph. (**A** from Barber, J. M., and Budassi, S. A.: Mosby's manual of emergency care, St. Louis, 1979, The C. V. Mosby Co.)

trauma in which the leg is extended before impact (Fig. 19-38). This is commonly seen in head-on collisions in which the leg is extended and the foot is on the brake peddle just before impact, or the knee jams into the dashboard (Fig. 19-39). This type of injury also occurs from falls and crush injuries. The dislocation may result in either anterior or posterior displacement. The patient complains of pain in the hip area and the knee area. The hip will be flexed, adducted, and internally rotated on posterior dislocation and flexed, abducted, and externally rotated on anterior dislocation. The joint will feel locked, and the patient will not be able to move his leg.

Splint the extremity in the position found or in the position of comfort. Be sure to check for neurovascular status and other associated in-juries. Apply a cold pack and transport the patient to an emergency department where the hip joint can be relocated. Necrosis of the femoral head may occur if the joint is not relocated within 24 hours.

Once the hip joint is relocated, the patient is usually placed on bed rest in traction. Children may be placed in a spica cast. Complications from this type of injury are femoral artery damage and nerve damage.

Leg dislocation

Knee dislocations. Knee dislocations are common to all age groups (Fig. 19-40). The mechanism of injury is usually a major trauma. The patient complains of severe pain in the knee area, inability to move the leg, much swelling, and deformity. Immediate therapeutic interven-

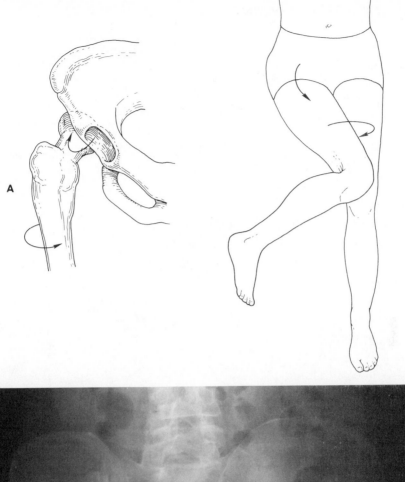

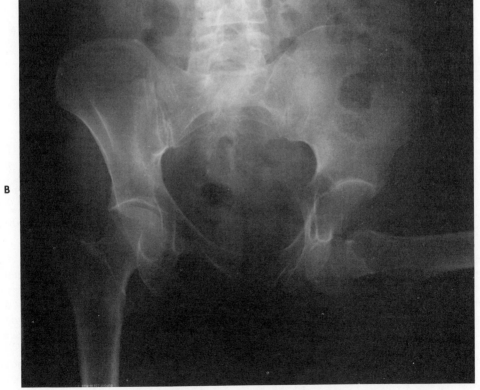

Fig. 19-38. A, Dislocation of hip; **B,** radiograph.

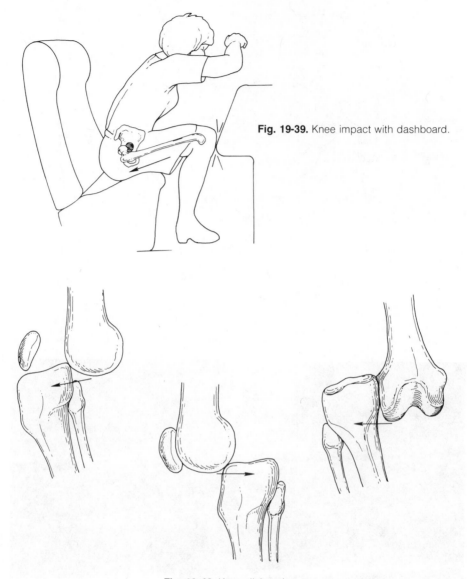

Fig. 19-39. Knee impact with dashboard.

Fig. 19-40. Knee dislocation.

tion includes splinting the limb in the position of comfort or in the position it is found. Check for distal neurovascular compromise, and apply a cold pack. When the patient arrives in the emergency department, after x-ray films are obtained to determine the extent of damage, the joint must be relocated. Early reduction is essential to avoid damage to the arteries and nerves. Complications include peroneal, popliteal, and tibial nerve damage. A fractured tibia is also frequently associated with knee dislocation. Almost all persons who suffer a dislocation of the knee joint have associated damage (usually severe) to the capsule (the muscles, ligaments, and tendons).

Following reduction, the patient is admitted

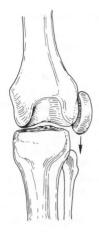

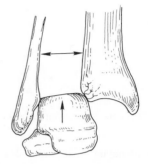

Fig. 19-41. Dislocation of patella.

Fig. 19-42. Dislocation of ankle.

to the hospital where he is placed on bed rest and his knee is kept elevated and in cold packs for 7 to 10 days. Following this period, the patient is usually casted.

Patellar dislocation. Dislocations of the patella are commonly seen in all age groups (Fig. 19-41). It is a common injury in athletes and in those individuals who have had a direct trauma to the lateral aspect of the knee or a rapid rotation on a planted foot. These patients usually demonstrate signs of pain, keep their knee in a flexed position, and are unable to use the knee. There is a great deal of tenderness and swelling in the patella area. Therapeutic intervention includes splinting the leg in the position found and applying a cold pack. Following x-ray films, the patient should have the patella reduced. This is usually accomplished spontaneously when the leg is placed in extension. Following relocation, the knee is placed in a compression bandage, and a cylinder cast is applied.

Ankle dislocation. An ankle dislocation is usually the result of an athletic injury and is commonly associated with a fracture (Fig. 19-42). They result from lateral stress motion in which the normal range of motion of the ankle is exceeded. The patient complains of severe pain in the ankle area and inability to move the joint. There will be much swelling and deformity. Therapeutic intervention includes splinting the ankle and foot in a position of comfort.

Neurovascular status distal to the injury should be checked. A cold pack should be applied. Further management includes obtaining x-ray films to determine the extent of injury. The ankle may be relocated either by closed or open method, depending upon the degree of injury and associated fractures. Complications of this type of injury are primarily neurovascular compromise.

Foot dislocation. Dislocations of the foot occur in all age groups. This is a rare injury and is usually the result of an automobile or motorcycle accident in which a combination of forces has acted at the same time. This type of dislocation is almost always associated with an open wound. The patient complains of severe pain in the foot region. There is point tenderness and an inability of the patient to use his foot. One will note much swelling and deformity. If there is an open wound, it should be covered with a sterile dressing. It should be splinted in a soft splint and one should check for neurovascular status. Apply a cold pack. Obtain x-ray films to determine the extent of injury. Once the foot is relocated, a cylinder cast is usually applied, and the patient is instructed to elevate the limb and apply cold packs for 24 hours. There should be no weight bearing on the foot.

Toe (metatarsophalangeal) dislocation. Dislocations of the metatarsophalangeal joints (toes) are rare. When they do occur, they are

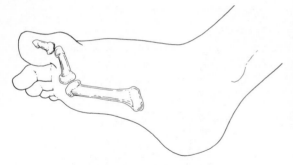

Fig. 19-43. Dislocation of metatarsophalangeal joint.

commonly associated with open fractures. It is important to reduce these dislocations immediately, as delay may result in inability to do a closed reduction of the dislocation (Fig. 19-43). The patient complains of pain and point tenderness in the area of the joint. There is a great deal of swelling and noticeable deformity. Therapeutic intervention is to cover the area with a bulky dressing to prevent further damage, elevate the extremity, and apply a cold pack. Following x-ray films, the dislocation should be reduced; the foot and toes should then be immobilized.

PEDIATRIC LIMB TRAUMA

If a fracture occurs at the epiphysis (growth center), early closure of the epiphyseal plate may occur. As the child continues to grow, there will be no growth of this particular bone in which a fracture at the epiphyseal plate has occurred. This results in the child having one extremity that is shorter than the other. If the fracture of the plate is only partial, there may be an angular deformity as the bone beneath the nonfractured section continues to grow while the section under the fracture segment does not grow. If an epiphyseal fracture does occur, these children should be followed closely by an orthopedic surgeon for several months, as it is difficult to predict the outcome at the time of the injury.

TRAUMATIC AMPUTATIONS

Traumatic amputations are common to farm workers as a result of heavy farm machine accidents, to factory workers as a result of a limb being caught by a heavy machine, and to motorcyclists, where a limb is amputated when the motorcycle and driver are involved in a collision with another vehicle. Body parts frequently amputated are the digits (the fingers and toes), the distal half of the foot (transmetatarsal), the lower leg, below the knee, the lower leg at the knee, the lower leg above the knee, the hand, the forearm, the arm, the ears, the nose, and the penis.

Therapeutic intervention for any type of amputation includes control of the ABCs, control of bleeding, support of the limb in a functional anatomic position if the part is only partially amputated, initiation of two large-bore IV lines, oxygen at high flow, usually by nasal cannula, and rapid transport to a facility where the patient can be further evaluated.

Preservation of the amputated part

Whenever possible, the amputated part should be preserved as though one were preparing it for reimplantation. The part should be kept at a hypothermic temperature of about 40° F. *Do not freeze the part.* This can be accomplished by immersing the part in normal saline solution in a container and placing the entire container in a bag filled with ice. *Do not place the part directly on ice.* If this type of equipment is not available, dress the part in a wrap saturated with normal saline solution or Ringer's lactate solution. Attempt to keep the limb in a correct anatomical position.

Reimplantation

Occasionally reimplantation is possible. Limiting factors are the availability of a reimplantation team, the amount of damage to the attached part and the amount of damage to the amputated part, the amount of time elapsed since the accident, the overall predicted outcome of the reimplantation, and the general physical condition of the victim. Historically, upper extremity reimplantations have been more successful than lower extremity reimplantations. Farrell (1977) has been treating fingertip amputations conservatively (without reimplantation) and has found that the fingertips have regenerated within 1 year.

SPLINTING

Splinting is done to prevent further damage to soft tissues; prevent damage to nerves, arteries, and veins; and decrease pain. One should always splint above and below the injury site. For example, when the elbow is injured, one should splint not only the elbow, but the forearm and the upper arm as well.

Application

When applying a splint, be sure to immobilize the injured part. If there is severe angulation, correct it only if it is impossible to splint or if neurovascular compromise is present. Whenever possible, do not try to splint an extremity alone; have the second rescuer place the padding and the splint while the first rescuer is supporting the extremity. Secure the injured part inside the splint but do not use an elastic bandage.

When applying an air splint, provided the splint is open at both ends, the rescuer should slip the splint over his own arm backwards. Grasp the distal portion of the injured limb with the hand of the arm that has the air splint on it. Then, slide the splint from the rescuer's arm onto the injured extremity. Once the splint is in the proper position, inflate it.

Always remember to recheck neurovascular status following splint placement.

Types of splints

There are four basic types of splints available. Those include soft splints, such as a pillow; hard splints, such as a board or other object that has a firm surface; air splints, which are inflatable and provide support without being hard; and traction splints, which provide support, decrease angulation, and provide traction.

There are many varieties of splints available to rescue personnel. These include the Thomas splint and the Hare traction splint (Fig. 19-44), which are used for fractures of the midshaft of the femur or upper third of the tibia. Note that these types of splints should *not* be used on hip, lower tibial or fibular or ankle fractures, or in fractures of the femur in which there is associated tibial or fibular fractures.

Other types of splints are shortboards (Fig. 19-45, *A*) and longboards (Fig. 19-45, *B*),

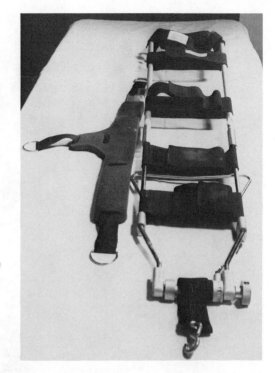

Fig. 19-44. Hare traction splint. (Photo by Richard Lazar.)

which are used for extrication or immobilization, particularly of those patients suspected of having a cervical spine or thoracic spine fracture. There are several commercial variations available on the market that perform the same functions as the shortboards and longboards.

Also available are aluminum long leg splints, cardboard splints, ladder splints, padded boards, air splints, vacuum splints, and a whole host of commercially available products, as well as improvised splints, which can be made by the creative rescuer.

PLASTER CASTS

This is simply a brief overview of casting and care of casts. Refer to a text for orthopedic assistants for a complete description of techniques and types of casts.

Applying the cast

Before the plaster is applied to the injured extremity, one should gather all needed equip-

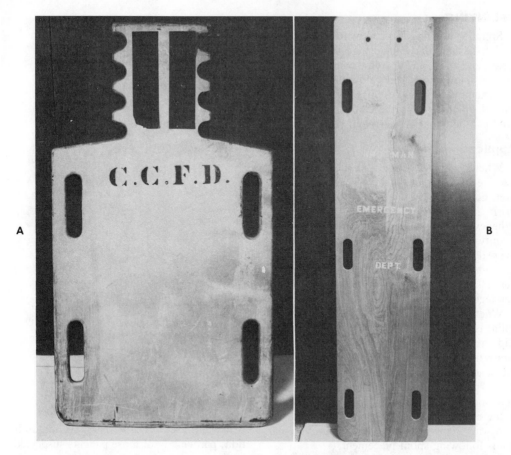

Fig. 19-45. A, Short spine board. **B,** Long spine board. (Photo by Richard Lazar.)

ment. The limb should be covered with stockinette, and bony prominences should be padded with cotton. Soak the plaster in cool to warm water and apply it rapidly, before it has a chance to harden.

Aftercare instructions for patients with casts

Return to the emergency department, the orthopedic clinic, or your private physician in 24 hours for follow-up care.

Keep the cast dry.

Keep the limb elevated above the level of the heart for 24 hours after the injury.

If any of these abnormalities is present, return to the follow-up clinic immediately:

Check the temperature of the digits; it is abnormal if they are very cold or very hot.

Check the color of the digits; it is abnormal if they are blue.

Check if there is feeling in the digits; it is abnormal if there is no feeling.

Wiggle the digits at least once each hour.

If a foreign object is dropped into the cast, return to the follow-up care facility immediately.

Return to the follow-up clinic if swelling recurs or if a foul odor is present.

Pressure sore

If a pressure sore is developing, the patient will develop an elevated temperature, he will continue to complain of pain after the first few days following the injury, and he will complain

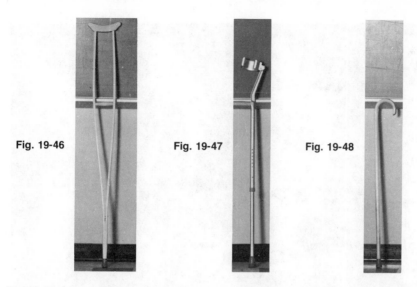

Fig. 19-46   Fig. 19-47   Fig. 19-48

Fig. 19-46. Axillary crutches. The underarm crutch illustrated is not adjustable but is lighter in weight than the adjustable crutch. (From Larson, C., and Gould, M.: Orthopedic nursing, ed. 9, St. Louis, 1978, The C. V. Mosby Co.)

Fig. 19-47. Loftstrand crutch. (From Larson, C., and Gould, M.: Orthopedic nursing, ed. 9, St. Louis, 1978, The C. V. Mosby Co.)

Fig. 19-48. Cane with half-circle handle is available in wood or metal. (From Larson, C., and Gould, M.: Orthopedic nursing, ed. 9, St. Louis, 1978, The C. V. Mosby Co.)

of not being able to get to sleep at night. If this occurs, the cast should be removed and the situation evaluated.

CRUTCH AND CANE FITTING

First of all, when measuring a patient for crutches or a cane, measure with the shoe he will be wearing when ambulating with the crutches or the cane. The shoe should fit well, have a 1-inch heel, and tie or buckle. Instruct the patient that he or she should not wear a slip-on shoe while ambulating.

Axillary crutches (Fig. 19-46). Axillary crutches should be fitted so that the armpiece is 2 inches from the axilla with no weight on the axilla. The tips of the crutches should be 6 to 8 inches to the side and the front of the foot at a 25° angle. The handpiece should be fitted so that the elbow will be at a 30° angle of flexion.

Loftstrand crutches (Fig. 19-47). Loftstrand crutches should be fitted so that the tips of the crutches are 6 inches to the side and the front of the foot at a 25° angle. The handpiece should

be fitted so that the elbow will be at a 30° angle of flexion.

Cane (Fig. 19-48). A cane should be fitted so that when the cane is held next to the heel, the elbow is at a 30° angle of flexion. A cane should be used for minimum support, particularly in hip injuries, and should be used to assist balance only.

GAIT TRAINING

1. Have the patient stand and balance (Fig. 19-49, *A*).
2. Have the patient hold the crutches 4 inches to the side of the foot and 4 inches in front of the foot (Fig. 19-49, *B*).
3. All weight is carried on the hands by straightening the elbows. Instruct the patient *not to place any weight* on the axillae, even while resting (Fig. 19-49, *C*).
4. In the emergency department, a three-point gait is usually taught, because this type of gait is used when little or no weight bearing is desired (Figs. 19-49, *D*, 19-50, and 19-51).

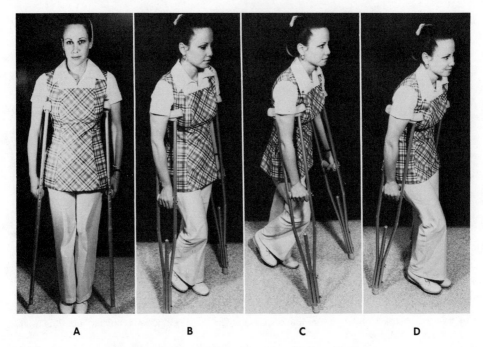

A   B   C   D

Fig. 19-49. Gait training series. (Photo by Richard Lazar.)

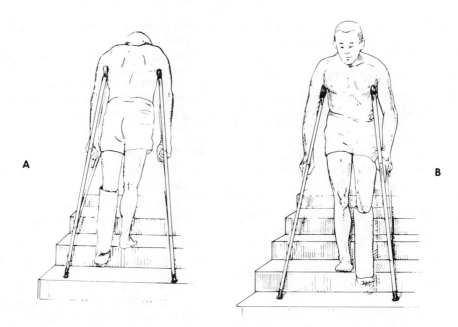

A

B

Fig. 19-50. Going upstairs, **A,** and downstairs, **B,** with crutches. (From Barber, J., Stokes, L., and Billings, D.: Adult and child care, ed. 2, St. Louis, 1977, The C. V. Mosby Co.)

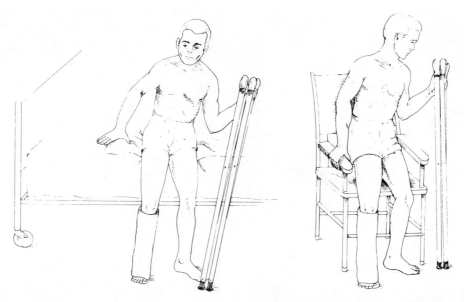

Fig. 19-51. Transferring from sitting to standing with crutches. (From Barber, J., Stokes, L., and Billings, D.: Adult and child care, ed. 2, St. Louis, 1977, The C. V. Mosby Co.)

BIBLIOGRAPHY

DePalma, A. F.: The management of fractures and dislocations, Vols. 1 and 2, Philadelphia, 1970, W. B. Saunders Co., p. 430.

Farrell, R. G.: Conservative management of fingertip amputations, J.A.C.E.P. **6:**6, June 1977.

ADDITIONAL READINGS

American Academy of Orthopedic Surgeons: Emergency care and transportation of athletic injuries, Chicago, 1970, The Academy.

American Academy of Orthopedic Surgeons: Symposium on sports medicine, St. Louis, 1969, The C. V. Mosby Co.

Badger, V. M., Conrad, M. B., Reynolds, F. C., and others: Fractures of the lower extremities. In Ballinger, W. F., Rutherford, R. B., and Zuidema, G. D., eds.: The management of trauma, ed. 2, Philadelphia, 1973, W. B. Saunders Co.

Barber, J. M., and Budassi, S. A.: Mosby's manual of emergency care, St. Louis, 1979, The C. V. Mosby Co.

Berg, E. W.: Fractures and dislocations: recognition and treatment. In McSwain, N. E., editor: Traumatic surgery, Flushing, N.Y., 1976, Medical Examination Publishing Co.

Cole, J. M., Cosgriff, J. H., Duarte, K. R., and Anderson, C. T.: Injuries of bones, joints, and related soft-tissue structures. In Cosgriff, J. H., and Anderson, D. L., editors: The practice of emergency nursing, Philadelphia, 1975, J. B. Lippincott Co.

Collins, H. R.: Acromioclavicular dislocations: mechanisms and treatments, J. Sports Med. **2:**11, January-February 1974.

Committee on Trauma, American College of Surgeons: Emergency care of the injured patient, Philadelphia, 1972, W. B. Saunders Co.

Corbitt, R. W.: Female athletes, J.A.M.A. **228:**1266-1267, 1974.

DePalma, A. F., and Flannery, G. F.: Acute anterior dislocations of the shoulder, J. Sports Med. **1:**2, January-February 1973.

DiStephano, V. J., and Nixon, J. E.: Rupture of the Achilles tendon, J. Sports Med. **1:**4, January-February 1973.

Hirato, I., Jr.: The doctor and the athlete, Philadelphia, 1968, J. B. Lippincott Co.

Hoopes, J. E., and Jabaly, M. E.: Soft tissue of the extremities. In Ballinger, W. F., Rutherford, R. B., and Zuidema, G. D., editors: The management of trauma, Philadelphia, 1973, W. B. Saunders Co.

Hughes, J. L.: Initial management of fractures and joint injuries: thoracic and lumbar spine, pelvis and hip. In Ballinger, W. F., Rutherford, R. B., and Zuidema, G. D., editors: The management of trauma, Philadelphia, 1973, W. B. Saunders Co.

Larson, R. R.: Fractures about the shoulder, J. Sports Med. **2:**48, January-February 1974.

Miller, R. H.: Textbook of basic emergency medicine, ed. 2, St. Louis, 1980, The C. V. Mosby Co.

Nicholas, J. A.: Ankle injuries in athletes, Orthop. Clin. North. Am. **5:**153-175, 1974.

Paradies, L. H., and Gregory, C. F.: Specific fractures and

dislocations. In Shires, G. T., editor: Care of the trauma patient, New York, 1966, McGraw-Hill Book Co.

Ralston, E. L.: Handbook of fractures, St. Louis, 1967, The C. V. Mosby Co.

Rang, M.: Children's fractures, Philadelphia, 1974, J. B. Lippincott Co.

Reid, D. C.: Ankle injuries in sports, J. Sports Med. **1:**3, March-April 1973.

Rockwood, C. A., Jr.: Posterior dislocations of the shoulder, J. Sports Med. **2:**47, January-February 1974.

Rockwood, C. A., Jr., and Green, D., editors: Fractures, Philadelphia, 1975, J. B. Lippincott Co.

Rodi, M. F.: Emergency orthopedics. In Warner, C. G., editor: Emergency care: assessment and intervention, ed. 2, St. Louis, 1978, The C. V. Mosby Co.

Ryan, J.: Musculoskeletal trauma. In Walt, A. J., and Wilson, R. F., editors: Management of trauma: pitfalls and practice, Philadelphia, 1978, Lea & Febiger.

Schmeisser, G., and Freidman, M.: Initial management of fractures and joint injuries: upper limbs. In Ballinger, W. F., Rutherford, R. B., and Zuidema, G. D., editors: The management of trauma, Philadelphia, 1973, W. B. Saunders Co.

Stephenson, H. E., Jr.: Immediate care of the acutely ill and injured, ed. 2, St. Louis, 1978, The C. V. Mosby Co.

Stewart, J. D. M.: Traction and orthopedic appliances, Edinburgh, 1975, Churchill Livingstone.

CHAPTER 20

Genitourinary emergencies

TRAUMA

The kidneys, ureters, and bladder are vulnerable to trauma involving the back, flank, pelvis, perineum, and abdomen, whether blunt or penetrating. Fractured ribs can also be implicated in trauma to the renal structures. It is important that emergency nurses suspect genitourinary injury when there is historical or physical evidence of impact or penetration involving any of these structures.

Renal trauma

Any individual who has suffered trauma to the back, flank, abdomen, or lower rib cage should be suspected of renal trauma (Fig. 20-1) (Table 20-1). Specific signs and symptoms include: hematuria, flank pain and/or ecchymosis of the flank, abdominal rigidity, flank mass, and possibly hypovolemic shock. Pain referred to the testes, groin, and shoulder also suggests renal trauma.

If there is evidence of foreign body penetration or a gunshot wound, radiopaque markers should be placed over the entrance and exit wounds. *Before* using contrast media, you must ascertain that there is no sensitivity to iodine. If there is any question, 250 mg methylprednisolone (SoluMedrol) may be given IV along with 50 mg diphenhydramine (Benadryl) before studies.

An excretory urogram is the diagnostic study of choice if the patient is not hypotensive or allergic to contrast media. A renal angiogram or an IVP may be desirable. An IVP is useless in shock states when renal perfusion is compromised.

Baseline blood studies to be drawn include a BUN and a serum creatinine.

Trauma of bladder and urethra

Trauma to the bladder and urethra should be suspected in abdominal trauma, fractured pelvis, or direct blows to the pubic area (Fig. 20-2) (Table 20-2). Rupture of the urethra is a classic occurrence associated with perineal straddle-type injuries. A straddle injury crushes the urethra between the pubic arch and the object on which the victim falls with force, creating a urethral tear.

Specific signs and symptoms of urethral trauma include urinary tenesmus and dysuria, hematuria, suprapubic pain, and possible hypovolemic shock.

If the patient with urethral trauma does void, the stream may be intermittent, or a sphincter spasm will cause sudden cessation of the stream. Blood may be noted at the external meatus.

The bladder may be ruptured, especially if it is distended by a force such as a seat belt or a blunt force to the lower abdomen. Shock, pain, near inability to void, and hematuria are common indicators. Some patients with a ruptured bladder will not experience pain or any other symptoms for several hours (Fig. 20-3).

A urethral catheter should never be used with suspected urethral trauma, because a catheter would increase the likelihood of infection and fibrosis at the site of injury. Suprapubic drainage is recommended for 2 to 3 weeks, to allow the urethra to heal.

Table 20-1. Renal trauma*

	Laceration	Contusion	Vascular injuries
Signs and symptoms Pain in involved upper abdominal quadrant or costovertebral angles is common in most renal trauma; abdominal tenderness and guarding may also be present	Extravasation of urine	Renal ecchymosis or subcapsular hematoma	Bruit heard in posterior midline near first and second lumbar vertebrae
Urine	Gross hematuria may be present	Slight hematuria, which usually is self-limiting	Lack of hematuria in the presence of renal injury
Diagnostic tests	Renal outline and psoas shadow on x-ray film obscurred; collecting system may be distorted or poorly visualized; extravasation of contrast medium may occur.		Excretory urography reveals no visualization of affected kidney; arteriography demonstrates blind arterial stump
Management	Hospitalize; observe for several days; penetrating renal injuries may require extensive surgery	Discharge with instructions to avoid physical exertion	

*From Barber, J. M., and Budassi, S. A.: Mosby's manual of emergency care, St. Louis, 1979, The C. V. Mosby Co.

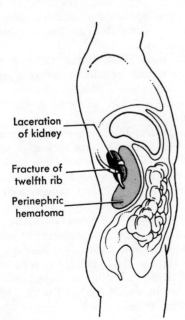

Laceration of kidney

Fracture of twelfth rib

Perinephric hematoma

Fig. 20-1. Fractured rib may lacerate kidney. Note hematoma resulting from hemorrhage from kidney into adjacent tissue.

Table 20-2. Other genitourinary trauma*

	Ureteral trauma	Bladder trauma	Urethra trauma
Signs and symptoms	Flank pain, urinary fistula	Suprapubic pain, possibly hypovolemic shock	Blood coming from urethra or presence of dried blood on meatus; suprapubic pain; possible hypovolemic shock; male patients may have high-riding prostate; perineal ecchymosis; proximal displacement of prostate noted on rectal examination; desire to urinate but inability to do so; bladder neck spasm; distended bladder
Urine	May have hematuria	Hematuria that is rapidly clearing or urine may be unobtainable due to extravasation	
Diagnostic tests	Excretory urography shows extravasation; retrograde pyelography may also be used	Retrograde cystogram	Pelvic x-ray films, retrograde urethrography
Management	Surgical reanastomosis of ureter	Hospitalization and surgery required	Do not ask patient to urinate; do not catheterize; divert urine via suprapubic catheter; hospitalization and surgery may be required

*From Barber, J. M., and Budassi, S. A.: Mosby's manual of emergency care, St. Louis, 1979, The C. V. Mosby Co.

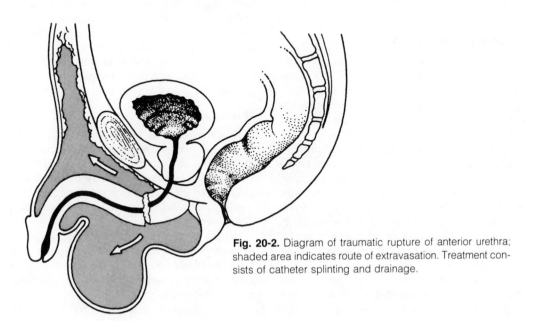

Fig. 20-2. Diagram of traumatic rupture of anterior urethra; shaded area indicates route of extravasation. Treatment consists of catheter splinting and drainage.

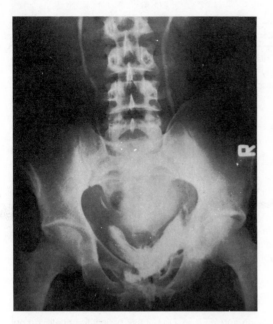

Fig. 20-3. Cystourethrogram with intravenous pyelogram showing rupture of posterior (prostatic) urethra with fractured pelvis. Note extravasation of contrast medium about base of bladder, which has been displaced upward. (From Schmidt, J. D., and Flocks, R. H. In Liechty, R. D., and Soper, R. T.: Synopsis of surgery, ed. 4, St. Louis, 1980, The C. V. Mosby Co.)

ZIPPER INJURIES

Occasionally a man or a child will come to the emergency department with his penis foreskin firmly entangled in the zipper of his trousers. This constitutes both an embarrassing circumstance for the victim and a real challenge for the staff.

A sedative or even a short inhalation anesthesia may be required to gain the patient's cooperation. A topical solution (for example, 2% lidocaine jelly) is satisfactory for some cases. A local anesthetic should not, however be injected or infiltrated, since it would only exaggerate edema and could cause a severe local reaction because of the tissue's extreme vascularity.

The zipper should *not* be cut, since it may damage it to the degree that it will not unlock teeth or slide; the skin should not be cut either, because a large laceration requiring extensive plastic repair would be created in the process, leaving the foreskin prone to contracture and scarring.

When the anesthesia has taken effect, the zipper should be held firmly and eased a notch or two, gently disentangling the skin concurrently. (There is no atraumatic way to accomplish this!) After the foreskin is freed, an antiseptic ointment and dressing should be applied. Iced compresses may be useful in reducing pain and edema. Scrotal suspensories are advisable for a man to relieve discomfort and to protect the delicate tissue during healing.

FOREIGN BODIES

Foreign bodies may damage the genitourinary tract when they are inserted into the urethra or if constricting devices are placed around the external structures (for example, a metal ring over the foreskin of the penis). Increasing numbers of such injuries are seen in emergency departments as behavioral results of inebriation, drug usage, senility, or eroticism.

Signs and symptoms

The manifestations depend on the nature of the foreign body, where it has been placed, and the site of its eventual lodgement. Urethral tears, hematuria, purulent urethral discharge, abdominal pain, acute retention, urinary tract infection, swelling and inflammation of external structures, and even necrosis may be exhibited.

Management

Hospitalization is indicated for the removal of foreign bodies and treatment of injuries to the involved structures. Internal foreign bodies are removed surgically, usually by a transurethral approach. Most external foreign bodies can be successfully removed in the emergency department.

It may be the role of the emergency nurse to provide required sedation, analgesia, and local anesthetic. Related infections and resultant trauma require specific management modes. Patients with foreign bodies in the urinary tract should be referred for follow-up care.

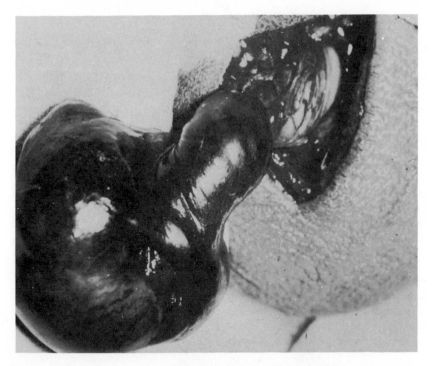

Fig. 20-4. Torsion of spermatic cord is demonstrated at surgery through scrotal incision; testical and its twisted cord are shown. Note dark or cyanotic appearance of testicle due to its blocked blood flow. (From Winter, C., and Morel, A.: Nursing care of patients with urologic diseases, ed. 4, St. Louis, 1977, The C. V. Mosby Co.)

TESTICULAR TORSION

Testicular torsion (Fig. 20-4) is a dire clinical emergency characterized by intense pain caused by twisting of the entire spermatic cord and twisting of a testicle in the tunica vaginalis. It is most common in children and adolescents.

Pain is paramount. There may be ipsilateral abdominal and back pain, nausea, vomiting, and fever. There is hyperemic and edematous skin over the area. The cord is thick and painful.

A urologist should be called at once for suspected testicular torsion. In the meantime, a urinalysis and complete blood count should be obtained.

The definitive management may be initiated by infiltrating lidocaine into the cord in the inguinal area. Additionally, an ice pack may be placed on the scrotum. Manual manipulation of the testicle may be attempted before surgery is performed to untwist or remove the affected testicle.

PENIS FRACTURE

The penis may be fractured by a direct blow resulting in hemorrhage, hematoma, and distortion. The erect penis is decidedly more vulnerable.

The emergency management consists of placing a Foley catheter, splinting the penis, and applying ice packs. Evacuation of the hematoma may be required in some instances.

ACUTE URINARY RETENTION

Acute urinary retention is an inability to pass urine through the urethra. It may stem from neurological, mechanical, or psychogenic causes. Among the more common causes are urethral stricture, phimosis, paraphimosis, benign prostatic hypertrophy, obstructing calculi, neurogenic bladder, and action of certain drugs. The only signs and symptoms are pain and a grossly distended bladder.

Emergency management

The patient may require sedation before catheterization. Intraurethral lidocaine or an IV anesthetic may be necessary to help the patient relax. If an obstruction is encountered, the catheter should not be forced. If an apparent impediment to catheterization is encountered, a urologist should be called, who will likely use a Coudé tip or stylet. If this method is not successful, a urethrogram may be indicated to detect any obstruction. An alternate procedure involves the use of a 22-gauge spinal needle. The physician enters the bladder suprapubically to aspirate the contents. (An intracatheter-type device [Cystocath] may be used instead.) The needle should enter two finger-widths above the symphysis pubis and be directed toward the anus.

No more than 500 to 750 ml urine should be removed at any one time (within 1 hour), however, since the sudden change in the intra-abdominal pressure can cause shock.

URINARY TRACT CALCULI

Urinary tract calculi can occur at any point in the genitourinary system. The resultant manifestations depend on the presence of obstruction, infection, local trauma, and edema of the structures.

Signs and symptoms

The patient with urinary calculi will come to the emergency department with flank or costovertebral pain that is excruciating and colicky. The pain may radiate to the abdomen, scrotum, or labia (Fig. 20-5). The patient's face may appear ashen, and it is likely that diaphoresis is marked. There is no position in which the individual can gain any comfort. A feeling of bladder fullness and a frequent urge to void is commonly associated with lower urethral stones. Nausea, vomiting, low-grade fever, paralytic ileus, hematura, tachycardia, and

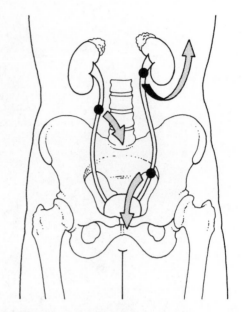

Fig. 20-5. Path of radiation of pain in renal colic is characteristic and serves to differentiate this problem from several other acute abdominal conditions.

hypotension complete the classic clinical presentation.

It is apparent that the signs and symptoms mimic many other abdominally-based conditions that must be ruled out, including acute appendicitis, pyelonephritis, ruptured ovarian cyst, ruptured or dissecting aneurysm, ectopic pregnancy, acute gallbladder disease, and renal artery thrombosis. It is important to note that individuals over 65 years old rarely have an initial episode of renal colic; so the physician must search for other causes to explain the symptoms.

Emergency management

The nurse should triage the patient to a treatment area where maximum privacy can be assured and where it is quiet. Allow the patient to be ambulatory if he desires, unless he is hypotensive. Monitor the room carefully, especially after analgesia, to ensure that accidents and injuries do not occur during ambulation.

A urine specimen should be obtained for

urinalysis, including pH. Ask the patient to void only in a bedpan, and strain the urine to search for granular particles or calculi.

The individual should be given analgesia such as meperidine or morphine. Half the total dose, at least, should be given IV push. An antiemetic may also be ordered for control of nausea and vomiting. Atropine is often used as a smooth muscle relaxant to aid in pain relief.

Radiological studies of the kidneys, ureters, and bladder (KUB) and an intravenous pyelogram (IVP) should be performed. (Be sure to check for iodine sensitivity before the IVP.) The radiologist will ensure that oblique, postvoiding, and delayed films at 1, 2, and 4 hours are taken.

An IV may be initiated for severely dehydrated patients or for those individuals whose nausea and vomiting preclude oral hydration. The patient with an acute calculi episode should be hospitalized if the pain is unrelenting, if there is fever or severe dehydration, if there is evidence of urinary tract infection, or if a stone (too large to pass) is detected, which would require surgery.

If the patient is discharged after the colicky pain is under control, or if the calculus has passed, follow-up care is mandatory and a referral to a urologist should be made. In the meantime, the patient should be instructed to strain all urine so any calculi or particulate matter can be carefully analyzed.

GROSS HEMATURIA

Gross hematuria can result from trauma or recent instrumentation of the urinary tract, as a side effect of anticoagulant therapy, or as an indication of a blood dyscrasia.

Patients who reach the emergency department with hematuria should be carefully questioned regarding a history of trauma, previous renal problems, medications taken regularly (especially anticoagulants), or long-term bleeding disorders.

The vital signs should be assessed and any evidence of hypovolemia noted. Venous blood samples should be obtained promptly for CBC, coagulation studies, hemoglobin and hemato-

crit, and a type and cross-match if the blood loss is thought to be severe. A urine specimen should be sent for analysis. The quantitative sample should be inspected thoroughly for clots, tissue, and stones. If a woman is menstruating, a catheterized urine specimen should be obtained.

Cystic (bladder) hemorrhage may be controlled by irrigation with a Foley catheter.

GENITOURINARY TRACT INFECTIONS

Patients come to the emergency department with infections of the genitourinary tract primarily because of associated pain and other discomforting symptoms. Upper urinary tract infections are classically marked by fever, flank pain, chills, and gastrointestinal distress. The lower urinary tract infection is probably involved if there is frequency, urgency, dysuria, suprapubic discomfort, and hematuria.

A detailed history is important, including the onset, location, description of pain, and its relationship to voiding. Any recent trauma should be explored, because it might potentially relate. It is important to obtain information about any previous history of urinary infections or trauma, too. Note chills, fever, nausea, or other symptoms of a generalized infection.

A clean-catch midstream urine specimen should be obtained for analysis and possibly for a culture and sensitivity. A culture and sensitivity is particularly indicated if the infection is recurrent or if the urinalysis did not confirm an infection. (Catheterization is usually requested if a female patient is menstruating.)

Draw blood for routine testing, including a CBC, electrolytes, hemoglobin and hematocrit, and blood sugar.

A physical examination is performed to detect point tenderness, to palpate the bladder, and to inspect the meatus. Female patients may require a pelvic examination if vaginal sources of infection are suspected. Male patients should have a rectal examination for prostatic palpation, and the penis and scrotal sac should be thoroughly examined. If renal trauma or calculi are suspected, a KUB and IVP may be ordered. Retrograde pyelograms, renal scintiscans, angiograms, and voiding cystograms may be indicated for more detailed study of the structures.

Specific management

A 10-day course of antibiotics is usually prescribed along with a referral for follow-up. If there is evidence of systemic involvement, hospitalization may be required. If bladder discomfort is severe, an antispasmodic or bladder analgesic such as phenazopyridine (Pyridium) may be ordered for symptomatic relief. The patient should be advised that phenazopyridine will cause the urine to be orange and that it may stain delicate underclothing.

The nurse may also choose to explain to the patient that coffee, tea, and highly seasoned foods may exaggerate bladder discomfort and thus should be avoided. Female patients should be instructed that sexual intercourse can aggravate the acute condition and that they may find it to their advantage to refrain from coitus for a few days and to empty the bladder before and after coitus. (Some clinicians think that it may be useful to provide a bacterial cream to lubricate the introitus to minimize trauma to the sensitive structures.) Since some people find that hot baths or a heating pad can help relieve abdominal discomfort, the nurse may want to suggest them.

EPIDIDYMITIS

Epididymitis is an infection of the male reproductive system usually originating from an infected prostate or the lower urinary tract. It is commonly associated with gonorrhea.

The man will complain of pain, tenderness, and swelling in the scrotum, which is very warm to the touch. Fever, malaise, and a characteristic "duck waddle" walk complete the classic presentation. It is important to rule out testicular torsion, since it can be sometimes confused with epididymitis.

Ordinarily the patient will be given instructions to rest at home with the scrotum elevated on a towel roll or with a Bellevue bridge (Fig. 20-6). Ice may be used to reduce the swelling but should not be used continually. Be certain that the man understands that it is to be removed at least for 15 minutes every hour to protect from prolonged drops in scrotal temperature that could possibly affect fertility. The necessity of ensuring a high fluid intake (at least 2,000 ml daily) should be stressed as a mode to reduce the risk of urinary tract infection. The wearing of a scrotal suspensory should be encouraged once ambulation is resumed. A few clinicians may prescribe antibiotics or steroids to manage epididymitis.

All men with this condition should be referred for follow-up, since unchecked bilateral epididymitis can lead to sterility, testicular necrosis, and even septicemia.

ORCHITIS

Orchitis is an infection of a testicle that is a common complication of mumps, especially when mumps occurs after puberty. The signs,

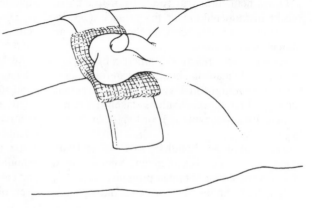

Fig. 20-6. Bellevue bridge for elevation of scrotum in treatment of epididymitis.

symptoms, and treatment are similar to epididymitis.

DIALYSIS-RELATED EMERGENCIES

The emergency department team may encounter patients experiencing dialysis-related emergencies including shunt clotting, shunt infections, and related cardiovascular phenomena. Here are a few helpful guidelines for emergency nurses for the management of these problems.

Shunt clotting

1. Assess the type of shunt. The external (Scribner) shunt, the bovine artegraft, and the Cimino-Brescia fistula (a surgically created fistula between the cephalic vein and the radial artery) are the most commonly used modes of access to circulation for dialysis. The Cimino-Brescia fistula is the most commonly employed. Only an *external* shunt can be declotted in the emergency department. All others must be referred to a vascular surgeon or members of the dialysis team familiar with the problem.
2. If an external shunt is clotted, a syringe should be used first in attempted aspiration. If the attempt is unsuccessful, a polyethylene catheter inserted into the lumen may be helpful. If not, a Fogarty catheter (No. 3 or 4) may be passed up arterial and venous limbs and *gently* retrieved by pulling back to remove the clot. Do not flush saline into the shunt, because this could cause embolization.

Shunt infections

1. If the *external* shunt appears infected or purulent drainage is present, culture the site and begin antibiotic therapy after consultation with the dialysis team. Since *Staphylococcus aureus* is the most likely organism responsible, oxacillin (parenterally) and cloxacillin (orally) are the drugs of choice.
2. Patients with Cimino-Brescia fistulas or bovine artegrafts may have signs and symptoms of systemic infection without external evidence of a shunt infection (see p. 240).

Cardiovascular phenomena

Cardiac dysrhythmias, hypotension, hypertension, and pericardial disease are commonly found in dialysis patients. There are a few exceptions to the usual emergency intervention.

Hypotension is usually dialysis related when too much extracellular fluid has been removed during the treatment or if antihypertensives have been taken on the day of dialysis. Nausea, vomiting, muscle cramps, general weakness, and an orthostatic drop in blood pressure will be evident. Normal saline is usually acceptable for fluid replacement, but the volume should be judiciously monitored to barely reattain normal body weight.

Hypertension in dialysis patients with peripheral edema and pulmonary congestion should not be treated with large doses of potent antihypertensives since dialysis is usually the key to the control of blood pressure elevation, which is largely from extracellular fluid expansion. However, antihypertensives are definitely indicated if the hypertension is renin related and the patient has a history of hypertension despite dialysis and other management (see p. 305). If headache is profound or other neurological phenomena are present, consider the possibility of intracranial bleeding caused by system heparinization.

SUMMARY

Emergency nurses may encounter trauma-related genitourinary problems and should be prepared to make appropriate assessments of injuries that could affect the kidneys, ureters, bladder, and urethra. Special attention should be given to blunt or high-impact trauma to the back and abdomen, as well as the classic straddle injures. Parameters related to catheterization should be clearly understood to prevent further damage to urinary tract structures after the injury.

The triage nurse should be alert to signs and symptoms of acute problems, including testicular torsion, acute urinary retention, urinary calculi, and gross hematuria, and be prepared to take prompt action.

Emergency nurses have a significant role in instruction and follow-up planning for patients with genitourinary tract infections or dialysis-related renal emergencies.

BIBLIOGRAPHY

Banowsky, L. H., Wolfel, D. A., and Lackner, L. H.: Considerations in diagnosis and management of renal trauma, J. Trauma **10:**587-597, 1970.

Brosman, S. A., and Fay, R.: Diagnosis and management of bladder trauma, J. Trauma. **13:**687-694, 1973.

Holcroft, J. W., Trunkey, D. D., Minagi, H., Korobkin, M. T., and Lim, R. C.: Renal trauma and retroperitoneal hematomas—indications for exploration, J. Trauma **15:** 1045-1052, 1975.

Kaufman, R. E., and Weisman, P. J.: Current concepts, N. Engl. J. Med. **291:**1175-1177, 1974.

McAllister, C. J.: Emergencies in dialysis patients, J.A.C.E.P. **7:**96-98, March, 1978.

Perksy, L.: Urethral injuries, Resident Staff **22:**1s-4s, 1975.

Perksy, L.: How we manage renal injuries, Resident Staff **100:**1s-9s, 1975.

Pontes, J. I.: Urologic injuries, Surg. Clin. North Am. **57:**77-95, 1977.

Smith, D. R.: General urology, Los Altos, Calif., 1972, Lange Medical Publications.

CHAPTER 21

Obstetrical and gynecological emergencies

Peggy McCall and Patricia Varvel

When a woman comes to the emergency department for an obstetrical or gynecological problem, she is often uncomfortable both physically and psychologically. She may have pain, vaginal bleeding, shocklike symptoms; she may have suffered trauma; or she may be pregnant or even in labor.

The emergency nurse, by a careful and sensitive approach to the individual woman, may help make this experience less frightening, less embarrassing, and less traumatic by following a few basic principles.

Information about the onset of signs and symptoms should be solicited in confidence, and privacy should be afforded for all aspects of the examination, as well as for the discussion of problems between members of the emergency department team. The nurse can further ensure the comfort needs of the woman by a careful explanation of all procedures, by assisting in appropriate positioning and draping, by instructing in techniques of relaxation, and by providing human support at the time of examination.

Before any procedures are actually begun, the woman should remove her underclothing and any constricting garments. It is important that the nurse carefully fold or place these belongings on hangers, as they are important parts of the woman's identity. Furthermore, time should be permitted to allow the patient to void,

so that the bladder is empty and does not interfere with digital examination of any of the pelvic or abdominal structures. When the pelvic exam is completed, it is important for the nurse to help the woman back into a comfortable position, to provide tissue paper or other cleansing agents to remove lubricants and secretion from the perianal area, and to provide time to regroom before being ushered back into a waiting or conference area, or to prepare for admission to an inpatient area.

This chapter has been organized according to symptoms that provoke a woman to come to the emergency department. Nursing care and medical management of common, recurring obstetrical and gynecological problems are incorporated into the discussion of signs and symptoms.

VAGINAL BLEEDING

One must realize that most cases of vaginal bleeding are seen by the ob-gyn physician in the office. It is hoped that the yearly check-up and the use of the Pap smear as a diagnostic and preventive tool for cancer of the genital tract will help prevent such medical emergencies as a woman coming to the emergency department with hemorrhage from an advanced carcinoma of the cervix.

Leiomyomata uteri (benign fibroid tumors of the uterus) can also cause sudden, dramatic hemorrhage as they grow large enough to begin to necrose or twist themselves, causing enough bleeding to create an emergency situation in which it is not unusual to see drops of as much as 3 and 4 gm of hemoglobin. In such cases, the patient may be in shock by the time she reaches the emergency department. The yearly examination, again, is the agent by which these severe cases are being seen early and treatment instituted before the situation deteriorates into an emergency. There will always be a few women who, for various reasons, decline to have a pelvic examination, and so there will always be a certain number of such cases seen in almost any emergency department in the country.

Other gynecological conditions that cause vaginal bleeding are those associated with disturbances in the hormonal control of the menstrual cycle and may be seen in all ages from the young girl who is just establishing her cycle to the woman who is menopausal; those associated with birth control pills or intrauterine devices; those associated with ovarian disease— polycystic ovaries, tumors, or infection; and those associated with systemic diseases, such as blood dyscrasias. Vaginal bleeding is the first symptom of leukemia in 10% of women. When all organic causes are ruled out, the diagnosis of dysfunctional uterine bleeding is made. In most cases, none of these will present an immediate threat to the patient's life and can be handled by referral to a private physician.

Endometrial biopsy

Occasionally, the physician may want to perform an endometrial biopsy in the emergency department to assist in the diagnosis. In this procedure, the lining of the uterus, or endometrium, is biopsied with forceps especially designed for this purpose. The nurse should prepare the patient for the examination by explaining the procedure to her and answering any questions she may have. The patient should then be placed in lithotomy position with drapes placed to afford the patient as much privacy as possible. Results from the following laboratory tests should be on the chart: CBC, urine, sedimentation rate and type, and Rh factor. Some physicians may order a type and cross-match for blood in case of hemorrhage but if not, a clot for type and cross-match should be in the blood bank. Equipment should include a vaginal examination tray with endometrial biopsy forceps, sterile gloves, water-soluble lubricant such as K-Y jelly, and culture swabs in case the physician requests them.

Bleeding associated with pregnancy and abortion

Because bleeding associated with pregnancy is probably the most commonly seen condition in the emergency department, any woman who has vaginal bleeding should be considered pregnant until proved otherwise.

Abortion is the number one cause for vaginal bleeding in the childbearing ages. Abortion is defined as the termination of a pregnancy at any time before the fetus has attained viability (24 weeks gestation). Types of abortion that the nurse should be familiar with include the following.

Threatened abortion. Vaginal bleeding or spotting with mild cramping but with a closed or only slightly dilated cervix indicates a threatened abortion.

Inevitable abortion. Bleeding is more profuse, the cervix is dilated, and there are contractions.

Habitual abortion. Spontaneous abortions that occur successively with three pregnancies or more are termed habitual abortions.

Incomplete abortion. The fetus is expelled, but the placenta and membranes are retained.

Missed abortion. The fetus dies in utero and is not expelled. The mother may not be aware that anything is wrong unless she becomes infected as the fetus begins to macerate. The first indication that something is wrong may very well be when the obstetrician notes a discrepancy in the size of the uterus as compared to dates. A definite diagnosis of fetal death is the conversion of the pregnancy test from positive to negative.

Septic abortion. An abortion that has become infected either with uterine contents intact (missed) or after they have been removed by surgical means. This may or may not mean that illegal intervention has occurred. Although the Supreme Court decision making therapeutic abortions legal before 6 months of gestation was hailed in some circles as a death-dealing blow to the criminal abortionist, it has not completely eradicated the problem, as not all septic abortions are caused by incompetence. A woman with a septic abortion can appear in a variety of ways, and it behooves the emergency department nurse to be alert to this possibility in the woman who has severe abdominal pain and high temperature and is in shock and possibly renal or cardiovascular failure. If she is indeed a patient with a septic abortion, speed of diagnosis and treatment can mean life or death.

Placental abnormalities are another condition in which vaginal bleeding is seen associated with pregnancy. These are an emergency for both mother and the fetus and will be discussed later in this chapter.

Postpartum bleeding

Excessive bleeding in the postpartum period is not only an emergency but can be very disquieting for a woman who has had a normal pregnancy and delivery, and has just begun to settle into her routine at home with her new baby when she suddenly hemorrhages and must return to the hospital. There are three main causes for postpartum bleeding. These are subinvolution of the uterus, retained secundinae (pieces of placenta or membranes present in the uterus), and vaginal or cervical tears suffered during delivery. Subinvolution usually occurs at 6 to 15 days postpartum when the thrombi detach from the placental sites and the sites begin to bleed. If the involutional process is not progressing as it should in returning the gravid uterus to its nonpregnant state, the bleeding may become excessive. The retention of membranes or placental fragments can also cause sudden hemorrhage as they interfere with the involutionary process. With the growing popularity of the home delivery, the emergency department nurse should also be aware of a condition known as *placenta accreta* in which the placenta fails to separate from the uterine wall following delivery because it has grown into the uterine muscle itself. If this is the case, immediate surgery is indicated. Cervical tears and vaginal lacerations may become more common if the present trend of home deliveries continues, because they preclude the use of the episiotomy as a means to deliver a relatively large head through a relatively small vaginal opening.

Assessment

When assessing the patient with vaginal bleeding, the nurse should survey the general condition, note presence or absence of pain, the color of skin (Is there cyanosis? Is she pale or flushed?) her posture, gait, motor activity, and facial expression. In obtaining a history of the present problem, the nurse should elicit:

1. Quantity, character, and duration of bleeding. How does it compare with a normal period for her? What is the number of pads used and how does it compare with the number she normally requires for a period?
2. Menstrual history. When was the date of her last period? Was it heavier or lighter than usual? Are her periods regular or irregular?
3. Does she think she might be pregnant? Does she use any contraception, and if so, what? Does she have any of the signs and symptoms of pregnancy, such as breast tenderness, lack of energy, or urinary frequency?
4. Does she have pain? What is the nature of the pain—is it dull, achy, cramping, constant, or radiating? Where is the pain? How long has she had it? Was its onset gradual or sudden?
5. Is there any history of trauma?
6. Gynecological history: Has she ever been pregnant? Has she ever had any infections of the reproductive system? Has she had previous episodes of bleeding? Has she ever had a miscarriage? (The word "abortion," although the correct word in medical terminology, has retained a certain illegal connotation and may elicit an immediate denial that may or may not be true).

When obtaining vital signs, include fetal heart tones if the patient is known to be at least 16 weeks pregnant. Check the pad she is wearing yourself in order to objectively evaluate the amount of bleeding. Note the presence or absence of clots or odor. Examine and save any clots or tissue the patient may have brought with her for laboratory examination if the doctor wishes. Note the condition of the abdomen—is it distended or flat, is there rebound tenderness, are there bowel sounds?

Evaluate the patient's condition, and institute appropriate measures for stabilization if necessary. If bleeding is profuse, an IV with a large-bore needle capable of delivering blood should be established. If respirations are labored, start oxygen to help blood saturation. On all patients, a complete blood count with sedimentation rate will be necessary for evaluation, and a clot should be drawn for type and cross-match for blood transfusions if they should become necessary. If the patient is aborting, the Rh factor will be very necessary in determining whether or not she should be given RhoGAM, a blood derivative given to Rh negative mothers after delivery of an Rh positive infant to prevent her from forming Rh positive antibodies that would be life-threatening to future pregnancies involving an Rh positive infant.

After collecting all data and stabilizing the patient's condition, the emergency department nurse should prepare the patient for a vaginal examination by the emergency physician. Explain each procedure and reassure her of your concern for her feelings by allowing her to express her fear, anger, or guilt to a sympathetic and open-minded nurse.

Most problems with vaginal bleeding caused by hormonal problems, IUDs, dysfunctional uterine bleeding, and ovarian disease other than ruptured ectopic pregnancies or cysts can be referred to the patient's personal physician. The nurse should assist in making appointments, inform the physician of the patient's chief complaint, and instruct the patient carefully in the need for follow-up.

Abortions will usually require hospitalization, sometimes for only several hours. The patient who is threatening to abort will be put to bed, sedated, and a pad count will be recorded. The inevitable and incomplete abortion will be treated by removing the products of conception from the uterus either by D and C (dilating the cervix and scraping the uterine lining) or by use of the suction curretage (a procedure considered much safer for the gravid uterus, as it avoids the use of a sharp instrument in removing the uterine contents). The immediate treatment of the habitual abortion is the same, but the nurse should also encourage the patient to have a good gynecological work-up to rule out any abnormalities of the uterus. Surgical treatment of such conditions as bicornuate uterus or a septate uterus have been very successful, and treatment of an incompetent cervix with a Shirodkar procedure or a McDonald suture have brought many women with these problems to term. In cases of missed abortion in which the uterus is less than 3 months in size and no sepsis is present, the suction curretage or D and C is the treatment of choice. In cases of pregnancy past the first trimester, or in the presence of infection, expulsion of the fetus through the use of oxytocins or, more recently, prostaglandins is the treatment of choice. In cases of septic abortion, the rapid institution of antibiotics such as cephalosporins, gentamicin, and clindamycin and the evacuation of the uterus as soon as the condition is stabilized is of utmost importance. The emergency department nurse as the history-taker and first-line assessor can mean the difference in immediate or delayed treatment for a woman who may confide certain details of her condition only to the sympathetic and nonjudgmental nurse.

Postpartum bleeding generally responds to the administration of IV oxytocin (Pitocin), bed rest, and fundal massage. Treatment of retained secundinae is removal of the offending piece by D and C and a thorough exploration of the uterus under general anesthesia. Suturing of vaginal lacerations can be done in the emergency department, but because of the possibility of damage occurring at the cervix as well, it is best done under general anesthesia when a good pelvic examination can also be done.

SHOCK

Shock, as seen in the ob-gyn patient, is usually associated with a loss of blood and therefore will be seen in a certain number of cases

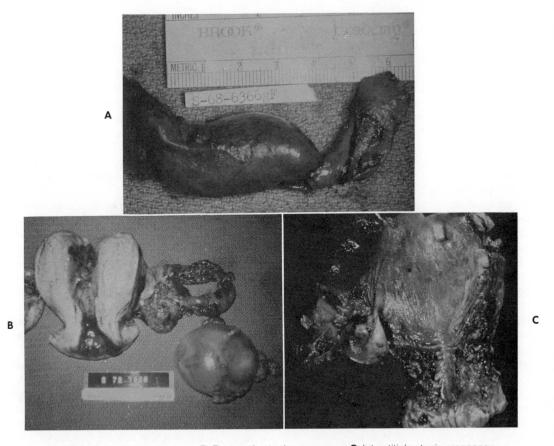

Fig. 21-1. **A,** Ectopic pregnancy. **B,** Ruptured ectopic pregnancy, **C,** Interstitial ectopic pregnancy.

of severe vaginal bleeding. It is also seen in cases of sepsis related to septic abortions or untreated infections.

Ectopic pregnancy

The most dramatic cases of shock in the female of childbearing age will be seen in the patient with the ruptured ectopic pregnancy (Fig. 21-1). Ectopic pregnancy occurs when the fertilized ovum implants anywhere other than the uterine cavity, such as the tube, ovary, cervix, or abdominal cavity. Ninety-five percent of all ectopic pregnancies involve the fallopian tube (where fertilization takes place) and occur in one out of every 150 pregnancies. Predisposing factors include previous tubal infections, adhesions from previous surgery, tubal ligations, and possibly, the presence of IUDs. The most common site for tubal implantations is the ampulla, and the next most common is the isthmus. Ectopic pregnancy is a condition that may confuse the best diagnostician. Being the great imitator, it may be mistaken as a ruptured ovarian cyst, appendicitis, pelvic inflammatory disease (PID), or incomplete abortion. Pelvic pain and vaginal bleeding or spotting in a woman of childbearing age should alway be treated as an ectopic pregnancy until ruled out. Pain, if present, will vary from mild to severe abdominal pain and, if the ectopic pregnancy is leaking or has ruptured, will include the classic Kehr sign—radiating shoulder pain that occurs when the diaphragm is irritated from blood loss in the peritoneum.

Ectopic pregnancies manifest in two forms: *acute* (or ruptured), with intraperitoneal hemorrhage, acute pain, and shock; and *chronic* (or unruptured), with less pain, and no shock. In either case, vaginal bleeding may be absent, spotty, or profuse. Ruptured ectopic pregnancy is often seen in the emergency department in a young woman complaining of severe abdominal pain radiating to one or both shoulders, with slight vaginal spotting and with a blood pressure of 70/0. The nurse should place her in the Trendelenberg position, start an IV of D/5/RL with a large bore needle and draw blood for CBC, sedimentation rate, and type and cross-match for possible blood transfusion. In many of the larger institutions now, it is possible to determine pregnancy at an early gestation with a blood sample for radioimmunoassay, but for those institutions without facilities to perform this test, the urine for pregnancy test is still used. It should be remembered however, that a negative urine for human chorionic gonadotropins (HCG) is not entirely reliable in ruling out an ectopic pregnancy, because not all ectopic pregnancies are fully enough established to produce sufficient levels of HCG to give a positive result. History taking is again of utmost importance for differential diagnosis of septic shock, PID, or ectopic pregnancy; sudden onset of pain, sexual exposure, missed or abnormal menstrual periods, and history of prior tubal infections or surgery are especially indicative of an ectopic pregnancy. The normal sedimentation rate and lack of a febrile course should rule out PID. Pelvic x-ray films are not helpful, but the pelvic sonogram is very specific for ectopic pregnancy. The patient needs no preparation for this use of ultrasonic waves to give a picture of pelvic structures other than hydration so that the full bladder can be used as a point of reference for the radiologist. Although still done in many areas of the country, culdocentesis (needle aspiration of the cul-de-sac of Douglas through the vagina) is not recommended, since the procedure is not infallible. Aspiration of blood from the cul-de-sac is diagnostic for intraperitoneal bleeding, but absence of blood does not rule out ectopic pregnancy. The use of laparoscopy as a safe and effective diagnostic tool is the usual course of action. If a tubal pregnancy is found, a salpingectomy is done. The laparoscopy involves a general anesthetic and a small incision (approximately 1 to 2 inches wide) at the umbilicus through which a slender tube containing a telescopic lens is passed into the peritoneal cavity. This permits the gynecologist to examine the ovaries, tubes, and the outside of the uterus without subjecting the patient to the trauma of the exploratory laparotomy and a prolonged hospital stay. The patient can usually be discharged as soon as recovered from anesthesia if no pathologic condition that would require surgery is found.

If the patient is in shock, the nurse should stabilize the shock with fluid or blood replacement as indicated, administer oxygen if blood loss is sufficient to cause respiratory difficulties, and transfer the patient to the operating room, if indicated. She must also recognize the patient's need and that of her family for emotional support. The patient may have fear not only for her life but for her future childbearing ability, sadness that the pregnancy is not intrauterine, or guilt if she had not wanted a baby. If single, she may fear that her parents and friends will find out about her sexual activity. The nurse must always keep in mind the patient's right to privacy. In some instances to protect the patient, the family may be told by the physician that the ectopic pregnancy was a ruptured ovarian cyst.

Other conditions that may cause the patient to come to the emergency department in shock are those related to placental accidents, ruptured ovarian cyst, and ruptured ovarian abscesses. Because placental accidents are related to complications of pregnancy, they will be covered in a later section.

Ovarian cyst

Patients with ruptured ovarian cysts can have the same symptoms as those with ectopic pregnancy except the pregnancy test will be negative. The corpus luteum cyst of the ovary arises as a result of hemorrhage in a mature corpus luteum, which causes cystic changes in the wall itself. It is of clinical significance, as it can become very large, causing menstrual irregularities, and, after several cycles, rupture with

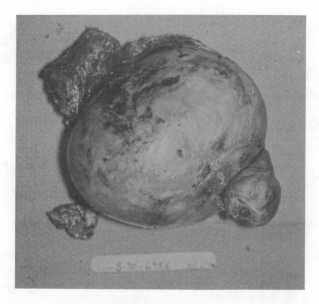

Fig. 21-2. Dermoid cyst.

additional bleeding and occasional massive intraperitoneal hemorrhage. When this occurs, it constitutes a surgical emergency in its own right. Nursing intervention includes all of those things discussed for ectopic pregnancy.

Dermoid cysts or benign cystic teratomas are those arising in the ovary from all three germ cell layers and most often contain hair, teeth, and sebaceous material, but can contain tissue from almost any structure in the body (Fig. 21-2). These represent 20% of all ovarian cysts and usually appear during active reproductive life. Dermoid cysts most commonly manifest as acute abdominal and pelvic pain when they become twisted on their pedicle (torsion) or begin to leak contents into the peritoneal cavity.

Ovarian endometriomas or "chocolate cysts" occur when actively growing and functioning endometrial tissue is present in the ovary. When this is so, the endometrial tissue cyclically bleeds with each menstrual period and forms a cyst that contains blood and blood clots (Fig. 21-3). This situation not only will cause menstrual irregularities and chronic pelvic pain, but can become an emergency if the cyst ruptures, causing hemorrhage and shock. Again, the nurse should stabilize the patient, and after evaluation, transfer her to the operating room for an emergency laparoscopy.

Ovarian abscess

A tuboovarian abscess is a complication of untreated pelvic inflammatory disease, and if ruptured, can bring the patient into the emergency department with gram-negative sepsis and septic shock. In this case, the differential diagnosis from ectopic pregnancy is a clear history of febrile illness, pelvic pain, foul vaginal discharge, increased white blood count, and elevated sedimentation rate. Culdocentesis is definitely contraindicated, because all treatment is aimed at bringing infection under control before any invasive procedures are attempted if possible. The rupture of the pus-filled tuboovarian abscess causes peritonitis, and large doses of a combination of antibiotics (usually penicillin, cephalosporin, clindamycin, kanamycin and/or gentamicin) are started by intravenous infusion immediately. A nasogastric tube is usually placed, because peristalsis will be slowed by the bowel irritation. If rupture has occurred, immediate surgery is indicated. If unruptured, the patient will be admitted to the hospital for at least 48 hours of

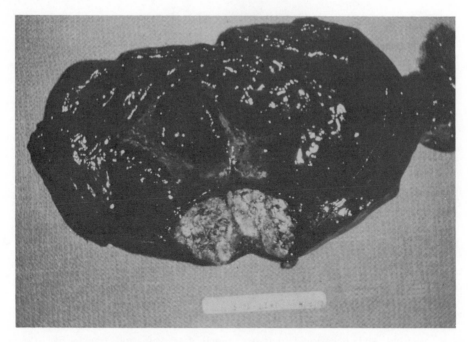

Fig. 21-3. Ovarian endometrioma or "chocolate cyst."

antibiotic therapy before surgery to remove the abscess is considered.

PAIN
Pelvic inflammatory disease

One of the most common and distressing gynecological conditions seen in the emergency department is pelvic inflammatory disease (PID). This is an acute or chronic infection that may involve the uterus, tubes, ovaries, and adjacent structures, such as the peritoneum and the intestines. The most frequent cause of PID is the *Neisseria gonococcus,* but it can also be caused by staphylococcus, streptococcus, the tubercle bacillus, or a variety of nonspecific organisms. The gonococcus usually causes acute salpingitis, which in turn causes the pain that brings the patient into the emergency department. The transmission of the disease is by sexual contact. The incubation period is 3 to 8 days. The organism primarily infects the urethra, the Skene ducts, and the Bartholin glands, with the fallopian tubes becoming involved by direct extension. The patient usually comes in following menses; symptoms include:

1. Acute generalized lower abdominal pain
2. Anorexia, nausea, and vomiting
3. Fever and chills
4. Pain on pelvic examination and movement of the cervix
5. A tense abdomen with rebound tenderness
6. Leukocytosis with white blood cell counts of 15,000 to 30,000
7. Purulent vaginal discharge

Diagnostic procedures should include a CBC with sedimentation rate, a urine specimen, and cervical smears and cultures for gram stain, anaerobes, and aerobes.

The nurse should place the patient in semi-Fowler position until the emergency department physician is ready to do the vaginal examination in order to facilitate drainage of the discharge. She should see that the blood work is done and the urine specimen collected. She should explain to the patient what is going to be done and position her for the vaginal exam, being sure that the speculum, gloves, and proper culture tubes are available. Careful

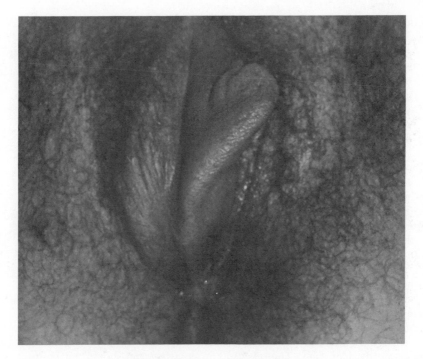

Fig. 21-4. Bartholin gland abscess.

handwashing technique and disposal of tissues and pads are especially important when dealing with a gynecological infection. In mild cases of PID, the treatment of confirmed cases will require only a prescription for antibiotics, and the patient can be released to be followed by a private physician. Again, it is important for the emergency department nurse to be aware that many patients who have symptoms of abdominal pain are incorrectly diagnosed as early PID, treated with penicillin, and sent home with an unruptured ectopic pregnancy. The nurse should be aware that a normal temperature, normal white count, and normal sedimentation rate *do not support* the diagnosis of PID. The attitude of the nurse as teacher and support for the patient is of great importance. If the nurse cannot accept the patient as a person of worth with a disease process, the patient may not be receptive to her instructions to see her physician for follow-up and to be sure that her sexual partner is treated. Inadequately treated or untreated PID with salpingitis will cause

scarring of the fallopian tubes, and the patient may be unable to conceive a child. With early diagnosis and treatment of PID, the prognosis is excellent, providing that the contact is treated so that reinfection does not occur. Other complications of untreated PID are endometritis, tuboovarian abscess, peritonitis, sepsis, shock, and death.

Bartholin gland abscess

A patient with a Bartholin gland abscess will have severe pain of the vulva and obvious swelling (Fig. 21-4). The treatment is incision and drainage of the abscess and treatment with antibiotics. The patient is usually hospitalized.

Vaginal infections

Vaginal infections will also be seen in the emergency department when pain becomes no longer tolerable for the sufferer. Trichomonal vaginitis causes a thin, watery discharge that is malodorous, burning, and itching and becomes worse after a period. Diagnosis is confirmed by recognition of the motile, flagellated *Trichomonas vaginalis* on a fresh smear of the discharge. The organism can also be found in the urine in some cases and will cause symptoms of urinary tract infection. Treatment of choice is the administration of metronidazole (Flagyl) orally to both the patient and her sexual partner. If he is not treated, the organism can remain in the male urethra and prostate asymptomatically and the patient will be reinfected with the next contact.

Intense itching with the presence of a thick, cheesy, white discharge and inflamed vaginal mucosa indicates monilial vaginitis. It is caused by *Candida albicans* and is frequently associated with diabetes, pregnancy, or broad-spectrum antibiotic therapy. Diagnosis is confirmed by culture or by special examination of a fresh smear of the discharge. Treatment is with nystatin (Mycostatin) and does not require treatment of the partner.

In recent years, the incidence of herpes progenitalis seen in the emergency department is increasing at an alarming rate. This disease, caused by herpesvirus hominis, or herpes genitalis 2 (HVH-2), is considered to be of venereal transmission. Multiple small vesicles appear on the labia, the clitoral prepuce, and along the vagina (Fig. 21-5). In 75% of cases, they are seen on the cervix as well. The presenting symptom is severe pain of the vulvovaginal area—often so severe that the patient is unable to void, or if able to void, holds urine in an attempt to avoid the scalding pain she experiences when urine passes over the affected area. She may therefore have a distended bladder, fever because of dehydration, and a waddling gait. The incubation period is usually 10 days to 2 weeks and can occur periodically after the initial infection. A specific diagnosis can be made on smear by recognition of viral inclusion bodies. The lesions may become infected secondarily with bacteria when scratched, and this may further cloud differential diagnosis. There is no specific treatment, and supportive care is given until the disease runs its course. Supportive therapy may include analgesics for pain, sitz baths, insertion of a Foley catheter, IV therapy to correct dehydration, and the use of

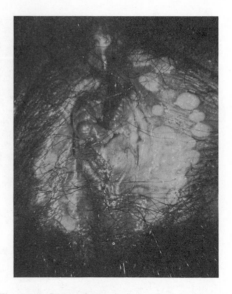

Fig. 21-5. Characteristic lesions of vaginal herpes.

compresses and drying agents. Antibiotics have no effect and should not be used unless there is a secondary infection.

Nursing intervention should include the use of good handwashing both for the nurse and the patient, the careful disposal and cleaning of used equipment, and emotional support and understanding. This disease tends to be recurrent and is not something that the patient can take lightly because it can change her life-style. It is particularly dangerous when it occurs during pregnancy. Infant mortality from herpes encephalitis is 95%. If active lesions are present at term, most obstetricians will perform a cesarean section to prevent exposure of the infant during vaginal delivery.

TRAUMAS

Trauma to genital organs will be seen in the emergency department as vaginal bleeding, a hematoma of the perineum, or as obvious laceration of the vagina. It can be caused accidentally (most often seen in children) or by sexual abuse. Careful examination of the external genitalia must be done in order to assess the extent of the injury. The entire vagina must also be visualized in order not to overlook an

OBSTETRICAL AND GYNECOLOGICAL EMERGENCIES

associated but separate vaginal injury. In addition to a CBC, a urine screen for hematuria should be done to rule out intraperitoneal injury. If, as is most often the case, the patient is a child, it is almost impossible to adequately examine her in the emergency department without the benefit of anesthesia. The preferred treatment is admission and a complete examination and repair under general anesthesia. In treating children, a working knowledge of growth and development is essential. It is important to

1. Gain their confidence
2. Be direct and honest
3. Be aware of age idiosyncrasies
4. Set limits for their behavior
5. Support the patient and her family

Emergency nursing interventions include preparing the patient mentally and physically for the examination and providing emotional support for the patient and family by listening attentively and calmly reassuring them. Be aware that most patients, and especially children, will pick up on the family member's fear, and that, in calming the family, you become much more effective in calming the patient. The nurse should be aware that there is always the possibility of abuse and that discrepancies in history as related to presenting symptoms should be noted. If abuse of a child is suspected, it must be reported to child welfare authorities; all 50 states now require it by law.

Another clinical condition that presents as trauma or infection in children is the presence of a foreign body in the vagina (paper clips, erasers, and so on). The chief symptom is a bloody, watery discharge secondary to vaginitis. These can occasionally be removed in the emergency department, but more often require admission for examination under anesthesia and treatment with antibiotics.

Sexual trauma

Sexual trauma or rape can cause deep vaginal lacerations that require admission for surgical repair and antibiotic therapy. The patient often brings herself into the emergency department or is brought in by police. The patient is frightened and humiliated, and seeing an understanding nurse is usually very comforting. Many areas now have a rape kit that allows the patient to be examined by her private doctor with the evidence placed in the kit and given to police for prosecution. The kit includes (1) slides for vaginal smears, (2) culture tubes, and (3) separate packets for collection of pubic hair belonging to the attacker and to the victim. There is a form on which is noted the state of the patient's clothes and her general condition that the patient, the doctor, and the nurse sign. As this is legal evidence, the kit is opened in front of the patient and sealed immediately after use. After the initial vaginal examination and the completion of the kit, vaginal smears and cultures are taken. If pregnancy is considered possible, the patient will be given stilbestrol to prevent implantation of a fertilized ovum. Treatment with penicillin for possible gonococcal infection is also instituted. The greatest injury to the patient is emotional.

Nursing intervention should include the initiation of emotional support and understanding. All procedures should be carefully explained in full before initiating them. Stay with the patient and talk with the family if the patient wishes. Many times the patient may need further counseling. There are a number of agencies that offer counseling and legal and emotional support to the victims of rape. Volunteers in many of these organizations have been rape victims themselves and are uniquely suited to offer the support these victims so desperately need. The nurse needs to be aware of these agencies and initiate a referral.

OBSTETRICAL EMERGENCIES

Before obstetrics in the emergency department is studied, the nurse should review some basic terms concerning childbirth. A nulligravida is a woman who has never been pregnant, and a nullipara is one who has never been delivered of a viable infant (greater than 24 weeks gestation). A primigravida is a woman who is pregnant for the first time, and a multigravida is one who is pregnant with her second (or subsequent) baby. Once she has been delivered of her first child, a woman is known as a primipara, and once she has delivered her second or

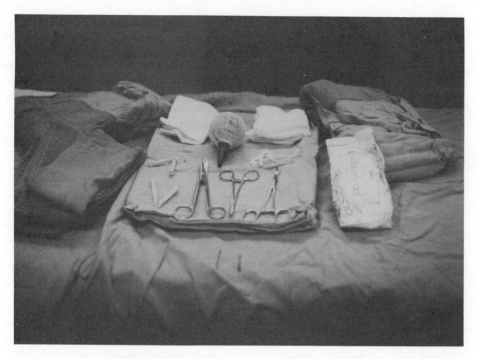

Fig. 21-6. Equipment used for emergency deliveries.

subsequent babies, she is then referred to as a multipara. It is important to know whether a woman is a nullipara, a primipara, or a multipara if she is admitted to the emergency department in labor, because labor time for most multiparas is much shorter than that for most primiparas or nulliparas. This is because a woman who has had a baby before will dilate her cervix more quickly once labor begins, and the perineal musculature is usually more relaxed. The average time required for the completion of the first three stages of labor in a primigravida is 13 hours and 8 hours for a multipara. However, do not forget that each individual is different, and that there are many primiparas that can and do deliver in much less time than average.

The first stage of labor is that time from onset of regular contractions until complete dilatation of the cervix is accomplished. This stage is much longer than either of the other two and may be completed before the patient comes to the emergency department, if the patient is unsure about whether she is in labor or not.

The second stage lasts from full dilatation of the cervix until delivery of the infant. The average time for this stage is 20 minutes to 1 hour. The third stage of labor is from delivery of the infant to delivery of the placenta, and duration is from 3 to 5 minutes. The placenta normally detaches from the uterine wall with the first few contractions following the delivery of the infant and is expelled with the next contraction. In unusual cases, the placenta may fail to separate and may need to be manually expressed by the physician. Under no circumstances should the cord ever be pulled on to force delivery of the placenta as this could cause hemorrhage if the cord should tear.

If a nurse works long enough in a busy emergency department, she will probably be faced with delivering a baby in the department (Fig. 21-6). Just remember, the mother usually accomplishes her task very well with just a little help from one of us. There are two things to keep in mind. They are (1) the baby must breathe, and (2) the mother needs reassurance. Use a clean or sterile towel to exert gentle pressure as the head crowns and control its progress to prevent tearing of the perineum. The mother should be encouraged to pant which helps her prevent bearing down. Holding the head in both hands, gently exert pressure downward to assist in delivery of the shoulders. If the cord is looped around the baby's neck, gently slip it over the head. Support the infant's body and head as it is born. Pick the baby up by the feet with head down to prevent aspiration and gently rub his back to stimulate breathing. After the baby cries, and the cord stops pulsating, place him on the mother's abdomen. This serves two purposes: (1) it reassures the mother, and (2) it places weight over the uterus, causing it to contract. Avoid touching the perineal area in order not to cause infection. Do not pull on the cord, because it could break and hemorrhage. Watch for signs of placental separation (a sudden gush of blood). When the cord stops pulsating, clamp the cord. If a clamp is not available, tie off the cord with some type of tie several inches from the infant's abdomen. Avoid cutting the cord in order to allow the physician to cut it under more sterile conditions. Wrap the infant in a blanket. Check the fundus—massage and putting the baby to breast helps the uterus contract and reduces bleeding. The patient should be transferred to the labor and delivery department for complete evaluation and further management. The baby should be transferred to an isolation area of the newborn nursery until cultures can be determined to be negative.

Evaluation of the newborn

The Apgar Score is a designation of the health of the infant at the time of delivery and should be evaluated at birth and at 5 minutes. The baby is scored for heart rate, respiratory effort, muscle activity, reflexes, and color. In a range of 0 to 10: 7 to 10 is considered good, 4 to 6 is moderately depressed, and 0 to 3 is severely depressed. It is easier to remember which observations to make when you remem-

ber: A for appearance, P for pulse, G for grimace, A for activity, and R for reflexes.

Resuscitation of the newborn

After the infant is born, he should cry immediately and remain pink. But if the infant has to be resuscitated, it is important that we know the tools of resuscitation. It is necessary to keep *TABS* on the infant. This is again a simple way to remember the important things to help a newborn adjust to his new environment.

T = temperature
Dry the infant as soon as possible to keep from further decreasing his temperature. Cover him, or if one is available, place him in a heated incubator.

A = airway
It is important to suction the nostrils first to clear the baby's airway before he breathes and aspirates blood or amniotic fluid. This is done with a bulb syringe or Delee mucous trap.

B = breathing
Breathing or the cry should be stimulated by rubbing his feet or gently slapping the buttocks. Do not slap the infant's back, as this may cause hemorrhage or injury to the adrenals.

S = sugar
If possible, the nurse should obtain a heel stick for glucose level, because any blood sugar in an infant that is below 40 mg/100 ml is considered critical. In such cases, the infant should be given 50% dextrose by IV.

Danger signs in a newborn include a low Apgar score, rapid difficult respirations, apnea, cyanosis, low birth weight, small head, fewer than three umbilical vessels, sweating, edema, petechiae, excessive salivation, an abnormal cry, and lethargy. Resuscitation of the newborn may include intubation. Equipment needed includes small bag resuscitator such as a Penlon or Ambu, oxygen at 3 to 4 liters/minute, a laryngoscope with a size 0-1 blade and a small endotracheal tube, usually 2.5 or 3.0. Dextrose (50%) may be needed for the infant if sugar is below 40 mg/100 ml. Warmth is the most essential thing in stabilizing an infant. Overhead heat is very desirable, as a baby with cold shock is unable to respond well to other resuscitative measures. If external cardiac massage is necessary, it should be done gently

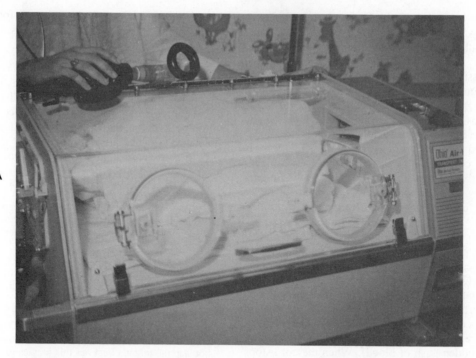

Fig. 21-7. A, Transfer incubator. **B,** Form, reprinted by permission of St. Luke's Episcopal and Texas Children's Hospital, Houston, Texas.

with the index and middle fingers. Small doses of sodium bicarbonate may be needed, and an umbilical catheter tray may be necessary. Other drugs that might be used for resuscitation include naloxone (Narcan), epinephrine, calcium chloride, and atropine, all available in pediatric doses. When the infant is transferred, he should be provided with a clear airway and warmth. If a transfer incubator is not available (Fig. 21-7, *A*), wrap him with plastic wrap or aluminum foil to prevent escape of body heat into the environment. Plastic wrap is the preferred agent as it allows the nurse to observe the color of the infant at all times. He should be transferred with a bulb syringe, cord blood (properly labeled), a copy of the birth record, and any x-ray films that have been taken (Fig. 21-7, *B*). If the receiving department or hospital receives a warm baby with a clear airway, his chances for survival are greatly increased.

A final word on deliveries: With the growing wish of parents to make the birth of their infant a family experience without institutional restrictions, home deliveries are becoming more frequent. For this reason, we will most likely be seeing more women in the emergency department who have already delivered their babies, but who have suffered a vaginal or cervical laceration at birth or who have postpartal hemorrhage as a result of retained placental pieces. Even with the attendance of a skilled nurse midwife, women can and do suffer tears as the baby's head delivers through the vaginal opening without an episiotomy. The mother is set up for infection in any setting, because the womb, which is designed to nurture an infant, can also act as a perfect incubator for bacteria. The preferred treatment is admission, antibiotics, and D and C and/or repair of the lacerations with the patient under anesthesia. The baby should be thoroughly evaluated for any of the danger signs and kept warm. The nurse's role is in teaching the mother what signs indicate distress in the newborn infant. She should

ST. LUKE'S EPISCOPAL HOSPITAL
TEXAS CHILDREN'S HOSPITAL
HOUSTON, TEXAS

DEPARTMENT OF NURSING
INFANT ADMISSION AND HISTORY FORM

Date: _____ Time: _____ Mode of Arrival: _____

Temp: _____ H.R.: _____ R.R.: _____ WT: _____ Gms. (____lbs.____oz) Length: _____ cm

FOC: _____ cm   Chest: _____ cm   Voided: _____ B.M.: _____

Dextrostix: _____ mg%   B/P: _____ Doppler/Palpated

Transferring unit or hospital _____ Reason for admission: _____

PHYSICIANS NOTIFIED (<u>NOTE</u> if office nurse or answering service took message):

NAME: _____ _____

_____ _____

On Admission:
Silverman Score _____

Upper Chest	Lower Chest	Xiphoid	Narea dilation	Expiratory grunt
Rises synchronously with abdomen	No intercostal sinking on inspiration	None	None (no movement of chin)	None heard
Lag or minimal sinking as abdomen rises	Just visible sinking of intercostal spaces on inspiration	Just visible	Minimal chin descends, lips closed)	Heard with stethoscope only
"Seesaw" sinking with rising abdomen	Marked sinking of intercostal spaces on inspiration	Marked	Marked (chin descends, lips part)	Heard with naked ear

Apgar Score _____

Sign	0	1	2
Heart rate	Absent	Slow (below 100)	Over 100
Respiratory effort	Absent	Slow, irregular	Good, crying
Reflex irritability (response to catheter in nostril tested after oropharynx is cleared)	No response	Grimaces	Cough or sneeze
Muscle tone	Limp	Some flexion of extremities	Active motion
Color	Blue, pale	Body pink, extremities blue	Completely pink

Gestational Age _____ wks.

COLOR: Pink _____ Pale _____ Jaundiced _____ Cyanotic _____

CYANOSIS: None noted _____ General _____ Peripheral _____ Central _____

REFLEXES & ACTIVITY: Moro _____ Suck _____ Appetite _____
   Cry _____ Awake and Alert _____ Lethargic _____ Jittery _____
   Irritable _____

PHYSICAL APPEARANCE (Include abnormalities, bruises, etc. noted) _____
_____
_____

Additional Remarks, Symptoms Noted & Parental Comments _____
_____
_____

Family Informed of: Routines _____ Visiting Hours _____

IF AVAILABLE, PLEASE COMPLETE THE FOLLOWING:
MATERNAL HISTORY: Blood type _____ Rh _____ List any prenatal, perinatal, past pregnancy problems. Include medications, illness, type of delivery. _____
_____
_____

DELIVERY: DATE: _____ TIME: _____ PLACE: _____
      Number of cord vessels _____

APGAR: 1 minute _____ 5 minute _____ Not done _____ Resuscitated _____
      Vitamin K _____ Eye Care _____ Birth Weight: _____
OBTAINED FROM TRANSFERRING HOSPITAL: X-Rays _____ EKG _____ Cord Blood _____
      Mother's Blood _____ Placenta _____

7/79

SIGNATURE AND TITLE _____

B

Fig. 21-7, cont'd. For legend see opposite page.

also be made aware that follow-up and immunization by a physician is important. The nurse will also need to reassure the patient that she and her baby will be all right, and to respect the right of the patient and her husband to choose this type of delivery. Do not be judgmental; many couples deliver at home, have no problems, and have a very rich and fulfilling experience.

Fetal emergencies

Occasionally when a pregnant patient is brought to the emergency department, she is a fetal rather than a maternal emergency. Prolapsed cord (descent of the cord before delivery of the baby) is among these. One of the causes is the rupture of the membranes when the presenting part is not engaged. Although the presenting part may be the head, a prolapsed cord is more commonly seen in shoulder and foot presentations. Other causes are prematurity and polyhydramnios (more fluid causes increased pressure when the membranes rupture). This condition is obvious when the cord can be seen protruding from the vagina or palpated in the vagina on examination. Fetal distress as indicated by meconium staining of the fluid indicates anoxia, which can be caused by prolapsed cord. Nursing management is to place the mother in a knee-chest or Trendelenberg position, start oxygen at 5 liters/minute, place a gloved hand in the vagina, and push up on the head to relieve compression and prepare for immediate delivery of the infant. Most often, the infant is delivered by cesarean section to prevent further cord compression. As the patient usually must be transferred to another area for delivery, the nurse should continue to push up on the presenting part with her gloved hand. Repositioning of the cord is no longer recommended because fetal mortality is increased when handling causes accelerated cooling of the cord and increases vasospasm. It is important for the nurse to keep as calm as possible, explain why and how each procedure is being done, and allow the patient to express her fears. Keep the patient and family informed of her and her baby's condition.

The prolapsed foot can also be considered a potential emergency and occurs in breech presentations when the bag of waters has ruptured. Listen for the fetal heart rate. If normal, do not perform a vaginal examination, but transfer immediately to the labor and delivery area. Do not stimulate the foot; if further movement occurs, the cord could prolapse.

Maternal complications

Placenta previa. Placenta previa occurs as painless bleeding usually around the eighth month of pregnancy with no evidence of contractions. The uterus feels soft and flaccid. This is caused by the implantation and development of the placenta in the lower uterine segment rather than at the normal implantation site in the upper uterine segment. This causes the placenta to partially or completely cover the internal cervical os. *Previa* literally means "in front of" or "in the way of" the presenting fetus. By implanting in the lower uterine segment instead of higher, the placenta is in the zone of effacement (thinning) and dilatation. The clinical course and outcome depend on the extent of placenta covering the internal os.

Placenta previae are classified as:
1. Total, in which the placenta completely covers the os
2. Partial, in which the placenta partially covers the os
3. Marginal, or low implantation, in which the placenta is adjacent, but does not extend beyond the margin of the os

Although total placenta previa is rare, low implants or partial placenta previa occurs in one of every 200 pregnancies. Seventy-five percent of previas occur in multiparous women. Multiparity with advancing age and a rapid succession of pregnancies are felt to be among predisposing factors.

The cause of placenta previa is not definitely known, but there are several theories. One of the theories is that the ovum implants in the area of the healthy endometrium which, in these patients, is found in the lower segment of the uterus. Another is that abnormal motility causes the ovum to pass through the uterus too quickly and to implant in the lower segment.

Hemorrhage is the first and most commonly

seen symptom, and, because it is not accompanied by contractions, there is no pain associated with it. Because the cervix begins to dilate and efface in the eighth month, maternal vessels tear while the patient is asleep and may cease spontaneously or continue, depending on how large the vessels are that are torn. After two or three hemorrhages, labor usually begins. There may also be premature rupture of membranes with the resulting possibility of infection. Premature labor and an abnormal presenting part can further complicate the delivery. With total placenta previa, bleeding occurs earlier and is more profuse. Placenta previa should always be suspected when painless uterine bleeding occurs in the last half of the pregnancy.

Diagnostic studies should include sonogram, if available, because sonogram is very specific in determining the position of the placenta. X-ray studies are still done in areas where the sonogram is not available. Complete blood count, type and cross-match for several units of blood, and clotting studies should be done immediately. The nurse should establish a good intravenous line with a solution such as D/5/ Ringer's lactate and transfer the patient to labor and delivery for monitoring and, if indicated, immediate cesarean section.

Vital signs should always include fetal heart rate on anyone with a viable fetus. This is not as much a part of routine for the emergency department nurses as taking blood pressure and is sometimes not done. The nurse must always remember that in the case of a pregnant woman, there are two patients to be taken care of. Although most hospitals have fetoscopes, we would also recommend use of a Doptone, as it is more accurate in picking up the heart tones of the 20- to 24-week-old fetus. If fetal heart tones are not heard, this should also be documented and reported to the physician immediately. Do not alarm the mother. If she asks about the fetal heart tones, you can always say you are having difficulty hearing them. The normal fetal heart rate is 120 to 160 beats/minute. Stay with the patient and encourage her to verbalize her fear. Provide necessary assistance for her significant other with admitting

procedures and in calling family. Maternal mortality for placenta previa is approximately 1.5%; fetal mortality depends on gestation and extent of anoxia experienced.

Abruptio placentae

Another major complication of pregnancy in the last trimester is the premature separation of the placenta from its uterine attachment. This is known as abruptio placentae. The primary cause is unknown, but there are several theories. One of these causes is thought to be related to preeclampsia, because 25% to 60% of all abruptions occur in preeclamptic mothers. Another suspected cause is the increased venous pressure that occurs when the vena cava is compressed in the supine position by the gravid uterus. Contributing factors such as advanced maternal age (35 and over), multiparity, a short cord, and trauma certainly play a large part. A partial separation can occur with either occult or frank hemorrhage. A complete separation occurs with occult hemorrhage. Although frank hemorrhage is always an emergency because of blood loss, the most dangerous of the two is occult hemorrhage, because it is not always immediately diagnosed, and the extent of the bleeding is not known without testing unless the patient experiences symptoms of shock. Occult hemorrhage can occur if:

1. The fetal head is engaged
2. The placenta is partially separated, but the margins are attached
3. Blood breaks through the membranes and effuses into the amniotic cavity

External hemorrhage usually accompanies partial separation and is considered more common and less severe. Clinical findings in abruptio placentae vary with the degree of separation and bleeding. Blood loss that is less than 500 ml is considered mild to moderate. Blood loss of over 500 ml and apparent is considered moderate. The complete abruptio placentae is considered severe, because the blood loss causes shock. The uterus is usually relaxed in mild to moderate cases and rigid in severe ones. Pain is usually mild or localized in partial separation and severe and generalized in a complete separation. Fetal heart tones will be normal to slow in partial separation and irregular to absent in complete separation. There may be excessive fetal movements or none at all. Treatment is prompt replacement of blood, clotting studies, replacement of fibrinogens as needed, and delivery by cesarean section as soon as possible. Maternal mortality is 1% unless accompanied by hypofibrinogenemia. Fetal mortality in a complete abruption is 100% and in partial abruption is 30% to 60%. Fetal death occurs as a result of anoxia.

Disseminated intravascular coagulation

Disseminated intravascular coagulation (DIC), in which the clotting mechanism is activated and accelerated, can occur as a complication of pregnancy. It is most often seen in severe cases of abruptio placentae in the form of hypofibrinogenemia but can also occur as a result of excessive blood loss during delivery, following amniotic fluid embolus at delivery, or following fetal death in utero. In this hypercoagulatory state, clotting factors are used up before the liver has time to manufacture and send in replacements. During pregnancy, the level of fibrinogen increases above 440 mg, compared with the normal fibrinogen level of 200 to 400 mg. When this level falls below 100 mg, the blood fails to clot. Causes of hypofibrinogenemia in abruptio placentae are not completely understood, but it is felt that the deposition of fibrin at the site of placental separation depletes the amount of circulating fibrinogen. This causes patches of fibrin to detach from the capillary space and reenter the maternal circulation as minute emboli, which can cause necrosis of the organs. The kidneys are most often affected, and acute renal failure may occur.

Treatment is aimed at correcting the cause. All cases of DIC are not caused by low fibrinogen levels and may be caused by low levels of any of the clotting factors. If possible, consultation by the laboratory pathologist is often the wisest and most efficient way to determine the affected factor. Replacement of the factor will often reverse the condition. Heparin is occasionally used to neutralize the circulating thromboplastin and slow down clot formation,

thereby slowing the depletion of the clotting factors. Platelets, fresh frozen plasma, and packed cells themselves may all be used in the management of DIC. The organs themselves may require support with dialysis. In the case of abruptio placentae, the baby should be delivered immediately.

Preeclampsia and eclampsia

Preeclampsia and eclampsia were formerly thought to be due to toxins in the blood stream and thus were referred to as toxemia of pregnancy. It is now known that there are no "toxins" present, other than the body's own breakdown products as a result of metabolic processes. Preeclampsia and eclampsia are hypertensive disorders specific to pregnancy that occur in the last trimester or soon after delivery. The nonconvulsive state is called preeclampsia and the convulsive state, eclampsia. They are manifested by hypertension, proteinuria, and edema, occurring singly or in a combination, and are major causes of maternal morbidity and mortality. In North America, preeclampsia or eclampsia occurs in 5% of all pregnancies, and 15% of all eclamptic patients die from the disease.

Severe preeclamptic states are characterized by:
1. Blood pressure over 160/110 mm Hg.
2. Proteinuria (5 gm or more/24 hours)
3. Oliguria (output) less than 400 ml/24 hours
4. Headaches
5. Visual disturbances
6. Abdominal pain
7. Pulmonary edema and cyanosis

Eclamptic symptoms can include all of the above plus convulsions or coma, or both. The cause of these disorders is unknown. Current theories include:
1. Impaired uteroplacental circulation as a result of uterine distention.
2. Overstimulation of the adrenal cortex by a hypertrophic anterior pituitary and/or the placenta itself.
3. Poor dietary habits, particularly those diets low in protein.
4. Loss of sodium during pregnancy, which causes hypovolemia and vasospasms.

Management of this disorder depends on the severity. Those mothers who are receiving good prenatal care will likely be monitored closely by their physicians and put to bed at home or in an antepartal unit of the hospital long before they require emergency treatment in the emergency department. For this reason, the mother seen in the emergency department is probably in a severe preeclamptic or eclamptic state. The recommended treatment is to stabilize the mother, place her in a room with constant nursing attendance, and monitor vital signs and fetal heart tones until she can be transferred to the labor and delivery suite where she will be either sedated or delivered. Diazepam (Valium) is usually used to treat the convulsions, and diuretics and vasopressors may be given to reduce the blood pressure. Close monitoring of the intake and output is very important, as the renal condition is significant.

When a pregnant woman appears in the emergency department with any of the above symptoms, the nurse assessing her should be particularly aware of any edema present and note its severity. Complete vital signs including fetal heart tones should be obtained and precautions taken for the patient's safety should she convulse—side rails up, a tongue blade available, and an airway or suction at hand. An IV at keep open rate should be established with a large-bore intracatheter. Blood should be drawn for a CBC, electrolytes, and coagulation and liver studies. A catheter should be placed in order to determine the status of renal output. Immediate transfer to the labor and delivery unit is recommended. The patient and family should be kept informed about each step in order to allay anxiety.

STRESS FACTORS THAT INFLUENCE EMERGENCY CARE

Anxiety is highly contagious. At any moment the emergency department staff can be forced to deal with anxiety in a patient, family members, or in themselves. Emergency department nurses must be able to understand, accept, and handle their own levels of anxiety and be able to intervene successfully with the patient's or family's anxious behavior. We have the responsibility of coping with and responding in a positive manner to this behavior. Keep calm, and do not add to the anxiety already present. Recognize and assess behaviors that are provoked by anxiety such as guilt, fear, and anger. Successfully intervene in the situation if possible. Learn from each situation how to deal with the next anxious patient or parent, but always realize that people are individuals.

Guilt is another feeling that we must deal with in some cases. Anger is another and may

Table 21-1. Major presenting symptoms of gynecological emergency and differential diagnosis

Clinical causes	Vaginal bleeding	Hemorrhage	Pain	Shock	Trauma	Differential diagnosis
Ectopic pregnancy		Internal	X	X		Positive pregnancy test
Ruptured ovarian cyst		Internal	X	X		Negative pregnancy test; admit for observation and/or laparoscopy
Dysfunctional uterine bleeding	X	X				Irregular periods Intermittent spotting
Incomplete abortion	X	X	X	Rare		History of missed periods or scanty periods Passage of tissue
Pelvic inflammatory disease			X			History of sexual exposure
Vaginal laceration	X		X		X	
Vulvar hematoma	X		X	Rare	X	

Table 21-2. Major presenting symptoms of obstetrical emergency and differential diagnosis

Clinical causes	Hemorrhage	Shock	Pain	Convulsions	Fetal distress	Differential diagnosis
Placenta previa	X	X			Decreased FHT	
Abruptio placentae	(Usually internal)	X	X		Decreased or absent FHT	
Ectopic pregnancy		X	X			Positive pregnancy test
Eclampsia and preeclampsia			X	X		
Prolapsed cord					Decreased or absent FHT	Visualize fetal cord

sometimes be the patient's or family's way of dealing with guilt or anxiety. Fear can be of the known or the unknown, of disfigurement, of loss, of death, or of the nurse herself. As nurses, we must learn to support each other in difficult circumstances. For instance, if you see that one of your colleagues is losing her patience, you might try relieving her for a while. Always remember that we see patients many times at their very worst—they are under stress, their coping mechanisms are out of balance, and we have little time to develop rapport.

Age is an important factor that must be kept in mind in order to be effective in many situations. A working knowledge of the growth and development patterns in children will help us obtain cooperation from many of our younger patients. The elderly and disabled often recognize the loss of control in their lives and fear further loss. We should try to allow them to maintain as much control as possible over what is happening to them in the emergency department.

Legal factors influence much of what we can do in the emergency situation. Therefore a working knowledge of the local laws are important. Permission for treatment must be obtained unless the state has special provisions for emergency care. It is our responsibility to know what should be reported, to whom, and how it should be done. We must know what is available for the rape victim in the way of coun-

seling and what our responsibility is in preserving legal evidence.

The emergency setting itself is stressful. The equipment, the activity, the trauma that is seen can be distressing to the healthy person; the ill individual sometimes is unable to cope.

We, as emergency department nurses, know that the days of the accident room or emergency room are over. The emergency center now plays a prominent role in the delivery of health care, and with that come responsibilities. Eighty percent of all emergency department visits are not clinically emergent, and 25% of all hospital admissions are made through the emergency department. Over 60 million people are seen in emergency departments annually. One reason for this is the population migration. Another is advances in medical technology. It may be found that the physician has failed to establish a professional relationship with a private patient. It is difficult to get an appointment, and house calls are a thing of the past. There has been a decrease in the number of family doctors. Many insurances will not pay unless the patient is in the hospital. It has become more convenient for the patient and the doctor for the patient to be seen in the emergency department.

The emergency department nurse has more of a responsibility now to initiate referrals. She must help the patient obtain a private doctor and try to encourage follow-up care. She must be able to inform the patient or family of special counseling services such as those for rape victims and for parents who are involved in child abuse. She must be able to keep the staff, patient, and family informed of changes in condition and findings. She is responsible for follow-up with a call to the family physician with results of laboratory findings or cultures if this is not done by the laboratory. She must be sure that the patient understands that she needs to see a gynecologist, that she is clear on instructions for treatment, and that the doctor is informed that she is coming in and what was done in the emergency department.

As a result of the effort to improve the quality of health care and make it available to all segments of the population, we are seeing the development of the regional system. Resources of the community or region are pooled and coordinated so that a complete range of services suited to the community need can be economically provided. This system increases the need for transfer of the patient in many cases. Properly done, the transfer should be accomplished with the patient warm and clinically stabilized, with established supportive measures such as an IV, with a nurse in attendance, and with complete records, including medications given. Notification of transfer and acceptance by the receiving hospital are required by the JCAH standards.

BIBLIOGRAPHY

Bates, B., A guide to physical examination. Philadelphia, 1974, J. B. Lippincott Co.

Brunner, L. S., and Suddarth, D. S.: The Lippincott Manual of Nursing Practice, Philadelphia, 1978, J. B. Lippincott Co.

Cosgriff, J. H., and Anderson, D. L.: The practice of emergency nursing, Philadelphia, 1975, J. B. Lippincott Co., pp. 332-351.

Eckert, C., and Pearl, M. J.: Emergency room care, Boston, 1976, Little, Brown and Co., pp. 177-202.

Green, T. H., Jr.: Gynecology: essentials of clinical practice, ed. 2, Boston, 1971, Little, Brown and Co.

Jensen, M. D., Benson, R. C., and Bobak, I. M.: Maternity care: the nurse and the family, Saint Louis, 1977, The C. V. Mosby Co.

Jones, G. S., Jones, H. W., Jr., and Novak, E. R.: Gynecology: condensed from Novak's textbook of gynecology, ed. 8, Baltimore, 1971, The Williams and Wilkins Co.

Tucker, S. M., Breeding, M. A., Cannobio, M. M., Paquette, E. H., Wells, M. E., and Willmann, M. E.: Patient care standards, ed. 2, St. Louis, 1980, The C. V. Mosby Co., pp. 417-466.

CHAPTER **22**

Pediatric emergencies

COMMUNICATING WITH CHILDREN

Sick or injured children in an emergency setting require an organized and consistent approach. The following are basic assumptions for effective interaction with children:

Children are not "little adults."

Children are individuals with certain rights and needs.

The present illness or injury and how it is handled by all concerned affect the future growth and development of the child.

Every child responds to stress uniquely, but an understanding of stages of growth and development is essential as a guide to helping the child cope with the present situation.

Care of the child includes relating to those important to him such as family, friends, people who have brought him to the emergency department.

Separation anxiety and fear of pain are the two major forces shaping the child's present behavior.

Some guilt is experienced by parents whenever illness or injury affects a child.

When the child's emergency health situation temporarily makes the parent unable to cope, both should be treated as clients.

Children are very "feeling" individuals who need to be allowed to express those feelings openly and appropriately. The parent also is more likely to be more emotional than he might ordinarily be if he were the patient himself. Emergency personnel can do much to help if

they recognize that they are treating a family and not just the child.

Techniques of relating to children

Speak in simple, direct language appropriate to the child's level.

Use the child's first name frequently.

Do not ask too many questions.

Answer questions, being aware of hidden meaning.

Give simple instructions as commands; avoid "don't" rules.

Use touch to communicate understanding and warmth.

Do not separate the child from his parent unless it is absolutely necessary.

Recognize that screaming, sobbing, and crying are defensive behaviors and are probably the highest level of coping possible at the moment.

Remain calm and authoritative to show control of yourself.

Do not force a child to choose. This increases anxiety. If you give alternatives, be willing to accept the consequence of the choice.

Pediatric history and examination

Injured or ill children are characteristically not only distraught, but fearful of anyone assisting him. The very young child who cannot express himself in specific terms will respond with generalized protesting, disorganized behavior, and perhaps loud protestations. Emergency nurses should remember that adults may share the child's confusion and fear and even attempt to assume some of the pain and discomfort. Interactions with injured and ill children can therefore be a volatile experience if not managed judiciously.

Until a child reaches the age of 4 or 5 years, most information about illness or injury must be elicited from parents or the adults. Older children however, can often provide much valuable data including referencing the specific part that "hurts." It is important that triage nurses evaluate the potential of the child to aid in history-taking. For example, a 13-year-old can be an excellent historian, and it may in some instances be valuable to continue history-gathering activities when parents are out of the room. This is particularly important if genitourinary complaints are involved, which tend to embarrass the teen-ager, particularly when they are discussed in front of parents and if they potentially could be related to sexual activity. Reliability may be much greater in such instances if parents are separated from the child.

Unless immediate action is indicated, triage nurses should gain the confidence of the child and his parents before touching an injured or painful body part. Always use a slow, gentle approach. Take time, too, to observe parent-child interaction and to establish rapport while eliciting the necessary data.

Very young children and those over 4 or 5 seldom present critical problems during examination unless they are unusually dependent. They should be permitted to remain near parents during the observations as much as possible. Often it is helpful if they sit on their mother's lap, stand close to her, or allow her to hold them during this time.

The first thing to do as the nurse begins the examination is handwashing, preferably in view. It conveys to the parent initially that there is genuine concern for the child's health protection, and furthermore it is good teaching for the child and his family.

Do not sweep the young child from a parents' arms and place him on an examining table before gaining rapport with both parties. Elicit assistance from the parent when feasible during the examination. Some children respond best when viewing what the examiner is doing; others prefer to look in another direction, perhaps at mother or grandma.

If struggling and crying interferes with examination, restraining procedures may need to be instituted (Figs. 22-1 and 22-2), and occasionally, if parents are aggravating the situation, they may be asked to leave the room.

Respect the modesty of the child and his parents. Underclothing should be removed only when necessary and replaced as soon as possible.

Physicians and nurses find that they usually gain more cooperation from the child if he is acquainted with the tools used in the examination and is allowed to manipulate them or relate them to a familiar object. Often, giving the child a simple object such as a tongue depressor or Band-Aid may direct his interests, at least momentarily, while a specific observation is made. Avoid anxiety-producing delays by having all equipment at hand as the examination begins.

When parents bring an injured child to the emergency department, they convey behavior that ranges from guilt to anger that their child "got hurt." Often their frustration with the episode of coming to the hospital is so overwhelming that they displace hostility onto others, especially nurses and physicians. Because they feel inadequate about coping with the injury, perhaps responsible for the accident, and generally powerless in the emergency department setting, it is not uncommon for them to respond with anger at any provocation. It is important that emergency personnel convey warmth and understanding and avoid judgmental statements that threaten and intimidate the parents, who already feel impotent.

Children who are hurt are strongly affected by the behavior of those about them. They may feel guilty about being a bother to parents, may fear punishment for the acts that led to the injury, and may assume they deserve the painful consequences. This child may appear passive and dissociated. Nurses should ensure the child of acceptance and behave with sensitivity, regardless of the circumstances. Do not overwhelm the child with power, because this may lead to an outright battle of nurse and

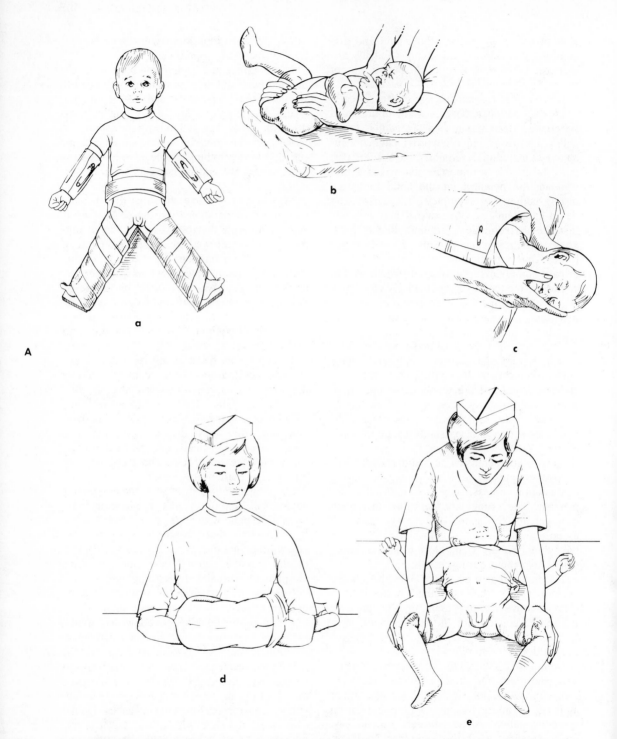

Fig. 22-1. A, Procedural restraints: **a,** Y-board (circumcision, exchange transfusion, and so forth); **b,** thigh flexion-abduction (perineal or rectal procedures); **c,** mummy (procedures involving head and neck); **d,** knee-neck flexion (lumbar puncture); **e,** frog position (femoral venipuncture).

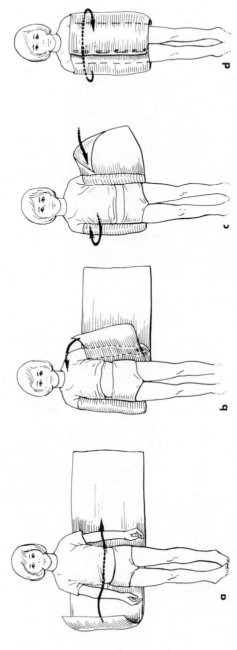

Fig. 22-1, cont'd. B. Body restraint, useful for procedures involving the head or perineum of a young child. **a,** Position child supine on treatment table covered with a sheet folded lengthwise. **B.** Body restraint, useful for procedures involving the head or perineum of a young child. **a,** Position child supine on treatment table covered with a sheet folded lengthwise, which extends from the axilla to the thighs. Arrange the positioning so that one third of the sheet extends from one side and two thirds from the opposite side. **b,** The shorter side of the sheet is brought (1) anterior to the proximal arm, (2) posterior to the trunk, and (3) anterior to the distal arm. The remaining length is carried posterior to the trunk. **c,** The remaining two thirds is brought (1) anterior to the extremities and then (2) on around the body until the length is exhausted. **d,** Completed restraint secured with safety pins.

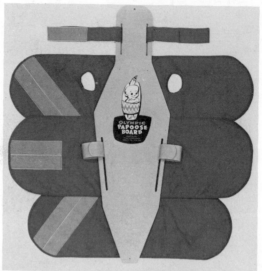

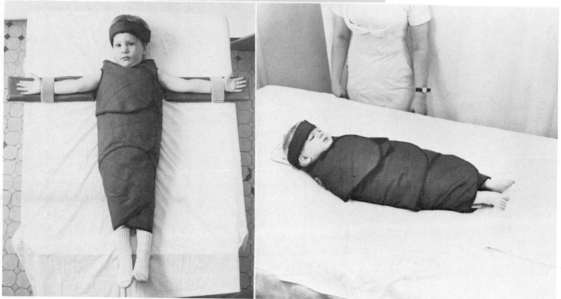

Fig. 22-2. Papoose board. (Courtesy Olympic Medical Co., Seattle, Wash.)

child. Rough, careless handling or conveying anger and disgust at parents only exaggerates the trauma of the emergency hospitalization.

Nurses should model behavior for parents that depicts caring and concern, and must take every precaution *not* to show anger or disgust at parents, because the child readily "tunes into" feelings of others.

It is usually helpful if parents of small children remain in the room while treatment is being given. They often can help in translating the emergency experience into the child's language. However, it is important to evaluate the ability and the desire of mothers and fathers to stay in the treatment area and to be able to visualize procedures without fainting, losing control, or making matters worse by verbalizing unhelpful comments, such as "What is that mean doctor doing to my precious little Missy?" Although thinking they are actually being supportive to the child, they are damaging the doctor-child trust relationship, so important for this and subsequent encounters with health personnel.

Children have the same fears in emergency settings as adults do—fear of needles and painful procedures, fear of loss or mutilation of a body part, fear of losing control, and fear of death.

Explanation of equipment, techniques, and activity should be offered at the level appropriate to the age of the child, being as honest as possible before the treatment activity is initiated; for example, "This is going to hurt—but it will be over as quickly as you can close and open your eyes." Honesty helps bring credibility to statements of the various health team members and eventually helps establish a bond of trust and confidence. Play therapy may be useful if time and circumstances permit. Books, puppets, and crayons, for example, should be kept in the emergency room for both diversional recreational and therapeutic play. Many studies have shown that drawing pictures is a helpful way for children to express their feelings about an accident and the hospital emergency department. They often can serve as a mode to help establish rapport among children and the staff and replace the injury as a focus of attention.

TRIAGING THE CHILD

Immediate attention should be given to any child with the following:

Airway problem

Dehydration

Seizures

High-impact trauma history

Unconsciousness

Fever (rectal temperature 103° F) with signs of sepsis (lethargy, petechiae) or meningeal irritation (nuchal rigidity, vomiting)

Anaphylaxis threat

Ingestions of toxic substances

Evidence of child abuse

Other conditions that result in a really "sick-looking" infant or child should also be managed properly. Apathy, lethargy, poor skin color, dull eyes, shallow respirations, or flaccidity are indices of significant illness.

Obtain a quick history of the present problem, asking questions while doing a head-to-toe assessment. If the child is under 2 years, a natal history including birth weight and health status during infancy is relevant. If the mother or father is present, permit her or him to undress and hold the small child during this portion of triage to mutually gain confidence in the emergency department process. Older children may be placed on an examining table. Be sure to assess fluid intake and output (by number of diapers or trips to the bathroom), and search the body for clues of injury as well as dehydration. Do not become distracted by a long-term problem (such as nutritional status or developmental delays) when the current problem is yet unassessed. Give careful attention to respira-

Table 22-1. Table of estimated weights*

Age	Kilograms	Pounds
Newborn	3-5	6-11
1 yr.	10	22
3 yr.	15	33
5 yr.	20	44
8 yr.	25	55
10 yr.	30	66
15 yr.	50	110

*Modified from Melker, R.: Resuscitation of the neonate, infant and child, Crit. Care. Q. **1**:49, May 1978.

tory status, peripheral perfusion, neuromuscular status, and indications of acute injury or child abuse (see pp. 41-42). When in doubt, triage the child in favor of immediate care. Remember to weigh (and record) all weights in pounds and kilograms, because medication dosages are calculated on a per-pound or per-kilogram basis. If weighing the child is impractical, Table 22-1 may be of value.

ACCIDENTS

Emergency personnel should learn to expect what accidents are likely to occur within certain age groups, because growth and developmental variables relate closely to cause. For example, when children are able to crawl and to walk, they can freely explore their environment, and these toddlers are prone to poisoning by ingestion and to falls. Table 22-2 outlines accidents by age groups and provides precautions that can be valuable in prevention.

Evening is the peak time for emergency visits. Children are usually injured in the late afternoon or evening, particularly right before dinner and bedtime. In addition, some parents do not seek emergency care until they complete their work day and have time to take the child to the hospital for treatment.

Common accidents include falls from bicycles, stepping on sharp objects while barefoot, fighting injuries, burns, lacerations, head trauma, human and animal bites, and dental injuries.

The triage nurse should assess all accidents with great care, always considering that resultant injuries might be the product of child abuse or neglect (see pp. 41-42). It is important that all factors associated with the accidents are included in the data gathering, because they could be valuable in confirming or ruling out abuse or neglect.

Trauma is a significant problem among the pediatric population, because accidents cause 1 out of 3 deaths in children up to 14 years of age. In addition to those killed each year, there are thousands more seriously injured or permanently disabled. Falls, vehicular accidents, and recreation-related injuries account for nearly half of these, but stabbings, gunshot wounds,

Table 22-2. Accident risks and precautions at various age levels*

Typical accidents	Normal behavior characteristics	Precautions
First year		
Falls, inhalation or ingestion of foreign objects, poisoning, burns, drowning	After several months of age, can squirm and roll, and later in year creeps and pulls self erect Places anything and everything in mouth Is helpless in water	Do not leave alone on tables, and so forth, where falls can occur Keep crib sides up Keep small objects and harmful substances out of reach Do not leave alone in tub
Second year		
Falls, drowning, motor vehicles, ingestion of poisonous substances, burns	Is able to roam about in erect posture Can go up and down stairs Has great curiosity Puts almost everything in mouth Is helpless in water	Keep screens in windows Place gate at top of stairs Cover unused electrical outlets; keep electric cords out of easy reach Keep in enclosed space when outdoors and not in company of an adult

2 to 4 years		
Falls, drowning, motor vehicles, ingestion of poisonous substances, burns	Is able to open doors Can run and climb Investigates closets and drawers Plays with mechanical gadgets Can throw ball and other objects	Keep medicines, household poisons, and small sharp objects out of sight and reach Keep handles of pots and pans on stove out of reach and containers of hot foods away from edge of table Protect from water in tub or yard Keep doors locked when there is danger of falls Place screen or guards in windows Teach about watching for automobiles in driveways and streets Keep firearms locked up Keep knives and electrical equipment out of reach Teach about risks of throwing sharp objects and about danger of following ball into street
5 to 9 years		
Motor vehicles, bicycle accidents, drowning, burns, firearms	Is daring and adventurous Control over large muscles is more advanced than control over small muscles Has increasing interest in group play; loyalty to group makes him willing to follow suggestions of leaders	Teach techniques and traffic rules for bicycling Encourage skills in swimming Keep firearms locked up except when adult can supervise their use
10 to 14 years		
Motor vehicles, drowning, burns, firearms, falls, bicycle accidents	Organic need for strenuous physical activity Plays in hazardous places (street, railroad tracks, near rivers) unless facilities for supervised, adequate recreation are provided Need for approval of age mates leads to daring or hazardous feats	Teach the rules of pedestrian safety Teach bicycling safety Instruct in safe use of firearms Provide safe and acceptable facilities for recreation and social activities Prepare for automobile driving by good example on part of adults and closely supervised instruction

*From Shaffer, T. E.: Accident prevention. Pediatr. Clin. North Am. **1:**421-432. May, 1954.

and child abuse are seen with increasing frequency in the emergency department. Emergency nurses should be familiar with the unique management aspects important in pediatric trauma.

Anatomical variations

There are a few important anatomical variables in children that should be reviewed, because they directly affect the vulnerability and response of organs to injury.

Head and neck. The infant's and small child's head is expandable because of the suture lines remaining open and the presence of fontanels. Although the brain is not protected with heavy bone as in the adult, head injury often may not produce serious sequelae, since the presence of intracranial pressure is tolerated well because of the expandable calvarium. Furthermore, the signs and symptoms are relatively easy to assess, in some instances; for example, bulging fontanels noted during crying.

The neck is short, and if hyperextended, can block the airway because of kinking as opposed to opening it (see p. 135).

Radiographs of the head may be of limited value in searching for skull fractures and midline shifts, since variations in suture line widths and the normal absence of a calcified pineal gland in the young child may obscure a definitive clinical picture.

The vertebral column is generally more vascular in the infant and young child because it is growing rapidly. Impact to the neck and spine can create hemorrhage at the site with relative ease.

Chest and abdomen. The chest and abdomen of the infant and young child provide less protection for underlying organs than do those of adults. For example, the ribs are soft and flexible, and the thin-walled abdomen has little muscular protection. The large liver of the young child is obviously less protected than if it were neatly tucked behind the ribs' protective barrier. The pancreas, liver, and spleen are frequently injured in blunt abdominal trauma. In young children, the spleen can be avulsed without hemorrhage, since the small but muscular splenic arteries contract vigorously, forming a lifesaving thrombus.

Gastric perforation occurs easily, especially if the organ is distended. The poorly developed rectus muscle permits the stomach, duodenum, and pancreas to be driven against the spine in response to blunt trauma of considerable force.

Kidneys. The kidneys are more vulnerable in children than in adults because they are poorly protected. They lie mainly within the abdomen, and their perirenal support tissues are poorly developed. The kidney itself, of course, is quite vascular and fragile.

SHOCK STATES IN CHILDREN

The principles of shock management in children are the same as for the adult: giving attention to cardiorespiratory efforts while taking specific measures to find and correct the cause. However, there are some special considerations with pediatric shock states that deserve attention.

Child shock states are often caused by poisonings, hypersensitivity reactions, septicemia, respiratory insufficiency, and fluid loss. Children rarely have cardiogenic shock. The most important rule to follow is to always suspect shock in relation to trauma or severe dehydration and manage the child accordingly.

Assessment and monitoring

The infant or small child in shock has a weak cry and is essentially unresponsive to stimulation. Pallor or frank cyanosis may be evident together with poor capillary filling. The core body temperature is subnormal, trending downward, with the extremities decidedly cooler than the abdomen. Respirations are likely to be shallow. In certain shock states when perfusion failure is far advanced, there may be necrotic lesions (intravascular coagulation) in oral and nasal mucosa, the anus, and at injection sites or surgical incisions. Hemorrhage may accompany or follow this phenomenon. A condition called *sclerema neonatorum* may be present, which is characterized by a tallowlike hardening of the arms and legs.

The assessment of the infant or child with

Table 22-3. Pediatric vital signs*

	Pulse	Respirations	Blood pressure
Newborn	120-160	60	60-90/20-60
1 yr	80-140	25	65-95/25-65
3 yrs	80-120	20	70-100/30-70
5 yrs	70-115	20	70-100/30-70
7 yrs	70-115	25	70-100/30-70
10 yrs	70-115	30-35	90-120/50-80
15 yrs	70-90	18	102-140/50-70

*From Barber, J. M.: EMT checkpoint: Tips on assessment and management of pediatric trauma, EMT J. **4:**66-71, March 1980.

shock depends on the knowledge of the normal vital sign values for specific age groups (Table 22-3).

Assume that shock is present or will quickly develop in every injured child. An IV should be established promptly in the largest accessible vein. The dorsum of the hand, the scalp, or the dorsum of the foot are suitable sites for butterfly devices. Catheters are best limited to the antecubital fossa or the saphenous vein—an ideal site unless the injury is in the abdomen or lower extremities (see p. 203). The application of antishock trousers may be helpful in distending a peripheral vein for percutaneous entry (see p. 247). Ringer's lactate is rapidly infused (20 ml/kg) and the response carefully monitored. (As soon as the IV is secured and before initiating the fluid infusion, the nurse should collect blood for hemoglobin and hematocrit and typing and cross-matching.)

Monitoring techniques are similar to those employed in adults with slight modifications. For example, tachycardia is not a reliable indicator of hypovolemia in children, and since heart rate varies from 100 to 160 beats/minute (and may reach 200 beats/minute during crying), it is clear that fluctuations such as these make trend following quite difficult. Bradycardia (less than 80 beats/minute) is often noted in severe anoxic states or heart block and requires prompt reversal for survival.

Blood gas monitoring is valuable as a guide to respiratory therapy, employing intermittent femoral punctures or capillary sampling. (Arterial lines are usually not placed in the emergency department setting and are reserved for the intensive care unit.) Assisted ventilation with supplemental *humidified* high-flow oxygen (using a face mask, endotracheal tube, or Isolette) is desirable. Of course, continuous monitoring of the inspired oxygen concentration is essential. Chest x-ray films should be used frequently to evaluate respiratory management. Controlled ventilation can be hazardous in the infant who has abnormal respiratory functioning and should not be used without an expert pulmonary clinician in attendance to supervise the process—especially in the emergency setting.

Since positioning greatly affects air exchange, a small rolled towel should be placed under a supine infant's shoulders to improve the airway. Frequent turning and position change are recommended—even in the emergency setting as a facet of pulmonary hygiene.

Body temperature (both core and surface) should be carefully monitored. Since infants lose heat readily, nurses should ensure that the infant is kept warm during emergency procedures. The use of the controlled radiant hood unit is ideal, since it permits easy access to the infant and facilitates constant observation of the skin.

Urine output and urine osmolality should be carefully observed with the aid of a fixed catheter and a urimeter. Some pediatricians do not approve of the use of a Foley catheter, since the balloon can irritate the trigone and even obstruct the ureteral orifices. The use of a fine No. 5 plastic feeding tube instead of the usual urethral catheter has been advocated.

Laboratory analyses of electrolytes, blood urea nitrogen, creatinine, complete blood count, and hemoglobin and hematocrit should be used to detect consequences of volume change and to serve as an index of the response to infection. Coagulation parameters should be assessed as a baseline and when disseminated intravascular coagulation (DIC) is suspected. Microsamples should be taken to prevent volume depletion from sampling alone.

Central venous pressure monitoring (preferably by the internal jugular vein) is sometimes useful, but should not be considered a routine procedure. Subclavian lines are not advised in the young infant. An antecubital approach may be successful in older children. Careful radiographic confirmation of tube placement is crucial, since false or misleading readings will be obtained if the catheter is malpositioned (see Chapter 12).

Blood pressure monitoring by a noninvasive route is unreliable in infants with constructed blood vessels; intraarterial monitoring is recommended in the intensive care setting. Older children can be monitored by the standard indirect cuff technique.

Bacteriological cultures are useful to manage certain types of septic shock states. Blood, urine, spinal fluid, tracheal aspiration, and wound drainage may be cultured as an adjunct to diagnosis and to guide antibiotic therapy (see pp. 240-244).

Fluid therapy

Fluid therapy in pediatric shock is guided by the same principles as in adult shock. Volume is supplemented to restore central and peripheral circulation, while guarding cautiously against overloading the heart. Continuous CVP monitoring is crucial, remembering that trends in direction, rather than absolute values, are the important parameters (see Chapter 12).

The type of fluid infused depends on the clinical course of the shock state, but generally, the considerations in choice of fluid and parameters of administration are similar to those of

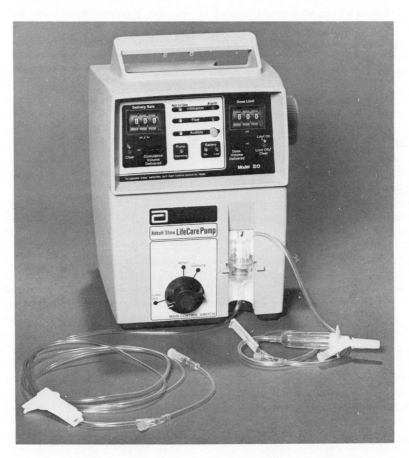

Fig. 22-3. Life Care Pump. (Courtesy Abbott Laboratories, Chicago.)

the adult (see pp. 244-250). Buffer therapy may also be required, based on serial blood pH samplings, and various pharmacological agents may be used to control vascular response, improve cardiac efficiency, or influence peripheral resistance. (See p. 247 for discussion of agents useful in shock states.) A controlled infusion pump is vital for all IV fluid and pharmacological therapy for infants and small children except during resuscitation (Fig. 22-3).

Parameters for pediatric fluid administration in shock management are variable, but here is one common set of guidelines. If the blood pressure returns to normal after the initial bolus, a ''maintenance only'' infusion should be continued while observing vital signs. Stability indicates that blood loss is not continuing and blood transfusion is an unlikely need. If the pulse remains elevated and the blood pressure reveals hypotension, a second loading dose of Ringer's lactate is given rapidly (20 ml/kg). In the meantime, preparations for blood administration should be underway.

Since crystalloids dilute the oxygen-carrying power of the blood, fresh whole blood should be infused after the child has received Ringer's lactate equal to half of his blood volume. The blood should be warmed and given in bolus doses bearing a definitive relationship to normal blood volume. The initial blood bolus is usually 20 ml/kg. CVP monitoring is usually unnecessary and a waste of precious time *unless* the child is not resuscitated adequately by the method described. In this latter case, the CVP line is an important adjunct to further management.

Bolus fluid administration is far more valuable than constant rate infusions since the cardiovascular response to fluid correlates with the severity of shock (see Chapter 12).

Calculating pediatric fluid therapy

Estimate the degree of dehydration
  (slight, 3% to 5%; moderate, 6% to 8%; severe, 10%).
Obtain the child's weight in kilograms.
Calculate *fluid loss* to produce the estimated percentage deficit in hydration.
Add maintenance fluid requirements.
  Over 2 years: 100 ml/kg
  Five to 24 months: 120 ml/kg

Small infants up to 6 months: 150 ml/kg
Estimate continuing loss from diarrhea or vomiting (50 to 100 ml is average.)
Total the estimated fluid requirements for 24 hours.
Give half the total in the first 8 hours and the remaining half over 16 hours.

RESPIRATORY DISTRESS

The emergency nurse should be aware that *all noisy breathing is obstructed breathing.* Coughing may accompany various airway obstructions in children and should arouse suspicion regarding the patency and efficiency of airway channels. Remember however that coughing and choking, apparent with acute aspiration, may subside when the foreign body migrates into small airways.

Infants and children in the first year or two of life usually become victims of respiratory distress caused by respiratory tract infections, such as bronchitis, pneumonia, bronchiolitis, and laryngotracheobronchitis. The pathogens include a wide variety of bacteria and viruses. Older children are more likely to have asthma, epiglottitis, or foreign bodies in the lower respiratory tract.

The triage nurse should obtain a careful history of the onset of the respiratory distress, including factors such as age, family history of asthma or tuberculosis, previous cardiac disease, or chest trauma. It is also important to determine if the child has experienced seizures or vomiting, because aspiration can often accompany such problems. The nutritional status can also provide clues to the presenting pattern of distress. For example, a marasmic child may be prone to rumination and regurgitation, and thus to aspirating of stomach contents.

Emergency nurses should carefully examine the infant or young child to determine how exhausted he is becoming from the work of breathing. Observe carefully for retractions, cyanosis, and a barrellike chest. Is there evidence of intercurrent infection manifested by signs and symptoms of fever, toxicity, increased pulse and respirations, and extreme restlessness or lethargy?

Auscultation of the chest is extremely important to detect wheezing, rales, and other adventitious sounds. Note a stridorous cough. Search for anatomical abnormalities such as trauma to the rib cage, mediastinal shift, and cardiac pathologic conditions. Be sure to obtain blood pressure and peripheral pulses. Do not ignore the abdominal examination in a child with respiratory distress. Is there hepatomegaly or abnormal bowel sounds? A paralytic ileus often accompanies pneumonia, for example.

Laboratory data indicated might include a complete blood count, a skin test for tuberculosis, a stool for parasites, various cultures, (such as oropharynx, nasopharynx, and blood), and arterial blood gases if there is any suspicion of respiratory decompensation. A posteroanterior and lateral chest film (both inspiratory and in full expiration if feasible) are very important to search for infiltrates,* to evaluate for cardiomegaly, free air, atelectasis, the presence of foreign bodies, and to detect a flattening of the diaphragm. If there are 10 or 11 ribs visible above the diaphragm on the posterior view and a decrease in cardiothoracic ratio, the emergency clinician should strongly suspect pneumonia, bronchiolitis, or asthma. In upper airway obstruction problems, anteroposterior and lateral cervical films,† a barium swallow, and laryngoscopy or bronchoscopy may be indicated in order to search for intraluminal foreign bodies or a narrowing of the upper airways because of a retropharyngeal abscess, epiglottitis, or other inflammatory disease. Such studies could also point out congenital structural defects such as a vascular ring, segmental bronchial stenosis, and similar anomalies. Perfusion lung scans may be used for selected problems.

Emergency department management for respiratory distress may include IV therapy (to increase fluid intake and to provide a vehicle for antibiotics, for example), administration of antihistamines and expectorants, and perhaps agents for hyposensitization to allergens. Hu-

*Infiltrates may not be evident in children with severe dehydration.

†In suspected epiglottitis, all films should be taken with the child in an upright position, because total respiratory obstruction can occur if the child is placed supine.

midified oxygen is often employed in cases of pediatric respiratory distress. Usually an ENT or chest consultation should be obtained when obscure or unusual respiratory distress problems appear in an emergency setting. It is advisable to reexamine most children in 24 to 48 hours if the decision is reached not to hospitalize. However it is usually recommended that infants with the following conditions be admitted: moderate to severe respiratory distress, any foreign body aspiration, noisy breathing or cough when accompanied by cyanosis, epiglottitis, asthma that does not respond to two or three doses of epinephrine, whooping cough, and any other cough with stridor.

Airway obstruction

There are four basic anatomical sites of airway obstruction: (1) the nasopharynx; (2) the oropharynx; including the hypopharynx and epiglottis; (3) the upper airway (the larynx and cervical trachea); and (4) the lower or intrathoracic airway. The causes of interruption to airflow include congenital anomalies, anatomical derangements due to trauma, foreign bodies, inflammation and infection, and allergic phenomena. It is important that emergency nurses promptly recognize any type of airway obstruction and take immediate, definitive steps to intervene.

Upper airway obstruction. Upper airway obstruction is associated primarily with inspiratory stridor (that is, a "crowing sound") a barklike cough, nasal flaring, and retractions in the supraclavicular and the chest wall regions. If stridor is loud, it can be assumed that the obstruction is partial, allowing a slight or even moderate amount of air passage. In complete, or near-complete obstruction, there may be no sounds of stridor; air-hunger and cyanosis are profound.

Emergency nurses should assess chest sounds bilaterally and attempt to detect diminished or absent sounds. Simultaneously with such assessment, obtain a careful history of the problem, including its onset in relation to other phenomena (such as activity, fever, ingestions), and determine if the situation is stable or worsening.

It is reasonable to assume that signs and symptoms of upper airway obstruction in a child over 6 months of age are due to aspiration of a foreign body. Attempt to link historical information to physical findings to confirm or rule out such aspiration accidents.

Nasopharyngeal obstruction. Nasopharyngeal obstruction can be promptly recognized by the inability of the victim to breathe through the nose. Since infants are essentially "mouth-breathers," they may become rapidly decompensated, with increasing dyspnea and hypoxia. An example of nasopharyngeal obstruction seen early after birth is *complete, bilateral, choanal atresia,* which results in rapid cyanosis. In some cases correction of this anomaly may be accomplished simply by passing a small catheter through obstructing membranes, others require more complicated surgical correction. Until the defect is repaired, an oropharyngeal airway should be used to facilitate ventilation, and an endogastric tube should be employed for feedings until satisfactory mouth-breathing can be learned. Enlarged adenoids, facial trauma, foreign bodies, and even tumors may also contribute to nasopharyngeal airway obstruction. A side-lying position, placement of an oropharyngeal airway, and provision of supplemental oxygen are useful modes to minimize the effects of this type of obstruction to ventilation.

Oropharyngeal obstruction. Oropharyngeal obstruction can be promptly identified by the gargling or snoring sounds that occur in conjunction with dyspnea. The victim may extend his neck and insist on sitting up. There may be a complete absence of breath sounds. An example of this may result from facial trauma (such as a swollen tongue) that obstructs the upper air passages. Correction can usually be accomplished by insertion of an oropharyngeal, nasopharyngeal, or other type of suitable airway device (see Chapter 8).

Oropharyngeal obstruction due to foreign bodies can be corrected by various manual maneuvers. However certain authorities advocate that you not attempt to remove the foreign body or change the victim's position as long as he is breathing adequately to support life processes *since any movement has the potential to make matters worse as well as better!* If, however, ventilation is inadequate, proceed with four back blows, four manual thrusts, finger probing, and attempts to ventilate (see pp. 134-136). Always be certain, too, that the head is in a dependent position.

Infectious causes of oropharyngeal airway obstruction include enlarged tonsils and peritonsilar abscesses. An oropharyngeal airway and supplemental oxygen are useful therapeutic modalities in these instances. (See Chapter 15 for other considerations.)

Epiglottitis. Epiglottitis is an acute, life-threatening emergency, usually due to an invasion of *Hemophilus influenzae,* type B. It can, however also be induced by ingestion of unusually hot beverages or inhalation of super-heated steam.

Epiglottitis is usually found in children 2 to 7 years old, although it can affect older individuals.

The onset is rapid, with a high fever, a sore throat, toxemia, and severe dyspnea. The victim will struggle to sit forward trying to breathe. Drooling is also prominent since dysphagia prevents swallowing of saliva. The epiglottis appears cherry red and swollen. An inspiratory stridor, hoarseness, a brassy cough, and irritability and restlessness due to hypoxia complete the clinical presentation.

The emergency nurse must respond to these signs and symptoms without delay and summon a physician who can intubate or perform a tracheotomy, which may be required emergently. The child and his parents should be placed in a shock room fully equipped for cardiopulmonary resuscitation. *Do not* use a tongue depressor or other means to examine the throat since any stimulation can create laryngospasm, resulting in complete airway obstruction. *Do not* separate the anxious child from his parents if at all possible, since allowing them to remain as support may reduce the child's struggling and anxiety, which can aggravate an already crucial situation.

Ready supplies for nasotracheal and endotracheal intubation, and ready a tracheotomy tray for immediate use. Be prepared to deliver well-humidified, supplemental oxygen by face mask. If it is necessary to transport the child to the x-ray department for the diagnostic lateral films of the neck, he should be accompanied by personnel and equipment for intubation if this has not yet been accomplished. Large doses of antibiotics by the intravenous route are indicated (such as ampicillin, 300 mg/kg/day) as soon as blood cultures have been obtained. A child with confirmed epiglottitis is admitted to an intensive care unit for constant monitoring and observation for signs of cervical tracheal obstruction.

Airway obstruction in the larynx or cervical trachea is marked by inspiratory stridor, an increased inspiratory-to-expiratory ratio, agitation from hypoxia, and no audible breath sounds.

Croup (laryngotracheobronchitis). Croup is a viral condition* that results in inflammation and edema of the lining of the larynx and the trachea. Victims of croup usually are between the ages of 6 months and 4 years, although older children are occasionally seen with the disorder. Croup is an allergy—equivalent condition that has its onset with 1 or 2 days of coryza followed in a day or so with nocturnal awakening of the child in a state of apprehension, inspiratory dyspnea, and an expiratory barking cough. At this point the parents may decide to seek emergency care. The reported history is usually an upper respiratory tract condition accompanied by low-grade fever, rhinitis, pharyngitis, bronchitis, and bronchiolitis that has persisted for several days.

Although a lateral neck x-ray film should be obtained to rule out epiglottitis, the emergency management is usually humidification with or without supplemental oxygen. Parents may be instructed to walk the child outdoors in cool, moist, night air or sit with him in a steamy bathroom for 15 minutes, both maneuvers that usually relieve the annoying symptoms.

In moderate or severe croup that threatens respiratory efficiency, 0.25% racemic epinephrine (Vaponefrin) may be given per nebulized oxygen while carefully monitoring the heart rate. (Antibiotics and steroids are of little or no value in the viral syndrome.) Hospitalization, endotracheal intubation, and tracheostomy are seldom required in the management of croup.

Laryngeal obstruction. Laryngeal obstruction is usually caused by edema secondary to anaphylaxis or an infectious process, although foreign bodies in the larygotracheal region account for over 2,000 deaths per year. Direct trauma, laryngospasm (secondary to foreign body aspiration, inhalation of noxious fumes, or water in near drowning) and congential malformations account for respiratory embarrassment related to laryngotracheal structures.

An emergency nurse must be able to differentiate laryngeal obstruction induced by foreign bodies from that due to anaphylaxis. The latter is characteristically accompanied by vomiting, urticaria, periorbital edema, hypotension, and bronchospasm, and requires epinephrine, antihistamines, steroids, and bronchodilators to supplement mechanical management of the airway (see pp. 142-156). A tracheotomy or cricothyrotomy, using a 14-gauge needle, may be required to manage the airway if a complete obstruction is evident (see pp. 148-150).

Intrathoracic airway obstruction. *Asthma* is the most frequently encountered course of intrathoracic airway obstruction; the symptoms are the result of contractions of smooth muscle, edema of mucous membranes, increased secretions, bronchial constrictions or spasms, and mucus plugging. Asthma may have a rapid onset precipitated by strong odors, noxious fumes, upper respiratory tract infection, stress, anger, and a series of other phenomena that are allergy-related.

Children with asthma have a decreased inspiratory-to-expiratory ratio. They may have prolonged expiratory wheezing, or they may have no expiratory sounds at all in severe cases. Lip pursing and retractions are not uncommon as the child struggles to breathe. Cyanosis and hypoxic agitation are likely accompaniments.

Emergency department assessment must

---

*Usually parainfluenza virus I, II, or III.

include details about any medications taken within the 24-hour period before the attack, because any inhalant or ingested agents may affect decisions regarding emergency drug management.

The emergency nurse should assist the asthmatic child and his parents to a room equipped for managing an eventual respiratory crisis. After initial arterial blood gases and venous blood samples are drawn,* 1:1000 epinephrine (0.01 ml/kg to maximum of 0.4 ml) is given subcutaneously. The dose may be repeated every 20 minutes for a total of 3 doses if necessary. Oxygen by mask or nasal prongs is initiated, allowing the child to sit upright. A chest x-ray film is also obtained. An IV of normal saline or Ringer's lactate is begun to assist with rehydration and to serve as a vehicle for delivering adjunctive medications. The drip should be regulated to deliver 10 ml/kg over 30 minutes. Oral fluids may be used in mild cases. If the initial epinephrine relieves the bronchospasm, an aqueous suspension (1:200 epinephrine [Susphrine] in a 0.005 ml/kg dose (to a maximum of 0.2 ml) is given subcutaneously for a longer acting sustained effect before discharge.

If initial therapy (three doses of epinephrine) does not allay the wheezing, hospitalization is mandatory. Other agents such as aminophylline (4 to 7 mg/kg IV over 20 minutes), dexamethasone sodium phosphate (Decadron) 0.3 mg/kg/day in four divided doses IV, and isoetherine hydrochloride with phenylephrine hydrocloride (Bronkosol) 0.5 ml diluted in 1.5 ml normal saline by nebulizer may be administered to relieve the asthmatic crisis. Antibiotics are reserved for cases in which bacterial infection is identified.

Occasionally hypercapnia may be so severe that assisted ventilation is required. In these unusual circumstances, the child must be admitted to an intensive care unit for constant monitoring.

Bronchiolitis. Bronchiolitis is a viral infection of the bronchioles marked by wheezing and dyspnea. There is bilateral hyperinflation of the lungs caused by air trapping. It occurs primarily in children under 18 months old. Interestingly, children who experience bronchiolitis at this age are likely to suffer from asthma in subsequent years. It is often difficult to distinguish bronchiolitis from asthma, although the former condition is characteristically caused by the respiratory syncytial virus and is not responsive to epinephrine. The syndrome begins with acute coryza and progresses in 3 to 7 days to a severe pattern of respiratory distress including wheezing. It can result in obliterative bronchiolitis or viral pneumonia. (Interstitial pneumonia can look like bronchiolitis.) The condition can be life-threatening in instances of underlying cardiac or pulmonary disease or if secondary bacterial infection develops.

Treatment of bronchiolitis consists of cool humidification, oxygen administration, bronchodilators, and occasionally, endotracheal intubation, and ventilatory assistance. Fluids may be restricted to prevent peribronchial edema and obstruction of bronchioles. If IV hydration is needed, normal saline or Ringer's lactate is administered (100 ml/kg/day). In severe cases, arterial blood gases should be closely monitored to assess the degree of hypoxemia in relation to the inspired concentration of oxygen.

Physicians may order bronchodilating agents because there is always a chance that asthma, rather than bronchiolitis, is responsible for the symptoms. Steroids and antibiotics are not useful in this viral syndrome.

Foreign bodies in intrathoracic structures. Foreign bodies aspirated by children under 4 years of age tend to lodge in a bronchus, creating unilateral wheezing. Half of these foreign bodies are peanuts. With the resultant airtrapping, there is a mediastinal shift away from the affected side. A tension pneumothorax may develop as a complication of foreign body aspiration, and this condition should be promptly managed by a flutter valve (see p. 355) and the administration of supplemental oxygen.

---

*Blood samples should be drawn before administration of epinephrine, since this drug falsely elevates the white blood count.

VOMITING AND DIARRHEA

Vomiting and diarrhea can be lethal to an infant or young child within a few debilitating days or even hours, as a result of dehydration and resultant electrolyte imbalances. The reasons for this phenomenon are manifold, but essentially they relate to these: (1) A greater percentage of the body weight of infants and young children is fluid (about 80%); (2) their body fluid behaves in an unstable manner because of a high metabolic rate, causing a rapid fluid turnover, and their kidneys are inefficient, resulting in a high output of dilute urine; and (3) there is a relatively high proportion of body fluid in interstitial spaces where exchanges and loss occur with considerable ease.

Since infants' water turnover is high in relation to their total body water supply, dehydration is much more common in infancy than in adulthood. It can result from inadequate intake or abnormal losses, especially through vomiting and diarrhea. Emergency nurses must be aware of the consequences of severe dehydration (fluid loss of about 5%) and electrolyte imbalances and be prepared to promptly recognize them during the triage process.

The results of prolonged infantile vomiting and diarrhea may include weight loss, sunken fontanels, ashen or mottled skin with poor turgor, and listlessness and unresponsiveness.

Parents or other caretakers may report that diapers remain dry longer than normal, indicating a decreased urinary output.

Vital signs may indicate a decreased cardiac output, with a weak and rapid pulse that is easily obliterated. The emergency clinician should obtain a careful history and rule out any trauma. Home remedies that have been used should be elicited, since they frequently have only aggravated the problems. Assess the nutritional status, and palpate the abdomen for tenderness. Inspect the oral mucosa for signs of toxic ingestions. Consider the possibility of infections that could result in gastrointestinal distress. Be particularly alert to the green, watery, "starvation" diarrhea and stools that contain pus or blood. Think also of cranial trauma or an inflammatory condition that could result in vomiting bouts.

Emergency nurses should assume that all diarrhea is infectious until proved otherwise and take precautions to "isolate" the problem in the department. Of course, scrupulous handwashing and linen precautions are essential to prevent the spread of organisms—viral, bacterial, or parasitic.

Laboratory tests may help determine the cause of vomiting and diarrhea and certainly will be valuable in fluid and electrolyte therapy and specific drug threapy if indicated. Among tests commonly used are complete blood count; sedimentation rate; urine for specific gravity, ketones, and coproporphyria-reducing substances; electrolytes; cultures; stool for guaiac, pH, and parasites; and possibly barium contrast studies.

Emergency management of diarrhea and vomiting is aimed at rehydration and establishing electrolyte balances. If there is severe vomiting, oral fluids and feedings are usually of little value. IV fluids may be indicated. Clear liquids such as juice or a carbonated beverage may be given in selected cases if a surgical problem has been ruled out previously. Antipyretics and antibiotics may be ordered for the management of specific infectious processes.

Infants or children with vomiting and diarrhea are usually admitted under the following circumstances: (1) if the vomiting contains blood or bile; (2) if the stool contains blood; (3) if dehydration over 5% exists; (4) if projectile vomiting creates suspicion of an intracranial pathologic condition, especially if accompanied by fever, lethargy, or seizures; or (5) if there is an abdominal mass.

Some children may be sent home with specific instructions regarding the management of vomiting and diarrhea. The BRAT diet (bananas, rice, apples, and tea) is still used by some clinicians to control dehydration and reestablish electrolyte balance in the infant and young child.

FEVER

Fever is the most common problem in the child up to 1 year of age. A fever is defined as an elevation of an oral temperature above 99.4°

F ($37.4°$ C). *Hyperpyrexia* refers to an elevation above $106°$ F ($40.6°$ C).

The most common causes of fever include infection, dehydration, and reactions to immunizations. There are a number of other causes, too, including pyelonephritis, drug toxicity, tuberculosis, adrenal insufficiency, congenital absence of sweat glands, high environmental temperature, hemolytic anemias, collagen diseases, and central nervous system disorders such as meningitis or trauma. Unusually high temperatures, in the hyperpyrexic range, may be due to central nervous system infections, adrenal hemorrhage, septicemia, drug poisoning, and heat stroke.

The triage nurse should be well aware of signs and symptoms of fever other than an elevated temperature, which may include a flushed face, increased restlessness, tachycardia, and diaphoresis. Delirium and seizures can occur with high fevers, especially in children aged 1 to 6 years.

When a child with a fever is encountered in the emergency department, various laboratory tests may be employed to identify the cause. Among them are urinalysis, complete blood count, lumbar puncture, chest x-ray films, blood cultures, nasopharyngeal cultures, and a tuberculin test.

The emergency management of fever may include forcing fluids, use of antipyretics, and modes for cooling, such as undressing, tepid sponging, and using fans. Alcohol sponging, ice water enemas, or icing the body are usually not recommended by most authorities as acceptable methods of reducing body temperature. Chlorpromazine (0.2 mg/kg) IM is advocated by some clinicians as an adjunct to therapy. With this drug it is important to watch for hypotension and to discontinue use of the agent if this side-effect occurs.

Most clinicians believe that aspirin and acetaminophen are more effective if given together, using half of each drug's dosage.

Ordinarily antibiotics are not given in febrile conditions until the causative organism is identified. Rather, in fevers of unknown origin (FUOs), the child is admitted for further study. Many clinicians routinely admit infants less than 1 month of age with any fever above $101°$ F and infants 2 to 6 months old, if the fever exceeds $103°$ F. Other standard criteria for admission are any fever with petechial rash that is not confined to the face and neck, or if seizures, hematuria, joint pain and swelling, or known cardiac disease accompany the febrile state.

BLEEDING
Rectal bleeding

Rectal bleeding in an infant or child can result in severe anemia if it continues for several days, even if the bleeding is modest. The problem can also contribute to dehydration if unchecked.

A child with rectal bleeding should be assessed carefully. Anal inspection or a probing rectal examination can be extremely traumatic, both physically and psychologically for the young child. (Infants should be examined with the thighs flexed onto the abdomen.) Many clinicians defer a rectal examination if fissures are evident.

Laboratory parameters of importance may include complete blood count; hemoglobin and hematocrit; stool for guaiac, ova, and parasites; coagulation studies; flat and upright x-ray films of the abdomen; and possibly an upper GI series and endoscopy.

Most children with rectal bleeding are not admitted but are managed conservatively at home. Severe anemia, dehydration, or an acute toxic state is usually reason for hospitalization. Outpatient or day surgery may be scheduled for excision of polyps.

Parents may be instructed to use sitz baths, enemas, or stool softeners in a regimen to manage rectal bleeding.

Hematuria

Hematuria can be quite serious in children and may go essentially unnoticed because accompanying signs and symptoms are vague and may include vomiting, fever, jaundice, failure to thrive, irritability, hyperbilirubinemia, and a range of other phenomena that seem largely unrelated to the renal system.

A suprapubic urinary tap may be done to aspirate a sample of urine for study, and an

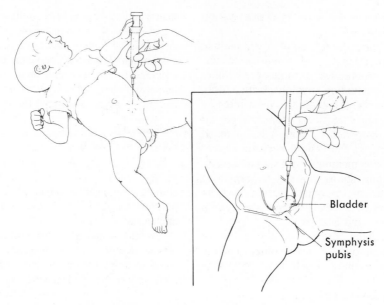

Fig. 22-4. Procedure for direct aspiration of bladder using suprapubic approach.

IVP may be scheduled to assess the functional pattern of the renal system.

Suprapubic bladder tap (Fig. 22-4)

1. Ascertain that the infant or child has not recently voided, and palpate the bladder to ensure that urine can be obtained from the bladder. *Do not proceed with the tap if the bladder cannot be palpated!*

2. Place the child supine. Restrain if necessary.

3. Cleanse the suprapubic area with an antiseptic solution. Infiltrate a local anesthetic if desired.

4. Assemble a 23-gauge, 1½-inch needle and a 10-ml syringe.

5. Palpate the superior border of the pubis, and introduce the needle in the midline of the border. Ensure that the needle is perpendicular to the abdomen upon entry.

6. Pull back slightly on the plunger while carefully advancing the needle (directing it slightly downward) until urine is obtained. If no urine is obtained, insert a gloved finger into the rectum and push up on the bladder while guiding the aspirating needle.

7. Withdraw the needle when the desired specimen is aspirated.

8. Optional: Apply a small dressing to the puncture site.

If there is a history of trauma, other assessments and therapeutic considerations are in order (see Chapters 18 and 20).

CHEST PAIN

Children ordinarily cannot identify and specifically complain of chest pain until they reach the age of 4 or 5. Therefore emergency nursing personnel should be alert to any assessments that could point to cardiorespiratory problems and should carefully probe if trauma or infection involves the chest region. A tension pneumothorax should be managed immediately with a needle aspiration.

Physical assessments should be carefully and systematically performed while laboratory data are being gathered. Oxygen should be given if there is cyanosis or dyspnea as soon as baseline arterial blood gases have been obtained. A complete blood count, chest x-ray film, and blood cultures may be requested. Herpes zoster can accompany chest pain, as well as a characteristic vesicular rash that tends to follow intercostal nerve distribution.

Children with chest pain complaints are usually admitted if there is a murmur detected, or if there are indices of dysrhythmias, muffled heart sounds, dyspnea, cyanosis, or pneumothorax/pneumomediastinum. (See also Chapter 17.)

ABDOMINAL PAIN

Children respond to abdominal pain with highly differentiated responses, depending on their stage of development. Small infants cry and draw up the legs onto the abdomen. Older children may exhibit guarding, abdominal wall rigidity, and often can at least define the zone of discomfort. It is important that emergency nurses remember that a systematic assessment can be most productive when the child cooperates and is not crying, since tension makes palpation and auscultation almost nonproductive.

BLOOD DYSCRASIAS

The most common blood dyscrasias that the emergency nurse may encounter include hemophilia and sickle cell disease in crisis. In both instances, initial data gathering should include historical antecedents, and management of acute symptoms should be prompt and definitive.

Hemophilia

Hemophilia is a genetically transmitted defect of intrinsic clotting mechanisms found almost exclusively in males. Even known hemophiliacs may be asymptomatic for years until stressed by trauma or surgery. A prolongation of the partial thromboplastin time helps confirm a diagnosis in the event of unexplained or difficult-to-control hemorrhage.

Emergency personnel should be alert to hemostatic defects, noting any prolonged bleeding after injections, multiple site bleeding, spontaneous hematomas, or any other hemorrhagic phenomena that cannot be otherwise explained.

General management of bleeding should include elevation of the part, local pressure to bleeding sites, and volume replacement. Specific therapy is the administration of cryoprecipitate or fresh frozen plasma, or both. If hemarthrosis is apparent by a distention of a joint capsule, the involved part should be immobilized and elevated. Ice and a light pressure dressing may also be employed to control the bleeding site. Later, after correction of the coagulation defect, the blood may be aspirated. All patients with hemarthrosis should be referred to an orthopedic specialist for follow-up.

Sickle cell disease

Sickle cell disease is an inherited blood disorder found almost exclusively in blacks. It is characterized by an abnormal hemoglobin, termed hemoglobin S. Although this hemoglobin can carry and release oxygen, it becomes relatively insoluble in its deoxygenated state and its shape is distorted into the "sickle" appearance. These cells clump together and block microcirculatory channels, resulting in stasis of blood, hypoxia, ischemic pain, vasospasm, and organ damage.

The sickled erythrocytes can be reoxygenated several times and regain a more normal shape. Eventually, since they are more fragile and are phagocytized more readily, their life span is as short as 15 to 30 days, compared with a 120-day life expectancy for a normal red blood cell. Thus, a chronic hemolytic anemia exists.

Sickle cell crisis. The sickle cell crisis may be precipitated by acid-base disturbances, infections, exposure to cold, high altitudes, dehydration, and stress (both physical and emotional). The emergency nurse should search for such clues when eliciting a history.

The patient usually has throbbing pain in selected sites affected by the tissue hypoxia. Bone and joint pain, fever, visual disturbances, priapism, respiratory distress, and pallor are among common complaints. Abdominal pain with rigidity and tenderness may be present, and thus sickle cell disease can easily be confused with an acute abdomen. Edema of the hands and feet (dactylitis) is sometimes seen in young children.

Emergency management includes a battery of

diagnostic tests to differentiate sickle cell disease from other entities commonly confused with the disorder. Tests often requested are arterial blood gases, CBC, serum bilirubin, x-ray studies, and urinalysis including culture and sensitivity.

Treatment of the painful crisis is symptomatic. Meperidine and promethazine hydrochloride are choice drugs for analgesia. Oxygen and intravenous fluids are employed to correct hypoxia and to expand vascular volumes, respectively.

The nurse should carefully monitor intake and output and utilize both physical and emotional comfort measures. Instruction regarding the pathogenesis of crises should be provided along with suggestions for curbing future painful episodes of the disease. Referral for follow-up must be accomplished for all patients who are not hospitalized for therapy.

CHRONIC ILLNESS IN EXACERBATION

For some children and their parents, a visit to the emergency department is prompted by the recurrence of a chronic illness that could result in another hospitalization in a series that may span several months or years. It is important that nurses convey their understanding to all family members and to handle the visit with as much efficiency as feasible within the emergency department setting. Although the problem may not seem life-threatening—or sometimes not even acute—it may signal to the child and his family another failure of at-home treatment and one step more into the process of termination of life. Much sorrow and other emotions are often wrapped into such episodes, and unless emergency staff are cognizant of the series of events that precipitated this episodic visit, they may not respond with the expedience and sensitivity that is appropriate.

THE WELL CHILD IN THE EMERGENCY DEPARTMENT

Nurses are sometimes disturbed by the fact that parents bring children to the emergency department for noncritical problems. It should

be remembered that parents may be unable to distinguish a minor from a major health problem. Furthermore, some parents need continuing reassurance that their child is *not* sick. Other instances of transporting an unsick child to the hospital may be symptomatic of a family crisis, social disorientation, inability to manage the child, and occasionally as a conscious or unconscious mode to hurt, reject, or punish the child by subjecting him to discomfort and fear associated with the hospital.

It is important that emergency nurses check their own feelings in such instances and capitalize on the opportunity to assist the family through appropriate modes of communication and referral processes.

SUDDEN INFANT DEATH SYNDROME

Sudden infant death syndrome (SIDS) or "crib death" accounts for 10% of all deaths in the first year of life. The child most often affected is between the ages of 5 weeks and 5 months; the incidence peaks between 9 weeks and 4 months. It occurs most often in late autumn, winter, and spring. It happens more often to nonwhite infants, to infants with a low birth weight, or to infants of lower socioeconomic class.

The history of SIDS usually reveals a good health history (except perhaps for a minor upper respiratory tract infection) and death during sleep. Parents are totally unprepared to cope with the sudden death of an essentially healthy infant. Often parents assume a great burden of guilt and feel that they somehow might have contributed to the death by acts of commission or omission.

Emergency personnel should begin the process of helping these parents deal with the crisis by offering essential facts about SIDS. For example, these deaths are not predictable, preventable, inherited, or due to faulty parenting. They are not due to suffocation, and the risk to other siblings over 6 or 8 months is minimal, if any.

See Chapter 3 for specific ways nurses can assist the acutely grieving family.)

Refer patients to SIDS parents groups for long-term support.

PARENT EDUCATION ABOUT EMERGENCY SERVICES

The nurse is in an excellent role to help parents understand the appropriate ways to utilize emergency services. It is also important to ascertain that they comprehend the distinction of when to *take* the child to the hospital and when to call for help to come to the child. It is also important to determine if they know how to assess various modes of assistance, such as a paramedic ambulance, rescue squad, and the poison control center. It is an excellent time to review what items they should try to remember to take or send to the emergency department—medicine containers, emesis, potentially poisonous berries the child has ingested, a record of immunizations, clinic card, and so on. Emergency nurses should alert parents to the importance of sharing such information with schoolteachers, babysitters, and the next-door neighbors, who may be present when the child becomes ill or injured.

REFERENCES

Dhar, G. J., and others: Principles of diarrhea therapy, Am. Fam. Physician **19:**164, January 1979.

Dube, S. K., and Pierog, S. H., editors: Immediate care of the sick and injured child, St. Louis, 1978, The C. V. Mosby Co.

Gaffney, K.: The pre-schooler in the ED, J.E.N. **2:**6, 1976.

Gorman, R. J., and others: Febrile seizures, Am. Fam. Physician **19:**101, January 1979.

Hansen, M.: Accident or child abuse? Challenge to the ED nurse, J.E.N. **2:**1, 1976.

Lanros, E.: Assessment and intervention in emergency nursing, Bowie, Md., 1978, Robert J. Brady Co.

Miles, M. S.: SIDS: parents are the patients, J.E.N. **3:**29-32, 1977.

Pascoe, D., and Grossman, M.: Quick reference to pediatric emergencies, Philadelphia, 1973, J. B. Lippincott Co.

Resnick, R., and Hergenroeder, E.: Children and the emergency room, Nurs. Digest **4:**37-40, November/December 1976.

Roskies, E., and others: Emergency hospitalization of young children, Nurs. Digest **4:**32-36, November/December 1976.

Rosman, N. P.: Pediatric head injuries, Pediatr. Ann. **7:**55-74, December 1978.

Schwartz, G. R., and others: Principles and practice of emergency medicine, Vols. I and II, Philadelphia, 1978, W. B. Saunders Co.

Singer, H. S., and others: Head trauma for the pediatrician, Pediatrics **62:**819, November 1978.

Smith, C. A.: The critically ill child: diagnosis and management, ed. 2, Philadelphia, 1977, W. B. Saunders Co.

Touloukian, R. J., editor: Pediatric trauma, New York, 1978, John Wiley and Sons.

Weller, C. M. R.: Assessing the non-accidental injury, J.E.N. **3:**17-26, 1977.

CHAPTER 23

Psychiatric emergencies

Gail Pisarcik

Emergency departments are based on the concept of quick assessment, intervention, and short-term management. The patient with a psychiatric complaint defies this concept. Quick assessment is difficult. The patient has taken a lifetime to acquire the personality and emotions that he brings to the emergency department, and the complexity of his responses to unknown precipitants presents a unique challenge. He may or may not respond to intervention, and keeping his management short-term is often difficult. History and physicals are time-consuming. The patient's social network must often be involved, discharge planning is much more elaborate, and intervention often consists of a time-consuming personal involvement by the practitioner.

These inherent conflicts, coupled with a tendency to "blame the victim," often make the psychiatric patient the hands-down least favorite patient in the emergency department. The problems, however, are not insurmountable. There is as much science as art to the treatment. What many practitioners will find in the end is that a successful intervention in a crisis or psychiatric situation is one of the most rewarding experiences of the emergency department. It is also a chance for nurses to become the primary caregiver that they may not be with an acutely medically sick individual.

COMMUNICATION

Webster's includes in its definition of communication "an exchange of information" and "personal rapport." Effective communication is basic to good medical care, more so to emergency department care, and particularly essential to psychiatric emergency department care. Communication is as much the *route* to diagnosis as it is the treatment. Good communication skills and the confidence that accompanies them come with time, certainly, but even more so with practice. These attributes are crucial when dealing with psychiatric illness. Many times management problems and escalation of crises in the emergency department are a result of ineffective communication.

Real communication is often based on a mutual respect. Respect denotes, in accordance with the root of the word (*respicere,* to look at), the ability to see a person as he is, and perhaps to see beneath a veneer of superficial behavior to the root of that behavior. All behavior has a purpose. Much of it is designed to communicate what cannot, or will not, be articulated verbally. Many times a person's extreme behavior is at least in part meant to impress upon others how extreme the pain he endures is, and/or the fear that he doesn't think he can bear it. (For example, after hearing the news of her son's being sentenced to life in jail, a mother's extreme emotional reaction was, to a degree, abated by the practitioner's acknowledgement of the pain she was experiencing and the active demonstration that other people were available to support her now and in the future.) Hers was a type of communication

516

that could, at least partly be translated into a verbal mode.

Respect and dignity accorded a patient set the stage for the patient's behavior to improve. People tend to behave in a way that is expected of them. Expect the best, and you'll often get it. Allow a patient to overhear you saying that he is crazy and he will be more disposed to fullfill your expectations. Tell him that he is a worthwhile individual who is obviously in distress because you know that he must be behaving the way he is for an awfully good reason, and you have the start of some valuable communication.

Communication with children and adolescents

Children present unique problems of communication. Less verbal, they may be more difficult to engage. Nonverbal communication may be one route. A tangible reward like a lollipop or an ice cream after the emergency department visit may be more appreciated than the long-range good of medicine. Having less self-control and being less subject to social pressure, they are less likely to cooperate because they "should," thus presenting a real challenge for the practitioner. Children's fears are larger and more irrational than those of adults because of a greater area of "unknowns." The child's familiarity with emergency department setting, especially those things that he will come in contact with, should enhance the interaction. Only one nurse and one doctor, if at all possible, should be involved with a child. Children are very sensitive to deceit and are suspicious of people who are "goody-goody" and fuss over them. An ideal approach to a child is one of matter-of-factness and honesty combined with warmth, and where possible, humor. The last, when used deftly, whether with children or adults can be the "best medicine." Children pick up their clues from you and their parents. The less anxiety they perceive, the less they will have. The reactions of children are harder to judge than those of adults. Some game playing or use of stuffed animals to demonstrate may induce a response where conversation does not. It is important to

practice trying to perceive a situation from the patient's eyes. Children may be less frightened, even untouched by something adults find very distressing. Victims of nonbrutal molestation, for example, may be unscathed except to see and react to their parent's consternation and behavior as the traumatic experience. Children's concerns revolve around pleasing or displeasing their parents and interacting with their peers. Talk in relation to these important aspects of their lives. Children may see illness, medicine, or being kept home as punishment in their good-and-bad-oriented world.

The adolescent patient in the emergency department for emotional problems is especially needy and vulnerable, but characteristically nonverbal, at least initially. Adolescents tend to experience feelings passionately. Unhappy feelings are often expressed as, "I wish I were dead"; happy ones as euphoria. If the initial nonverbal hurdle is overcome, the adolescent presents a fertile field for mental health work. Impressionable, the adolescent who has no one to talk to or turn to may be quite affected by the interaction that takes place with the professional who "understands." The experience may represent a turning point in his life.

Communicating with the elderly

Communication with the elderly involves no less respect than any other interview. Our concepts of old age and stereotypes must be discarded in favor of dealing with the uniqueness of each individual. Current research does not support such stereotypes as the older person who responds with, "you have no business asking such personal questions, you're young enough to be my . . ." Older people are often anxious to interact with younger people, but fear rejection. Automatically calling older people by their first names implies a lack of respect, as does automatically talking too loud. Speaking in a slow, clear, low-pitched voice is sometimes helpful, as is limiting the use of new slang words or colloquial expressions. Since a universal concern of older persons is a life review and integration of past events with current situations, one question may lead to a chain of thoughts that veers from the topic. A technique used by comedians called a "blend" is helpful here or in other situations where a patient gets "off the track." For example, if a person is asked about what precipitated his coming here and he ends up talking about a death in the family 10 years ago, the practitioner might interrupt very gently and, with genuine interest, say, "Speaking of stressful crises, nothing like that has happened recently to you, has it?"

Commonly found among older persons is a memory loss for recent rather than remote events, a decrease in ability of concentration, paranoid thinking, and depression (often confused with organic brain syndrome). The elderly may be less accustomed to a verbal tradition (they may be foreign-born, may not have completed high school, or may be isolated and have little conversation with others). They may be slower in responding to questions. Attempts to hurry them may lead to increased anxiety and confusion. The elderly may take poor health for granted as being part of getting older. They may not complain about the pain of arthritis, for example. Those who desire to see life from the perspective of the aged will soon appreciate that safety is of paramount concern. Staying home and missing a clinic appointment on an inclement slippery day, and being unable to go to get a prescription because it is after dark are more easily understood in this light. By the same token, very basic concerns for food, shelter, and the like are more important, as the older person might be worrying increasingly about what will become of him or her.

Anxiety has been viewed as qualitatively and quantitatively different in the aged, related to the threat of emotional isolation and eventual total annihilation, calling forth more primitive defenses and regression. Loss and depletion are important issues in the life crisis of old age.

THE PSYCHIATRIC INTERVIEW PROCESS

The psychiatric interview is especially important. It is the main tool by which the practitioner gains knowledge of the patient and what is wrong with him. A perceptively conducted interview elicits a mental status and a history of past and present illnesses as well as establishing a therapeutic alliance that allows for effective intervention. The following are general considerations that apply to interviews with all patients.

Begin the interview by making the patient comfortable and relieving as much stress as possible. The patient has come to the emergency department with the anxiety of some emotional crisis. He does not need any additional stress. Make yourself and the emergency department environment as familiar as possible. Be courteous, respectful, interested, considerate and tolerant, and give the patient your undivided attention. Put yourself in the patient's place, and pay attention to such things as the fact that the patient may have been waiting some time. He may be hostile. Addressing this early will preclude the necessity of having to act out his anger.

Despite time exigencies in the emergency department, try not to rush the interview. Allot a certain amount of time and share with the patient how long that will be. Maintain eye contact rather than paying undue attention to the chart or distractions. The patient might be put at ease by establishing common ground ("I see you're from the town I grew up in.") This sets the tone for approaching the patient as a person. The interview should be structured enough so that the practitioner, as well as the patient, feels comfortable and has a sense of purpose. The interview is basically conducted to determine the following:

Is something wrong?

How urgent is the situation?

Must I take action?

To determine these, it is helpful to direct your attention to the patient's *chief complaint and chief request:* Why now? and, "What does he want from this emergency department?" The emergency department interview is less concerned with accumulating a complete and detailed history than in gathering meaningful information on salient points. What has *led* to a person's being suicidal is important, but more important in the emergency department is how suicidal that patient is at that particular time and what might attenuate that intent. The interview might begin by first allowing a spontaneous elaboration in response to a nondirective open question, and follow with specific questions regarding key features and facts. Early on, the patient should be advised of the "rules" of the interview. Patients want to answer questions in the right way, but often don't know how. Know what it is you're looking for (feelings, for example) and whether you want a brief, general answer or a more elaborate one. Give examples of questions and the type of answer that you might expect, instead of quietly enduring a much too long or too short answer. If you want to know how long something has been going on and the patient appears confused, ask him, for example, whether it has been 2 days, 2 weeks, or 2 years.

Validation of nonverbal behavior throughout the interview is often valuable. Don't *assume* that a patient's behavior means something. Ask. Validating information and behavior is very revealing. If a patient says he drinks "a little," don't assume that he means once a week. Ask him in terms of pints or cans of beer per day or week, and so on. Validate behavior with such questions as "you look a little angry. Is it because of the long wait?" or "Are you feeling sad as you look?" Rather than being rude or unkind, they are welcomed chances for the patient to express in words, rather than actions, what he is feeling. The practitioner should trust intuition and learn to openly discuss what is perceived. By validating, the practitioner will also find, with experience, that asking patients even the most awkward questions can be done easily with skillful phrasing. For example, to the possibly suicidal person: "You look so sad. Have you reached the point where you feel as though you just don't care anymore? Has it ever crossed your mind to hurt yourself?" To the person who may be having problems with his sexuality: "How would you describe your relationship with your wife/girlfriend? Are the physical aspects of the relationship at all a problem? Can you relate the physical problems to any feelings or things that are going on in your life?" There is no subject that is too awkward for professionals who believe they can help and desire to do so.

To the woman with a basket of flowers on her head who is dressed very inappropriately:

"What you are wearing is very different, and I can't help noticing and wondering about it. I'm sure you won't mind my asking about it."

To the person who is unaware of what the problem is or that there is any problem, it is sometimes helpful in determining how much, if any, insight there is by sharing with the patient your perceptions of the problem. If he agrees, you can move on to what can be done about the situation. If he disagrees, you can discuss your differing perceptions and ask why he thinks it is that the perceptions are so different. When a patient draws a conclusion that doesn't make perfect sense to the practitioner, she or he should ask the patient "Why is that?" or "Can you elaborate on that a little?"

Mirroring what the patient says with different words shows that you understand him. If he's saying that he's suicidal, you might say, "You really feel that you don't want to live." You want to be involved in the conversation without veering the patient away from his train of thought. Pausing after questions, looking expectantly, and casually interjecting phrases such as "I see," or repeating the patients last phrase or statement with your voice slightly raised encourages the patient to speak on. This helps prevent disconcerting silences that aren't particularly useful in the emergency department settting and may provoke more anxiety. The practitioner is well-advised to pay attention to what the *patient* thinks is important. What might seem an insignificant and trivial experience may be the cause of a great deal of distress to another person.

The patient who is being interviewed may be in the emergency department under duress, brought by relatives, friends, or the police. Initially, the patient may be angry, inhibited, and unreceptive. Tact and understanding can win the patient over, despite the inauspicious circumstances. Helpful here, as in many emergency department situations, is the therapeutic alliance: the development of a "you and I against the world" feeling of mutual trust and respect between practitioner and patient.

An adjunctive interview with the family, friends, landlord, and police is often invaluable, especially in the case of the patient who is retarded, psychotic, or in a toxic condition. Interviews with others are also useful with patients having character disorders. These patients are notorious in their distortions, as are patients with alcoholism and other addictions, who may deny or underestimate the problem. Patients involved in marital or family conflict may relate differing stories than other family members.

Though nondirective interviewing is desirable, especially initially, there are many times when this style is an unaffordable luxury. Patients from lower socioeconomic backgrounds may not know what to say unless asked more direct questions. They may be confused by a question such as "What are your feelings right now?" Similarly, problems arise with the old or young patient, or when time is a pressing consideration. Whatever the style of questions, most important is that the interviewer be a calm, steady, reassuring, attentive, and empathetic professional who says, in effect, "Even though I'm not you, I try to feel your feelings. I can help you. I have the expertise."

CRISIS INTERVENTION

It is widely recognized that persons undergoing a crisis are amenable to influence when a professional offers skilled and caring intervention. The potential for that intervention in the emergency department is limitless. The countless unique opportunities for the emergency department nurse to do preventive mental health work should not be lost.

Crisis may be defined as a period of disequilibrium in a steady state. The hazardous event precipitating the crisis may be seen as a threat, a loss, or a challenge. A threat to the integrity or needs of the individual meets with an anxious response; a loss is met with depression; and a situation viewed as a challenge is likely to be met with increased energy and problem-solving. The same irritant may erode one surface and generate a pearl from another. A crisis can also be seen as a turning point from which there is no escape and for which habitual problem-solving techniques are not adequate to return the individual quickly to the precrisis equilibrium. Patients in the emergency department are frequently in crisis. Some may be experiencing a normal maturational crisis that one expects at some time, such

as marriage, children leaving the home, or the death of a spouse. For others, the crisis is completely unexpected, for example: severe trauma or medical illness, sudden death, admission to the hospital, or assault. Concurrent developmental crises, such as adjustment to adolescense or old age may also be present. The older patient may be in the midst of asking himself how much of a burden he is, how capable he is, what respect is due him, and how self-sustaining he is. When an acute crisis strikes someone with such a significant concurrent crisis, the result is often a prolonged period of resolution or a less than optimal one if extra support is not forthcoming.

If the person in crisis is helped to ameliorate the psychic trauma, the result for the individual may be a shorter period of disequilibrium. If the stresses associated with the crisis are *not* well met and the person has no supportive system, irreparable damage may be done, leaving the individual in a poorer state of mental health.

What does the emergency department nurse do first in a crisis situation? A quick assessment to make sure that the patient is safe and that the disorganization does not progress is in order. The nurse should immediately relieve as much anxiety or guilt as possible. A more in-depth assessment of the patient to determine the hazardous situations is done next, with attention to what they mean to the patient and how he feels (afraid, overwhelmed, and so on). As nurses begin to assess, they are, at the same time, conveying empathy and caring. Demeanor should be calm and communicate to the patient control of the situation. The patient should be allowed to ventilate. He may be reluctant to begin talking, but will do so with encouragement. Invariably, patients feel relieved after this ventilation.

The nurse helps with practical problem solving and acts as a reality tester. When the patient says that everything is lost, that no one cares, or that he's never been happy, the nurse might point out that his observations might be colored by the circumstances of that moment, pointing out objective facts that may contradict his skewed perceptions.

The nurse helps the patient mobilize his personal resources and those of family and friends. Indirectly reminding the person in crisis of strengths and supports may help. Respect is contagious. It may be helpful to focus at times on the individual rather than on the traumatic episode, thereby periodically diminishing the intensity of the reaction while reinforcing the person's own integrity and sense of worth.

Good communication with the patient is the key to *any* therapeutic intervention. A sharing of words allows a sharing of feelings that, in turn, creates the therapeutic "bonding" necessary for most effective intervention. There are many instances in which the reaction to loss or threat of loss occurs in the emergency department (see Chapter 3). When a patient has just suffered a significant loss or devastating psychic blow, what can the nurse possibly say to the distraught person? It does not have to be profound. A comforting touch, followed by quiet validation of the shock and horror, decreasing the necessity to act it out, and putting into words what is so far unspeakable, all help begin the process of resolution. Nothing can be as damaging as the unconceptualized, unarticulated, unspoken, unknown that creates the unbearable apprehension we call anxiety. This feeling is often what precipitates behavior that confronts staff in the emergency department. Simply naming the fear and putting it into words is often a great relief. Many nurses are afraid to say something for fear that it will "upset the patient." In fact, by the time the nurse's concern has been aroused, the patient is probably experiencing far more discomfort than the nurse could possibly induce. Whether patient's fears are irrational or very rational (as is the case with a terminally ill patient), the response to the threat is positively attenuated when they share their thoughts and their burden with a supportive professional. The nurse can be used by the patient as a sounding board when social supports may not be able to emotionally tolerate the painful exchange or may be too close to the situation to remain objective. Besides objectivity, nurses bring with them the authority and dignity of their profession and the hospital setting, which enhance their observations and esteem in the eyes of the patient. Also, when the patient learns that there is someone available for consultation by phone or that a return visit to the emergency department is possible, if necessary, the urgency of the situation often seems to abate.

The immediate crisis reaction may last from a few moments to a few hours. The process of crisis resolution may last up to 4 to 6 weeks. If it seems appropriate, the patient can be reassured that crises are usually self-limiting. If the nurse feels uncomfortable about the patient upon discharge, he or she may want to refer the patient to a psychiatric nurse or other professional within the hospital or at a neighborhood facility for ongoing support and continued assessment.

RAPE VICTIMS

The rape victim in the emergency department is a crisis intervention situation in which the nurse can be an absolutely invaluable resource for a patient, but all too often is not. Aspects of intervention in this case can be applied to other crisis situations and therefore deserve extra attention. Rape victims still suffer as a result of society's awkwardness and shame about sexual matters and ambivalences toward women. In this, as in other unfortunate circumstances, blaming the victim is as common as it is subtle. The myths surrounding the crime abound, one such myth being that rape victims only *say* that they have been raped. Nurses experienced in victim counselling, however, know that virtually *all* victims who come to an emergency department with a chief complaint of rape, have, indeed been raped. They know, too, that it is basically an overwhelming, terrifying, debasing experience, involving an aggressive, rather than a sexual act. The victim will, in the following weeks and months, be likely to meet with the confusion, shame, distrust, misplaced anger, and misunderstanding of those close to her and society at large. She will assume the label of "the one who was raped"; the long, tedious court process will be openly hostile to her.

The nurse is in a most opportune place to effect a positive influence on the victim's resolution of the experience very early on. She should begin by looking at the victim as a normal person in crisis. She should then determine the victim's request—thereby beginning to return to her some of the control she completely lost during the assault. Is her concern medical, legal, emotional, a combination, or undetermined? The victim's request should be met. She should be allowed to make informed choices as to her treatment. The patient may not want an examination and simply request a tranquilizer.

If the crime can be prosecuted, the documentation of the hospital record is very valuable, but the victim makes the choice. (See also Chapter 4.)

The victim will, even with the most supportive response from those around her, experience a syndrome of symptomatology—physical and psychosocial—that is predictable, as delineated by Burgess and Holmstrom, 1974. The victim can be helped by anticipatory guidance. In the acute phase of disorganization, somatic reactions include skeletal muscle tension, headache, GI irritability, stomach pain, nausea and vomiting, genitourinary disturbances, vaginal discharge, itching, burning, generalized pain, and so on. Some of these symptoms have to do with the trauma of the rape itself, the medications for pregnancy and infection prevention, and the person's psychosomatic reactions. (Some may be brought on by the victim's somatic reactions to the psychic stress.) The victim will invariably experience some signs and symptoms of a clinical depression. She may report disturbances of eating and sleeping; fatigue, lack of motivation, anhedonia, emotional lability, and an anxiety reported as jumpiness or edginess. Emotional reactions can run the gamut. Victims frequently blame themselves for finding themselves in a position to be assaulted, blame themselves for not escaping the assault—in the beginning, or sooner than they did—or wonder if they deserved what happened. They wonder, "Why me?" and thank God they are alive, only to wonder *why* they are, or why they should *want* to be alive in an unfair world in which they are so vulnerable and powerless. The victim may feel an intense, frustrated anger and wish for retaliation. They may feel an intense fear of the assailant returning and attacking them again. The victim's reaction will be affected by the type of rapist and the circumstances of the assault. In exploring the "why" of the assault, the nurse should reinforce the fact that the victim did not, for any reason, deserve the assault and that the motivation for the rape stems solely from the rapist's characteristics—sociological, emotional, and mental problems.

The rape victim often looks at her experience through glasses colored by her concurrent, maturational, and historical stresses, as do all victims of crisis. A person with a disorganized developmental background who is experiencing an adjustment to adult life and questioning who she is, and who is in a transitional period with a new job or living situation will experience the trauma differently from someone with a very stable, supportive background and current situation. The victim should be asked if something like this has ever happened before, and what the resolution of the event was like.

It is helpful to speak to a spouse, boyfriend, or significant other alone, and then together with the victim. A reassessment of relationships with loved ones often follows a rape, as well as a disruption of normal sexual and social interaction. Feelings of vague paranoia, distrust, thinking the worst of people, or the victim's realization that she would be capable of punitive violence can confuse and dismay the victim. Since the nurse can only support the victim for a few hours and, afterward, only intermittently, the seeds to a positive resolution need to be planted in the minds of the victim's significant others. Does her spouse blame the victim? Is his main concern *his* pride and feeling of frustration? Difficulty in the psychosocial and sexual adjustment will be met with more understanding if it is anticipated. Much preventive mental health teaching and general consciousness raising can be done in the emergency department. It will go a long way toward helping someone who might not ordinarily go to a mental health resource for guidance. The basic support, exploration of feelings, and anticipatory guidance hold true for male victims or children. With children, more work may need to be done with the parents, since it is their reactions that are so important in determining the child's reaction. Supporting them enables them to, in turn, support the child. If chronic abuse or neglect is involved, the nurse may want to involve other agencies in order to prevent a continuing or chronic situation.

Some victims may benefit from the nurse's follow-up by telephone and/or accompaniment them to court. A phone call within a few days and then as necessary is very helpful.

ANXIETY

At best, anxiety can make a person alert, sensitive, perceptive, and more spirited than he usually is, better prepared to meet a crisis than if he were relaxed and inattentive. At worst, anxiety can precipitate and perpetuate terrifying ego distortions in which the adult patient experiences something like the objectless world of infancy. The most important symptoms in neuroses and psychoses are attempts to defend against anxiety, attempts to discharge its intolerable tensions, or signs that the threat inherent in anxiety has already been realized and that the ego has at least in part disintegrated. Anxiety is directly involved in producing "psychosomatic" disorders (such as cardiac disease, hypertension, ulcers, and so on) by virtue of its triggering "fight or flight" responses on a more chronic level. It is a major factor in structuring early personality development.

What is anxiety? It can be conceptualized as a type of fear but, unlike fear, not having an easily definable cause. Although anxiety is almost indistinguishable from fear in quality, it may arise from dangers in the environment, or threats emanating from within oneself. The perceived threat may be related to biological, psychological, or social integrity, as well as to a threat of bodily harm. For example, the elderly person with minor illness feels an anxiety associated with the reminder of the relatively imminent threat of death (biological, psychological, and social integrity).

Patients in the emergency department may experience anxiety arising from feelings of loss of control, vague unfamiliarity, frustration, unwilling dependence, and a feeling of rejection from the staff. Their amount of anxiety is not necessarily correlated with severity of stress or illness. An analogy might be drawn with the following situations.

A commuter traveling a further distance will be less likely to experience stress or anxiety if he enters the train or bus at the beginning of its run and is able to "stake out" his territory, arrange his things, make himself comfortable, and feel that he "belongs." The commuter who has only a very short distance to travel, but enters a car that is already "inhabited" by those who seem to belong and who are probably not particularly glad to see him will probably experience more stress and anxiety. A person with a cut finger may react far more anxiously than a person with a serious chest wound, depending on many factors, including his baseline ego functioning and how well it maintains an adaptive balance between both his internal and external worlds. The person with a cut finger may perceive the vague, ubiquitous threats of pain and intrusion in the emergency department setting as intolerable in light of an unstable and poorly integrated ego, concomitant stresses, and previous negative experience with hospitals. The patient with the chest wound, on the other hand, may be familiar with the emergency department setting, feel confident that he is in competent hands, and experience minimal anxiety, having a well-integrated ego and stable emotional background.

Anxiety is normal when its intensity and character are appropriate in a given situation and when its effects are not disorganizing and maladaptive. It increases a person's readiness for prompt and vigorous action. Anxiety is even sought after for recreation (such as tense movies or carnival rides). One of the most important functions of normal anxiety is the defensive preparation it affords a person who faces a probable or certain assault. The anxious preparation often takes the form of rehearsing the anticipated danger, so that when it finally materializes, the person has already organized his defenses in advance. Anyone who deals with the acute grief in the emergency department know that even the smallest amount of time in which the family is prepared for the worst makes a tremendous difference in their ability to cope when finally told of the death of a loved one. In some instances, even momentary anticipation seems to act as a protection against being overwhelmed by a sense of helplessness and anguish. In light of this, the emergency department nurse should, whenever possible, let the family know of any "turn for the worse" or foreboding signs and symptoms that point to a patient's becoming gravely ill. The family of a cardiac arrest patient should be kept abreast of the fact that the patient is *not* responding to medical efforts as well as any encouraging signs.

Anxiety actually exists simultaneously at three levels—a neuroendocrine level, a motor-visceral level, and a level of conscious awareness. Generally, the person is conscious of a disagreeable feeling, and more rarely, of intense discomfort, but he is not usually aware of the cause of his anxiety. The disagreeable feeling has two components—the awareness of the physiological sensations and the realization of being nervous or frightened. Recognizable clues of mild to moderate anxiety in a patient are: a tense facial expression or affect that is appropriate but forced, tremors of the extremities, rapid speech, restlessness, hyperactivity, tense and awkward movement, unreasonable demands, irritability, preoccupation, increased pulse and blood pressure, decreased respirations, dry mouth, constricted pupils, and inability to perform simple tasks quickly. The patient experiencing moderate anxiety needs guidance in the process of logical thinking and problem solving. The patient in serious and severe anxiety exhibits an increased respiratory rate and decreased depth, marginal control, dilated pupils, startled expression, a rigid or inappropriate affect, and obvious bewilderment. They experience fragmented thought processes, loss of reality, and may focus on minor or distorted details. Anxiety may progress to a state of terror in which the patient is totally immobilized and incapable of attending to himself or his environment. When loss of control seems imminent, chemical or physical restraints, and possibly a brief hospitalization may be necessary to prevent harm.

Ideally, the patient's anxiety can be attenuated long before it reaches this peak. Unfortunately, emergency department staff is notorious, not only for not recognizing escalating anxiety, but often for contributing to it. An example is the young female patient with an undiagnosed abdominal pain who is in considerable discomfort and is terrified. The first thing that happens upon arriving in the emergency department is that her relative is told to wait in the waiting room. She is anxious and crying as she desperately tries to make the emergency department staff know how terrible her situation is. She wants them to be concerned enough to be on the alert to help her— possibly to save her life. She looks to see that the emergency department staff are sympathetic and will help her. A busy staff member avoids eye contact since her mind is on a priority patient she wants to get back to. It is difficult for the patient to express her feelings. How does one ask others to care? The staff may next tell her that there is nothing to worry about and that she'll be fine. Instead of being reassured, the patient hears only that the *staff* is not worried (that is, concerned) about her, not that *she* shouldn't worry. Staff may eventually look at her in a way that suggests that she couldn't be in *that* much pain. At this point, she is *really* afraid, and her task, to make people appreciate how sick she is, is more imperative than ever. By this time, she is crying out in pain, and moving toward a panic state. How much *more* helpful it would be to tell the patient that the severity of her pain is appreciated, offer to make her more comfortable as soon as time allows, tell her what is being done to determine the origin of the pain, and let her know how often someone will be by. Letting one family member unobtrusively stay close by (perhaps sitting on a stool or small chair at the foot of the stretcher) or visit for short, regular periods of time also helps relieve the anxiety of both parties.

The chief function of any organism is the maintenance of its organization. When an organism perceives a threat to its integrity—whether psychological or physiological—it moves toward alleviating anxiety in two ways —conscious and unconscious. If the action is largely a conscious, deliberately selected one, it can be considered a coping mechanism. Escaping to an "anxiety nap," studying for an exam, redirecting energies, or going home to mother are examples of coping. It is important to determine how a person has coped in the past in order to suggest helping behavior at a time of stress or anxiety. Unconscious forces that largely determine a person's behavior are called defense mechanisms. Defense mechanisms include introjection, projection, identification, repression, denial, reaction formation, displacement, turning against oneself, isolation, intellectualization, rationalization, ritual, and undoing. The two most commonly observable mechanisms in the emergency department are denial and displacement, although others become apparent with increasing sensitivity.

To allay anxiety in the emergency department, the following six points may be helpful.

1. Give support. An admonishment to physicians in the early 1900s reads: "Your patients do not come to you to be cured: they come to be relieved of their pains and other symptoms and to be comforted. Forced to choose, they would usually prefer a kind doctor to an efficient one. Never forget that the patient and his relations are usually frightened and anxious, upset in their normal life to such an extent that they are prepared to call you into their lives and to tell you the most intimate facts about themselves, though you may be unknown to them except as a member of an honorable profession." This admonition applies no less to the nurse in the emergency department in 1980 than to the physician at the turn of the century. The best "medicine" takes place in the atmosphere of trust, mutual respect, relaxed confidence, and empathy. If anxiety is fear without an object, then there is safety in numbers. Alerting other staff members to an anxious patient and increasing staff time with the patient

if possible seem to help. An aide may be enlisted to stay with the patient for periods of time.

2. Allow for verbalization. Anxious persons often feel the need to "talk to someone."

3. Be calm and in control of yourself. Anxiety is contagious. Fortunately, so is confidence.

4. Help the patient focus on reality, set priorities, and organize. Anxiety tends to produce confusion and distortion of perceptions. Lend your more objective observations and thinking to the situation.

5. Try to identify the object of the patient's anxiety. Put yourself in the patient's place. What is his cultural background? What have his past experiences with hospitals been like? What has the patient seen in the emergency department so far? What would most persons with the symptoms of a particular patient be thinking? Mention the unmentionable: ask if the patient is afraid that it is something very serious, or perhaps life-threatening. Also encourage the patient to ask any questions that may arise, even if they seem silly.

6. Allow the patient some degree of control to bolster his ego.

The patient whose anxiety becomes overwhelming may need further assessment before discharge by a psychiatric nurse or other professional, and/or referral to another resource if it seems appropriate.

Panic reactions in anxiety

Patients entering the emergency department with anxiety attacks will appear agitated and terrified. The patient may experience cardiac-related symptoms such as palpitations, precordial pain, and shortness of breath. He may experience disturbances of respiration (nervous dyspnea, hyperventilation, and pseudoasthma), GI disturbances (nausea, diarrhea, and abdominal pain), trembling, diaphoresis, and paresthesias. The characteristic psychological symptom is a feeling of apprehension that something terrible is going to happen. Attacks may last for a few minutes to a few hours.

Anxiety is a form of fearful reaction that is without a tangible object for that fear. It differs from object-related fear in the following ways.

1. It is "free-floating" and not restricted to definite situations or objects.
2. It is not accompanied by any degree of insight into its immediate cause.
3. It tends to be experienced in terms of its physical manifestations, although the individual does not recognize them as such.
4. It is prompted by anticipation of future threats against which current avoidance responses would not be effective.
5. It is not controlled by a specific psychological defense mechanisms.

The psychodynamics of anxiety attacks include such things as the need to ward off indefinite formless anxiety by the adoption of a definite form of sickness that might be cured: a "flight into sickness," to avoid threatening situations or pressures, or a reactivation of the sickness role that once obtained for the child a suspension from regular routine and the loving solicitude of the parents. It is usually the case with such patients that a recent history of disturbing events has precipitated the attack (such as marital discord and threatened divorce, failure or impending failure at significant work, homosexual panic, and so on). It is not necessarily the function of the emergency department visit to fully address or treat these problems, even if the patient is able to pinpoint them, which is often not the case. In fact, uncovering conflicts that are too painful to confront directly at that time may be counterproductive and prolong the acute discomfort of the attack. Health teaching about the causes of anxiety attacks in general will begin to expand the patient's awareness and insight. It is often more helpful to concentrate on the concrete, having someone stay with the patient at all times (if the nurse is unable, then a relative or an aide), being very reassuring (patients are often helped by such concrete signs as good vital signs or ECG) and explanations that this is a familiar syndrome that is encountered often in the emergency department and is not life-threatening. *Too* much false reassurance may make the patient feel that the nurse doesn't fully appreciate the urgency of his situation and make him more anxious, however. Touching the patient (taking his pulse while eliciting a history, wiping his brow, or holding the hand of a patient whose panic is unbearable) is often comforting and anxiety reducing. Patients experiencing an anxiety attack seem to be readily influenced by suggestion. Care should be taken not to indicate physical abnormalities or concerns about the patient's physical condition. The patient has little retentive memory and may ask the same question repeatedly. Rather, a suggestive expectation that the patient should be starting to feel better should be conveyed.

It is important that the emergency department nurse also convey concern. Since the patient feels he is literally depending upon the emergency department for his life, a negative attitude on the part of the nurse could lead to more anxiety and a prolonged attack. Diazepam (Valium) or other tranquilizer may be helpful, as are relaxation exercises. Hyperventilation is often a symptom of primary anxiety and occurs with the above symptoms, or it may occur as a symptom of anxiety secondary to a physical disorder. The simple treatment for hyperventilation is to have the patient rebreathe into a paper bag. This relieves symptoms that result from loss of carbon dioxide and accompanying alkalosis and gives the patient a concrete task that distracts his thinking away from the source of his anxiety and physical symptoms (see also p. 375).

In general, the patient with anxiety reaction should be given the feeling that he is in "good hands." With such patients, referrals should be made to resources for psychological counselling and support to explore sources of anxiety and preclude attacks in the future.

PSYCHIATRIC EMERGENCIES

There is little agreement as to what constitutes a psychiatric emergency, or whether such an entity exists at all, in psychiatric circles. In emergency department circles, the psychiatric emergency is routinely and empirically identified for us by the patient and/or those who bring him to the hospital. Whether the emergency involves an objectively suicidal or severely psychotic patient or a subjectively tormented patient who feels he can no longer "cope," suffice it to say that a psychiatric emergency occurs when a patient is unable to adapt to and cope with severe and overwhelming stress from within or without, and will suffer damaging emotional sequelae if intervention is not soon forthcoming.

Psychiatric emergencies are often less clear-cut in their diagnosis and treatment than medical emergencies and have a tendency to elicit negative responses and precipitate confusion in emergency department staff. A few methodic guidelines can help reduce that confusion and reduce staff's anxiety. Begin by determining the patient's chief complaint and chief request—a good way to begin with *any* emergency department assessment. A patient with the most apparent and seemingly severe psychiatric disorder may be exhibiting nothing more than a chronic state that is "normal" for that individual and which does not require emergency treatment. The patient may actually have a medical complaint, or his chief complaint may differ from that of his family or of the police who brought him in. The patient may have *no* complaint, perhaps indicative of a lack of insight into the gravity of his situation.

There may be a hidden or implicit chief complaint behind a stated chief complaint of vague somatic distress or multiple accidents. The patient may actually be depressed, without a place to stay, or experiencing domestic violence and not know where to turn. Has the patient suddenly been cut off from his usual source of income or gratification? Has his family decided that they can no longer care for the patient, given behavior exhibited that day, or the night before, that they consider to be "the last straw"? Has the patient come to the emergency department today because of a well-meaning passer-by who found a chronically eccentric person who seems strange, yet turns out to be someone who is neither commitable, nor amenable to treatment? If the patient is seeing someone in psychiatric therapy, the patient's visit quite probably has to do with problems in that therapy. Is his psychiatrist on vacation, or is he refusing the patient medication because it

is contraindicated? Determining what is troubling the individual *at this time* is half the battle, and addresses the acute nature of the emergency service. "At this time" is an important phrase. The answer to this question supplies the emergency department nurse with what the acute problem is, and most often determines what, if anything, the emergency department can do to mitigate the situation. Exhaustive exploration of a patient's history may be exasperating and prove fruitless.

When the chief request seems to be different from what first seemed apparent, the best way to decipher the actual request is to ask the patient what he thought the emergency department might be able to do for him when he decided to come to the emergency department. His request may stem from personal experiences or the experiences of friends who have used the emergency department in the past, or his request may be unclear even to himself and his knowledge of resources limited. The patient's request may or may not be legitimate. The request may be for support and confirmation of concern and ventilation of guidance and advice; it may be for medications; it may be for hospitalization or referral to an appropriate resource; or, it may be more complex. The female patient who overdoses may have as her implicit request that the emergency department somehow make her husband who is leaving her understand how much she is hurt and needs him.

After the chief complaint and chief request become clear, the next question is, "How can the emergency department be helpful?" In the case of the woman who has overdosed, the nurse might (ideally) try to enhance the communication between the couple after each has been given individual support during or after her medical treatment. Chief requests may or may not be able to be met by the emergency department, depending on the propriety of the request and the emergency department's ability to meet it. The emergency department must resist the temptation to be all things to all people. There will be some patients who will not be helped during their emergency department visit. For example, the patient who says that he needs drugs to detoxify himself might be better helped by a referral to a resource for that purpose. A patient who requests hospitalization for rest and relaxation might be helped by exploring what is causing the need to "get away" and how he might effect this outside the hospital. The patient who is in need of antidepressants might be better advised to seek them at a more comprehensive resource where the effects of the medication can be monitored and the patient can obtain ongoing therapy.

With any patient the emergency department nurse is assessing (but most especially with the psychiatric patient), what is seen and heard and thought about the patient must be validated. Decisions are necessarily made with limited information in a limited amount of time in the emergency department, and every scrap of available knowledge must be used. Nurses should always ask the patient if their observations are correct. If the patient is wearing a bizarre outfit, don't be too timid to ask. The nurse might say simply, "I hope you'll understand that I'd like to understand more about you, and that I need to ask about your clothes. They are unusual and I'm not sure what to make of them." If the patient looks as though he is frightened, anxious, angry, or euphoric, tell him how he seems to you, and ask how valid those observations are. Invariably, revelations occur when time is taken to listen to a patient. It is very easy to misinterpret behavior. Acting on those misinterpretations could result in an escalation of the situation or even bring harm to the patient.

An abbreviated, informal mental status exam should be done almost automatically with any patient having significant emotional problems. Following is a mental status evaluation tool. It may not be needed in its entirety for every patient. Reading through it, the nurse should keep in mind that if those appearances and functions do not seem appropriate, the patient should be asked about it. If the patient has poor hygiene, he should be asked if it has been difficult to care for himself lately. If affect seems unusual, this, too, should be clarified with the patient. The nurse should not assume the reason for anything. If the patient feels that the nurse's questions are borne of genuine interest and asked kindly, tactfully, even euphemistically, there should be no problem in eliciting helpful explanations.

1. *Appearance and grooming.* Is the patient's attire appropriate to the time, place, season, occasion? Is he clean-shaven, groomed, and so on?

2. *Behavior.* Is the patient's affect generally sad? Is it inappropriate in intensity or incongruent with what the patient is saying? Is the patient moving slower or faster than normal? Does he seem agitated? Are his movements purposeful, inappropriate, or different (for example, cogwheel rigidity or waxy flexibility)? Note the patient's posture, gait, and carriage. Notice voice and speech. Is he speaking in a monotone? Is his speech "pushed?" Are his answers organized? Relevant? Are there deviations such as neologisms or echolalia? Is his vocabulary appropriate for his background?

3. *Emotional reactions.* Is the patient sad, worried, fearful?

4. *Content of thought.* Are there persecutory, hypochondriacal, schizophrenic, depressive, or grandiose trends? Are there obsessions, compulsions, phobias, or hallucinations? Is his thought process logical, relevant?

5. *Sensorium.* Is the patient oriented to time, place, and person? Does he have recent memory, remote memory? Is he able to calculate figures and think abstractly?

6. *Insight.* Does the patient appreciate his own situation and its relationship to others and his environment?

7. *Judgment.* Is the patient able to make decisions? Does he have trouble deciding whether to undress for an exam? Does he have an appreciation for situations that may be dangerous for him?

Psychosis

Psychosis occurs when a person's mental capacity, affective response, and capacity to recognize reality, communicate, and relate to others is impaired enough to interfere with his capacity to deal with ordinary daily life. The psychotic patient is often brought to the emergency department by concerned family or police. Occasionally, the patient will appear by himself, with minor, vague, or no complaints. He may be, or become, out of control to the point where he may hurt himself or others. This, coupled with the fact that acute psychosis is extremely uncomfortable, makes this an emergency that should be treated with immediate consideration.

When the very disturbed patient is first brought in, he should be immediately brought to a quiet, sparsely furnished room—preferably including just a sturdy stretcher and heavy desk, with perhaps one chair. Nothing should be left in the room that can be thrown or prove dangerous. Police and/or family should quickly be asked for a brief account of his behavior before coming to the hospital to determine such things as how much protection he needs, and whether a family member staying with the patient helps or hinders. Probably the two most ''dangerous'' types of patients are the paranoid psychotic and the patient in a toxic condition. When someone is intensely paranoid, he may feel as though he is fighting for his life, and any behavior is rationalized as self-defense. When a patient is in a toxic condition, his emotionality is increased at the same time that his normal inhibitions to aggressive or self-destructive behavior are stripped away.

If there is any reason to think that the patient may be dangerous (for example, if police tell the nurse that the patient attacked someone without provocation, or that he made a determined effort to escape en route), a locked room or restraints may be in order. It is invariably better to be safe than sorry. It is necessary to create as controlled and safe an environment as possible for the time-consuming task of evaluating, treating, and planning and implementing hospitalization or other disposition for such patients. The patient should be advised of what is being done and have any fears allayed. Emergency department nurses should pay attention to their first gut reactions to a patient and never underestimate or disregard their intuition. Since there are many things on a pa-

tient's person, from a nail file in a purse to a concealed razor blade, it is a good policy to have all patients undress and get into hospital clothing. Their effects should be gathered together and put into safe-keeping. The patient is told very matter-of-factly that this is policy and necessary for the doctor to examine any patient. He should be reminded that he is in a hospital and that he is safe. The restraints, he might be told, are to give him some of the control he will regain soon. He should be told that while he is experiencing difficult and frightening feelings that are very painful, it is to be expected that he will be confused about making decisions. He should be reminded that the staff is there to help make decisions *for* him until he can do so for himself. This is sometimes reassuring and lifts some of the burden of decisions from someone who may be very ambivalent about *any* decision. Optimally, a family member, aide, or security guard should stand by and watch the patient.

If the legalities of detaining a patient against his will is a concern, the emergency department staff should be guided by the fact that courts are less concerned with the absolute right or wrong of an action than how *justifiable* it is. If the nurse can *justify* such precautions in light of the patient's past or present behavior and the reasonable possibility of harm to himself or others, the action is usually well advised. Nurses might ask themselves if it would be more difficult to justify why they did *not* treat the patient and let him leave.

Every patient who seems ''bizarre'' deserves as complete a medical workup as possible. The patient's unwillingness to cooperate and refusal of treatment are usually symptoms of his illness, and not reasons to dispense with the examination or allow the patient to go. This is the philosophy of most knowledgeable medical practitioners and the courts as well. The emergency department has a responsibility to treat someone who is not competent to refuse that treatment and in need of it just as thoroughly as it would a pleasant, cooperative patient.

As soon as the patient is brought under control and is as comfortable as possible, the diagnostic detective work begins. The first task is to decide if there is any question that the behavior is organic (see pp. 539-549), that is, caused by chemical or physiological sources. It is often helpful to gather information before talking to the patient. In this way, the nurse is more knowledgeable about the patient's situation before speaking with him, and if the patient denies any problem, the nurse can gently remind him of why others are concerned. A nurse might ask him about how he perceives certain events that others have told her about. When patients are unaccompanied or unable to communicate, names and telephone numbers are especially helpful and may be furnished by police or ambulance attendants or found in a patient's wallet or address book. Neighbors and landlords may help, in lieu of relatives. It is important to know how acute this state of mind is and what the progression of symptoms have been in order to predict the patient's course. When left with no information but a name, calling nearby state and private psychiatric hospitals may be helpful. The patient may have left that facility or wandered from a group of patients on an outing in the area. In the aftermath of ''deinstitutionalization,'' many former back wards' patients are without structure and may decompensate or wander from emergency department to emergency department. Without resources, these patients seem to fall into the cracks between inpatient and outpatient facilities. The nurse should ask about previous hospitalizations and medications and try to learn about the pattern of illness characteristic of this patient. These patients, as well as others without financial or social supports may appear often enough to make a simple, informative ''Repeater File'' system helpful. Current treatment plans, effective approaches, and names and numbers of those who know the patient might be included on 5 × 8 inch cards.

When *any* patient is interviewed, there should be only *one* anxious person in the room. Therefore, the nurse should begin by arranging the environment in order to feel as safe and comfortable as possible. The patient may exhibit pressured speech, the content of which may be tangential or ''word salad.'' If the nurse listens well, themes such as fear and vulnerability become apparent. Patients are often very sensitive and alert to the feelings and actions of others around them and may quickly sense feelings of negativity or insecurity in staff. Nurses should appear calm, competent, and genuinely interested. They should not become angry if the patient's behavior is disagreeable. Patients may overreact to perceived anger. The nurse might instead appear disappointed and convey to the patient a respect for him and that more is expected form him. People often live up to others' expectations. If a patient overhears that he is being called crazy, he may be more likely to act that way. The nurse should not directly challenge what the delusional patient is saying, should ask more questions about his thoughts, and explore them further. If the patient demands to know if the nurses agree with him, they can honestly answer by saying that they are trying to understand and are sure that he realizes how difficult it is, and would he explain more. They may tell the patient that they do believe that he would not mislead others intentionally.

It is sometimes anxiety-reducing to offer the patient a cup of coffee, cigarette, or drink of water, although this should be done only if the nurse feels comfortable with it. (Matches should be kept, coffee should be cooled, and water and cigarettes might need to be held for the patient.)

Some type of mental status examination should always be done. The patient should be asked about frightening voices. Auditory hallucinations are more common in functional psychosis. Men will report voices saying that they are homosexual, women will say they are being called prostitutes, both will describe voices that tell them to kill themselves or that they are better off dead. The patient with an acute schizophrenic psychosis will usually have a flat or shallow affect, with an ambivalent, constricted, and inappropriate responsiveness and loss of empathy with others. He may exhibit pushed speech, lack of speech, or blocking. His thinking may be disturbed and he may misinterpret reality. Disordered thought with clear sensorium is common. The schizophrenic patient will classically say that his mind is being controlled—electronically or otherwise. The patient may be combative, withdrawn, regressive, or catatonic. The patient may be a late adolescent or young adult having his first psychotic episode or a chronic schizophrenic who is experiencing stress.

Careful observation of the patient will provide clues as to his history. For example, the nurse might notice that an incoherent patient who appears not to have shaved for a few days has a receipt for a bank deposit dated 1 week ago. If the person has deteriorated in the space of one week, his condition might be fairly acute.

Acute paranoid schizophrenia is characterized by persecutory or grandiose delusions and sometimes by hallucinations or excessive religiosity. This patient, as previously noted, is often hostile. A systematized delusion, sometimes built upon actual situations but carried to outlandish lengths may be present. The patient may carry a notebook with handwritten, loosely associated themes. Some patients will have religious objects on their person. The paranoid psychotic patient should be managed with the utmost care. He presents a high risk and a difficult challenge.

Hypomania and manic psychosis are occasionally encountered in the emergency department. Hypomania involves a classic triad of symptoms: elated but unstable mood, pressure of speech, and increased motor activity. This patient talks easily, humorously, and endlessly. He is friendly, then uninvitedly personal. Beneath his thin veneer of well-being, however, is an intolerance for frustration, impulsive, ill-considered actions, and blatant disregard of obvious difficulties. In acute mania, all of the above are present, but they are more intense and more disturbing. Propriety and discretion are painfully absent. The content of the patient's conversation is frequently sexual and often loud. Manic patients may have recurrent episodes of mood elevation. They may also experience periods of depression. Lithium carbonate is a specific drug in the treatment of manic-depressive illness. The manic patient should not be encouraged to talk and should be asked to very succinct in giving a history, in the interests of effecting his best care. Physical restraints are often more agitating and should be avoided. The patient should be given a private room or area in which he can pace if he feels the need.

Whatever the type of psychosis, an appropriate disposition will need to be decided. If family is willing, and the patient is thought to be able, a relatively disturbed person may go home with medication and solid follow-up, and the option of returning to the emergency department or a more appropriate place if the patient becomes worse or worries the family. If the patient is clearly unmanageable in any other setting, inpatient hospitalization will have to be arranged. The determination of where he will go depends on such factors as the patient's willingness to be admitted, insurance status, and the availability of beds. If the patient is extremely agitated and self-destructive, even when restrained, some medication may have to be given. However, if the patient is going to be hospitalized, and most particularly if he is going to be committed to another hospital where the concurrence of the accepting physician will decide whether or not he will be admitted, the emergency department should use drugs sparingly, if at all. Ideally, the person at the accepting facility should clearly see the pathological condition or trust in the judgement of the referring agency. Medication may miraculously "cure" the patient or make him so sleepy as to preclude an interview. Family or friends should accompany the patient to enhance the transition and facilitate any further history taking. Even if the patient is willing to go to the hospital, the emergency department may want to send the patient with a commitment paper, in the event that the patient changes his mind en route and ambulance drivers are left without the legal right to restrain.

Violence

Although violence is not necessarily the product of one diagnosis, it is usually associated with either functional illnesses such as characterological disorders and paranoid schizophrenia, and organic disorders such as toxicity and temporal lobe epilepsy. Psychodynamically, violent behavior can be seen as a defense mechanism by which the individual protects himself from unbearable and overwhelming feelings of helplessness. Organically, it can be seen as a disorder of a specific cerebral anatomic structure and/or electrical or metabolic function.

If psychological or functional causes are inducing the behavior, the nurse looks for events, feelings, and conflicts that may help explain outbursts. If organicity is at the root of the behavior, it might involve such sources as electrical disturbances of the brain (temporal lobe epilepsy) or metabolic abnormalities such as barbiturate or alcohol use or withdrawal, electrolyte imbalance, or hypoxia.

In the emergency department, it is often necessary to quickly decide what to do when a patient has, or escalates to, violent behavior. If the patient is so out of control that there seems to be imminent danger to himself or others, restraints may need to be used. Attempts to subdue a patient with inadequate personnel should not be attempted. Usually not fewer than five strong persons should approach the person—one for each limb, plus one. They should plan their actions beforehand and act quickly and decisively. If the patient requires restraints, he requires ones that stay on. Personnel may tend to watch a patient less once he is restrained (they should watch him *more* closely), and experienced emergency department personnel know that a patient who gets partially or fully out of restraints represents a high-risk situation. If leather or specifically designed restraints are not available, soft material—Kerlix or stockinette—may be used and should be knotted as securely as possible without interfering with blood and nerve supply. A securely tied restraint will defy the quick, easy extrication by determined patients that often occurs when ''loops'' are used. (Looping restraints around extremities may be more useful for the senile, mildly disoriented, and combative patient.) If the patient is extremely intoxicated, supine positioning might be considered to guard against aspiration. Side rails should be up and the stretcher locked. If possible, the stretcher should be positioned in such a way as to make tipping it over by rocking less likely. Many

very psychotic patients will seem to feel relieved after being restrained—perhaps because they feel that they are being given the control that they lack, and decisions (even the smallest of which are often very difficult for the patient) are being made for them. A patient who is restrained should be reassured that it is primarily for his safety, that no one will harm him in any way, and that the restraints will be on for a very short time until he regains his own control.

Even with restraints, some patients may still present a significant risk of danger to themselves. Patients may hit their head or bite or pull dangerously at restraints. In this case, the benefits of chemical intervention may outweigh the risks of confusing the toxic picture, potentiating the effects of other drugs, or clouding the clinical picture.

Abusive, angry patient

The abusive, angry patient is a more frequent problem in the emergency department than the violent patient. Although prevention is the best answer to alleviating the problem of the angry patient, the key to secondary prevention is remaining calm and professional. Nurses should refuse to become embroiled in a personal struggle. Nurses are professionals. They should remain on the substance of the issues or point out objectively how they see the situation. They should also listen to what the patient is saying and allow him to ventilate. Ventilation relieves the pressure of an angry drive. If the patient is not talking, but acting out his anger, the nurse should try to understand the need prompting the behavior, what the patient is trying to express, and how the environment and the nurse might be influencing the patient's behavior. The nurse might explain that it would be more helpful for the patient to *explain* what he needs rather than *showing*, because it is so hard to know everything a person is feeling and thinking.

The anger being expressed may actually be displaced (misdirected) when the object of that anger is not the emergency department. The patient may be feeling rage at a terminal diagnosis or the tension and frustration of a lifetime.

The nurse might ask if it is the emergency department or staff that the patient's anger is really directed at. It is important not to feed into the patient's "angry system" by fueling potential fires. The nurse should do nothing that the patient can direct his ready anger at, and should be a "reality tester" for the patient, asking whether his anger is really appropriate in intensity, despite the legitimacy of his complaint.

Depression

There is probably more human suffering caused by depression than from any other single disease affecting mankind. Depression has been recognized as a clinical syndrome for over 2,000 years. Although there are differing opinions as to whether depression is just an exaggerated normal mood or reaction, a well-defined disease entity, or a catch-all category, it is wrong to think of depression as only a mood disorder any more than scarlet fever should be thought of as a skin disorder. There is a constellation of attributes that defines depression.

1. A specific alteration in mood: sadness, loneliness, apathy, anhedonia, or alteration of mood according to different times of day.
2. A negative self-concept associated with self-reproaches and self-blame, guilt and remorse.
3. Regression and self-punitive wishes: desires to escape or hide; thoughts of illness, death, and suicide.
4. Vegetative changes: anorexia and weight loss, difficulty in initiating and maintaining sleep, loss of libido, vague somatic complaints, and constipation.
5. Change in activity level: lack of energy or agitation, inability to concentrate.

Depression may be mild or severe. It may occur as a reaction to a loss (death, separation, and so on) or illness, in which case it is called a reactive depression; or it may be an endogenous depression—one coming from within with no discernable outside precipitant. Some patients, by virtue of situational, environmental, or genetic factors, are more predisposed to depressions than others. Patients may come to the emergency department with physical complaints that are depression-related because they don't know whether there are physical causes or because they simply don't know where else to go. If the patient says that he is depressed, it is important to explore what he means by depressed. Is it a clinical depression, as described above, or does the patient mean, instead, that he is angry, sick, unhappy, anxious, or tired of a situation? Every depressed patient should be asked about suicidal ideation. If the patient seems to be suffering from a significant clinical depression that has lasted a month, he may require medication and therapy and should be referred to a resource that will be able to evaluate him soon. The presence of severe psychomotor retardation or severe agitation, or that of suicidal ideation may require inpatient treatment, whereas most depressions can be handled on an outpatient basis and should be referred.

The emergency department may be the first place the depressed person comes for help. If he is met with warm, humanistic treatment, he is more likely to seek further help. Emergency department nurses should be exquisitely aware of the vulnerable state the depressed patient is in and should address themselves to his lowered self-esteem, which has probably taken a further blow in coming to seek help, and treat him with the utmost respect and deference. Allow the patient to ventilate in a sympathetic atmosphere, letting him know, in effect, that someone is aware of the suffering he is experiencing and cares; and reassure the patient—especially someone experiencing his first depression—that depressions are experienced by many people, that they are usually self-limiting, and that there is help (such as therapy, treatments, antidepressants). Refer depressed patients as you would any patient—only after discussing with the patient what type of resource would best meet his needs and what he would be most likely to actually take advantage of. The patient might like to avail himself of the services of a private physician, a clinic, neighborhood facility, or an urban facility with more anonymity. The most complete and well-intentioned referral plans are useless if the patient does not follow through with them because of some reservation about them that he might have been too shy to mention—making it imperative that the nurse discuss the referral with the patient.

Suicide

A sociological composite of a high suicidal risk person consists of a 50-year-old white, jobless male, living alone because of a disrupted marriage, and in poor physical or mental health. He drinks heavily, is likely to use a gun or rope or carbon monoxide from a car's exhaust, and usually leaves a suicide note. In contrast, a picture of a high-risk suicide attempter shows a white married woman under 45 years of age who handles domestic frustrations with drug overdoses, cooking gas, or wrist-slashing. She more often than not survives her ambivalent attempts, with exceptions occurring with miscalculations concerning lethality or the expected appearance of someone who should have found her in time.

Unfortunately, in the emergency department, typical pictures such as these are only partially helpful in determining whether or not a person is a significant suicidal risk. The person who gestures and the person who successfully completes a suicide are not two distinct entities. Often, the case is very much to the contrary. The importance of someone's accepting the responsibility for exploring a patient's suicidal potential is underscored by the fact that in a group of seriously suicidal people, two thirds had communicated their intentions to someone, and over half had sought professional help for depressive symptomatology within 1 month of the act. Given the fact that psychiatric as well as medical emergencies occur "after hours" and the fact that emergency departments are chosen for expedient care by many who are unable or unwilling to wade through the quagmire of red tape that often precedes someone's obtaining psychiatric help, the emergency departments are many times (willingly or unwillingly) left with the burden of the enormous task of deciding whether someone is "suicidal." The answer is never very clear-cut.

Despite popular thinking to the contrary, the capacity for self-destruction is universal, given particular situations. Any psychiatric clinician knows that suicidal thoughts are ubiquitous—from the child who daydreams of how sorry her mother would be for punishing her if she were dead, to the older person who thinks at times of freeing his children of the burden he has become. To complicate the picture, the lethality of suicidal behavior seems to exist on a continuum, not an either/or basis. On the one end is the person who rides a fast motorcycle or the somewhat depressed person who, preoccupied, crosses the street without looking carefully. On the other end is the person who takes what he knows is a lethal dose of drugs at a place and time when he knows no one will find him. Suicidal behavior is described by many patients as a sort of gamble. They may perpetrate suicidal behavior that may or may not be lethal and let the deciding factor be fate, God, or their loved ones. Patients may say that they don't care if they live or die and are hoping for something outside themselves to make that decision for them.

Notwithstanding this gray picture of suicide, there are guidelines to the assessment process.

Demographic data

AGE: Generally, age and rate of suicidal activity are positively correlated. Although younger persons attempt more often, older persons are more successful in their first attempt. Childhood, adolescence, and senility are characterized by emotional lability, low frustration, tolerance, high impulsivity, and, especially in children, the inability to see death as qualitatively different from running away. Consequently, the suicide situation might be reached without the warning of an overt depression.

SEX: Females have higher numbers of attempts at suicide and tend to use available pills. Males succeed two to four times as often.

RELIGION: Those persons who are "very religious" are less likely to commit suicide. More ingrained organized faiths that people can fall back on and that forbid suicide may more frequently preclude suicide.

LIVING ARRANGEMENTS: Persons who live alone or are temporarily separated without a stable living arrangement are at higher risk.

OCCUPATION: Those persons without work that they perceive as worthwhile and gratifying are at greater risk.

TIME: Holidays, anniversary dates, and the spring season seem to increase the incidence of suicidal behavior.

Clinical characteristics

CRISIS: Suicides are often triggered by a loss of social cohesiveness (*someone* to live for) and/or disturbance in social status (*something* to live for). Death, divorce, separation, chronic illness, unemployment, and drop in socioeconomic status are often precipitants to suicidal behavior.

FEELINGS AND THOUGHTS: Feelings of low self-esteem, despondency, guilt, and shame are common. Anger—unvented or misdirected toward the self—might predominate. Patients may express it the following way: "I'm so angry. You shouldn't have treated me like that. I'll show you. You'll be sorry when I'm gone. I'll kill myself."

COPING STRATEGIES: Does the patient have any? Have they been effective in the past? Might they be now?

SIGNIFICANT OTHERS: Spouses, lovers, parents, and best friends are usually the "significant others" whom people literally live for. Has the patient lost these—figuratively, literally, or in the patient's perception?

RESOURCES: Does the patient have social and personal resources available to call upon? Has the patient a baseline, healthy, well-integrated personality and concerned invested social supports? Dissatisfied passive-dependent personality increases suicidal risk.

PAST SUICIDE ATTEMPTS: Many people who commit successful suicides have made attempts or gestured in the past. Past unsuccessful attempts after which help was not forthcoming may confirm the patient's sense of worthlessness, leave him embarrassed with no other alternative, or act as a "rehearsal" for the more lethal attempt. The seriousness of the past attempts should be gauged.

MEDICAL HISTORY: Have others in the patient's family committed suicide? This may make it less forbidden behavior. Does the patient have a newly diagnosed cancer or any organic or chemical facets that might predispose to suicide? For women, the premenstrual and menstrual period seems to increase accidental and suicidal behaviors (Mandell and Mandell, 1967).

LIFESTYLE: Is the patient impulsive? Does he live recklessly? Does he have a history of accidents and illnesses?

PLAN: Explore whether or not the patient has a plan, what the method is, and if he has access to the method. Pay attention to the specificity and lethality of the plan.

High-risk factors

MULTIPLE HIGH-LETHALITY SUICIDE ATTEMPTS: Especially recent ones that are precipitated by a situation that remains unresolved and especially attempts that are increasing in intensity.

ALCOHOL ABUSE: Acute intoxication is countless times associated with suicide; chronic alcoholism even more so.

ISOLATION AND WITHDRAWAL: W. H. Auden once said that "We must love one another or die."

DISORIENTED AND DISORGANIZED BEHAVIOR: A mental status appraisal with particular attention to possible psychotic process is in order.

How will the nurse know whether the patient presents a low or high, emergency or chronic suicidal risk? Although no one can predict with certainty, not even psychiatrists, what an individual will do, information obtained by using the above guidelines should lead you to a fully informed opinion. Three fourths of all suicides fall into the clinically identifiable categories of chronic alcoholism and psychotic depression (Robins and Murphy, 1967).

Many professionals are reluctant to ask a person if he tried to kill himself, even after the most serious attempts, fearing they will be intruding. However, if nurses accept the responsibility to help a patient as comprehensively as they can, it is clear that they need to know. The only way to know is to ask. Ask the primary question and those relevant to the guidelines. The nurse who has a genuine concern for the patient will convey this, no matter how the patient feels or what is worrying him. Direct questioning will not precipitate a suicide. To the contrary, a patient who can bring himself to talk about suicide in a therapeutic setting is under significantly less internal pressure to act on the feeling. The ventilation and sharing of a painful affect can reduce its intensity. Patients probably often wonder why the emergency department staff *doesn't* ask, given sometimes obvious circumstances. Is it that the staff doesn't care or feel that the situation is hopeless?

The nurse should ask questions in a natural and relaxed manner that gives the patient complete permission to discuss feelings, plans, and so on. The nurse might ask what led to an attempt: "What's been happening? It must be pretty awful." After an attempt of suicide, the nurse needs to know if the attempt has changed things in any way. One might ask the patient what his significant others think about what happened. Has a husband who was threatening to leave decided to stay and be supportive? How does the patient feel in retrospect about the attempt? Are there significant others who can care for the person? Does the patient have plans for and concerns about the future? The patient should be asked if *he* perceives any way out, any hope. He may not, contrary to how things look to the nurse.

A good interview is both diagnostic and therapeutic. It is the interview that will lead to a human bond that, in the final analysis, is probably the chief antidote to the suicidal situation. The treatment of the suicidal patient includes reality testing—giving the patient an objective perspective on his situation, searching for latent sustaining affectionate feelings toward others and vice versa (nurses use their status to bring patient and family together as much as possible, identifying the patient as a "patient" to the family, who may see him as an antagonist), and offering themselves, the emergency department, or therapist who will be suggested as a transitional object throughout the bad time.

The significant others should be advised, supported, and directed. Couple's or family's communication may need to be enhanced. The patient's isolation should be minimized. There are only two dispositions from which to choose for this patient—hospitalization or referral to an outpatient resource. If there was an expectation of hospitalization that hasn't changed during this interview, it should be considered. If hospitalization is neither anticipated nor desired, and the patient is seriously suicidal, it is an especially difficult situation. The emergency department staff must remain firm if the decision is to hospitalize, and the concern behind their decision conveyed. Referrals should be made thoughtfully and arrangements for attendance and support made for the patient who will be discharged from the emergency department. Contingency plans should be made for the event

of the patient's again becoming actively suicidal.

Psychosomatic illness

The term "psychosomatic" (from the Greek, "psyche," meaning mind and "soma," meaning body) conjures up the age-old question of a relationship between mind and body, and, for the emergency department nurse, awakens the negativity expressed in the phrase, "it's all in your head." The emergency department nurse needs to be aware, as do all health professionals and the public at large, that *all* illness is psychosomatic, if that phrase is fully appreciated, as it should be, to mean that mind and body have a concomitant effect, each upon the other, and constantly, intricately work as an integrated machine. Most people will accept the fact that ulcers, cardiac conditions, asthma, and psoriasis may be stress-related. They may not see, however, that generalized stress and anxiety, leading to lack of sleep, appetite disturbance, and so on, in turn leading to a lowered resistance and followed by the onset of whatever an individual may be genetically or environmentally predisposed to—from cancer to the flu—might also be called "psychosomatic." Some seizures can be brought on by different purposeful or semipurposeful behaviors (from exposure to flashing lights, to continued alcohol consumption) as surely as a chronic seizure disorder may precipitate a depression. The effect of illness upon the psyche is the other side of the psychosomatic "coin."

Health teaching in the realm of psychosomatics should be done routinely. It is sometimes helpful to explain simple interactions of mind and body for the patient to demonstrate the integration. They can be reminded of how a person blushes when told an off-color joke, how his stomach feels like "butterflies" when he is excited, or how his heart pounds when a dog barks suddenly.

The nurse can be invaluable in intervening when a situation arises in which a patient is upset because the doctor has told her that "there is nothing wrong." If the patient has pain, the nurse can convey an understanding of how much that pain is affecting the patient, and allow for the fact that not all disease entities can be determined by an episodic examination by a house officer in an emergency room. The experience of pain is subject to wide alterations even within the same individual. Pain that comes from an unknown source perceived as potentially fatal (such as severe, undiagnosed abdominal pain) might be felt more than pain that is stronger in intensity but purposeful and understood to be without serious consequences.

The use of placebos to separate out "real pain" is often borne of ignorance. Abundant, though little-appreciated research on the subject shows us that about one third of this country's population are "placebo reactors." That is to say, they would obtain relief from an inactive substance, no matter what the cause of the pain. Given that there are so many variables (such as the degree of concern of the caretaker and the confidence the patient has in this caretaker), all the "test" proves is whether or not the patient is "placebo positive" (Hackett, 1971). Some patients focus on pain and illness that they may *need* rather than facing their real source of anguish.

Whatever the cause of the patient's pain or malady, the nurse is best advised to be sympathetic and understanding and validate the patient's pain. If the patient does have related concerns, it is in an atmosphere of acceptance, not criticism, that they will be most permitted to open up, rather than struggle over whether or not there is pain.

Valuable health teaching can and should be done in the emergency department about the chronic physiological effects of stress on the body's systems (cardiovascular, gastrointestinal, and so on). Patients should be encouraged to be in touch with their emotional and physical selves, their effects on each other, and how to help control these effects.

Manipulative patient

The first step for the nurse dealing with the manipulative patient is to identify the fact that he is being manipulative. Trying to understand the needs that prompt the behavior and what the patient is expressing through the behavior is a good beginning. Is the patient feeling hostility, dependency, anxiety? Is he seeking infinite love? The nurse might confront the patient *be-*

fore becoming angry, rather than *after,* while still remaining objective. Is the constant demand for attention motivated by fear? It is helpful to take a positive approach. Giving the patient respect and the benefit of the doubt, the nurse can be firm in limit setting if not doing it with anger. One might say to the patient, "Surely you can understand why I can't spend too much time in this room, although I'd like to," or, "You understand, of course, that this is an emergency department, and it's simply impossible for us to be prescribing anything but emergency drugs." Nurses should identify their own feelings. A patient who feels he has been wronged might strike out and find an Achilles heel in a nurse, who should keep in mind that the nurse is a target, not the source, of the patient's anger.

If the patient is extremely unreasonable, the nurse might say that although respecting the patient's right to his own feelings and opinions, she or he disagrees. When all efforts are exhausted, and a patient does not seem to have an urgent condition, but is detrimental to the treatment of the other patients in the emergency department, he may have to be asked to leave. The fact that a person comes to the emergency department does not necessarily mean that something can (or should) be done, our idealism notwithstanding.

Homosexual panic

Freud developed the thesis that paranoia arises when homosexual trends escape repression. Cases of homosexual panic, although infrequent, are seen in the emergency department. The reaction seems to occur in a latent homosexual who is exposed to dormitories or barracks with other men for the first time, and whose already overburdened ego renders him incapable of coping with the situation. He fears that the latent wishes will become conscious, and such fear may result in the individual's becoming extremely anxious and confused to the point of hallucinations. The patient may make agitated attempts to escape the inarticulated fears. Removing the stress situation, bolstering the ego through reassuring human conversation, sedation, and rest may or may not cause the episode to subside. Hospitalization may need to be considered. While in the emergency department, physical contact should be limited, and when it is necessary, prefaced with warning and reassurance, as the patient may overreact, thinking that he is being assaulted. He should be cared for by female personnel as much as possible. Medication should be given orally, avoiding injections and anxiety-provoking intrusive procedures.

PSYCHIATRIC MEDICATIONS IN THE EMERGENCY DEPARTMENT

The best advice concerning the use of psychiatric drugs in the emergency department is *not* to use them. Whenever possible, medicating patients in, or dispensing prescriptions from, such a transient and episodic area as the emergency department should be avoided. Very often, interpersonal intervention can accomplish much more good and do far less harm than drugs. However, medications to manage and afford relief to the severely disturbed patient in the emergency department are sometimes necessary. When, and if, to medicate are often difficult decisions, especially in light of the fact that diagnoses are seldom clear-cut and reliable. If diagnostic certainty is not possible, the risk of medicating the patient must be carefully weighed against the consequences of *not* medicating the patient.

Haloperidol (Haldol) is, in many emergency department situations, the drug of choice for attenuation of the commonly problematic severe agitation, psychomotor hyperactivity, assaultiveness, mania, and the extreme mental anguish of an acute psychosis. It seems to be the safest medication for these purposes, with rare instances of the hypotension that is a more common occurrence with chlorpromazine (Thorazine), which is also an effective antipsychotic with a more sedative effect. Because of this lack of pronounced sedation, haloperidol seems to be less threatening to the paranoid patient, who may be afraid of being "put to sleep." Dystonic reactions (see pp. 547-548) are infrequent and seem to occur more often and become problematic when the patient is given lowest oral doses rather than IM doses. Inasmuch as it is possible, the nurse should check

for allergies to medication; obtain baseline vital signs—in particular, the blood pressure; and determine and report suspicion of any other drugs or alcohol that the patient may have ingested—even days or weeks before admission, with special attention given to a positive history of using CNS depressants. Blood pressure and general patient condition should be monitored carefully and frequently after administration of medication to any patient, but particularly those whose mental and emotional status is compromised. These patients may not be able to give feedback regarding the effect of the medication nor understand its purpose. The initial IM dose of haloperidol is 0.5 to 5.0 mg, with subsequent doses in the same range every 30 to 60 minutes. It is my experience that a 40-minute interval between doses prevents unnecessary somnolence due to the rapid administration of additional doses, and should be observed unless the patient's safety demands that a dose be administered slightly sooner. Infrequent side effects of lowered seizure threshold and cholinergic blocking can occur. Contraindications to using haloperidol are pregnancy, hypersensitivity, narrow-angle glaucoma, CNS depression, and severe cardiac disease with arrhythmia. It is commonly in the emergency department for acute schizophrenia, alcoholic hallucinosis, and emergency sedation with uncertain diagnosis. Results with those with whom the drug is appropriately used are often dramatic. Thought disorders improve significantly with few and minimal side effects. The danger involved with this drug is that it often works *so* well that emergency department staff see the patient as cured. They may be more inclined to discharge a patient who does not have social supports or ability to continue with the medication, and who will probably again become sick when the medication wears off.

Two commonly used minor tranquilizers, or antianxiety agents are chlordiazepoxide (Librium) and diazepam (Valium). The initial IM adult dose of chlordiazepoxide is 25 to 50 mg, with 25- to 100-mg subsequent doses every 1 to 2 hours. Doses given orally range from 5 to 25 mg, with 5- to 25-mg subsequent doses, up to 100 mg daily. Initial IM doses of diazepam range from 5 to 10 mg, with 5- to 10-mg doses every 1 to 2 hours. The oral dosage ranges from 2 to 10 mg, up to 40 mg daily. When chlordiazepoxide or diazepam are used for the management of acute withdrawal from alcohol, higher doses may be required, depending on the severity of the withdrawal. Chlordiazepoxide, 50 to 100 mg, may be followed by repeated doses, as needed, until agitation is controlled, up to 300 mg per day. Diazepam 10 mg 3 to 4 times daily during the first 24 hours is also recommended. With both medications, drowsiness and ataxia are frequently encountered side effects. Confusion, hypotension, prolonged sedation, and paradoxical excitement are less common. The last, called "Valium rage" when induced by that drug, is a distinct emergency department management problem.

Oxazepam (Serax) has been found efficacious in the treatment of a wide variety of disorders—anxiety, tension, agitation and irritability, and anxiety associated with depression. An oral medication, oxazepam seems to be safer in terms of tolerance and toxicity than other related compounds such as chlordiazepoxide and diazepam. Dosages of 10 to 30 mg, up to 120 mg per day, are suggested. This drug might be considered when a prescription is being given a patient in the emergency department. As with all prescriptions given in the emergency department, the number should be limited to less than would produce serious consequences if taken together at one time. Before being given a sizeable prescription, the patient should be asked honestly and with concern if he has experienced any suicidal ideation or if self-destructive behavior is a possibility. The patient should then be referred to a less episodic resource to further medication and other support, if necessary.

TOXIC REACTIONS: ORGANIC AND CHEMICAL

To arrive at a differential diagnosis with a patient who exhibits bizarre or exaggerated emotional behavior, it is essential to consider organic and chemical precipitants before deciding that it's "all in the patient's head" or that he is "strictly psychotic." The more experienced emergency nurses become, the more instances they will recall in which an intoxicated or organically poisoned patient, dubbed a "psychiatric patient," suffered because of the hastily applied label. It is a disservice to any patient to regard different or exaggerated behavior as anything but physiologically based until proved otherwise. Too often, it works the opposite way. Every patient deserves a thorough physical examination, a full set of vital signs, blood work for toxic screen as well as routine studies, and a good history from relatives and friends and other institutions, as well as the patient himself—even if he does not appreciate the need or is unable to fully cooperate with the procedures because of an organic or "functional" disease process.

Alcohol-related emergencies

Alcohol-related emergencies are common in most emergency departments and have become more so since the recognition of alcohol as a disease rather than a criminal offense. Police in many parts of the country now are mandated to bring an alcoholic to an emergency unit or detoxification center rather than to jail. Although the alcohol is a psychiatric illness from one vantage point, it should always be considered first and foremost in the emergency department setting as a medical emergency. Acute alcohol intoxication may result in death. An acutely intoxicated person is more likely to sustain a head injury and less likely to relate an accurate history or present a clearcut diagnostic picture. Chronically intoxicated persons are often chronically sick. They often have many medical conditions. Nutritional deficiencies with mental sequelae—such as Wernicke and Korsakoff syndromes—seizure disorders, tuberculosis, hepatic coma, alcoholic hallucinosis, and delirium tremens are frequently seen and should be kept in mind.

As much history as possible should be obtained about every intoxicated patient. If the patient is not able to relate information, whoever brings the patient to the emergency department should be asked about the patient. Obtaining telephone numbers of the patient's relatives, friends, landlord, and so on is particularly helpful. These people may be able to tell you what and how much the patient drinks, what his behavior baseline is like, whether he has currently stopped drinking, what his behavior is like when he drinks, when he stops, and when he involuntarily withdraws. The presence of blackouts (periods during which the patient is drinking when he continues to function, but later does not recall) is particularly indicative of chronic severe alcoholism. A particularly helpful question is whether the patient has been "sick" lately. Has he, in particular, been vomiting for the past couple days, and consequently been unable to keep down the normal amount of liquor? The patient may be in withdrawal, although he may deny that he has stopped drinking. The possibility of drugs taken in combination with alcohol should always be suspected at the beginning of the patient's emergency department visit—not 5 hours later when the patient is obtunded as a result of a serious overdose that went without consideration.

At the same time the emergency department is assessing the alcohol-affected patient, there is often the question of immediate management of a potentially disruptive and possibly dangerous patient. Intoxication produces confusion, moroseness, combativeness, regression, and generalized lack of inhibitions.

A safe environment must be provided while the patient is being evaluated and subsequently sobering. He should be positioned on his stomach or side, especially if restraints are required, to prevent aspiration. The possibility of the patient's vomiting or seizing should always be kept in mind. Accordingly, the patient's restraints should be kept loose to prevent injuries to soft tissue or bones in the event of a seizure.

After an initial evaluation, watchful waiting while the patient ideally has some restorative sleep without unnecessary active intervention is the safest and most desirable approach. Caffeine in any form may precipitate seizures, and sedatives may potentiate the alcohol. The patient's behavior may be such that he presents an imminent danger to himself or others. Occasionally, a patient will be extremely "bounc-ing off the walls" hopelessly suicidal, and actively self-destructive. In the event that the patient does not respond to the structure and intervention of the emergency department after a reasonable amount of time, a very small, almost subtherapeutic dose of haloperidol has been used very effectively with a resultant calm, rational, apologetic patient. With this, as with other medications, the desired effects must be weighed against the possibilities of respiratory depression and coma in the situation of excessive alcohol intoxication. Haloperidol seems to have much less an effect of CNS depression than other tranquilizers.

A very objective, sympathetic approach should be used with every intoxicated person. A punitive approach is counterproductive and may result in the patient's becoming a greater management problem or finding reinforcement for his already negative self-image. Nurses' responses to the verbal abuse of an intoxicated patient are indicative not only of their maturity, self-confidence, and level of professionalism, but also of their understanding of the disease of alcoholism and an appreciation of the alcoholic's past and present psychic pain.

An alcoholic's affect may range from the morose to the euphoric—the latter often belying his true feelings.

The nurse should remain kind and supportive, indicating a belief in his basic good worthiness and expecting the best behavior possible from the patient. Serious consideration should be given to what the patient says while intoxicated, whether it be suicidal ideation or information about situational stresses. However, it is often not productive to spend long periods of time talking with a patient who is very intoxicated. Although he may feel uninhibited enough to divulge painful information, the very intoxicated individual may not remember what was said and may feel very differently upon sobering. A case in point is the patient who arrives in an agitated, suicidal state lamenting that there is nothing to live for, only to leave 4 hours later wondering what happened and quite surprised when asked if he'd like to talk to someone about the way he's feeling.

Ideally, every intoxicated patient should have

at least some evaluation of the circumstances that led to his intoxication and the overall pattern of his use of the drug. A good way to being with a patient who may dismiss, understate, or deny the incident is to gently, positively, in the least threatening way possible, make such commentary as the following:

"I'm sure finding yourself in the emergency department is not an everyday occurrence for you. You must be surprised."

"Although the emergency department is glad to help you, there might be something that could be done to prevent further such visits."

"Is drinking giving you more bad feelings than good ones lately?"

"I'm concerned that during your period of intoxication you could have been seriously hurt from all reports of your activity."

"Does this worry you at all?"

The person with an alcohol problem may be more likely to return for follow-up treatment to the same institution with which he has become familiar through his emergency department visit, and which he sees as "knowing his situation" more than another. The first and the biggest step for any person with alcoholism is admitting that the problem exists. It may take less courage to do that if a foundation and tone of trust and help are set during the emergency department visit—perhaps the patient's only contact with helping professionals.

If what the patient says is at variance with what others have said about his drinking, he should be matter-of-factly told, but the nurse should be careful not to engage in a battle as to whether the patient had three or four drinks or whether or not he has a problem. It only puts the patient on the defensive and just increases his denial. If there is time, an exploration of ways in which harmful drinking behavior can be modified might be helpful. The important message is that there is genuine concern on the nurse's part, not an effort to get the patient out of the emergency department as fast as possible. (Depending on the patient, referrals to AA, alcohol clinics, individual therapists, detoxification centers, or halfway houses may be in order. The families of such patients may need support, ventilation, reality testing, and referral themselves. There is usually an alcoholism information and referral source available if where to refer someone is a problem.)

If there is alcoholism within the patient's family, there is greater likelihood, whether because of genetic or environmental factors, of the patient's becoming an alcoholic. This should be presented in a matter-of-fact way, much as you would caution a patient with diabetes in his family.

Alcohol-induced states that may be confused with psychiatric illness per se are delirium tremens, alcoholic hallucinosis, alcohol paranoid state, Wernicke syndrome, and Korsakoff syndrome.

Delirium tremens is an acute, potentially fatal medical emergency. Although the patient's behavior is psychotic, the differential diagnosis can be made quickly on the basis of history, physical appearance, and behavior. The patient is often anxious, extremely agitated, and diaphoretic, and has fine tremors, visual hallucinations, a "picking motion" of the fingers, and elevated vital signs. The delirium is usually preceded by restlessness, irritability, an aversion to food, tremulousness, and disturbed sleep.

Alcoholic hallucinosis exists on a continuum with delirium tremens. The patient is often oriented to time, place, and person and may not be tremulous. This particular patient may resemble a schizophrenic. A differential diagnosis is important since the patient requires prompt and careful medical evaluation and hospitalization, rather than psychiatric hospitalization. A medical admission is necessary, as many psychiatric facilities are ill equipped and unable to deliver medical care, even though many doctors are reluctant to hospitalize someone they see as a psychiatric case who presents many potential management problems. The patient may experience auditory hallucinations of a threatening nature with ideas of reference and an elaborate delusional system.

The patient is likely to respond to his hallucinations and ideas, conversing with and acting upon them. The symptoms may wax and wane in the emergency department, giving a clue to the toxic nature of the situation. Wernicke syndrome and Korsakoff syndrome are due to the nutritional deficit, especially of thiamine and niacin, often accompanying alcoholism. Wernicke syndrome involves brainstem destruction, whereas in Korsakoff syndrome, degeneration is mainly in the cerebrum and peripheral nerves.

Signs and symptoms of Wernicke syndrome include ophthalmoplegia, apathy or apprehension, clouding of consciousness, and even coma. Korsakoff syndrome involves disorientation to time and place and peripheral neuropathy. An especially helpful diagnostic clue in both conditions is the presence of memory impairment (especially recent memory) and confabulation (covering up for memory deficit by "filling in false details").

Drug-related problems

There are many theories and postulations about drug-dependence, which are beyond the scope of this chapter. Whether the psychodynamics includes regression, fixations at pregenital levels of psychosexual development, passive dependency, passive aggression, preferred modes of dealing with stress such as indifference and withdrawal, peer acceptance of pressure; or, whether the patient is medicating an illness that is more than characterological in nature, such as depresson or schizophrenia; or whether he seeks relief from unbearable tensions, two points should be remembered:

1. The patient is usually emotionally needy and vulnerable and has suffered, or felt he has suffered, to the point where he feels he deserves help.
2. The patient may be emotionally draining and/or manipulative, and may evoke mixed feelings from the emergency department practitioner.

The practitioner therefore must combine self-confidence with kindness and set reasonable but firm limits with such patients.

In planning for referral or individual or family counseling in the emergency department, the nurses should keep in mind the individual needs of the particular type of patient they are

dealing with: The needs of the young include peer support, a sense of identity, self-esteem, purpose, involvement, a place to go, people to "fit in with," and a positive role in society. The needs for the elderly patient might include company, purpose, activity, and better medical care. Women might need the means to obtain a life outside the home such as day care, transportation, and vocational skills. Homophiles may need social acceptance, self-understanding, acceptance of their sexual orientation, and perhaps the peer-counselor support from a homophile resource. Veterans may need help with the social, economic, and mental adjustment of leaving the service or help with an addiction developed while in the military. Referrals and advice, then, would differ according to the individuals and their situations (Tyler, 1977).

Addicted patients seeking drugs in the emergency department are a fairly common situation, especially in larger urban hospitals. Patients may request paregoric for a teething child or mimic the symptoms of kidney stones, even pricking their finger to drop blood in their urine sample. They may say they are allergic to codeine and pentazocine lactate (Talwin) and ask specifically for oxycodone (Percodan) or meperidine (Demerol) when being treated for a whiplash. They may be desperate enough to steal prescription blanks from the hospital or change a prescription given them.

Emergency department practitioners should be alert, though not suspicious or punitive when treating possible drug-addicted patients. Needle marks can be observed while taking blood pressure. (Take it in the arm that the patient *doesn't* offer.) Yawning, pinpoint or enlarged pupils, sneezing and nervousness, reddened nose from scratching or rubbing, unusual thirst, slurred speech, and a general physically run-down appearance (weight loss, unkempt appearance, dental caries) might point to drug dependence.

Heroin and methadone. With the popularity of heroin and the number of methadone-dependent persons maintained at outpatient clinics, the emergency department encounters many patients who are specifically requesting relief from withdrawal symptoms or the possibility thereof. It has been the policy of many larger hospitals confronted with this problem to be firm in not giving anything but symptomatic relief from symptoms, that is, prochlorperazine (Compazine) for nausea and vomiting, Kaopectate for diarrhea, diazepam (Valium) for agitation, and referral to other facilities for maintenance or detoxification. Oftentimes, patients may be more afraid of possibly withdrawing than actually suffering from the withdrawal itself. They may experience acute anxiety around their need for drugs. An abuser may come to the emergency department on a weekend evening saying that he is on a program in another state and in need of his methadone dose. Three things should be kept in mind in such situations:

1. The drug-dependent person did not become that overnight, and the urgency and anxiety he may create about the situation may not belong there.
2. Most maintenance programs have rules and regulations and contingency plans (such as planning for a patient to get his medication in another state if he is traveling, or another center in the area if it is necessary) with which the patient is very familiar.
3. Methadone stays in the patient's system for approximately 48 hours. It is not until 24 to 36 hours that withdrawal symptoms begin, so that there is a sufficient period of grace to allow a patient to skip a day if unavoidable.

Methadone patients usually do not know their dose, and the history of how many bags of heroin is used per day is unreliable for many reasons. Therefore the individual and symptomatic treatment in the emergency department is best. Patients who are exhibiting withdrawal usually manifest symptoms of pupil dilatation, increased blood pressure, pulse, and respirations (upwards of 24), restlessness, stomach cramps, nausea and vomiting, diaphoresis, low back pain, yawning, and tearing. If significant withdrawal is present and the need to treat the patient specifically is in order, it might be best to give methadone rather than meperidine

(Demerol) or other such drug. Meperidine or morphine is needed in fairly large doses every 4 hours, whereas methadone relieves the symptoms for some time. The methadone should be given in 5- or 10-mg increments, titrating the medication while closely watching the pupil size become smaller, the vital signs come down, and the other symptoms abate.

Resources available for drug-addicted persons, or at least a number for a drug-referral source, should be listed in the emergency department. Before making referrals, determine what facilities the patient already knows about and/or has used and which he can or can't use at this time. Members of the drug community may be better informed than the nurse in many instances, and valuable time spent in phone-calling may be eliminated with careful interviewing.

Barbiturates. Barbiturate dependence is an increasing problem in our society. Our emergency departments see patients with barbiturate intoxication or withdrawal problems frequently. Long-acting barbiturates such as phenobarbital (Luminal) are generally less toxic and have less dramatic withdrawal effects than the shorter-acting amobarbital (Amytal), pentobarbital (Nembutal), or secobarbital (Seconal). Other sedatives and the so-called "minor tranquilizers" may also produce barbiturate-type dependence to a lesser degree. These include diazepam (Valium), chlordiazepoxide (Librium), meprobamate (Miltown), methyprylon (Noludar), and glutethimide (Doriden). Diminished alertness, confusion, lateral gaze, nystagmus, dysarthria, ataxia, and emotional instability are seen in patients who are barbiturate-intoxicated. The emotional instability of these patients frequently has a paranoid aggressive character, and their tendency toward destructiveness and combativeness in the emergency department makes them a particularly difficult management problem. The successful control of this type of patient requires a very neutral, objective approach to their care. Negative verbal and nonverbal communications by emergency department personnel can be blown out of proportion and overreacted to by the patient. The drug has the effect of removing inhibitions and bringing to the surface an intense affectual component of unresolved feelings. People who might otherwise glibly and without emotion talk of problems, when intoxicated weep bitterly, exhibit aggression, and vent anger and frustration. Since barbiturates are one of the most frequently used drugs in suicide attempts and the most common cause of drug fatalities, the emergency department practitioner should be very aware of the potential for abuse when patients are given prescriptions in the emergency department, and make sure prescriptions are limited.

Hallucinogens. LSD "bad trips" seem to be an increasingly rare phenomenon in emergency departments today. However, the frightening and dangerous effects of other hallucinogens—mescaline, tetrahydrocannabinol (THC), and combinations including these and others are not at all uncommon. The patients who come to the emergency department usually have anxiety, hyperactivity, and sympathetic nervous system signs—pupil dilation and increased vital signs. Symptoms seem to be a function of dose; low doses produce euphoric responses, and high doses produce a hallucinatory psychosis.

With this and other drug-induced psychosis, patients seem more disorganized, have less motor retardation, and are more excited than their counterparts suffering from schizophrenia. They also show better histories of socialization, more intelligence and have better premorbid work records (Cole, Freedman, and Friedhoff, 1973). These factors should be kept in mind when gathering a history about a patient with a questionable diagnosis. The patient usually has some insight to help the practitioner. Supportive care in a reassuring environment is helpful. One familiar person who is unquestionably trusted by the patient staying with that patient continuously is invaluable, and lends an aspect of reality testing to the patient's condition. Diazepam (Valium) orally is the medication most generally accepted. Phenothiazine compounds may exaggerate the psychotic reaction in some instances.

Belladonna alkaloids. Drugs of the belladonna group can cause severe delirium and psychotic manifestations. Associated symptoms include blurred vision, dry mouth, and difficult urination. Weakness, hallucinations, acute disturbances of the sensorism, rapid, weak pulse, flushing and dryness of skin, widely dilated pupils, and an extremely elevated temperature are signs of toxicity. As in all toxic reactions to drugs, attempts at sedation with more drugs is always best avoided because of the possibility of potentiating CNS depression, causing an idiosyncratic reaction, and/or clouding the clinical picture. If absolutely necessary, small doses of sedatives should be given. Physostigmine salicylate given IM is a specific antidote. Suspect belladonna toxicity when drugs including atropine (such as Donnatal and Donnagel) or scopolamine (such as Nytol and Sominex) are involved. Some plants contain belladonna alkaloids and, when ingested, cause atropine-like effects (see p. 623). The patient should be given fluids, catheterized if necessary, and provided a quiet atmosphere with minimal stimulation.

Bromide toxicity. Although an infrequent problem, bromide toxicity (from potassium, sodium, ammonium) is one that the emergency department practitioner should be aware of. The effects can be similar to psychiatric symptomatology. The sequelae comprise four distinct entities: simple bromide intoxication, hallucinosis, delirium, and transitory schizophrenia associated with paranoid symptomatology.

SIMPLE BROMIDE INTOXICATION. Though oriented, the patient lacks coordination and seems sluggish, forgetful, irritable, and exhibits irregular pupils that may be slow to react or be fixed to light.

DELIRIUM. The most common manifestation of toxicity, it characteristically includes disorientation. There may be mood disturbances, restlessness, inability to sleep, delusions, and hallucinations.

TRANSITORY SCHIZOPHRENIA. Associated with paranoid symptomatology and disturbed rapport and affect, the patient may have had a schizoid premorbid personality and have taken bromides over a period of time for some neurotic symptom. There may or may not be disorientation.

BROMIDE HALLUCINOSIS. The patient remains well oriented in spite of his hallucinations.

Whenever an acute, "unusual" psychiatric presentation is encountered, careful history taking (well water was the source of bromide in one particular case familiar to me) and attention to physical findings and bromide level (150 to 200 mg/100 ml is considered toxic) are in order to afford the patient the benefit of definitive therapy.

Marijuana. Marijuana popularity is second only to alcohol for a sizable portion of our society, and its use is widely condoned. Its psychological dependence and physiologically negative effects create a potential for distraction from school/work and so on that cannot be overlooked, however. Problems arising from marijuana use are often in the form of anxiety attacks. The patient may have increased vital signs, palpitations, hyperventilation, apprehension, restlessness, preoccupation, and the feeling of imminent death. These patients are often helped to a great degree by a nurse or designate staying with the patient. He may be given diazepam by mouth and reassurance as to physical symptoms. Though the reaction may be immediately precipitated by the marijuana, the patient's problems often include current overwhelming stresses and a predisposition toward anxiety attacks.

Conversely, when a patient enters with what appears to be an anxiety attack, he should be questioned as to drug use (being reminded that police will not be given the information). Other drugs (cocaine, for example) may trigger an anxiety reaction in a patient who might be reluctant to mention using it. Without that information, we are unable to reassure the patient that the particular substance will not be lethal, and he remains inexplicably frightened after all our calming measures are exhausted.

Phencyclidine. PCP, or phencyclidine, warrants a few words in light of its popularity (it is the third most widely abused drug in many sections of our country) and its attendant dangers are different in quality and quantity from any other widely abused drug.

Originally developed in the late 1950s as an anesthetic for humans, its use was discontinued because of untoward psychological sequelae, and it is now used infrequently with animals. On the street, the drug soon earned a reputation for bad side-effects, which led to its being passed off as, or combined with, other drugs such as THC and mescaline. Differential diagnosis of PCP poisoning in the emergency department is difficult, since phencyclidine is thought to mimic, precipitate, and/or exaggerate psychiatric illness. A patient may present a picture of anxiety, psychosis, toxicity, or organicity. The degree of severity of the pictures vary greatly. Pharmacologically, PCP is an analgesic, with sympathomimetic and central nervous system stimulant and depressant properties. A constellation of signs I find particularly helpful in identifying a PCP poisoning include acute onset of unusual behavior in a young patient with history of intermittent drug abuse, elevated systolic and diastolic blood pressure, small pupils, and vertical nystagmus.

Signs also include, in low to moderate doses, ataxia, increased deep tendon reflexes, clonus, tremors, amnesia, anxiety/agitation, image distortion, euphoria, increased pulse and blood pressure, nausea and vomiting, and increased urine output. In high doses, signs include slurred speech, drowsiness, decreased deep tendon reflexes, convulsions, opisthotonus, coma, decreased respiratory rate, respiratory arrest, depersonalization, disordered thought processes, hallucinations, psychopathology, arrhythmias, decreased blood pressure, and decreased urine output. Fatalities seem to be related to seizures and respiratory arrest.

The history of a person who abuses drugs may be consistent with that of someone likely to manifest psychiatric problems. PCP may come in many forms—tablet, powder, leaf mixture for making cigarettes, and rock crystal. The patient may think he has smoked pot when it actually has been laced with PCP. Add to this the fact that symptoms may appear, and often do, up to many days later, and the difficulty of a definite diagnosis becomes apparent.

There is a tendency to treat PCP toxicity similarly to the way a bad LSD trip is treated; this can be a disservice to the patient. Whereas reassurance may be helpful with someone who is on a bad LSD trip, persons with PCP poisoning respond better to the least amount of stimulation—visual, auditory, and tactile. Caretakers should be limited to one person; the patient should be placed in a dimly lit room that is as quiet as possible. Constant observation or restraints may be in order for those significant reactions. LSD users will usually report ingesting the drug under 12 hours before admission, and usually follow a predictably improving course, recovering within 1 to 2 days. The sequelae of PCP poisoning may culminate in an emergency department presentation days after its ingestion. Its course is unpredictable and may manifest itself intermittently for days, weeks, or longer.

Blood and urine (urine is more desirable for detection purposes) should be obtained for toxicological studies. Calculated blood levels as low as 0.06 mg/100 ml caused toxic psychosis and hallucinations in over 50% of patients tested in one study.

Phenothiazines (Thorazine and so on) should be avoided as they are chemically similar to phencyclidine, and may potentiate its effect or produce an anticholinergic crisis. Haloperidol, however, has been found useful by many practitioners, its composition differing significantly from that of PCP. The response to the drug is often a relief of symptoms so dramatic that the patient may be thought cured and be released, when, in fact, symptoms are likely to return as the medication wears off. Diazepam is also recommended to control agitation and may be helpful in the control of seizures associated with larger doses of PCP. An emerging concept of PCP management theorizes that since the drug is a weak electrolyte (base) that is readily ionized in an acid medium, there is extensive secretion into the gastric acidity where it becomes trapped because of the impenetrability of membranes to ions. Management with gastric suction, saline laxative, and acidification of urine and serum by this group of researchers has shown successful results.

The possibility for the need of hospitalization should always be kept in mind with cases of PCP toxicity.

Also to be remembered is the opportunity for preventive health teaching in the emergency department. The emergency department practitioner should convey, without blanketly condemning drug use per se, that the PCP chemical is a *relatively* dangerous choice.

Opiates and related compounds. When subcutaneously administered doses are compared for analgesic activity, the opiates and related compounds are listed, in order of ascending strength, as follows: codeine (Darvon roughly equivalent), meperidine (Demerol), morphine (Dolophine roughly equivalent), heroin, and dihydromorphinone (Dilaudid). The effects of these drugs, and morphine in particular, that are of major clinical interest are those mediated by actions on the CNS, although certain side effects are produced by actions on other structures: flushing and itching of the skin by release of histamine, constipation by decrease of propulsive movements of the intestines coupled with spasmogenic actions on contractile movements of the intestinal tract and on sphincters.

In mild cases, opiate poisoning may be treated by vigorous and continued sensory stimulation and gastric lavage if the drug has recently been taken orally. In more severe cases, airway and support of respirations are the primary focus. When heroin overdose is strongly suspected in the comatose patient, naloxone (Narcan) is usually the narcotic antagonist of choice, because it does not add to the respiratory depression. Naloxone is diagnostic as well as therapeutic in its often dramatic treatment of opiate overdoses. Relatively small doses of this and other antagonists to opiates precipitate violent abstinence phenomena.

The seasoned emergency department practitioner is all too familiar with the scenario that transpires when the drug-addicted person who is brought in comatose is given naloxone. Within seconds, the patient is awake and flailing, acutely dysphoric, uncomfortable, and confused, with emergency department personnel on each extremity. Anticipation of this occurrence and intervention can preclude injuries and/or a patient who abruptly leaves. Side rails on the stretcher should be quickly brought up as the naloxone is being given, and personnel should be designated to control the patient. Loose restraints may be applied if there is time. As soon as the medication is administered and the patient is alert, the staff should make it clear to the patient that his discomfort is appreciated and that it will be time-limited. Explanation of how the patient got to the hospital and what is being done for him is in order. Especially in the case of the person taking methadone, the naloxone will wear off within a few hours, and the methadone still in his system will offer relief. The danger of respiratory depression returning as the naloxone wears off is a very real threat, and patients should be kept well beyond 4 hours after administering the antidote. Precipitous departures should be discouraged with simple but compelling explanation. If the patient is insistent, arrangements with friends and relatives should be arranged. With some show of concern and a few measures of comfort for the patient (a cup of coffee or a supervised cigarette smoke), cooperation can usually be attained.

Dystonic reactions to phenothiazines. Dystonic reactions can be easily mistaken for tetanus, calcium deficiency, seizures, and a host of other misdiagnoses. Most often, however, a dystonic reaction is seen as a hysterical conversion or posturing in the psychiatric patient or a malingering for drugs or other secondary benefit by a drug abuser. The psychiatric patient is often unable to relate an articulate history and symptomatology, and may even regress under the stress of the interview and the frightening and painful effects of the antipsychotic—perhaps haloperidol. The vascillating nature of the symptomatology is typical, but often causes staff to pass the symptoms off. For the young person who has bought a pill on the street he thought to be Valium or a hallucinogenic, it may seem unsafe to tell the staff what has happened for fear that his family or the police will be notified. Or, he may have taken the pill 4 or 5 days before and not even associated the two. In a large percentage of cases, the symptoms do not appear for 4 to 5 days after an oral dose. Thus, the history makes the diagnosis of a relatively clear-cut reaction often confusing.

It behooves the emergency department nurse to learn what Haldol, Prolixin, Compazine, Stelazine, and Thorazine (common offenders) pills look like and to show patients a *Physician's Desk Reference* for positive identification, since many patients don't know pills by name. Even if the history is not clear, when the following signs and symptoms are present, treatment might be considered (Lee, 1977).

1. Oculogyric crisis—upward rotation of the eyes into the head.
2. Buccolingual crisis—protruding or retracting of the tongue, facial grimacing; patient feels as though his tongue is being pulled back.
3. Torticollic crisis—severe contractions of neck muscles, retrocollic or torticollic.

The first three are often seen in combination.

4. Opisthotonic crisis—opisthotonic reaction, scoliosis, lordosis.
5. Tortipelvic crisis—spasm of abdominal wall, abdominal pain, bizarre gait, lordosis, kyphosis.

Results of treatment are usually fast and dramatic; diphenhydramine (Benadryl), benztropine (Cogentin), or trihexyphenidyl (Artane) may be used. Since the half-life of phenothiazines is 24 hours, the patient must be given medication orally to prevent the return of symptoms for the next 2 or 3 days.

Nursing considerations should include early anxiety reduction to facilitate an accurate history initially. The drug abuser might be reminded that personnel will not divulge his story to anyone else. The patient should be reassured that the symptoms are easily and completely reversible. The nurse should convey her ability to handle the situation and let the patient know that this happens to many people. The symptoms are terrifying especially to those patients who are normally unable to cope and susceptible to delusions. The temptation to tell a psychiatric patient to stop taking the medication should be considered carefully. The particular medication may be the drug of choice for the patient who might become very psychotic without it. Ideally, the patient's physician should be notified and the patient told to contact that physician for advice as soon as possible. The patient should be told that his medication is a good one with controllable side effects that many medications have. This reinforces the patient's faith in his doctor and the medications he prescribes and reassures the patient.

ACUTE BRAIN SYNDROME

There is a tendency among emergency department personnel to view bizarre behavior negatively. It is often considered functional rather than organic in cause until proved otherwise. If the patient *looks* crazy, then he *is*. If he doesn't want help, then he shouldn't be given it. That help may, indeed, be given reluctantly. In many instances, however, the nature of the organic (or functional) illness is such that the patient is not capable of good judgment or decision making. Whether the patient has a psychiatric history or not, he deserves to have emergency department personnel search out, methodically and logically, all possible causes for his illness. He should be given the benefit of blood work for CBC, electrolytes, sugar, toxic screen, a neurological workup, etc. The rationale for a thorough investigation of causes of abnormal behavior is that many times, as in the case of acute organic brain syndrome, the pathologic condition is transient and reversible.

With acute organic brain syndrome (AOBS) there is usually biochemical or structural impairment. Characteristics include disturbed level of consciousness and cognition, clouding, physical abnormalities including the pulse and focal reflexes, and presence of delirium. Symptoms include:

1. Behavioral changes—dependent on premorbid personality (that is, the normally suspicious person becomes paranoid)
2. Vascillating symptomatology—sometimes leading the professional to think that the patient is ''fooling'' or that he is better and can be released.
3. Appearance—the patient's affect may be vacant. He may be disheveled, preoccupied, inappropriate, and weird, with purposeless movements (picking or itch-

ing), general agitation, lethargy, darting eyes that are glossy or dull.
4. Speech—slurring, perseveration, and echolalia may be present.
5. Affect—may be variable, labile.
6. Thought content—major diagnostic differentiator between organic and functional illness, includes a continuum of wakefulness or somnolence, inability to focus attention, distractibility by exogenous or endogenous things, inability to grasp meanings, and disorientation that depends on the severity and progression of the illness. The patient will be disoriented to time first, then place, then person. A great proportion of patients with acute organic brain syndrome will be disoriented.
7. Visual hallucinations—sometimes mere distortions of what the patient actually sees; visual hallucinations are more common than auditory ones.

Probably most common among the acute organic brain syndromes are those associated with drug or poison intoxication (see Chapter 27). Other acute brain syndromes are associated with the following:

1. Circulatory disturbances producing cerebral vascular insufficiency.
2. Disturbances in metabolism or nutrition, such as hypoglycemia or hypokalemia. The latter, for example, might develop as a result of hyperemesis gravidarum and can result in delusional or depressive mental changes.
3. Brain trauma, such as concussion.
4. Infections, such as meningitis, syphilis, hepatitis.
5. Intracranial neoplasms—gliomas, metastatic carcinomas, and meningiomas.
6. Epilepsy—grand mal, petit mal, and focal seizures.

There are many instances of organic brain syndromes that have psychiatric symptomatology. Classical catatonic states are sometimes encountered in patients with AOBS, produced by frontal lobe lesions, tumors, vascular lesions, encephalitis, and degenerative states of poisons. There are most often multiple, possibly interacting etiological factors that influence a particular case of AOBS, and the patient's response depends on the degree of the insult and the person's premorbid ego strengths, making the differential diagnosis sometimes difficult and confusing, but certainly worth the effort, given the treatable and potentially harmful nature of the illness. Medical management is dictated by the cause of the symptoms. Nursing management, in general, includes simplifying and familiarizing the environment. The nurse should decrease the number of objects or shadows in the room that can be misinterpreted, keep consistent personnel or family members in the room, orient to reality by simple statements, and keep lights on. Avoiding physical restraints is optimal if available personnel are able to stay with the patient, as the restraints only increase confusion and agitation. It is often very helpful to reassure the patient regarding this temporary confusional state, telling the patient that even though *he* doesn't remember at that particular moment, he need not worry because the *nurses* will remember *for* him until his memory improves.

BIBLIOGRAPHY

Bellak, L., and Small, L.: Emergency psychotherapy and brief psychotherapy, New York, 1972, Grune & Stratton, Inc.

Burgess, A. W., and Holstrom, L. L.: Rape: victims of crisis, Bowie, Md. 1974, Robert J. Brady Co.

Cole, J. O., Freedman, A. M., and Freidhoff, A. J., editors: Psychopathology and psychopharmacology, Baltimore, 1973, The John Hopkins University Press.

Freedman, A. M., and Kaplan, H. I., editors: Comprehensive textbook of psychiatry, Baltimore, 1978, The Williams and Wilkins Co.

Griffith, J. D., Cavanaugh, J. H., and Oates, J. A.: Psychosis induced by the administration of amphetamine to human volunteers. In Efron, D. H., editor: Psychotomimetic drugs, New York, 1970, Raven Press.

Hackett, T. P.: Pain and prejudice: why do we doubt that the patient has pain? Med. Times February 1971.

Lee, A.: Drug induced dystonic reactions, J.A.C.E.P. **6:**351-354, 1977.

Mandell, A. J., and Mandell, M. P.: Suicide and the menstrual cycle, J.A.M.A. **200:**792-793, 1967.

Mills, J.: Dystonic reactions to phenothiazines, J.E.N. November/December 1978.

Parad, H. J., editor: Crisis intervention: selected readings, New York, 1972, Family Service Association of America.

Resnick, H. L. P., and Ruben, H. L.: Emergency psychiatric care. Bowie, Md., 1975, The Charles Press Publishers, Inc.

Rivera-Camlin, L.: The pharmacology and therapeutic application of phenothiazines, Ration. Drug. Ther. **11:**4, 1977.

Robins, E., and Murphy, G. E.: The physician's role in the prevention of suicide. In Yochelson, L., editor: Symposium on suicide. Washington, D.C., 1967, George Washington University.

Tyler, S.: An assessment of substance abuse related needs: high risk populations, Boston, Fall 1977, Mimeographed report of the City of Boston Coordinating Council on drug abuse.

CHAPTER 24

Metabolic emergencies

The emergency nurse often encounters a patient with a metabolic-related crisis who is initially an "unknown case" of depressed level of consciousness, coma, or bizarre behavioral disturbance. Frequently there are associated neurological impairment and alcohol-related phenomena occurring with metabolic disorders, which further confuse the clinical signs and symptoms that the triage nurse notes upon the patient's arrival. It is important, therefore that a metabolic (or endocrine) problem be systematically considered as cause to explain any clinical presentation that is less than obvious.

The most common metabolic problems are alcohol- and diabetic-related emergencies. However, acute adrenal and thyroid crises should not be overlooked, since they can be life-threatening if not managed aggressively. Finally, the emergency nurse should also consider fluid and electrolyte imbalances as a metabolic problem, because they create a wide range of signs and symptoms and potentially endanger life (see Table 24-5). The mere association of their classic manifestations and associated causes can alert emergency personnel to their existence and ensure prompt, definitive therapy.

ALCOHOL-RELATED EMERGENCIES

The emergency nurse is likely to encounter alcohol-related emergencies (see also pp. 539-542) on a daily basis and should have a clear understanding of which problems are *true* medical emergencies and take care not to permit the behavioral manifestations to overshadow the underlying metabolic threat to life. There are a few general guidelines that should be carefully considered by all emergency personnel.

Alcohol intoxication and alcohol withdrawal can be fatal.

The patient with acute alcohol problems should not be punished. It will not deter future involvement with the substance.

Differentiate alcoholic problems from head injury, drug overdose, and diabetic reactions.

Do not be misled by the appearance of the patient in acute alcoholic crisis (that is, a well-dressed, refined, elderly lady can be intoxicated too)!

It is the amount of alcohol consumed, not the type of beverage, that determines the level of intoxication.

Always obtain a careful history. Be aware of differences between denial and lying about alcohol consumption.

Consider psychiatric referral for patients seen in the emergency department with alcohol-related problems.

History and assessment

There are several alcohol-related emergencies that by their very nature do not lend the patient to participation in a meaningful dialogue for history-taking purposes, such as coma, acute intoxication, delirium tremens. In these instances the course of treatment should follow that for the unconscious victim (see pp. 277-283) until meaningful information can be obtained. If the patient is conscious and can cooperate, or if there are friends, bystanders, or relatives who can provide information, the following questions should be asked:

When did you drink last? How much? What kind of beverage?

What is the average amount you usually drink? Daily? Weekly?

How long has it been since you have eaten?

Are you taking (or have you taken) any drugs such as disulfiram (Antabuse) or metronidazole (Flagyl)? (See p. 554.)

Have you ever felt like this before? Have you been hospitalized with symptoms such as the ones you're having today?

What is your general level of health? Any serious medical or surgical problems? (Be sure to look for surgical scars on the chest and abdomen.)

Ethanol intoxication

Alcohol intoxication is precipitated by short-term consumption of a large amount of alcohol. The inexperienced drinker, the individual who drinks heavily and does not eat, or the one with a low physiological tolerance for alcohol may become intoxicated from considerably less than the one who has a long-term pattern of heavy consumption.

Be sure to determine if alcohol is the precipitating factor of the condition. Assess for concurrent drug ingestion, head injury, or metabolic disease, which can appear similar to intoxication (Table 24-1).

Be prepared to deal with behavioral manifestations that can vary widely, depending upon the amount of alcohol consumption and the individual's basic personality type (Table 24-2).

Table 24-1. Assessment and management in brain injuries and alcohol intoxication*

Assessment	Signs and symptoms		Treatment
	Brain injuries	**Intoxication**	
Respirations	Underventilation	Slow, stertorous breathing	Oxygen therapy or endotracheal intubation
Arterial blood gases	Increased pCO_2, decreased pO_2	Changes at blood levels of 0.30%	Oxygen therapy or endotracheal intubation
Vital signs	Bradycardia, hypothermia, hypertension (late sign)	Tachycardia, hypothermia, hypotension (0.30%)	ECG monitoring; provide extra warmth; treat for shock if necessary
Level of consciousness	Fluctuations, worsening	Improvement (may occur very slowly)†	Monitor continually
Pupils	Unequal, unreactive	Dilated, equal	Monitor continually for changes
Motor ability	Nonpurposeful, nonreactive, uncoordinated	Depends on blood alcohol levels (Table 24-2)	Monitor continually
Reflexes	Absent in fifth cranial nerve damage, absent gag reflex in ninth cranial nerve damage	May be absent if patient is comatose	Provide artificial tears with normal saline; protect airway by proper positioning and suctioning of secretions
Vomiting	Projectile	Occurs normally with nausea at blood levels of 0.20%	Protect airway by positioning and suctioning secretions
Urinary output	Diuresis	Diuresis	Monitor closely; prevent dehydration from diabetes insipidus with proper use of IV fluids

*From Ansbaugh, P.: J.E.N. **3**:9-13, May-June, 1977.

†Remember that blood alcohol levels do not peak until 45 minutes following ingestion. You may see worsening symptoms in the intoxicated patient for a short time while blood levels are peaking. A good history of the patient's immediate drinking pattern may explain the worsening symptoms.

Table 24-2. Approximate correlation of blood alcohol levels and symptoms*

Blood alcohol level	Signs and symptoms
50 mg/100 ml	Rarely produces symptoms
100-200 mg/100 ml	Emotional and affective changes, such as exhilaration, talkativeness, boastfulness, belligerence, remorse, sentimentality Slurred speech Ataxia Decreased inhibitions Slowed reaction time Confusion
250 mg/100 ml	Sedation Decreased response to stimuli Nausea and vomiting Muscular incoordination Appears "acutely intoxicated"
300-400 mg/100 ml	Stupor or even coma Impaired deep tendon reflexes Peripheral vascular collapse Seizures Nystagmus Hypoventilation
Above 500 mg/100 ml	Usually fatal as a result of cardiac or respiratory arrest

*Chronic users of alcohol require higher blood levels before associated symptoms are noted; the lethal dose, however, is approximately the same.

Emergency management. The prime concern in acute intoxication is to prevent death from respiratory depression. Intubate the patient if he is comatose. Consider airway protection. Aspiration of vomitus is a major cause of death in acute intoxication. Use a left lateral, head-down position. The nurse will be asked to obtain blood specimens: glucose, electrolytes, serum amylase, hematocrit and hemoglobin, BUN, liver profile, serum osmolality, complete blood count, toxicology screening, and arterial blood gases. The blood alcohol level may be valuable as a baseline for later serial determination of increases or decreases in relation to clinical signs and symptoms. Know legal parameters of obtaining blood alcohol specimens (see p. 44).

The respirations must be assessed regularly. Note the rate, depth, rhythm, and the muscles involved in chest excursions (abdominal, diaphragmatic, intercostal). Ascertain if movements are symmetrical. If the respiratory effort is not adequate or if there is poor air exchange, mechanical ventilatory assistance may be required.

The level of consciousness should be noted. Is it increasing or decreasing? (Peak blood alcohol levels are reached within 30 minute to 3 hours after alcohol intake has ceased.) If the level of consciousness is decreasing, the circumstances may be more grave than originally perceived. Vomiting may be induced or lavage may be performed to empty the stomach if a large volume of alcohol has been consumed recently (less than 1 to 2 hours) provided that airway integrity is maintained (see Chapter 8). A nasogastric tube attached to continuous suction may be a desirable adjunct. Collect gastric contents if vomiting does occur, and save all other aspirate for quantitative and qualitative laboratory analysis.

Heavy sedation is not appropriate to control behavior; however, mild tranquilizers such as diazepam (Valium), chlordiazepoxide (Librium), or hydroxyzine pamoate (Vistaril) may be used. Barbiturates or phenothiazines are not judicious selections for sedation because they potentiate previously ingested sedatives.

If seizures occur, they should be controlled with diazepam or amobarbital (Amytal) sodium. Of course, all resuscitation equipment should be at hand.

Some physicians prefer that the seriously intoxicated patient have a patent IV infusion route for administration of emergency drugs. An IV of D/5/W may be ordered, especially in the event of coma or impending seizure activity. Glucose and insulin as well as analeptic drugs may be indicated in selected circumstances.

Thiamine (100 mg IM) and multivitamins are indicated for acutely intoxicated patients and individuals with a long-term history of alcoholism to improve the general nutritional state.

If it is suspected that traumatic injuries could have resulted from the intoxicated state, further x-ray studies should be done, including chest, skull, and abdominal films.

The emergency nurse will need to monitor urinary output. A Foley catheter may be inserted in the unconscious patient to facilitate this process.

Occasionally in dire circumstances when the blood alcohol level nears 400 to 600 mg/100 ml or if severe acidosis is evident, dialysis may be considered. Dialysis is usually utilized in severe pediatric intoxications or if there is evidence of methanol or ethylene glycol ingestion.

Other alcohol-related phenomena

Rum fits. Seizure activity that occurs while the individual is still drinking or during the first few days of abstinence may be the result of declining blood alcohol level or to abnormal physiology related to electrolytes or blood glucose. Traumatic foci may also be responsible in some cases. Seizures may progress to status epilepticus (see pp. 303-305).

Alcohol withdrawal. Alcohol withdrawal syndromes may include tremors, seizures, and hallucinations. Any or all of these may be evident as the blood alcohol level declines and resultant metabolic adjustment phenomena occur.

MILD ALCOHOL WITHDRAWAL. Mild alcohol withdrawal ("morning after" syndrome) may occur within hours after cessation of alcohol intake. Signs and symptoms include headache, tremors, irritability, nausea, and generalized lethargy. Hydration, rest, aspirin, and time are usually the only therapy.

SERIOUS ALCOHOL WITHDRAWAL. Serious alcohol withdrawal occurs from 7 to 24 hours after cessation of alcohol intake. A person with chronic alcohol abuse may still be drinking but have a blood alcohol level below the usual level for that person. Individuals with pancreatitis, recent surgery, diabetes, or infections have an increased vulnerability to alcohol withdrawal. The symptoms should be differentiated from delirium tremens (p. 541). Signs and symptoms include insomnia; nausea and vomiting; shakes (tremors peaking 24 hours after withdrawal); seizures (most seizure activity occurs 7 to 48 hours after withdrawal); photophobia; rapid, fine lateral nystagmus (24 to 72 hours after withdrawal); sweating; confusion; ataxia; and auditory or visual hallucinations (peaking at 24 hours).

Delirium tremens. Delirium tremens (DTs) is a major syndrome of alcohol withdrawal that begins at about 72 hours after withdrawal and may continue for several days. The mortality is high (10% to 20%). Careful clinical management of alcohol withdrawal is imperative to prevent progression to delirium tremens. Haloperidol and chlordiazepoxide are the drugs of choice to consider for symptomatic management.

The first concern is to assure the airway and breathing. Blood samples should be obtained as the IV is established and specimens sent to the laboratory for complete blood count, blood sugar, electrolytes, liver function, alcohol level, toxicology screening (if indicated), serum ketones, and blood smears. An arterial blood gas may also be requested. The IV should be infusing D/5/W or D/10/W—half-normal saline. Magnesium sulfate may be ordered as an additive (50% solution, 2 ml IV every 6 hours). Since hypoglycemia often accompanies DTs, supplemental glucose may also be administered. Fluid administration is of vital importance in the management of delirium tremens because of the extreme dehydration that may require up to 6 liters of fluid for correction over 24 hours. At least one fourth of the fluid should consist of normal saline. Serial electrolyte studies should be done to monitor any abberations that deserve correction. The 100 mg IM thiamine should be administered with 10 mg folate unless pernicious anemia is suspected. A vitamin B complex may also be ordered.

The following tests and x-ray studies should be obtained in the meantime: urinalysis, stool guaiac, chest and skull films, including a CAT scan, EEG, and brain scan. A 12-lead ECG should be recorded as a baseline, and monitoring should ensue for the duration of the acute phase. Temperature should also be closely followed, since hyperthermia is second only to shock as a lethal complication of DTs; antipyretics and a cooling blanket may be required. If seizures occur, they should be managed with diazepam or phenytoin (Dilantin). Phenytoin may be combined with chlordiazepoxide to take advantage of lower doses to achieve a therapeutic blood level. (Ordinarily up to one gm phenytoin is required for a therapeutic effect.*)

The emergency nurse's most important role in managing DTs is to provide a supportive environment (see p. 541). Individuals having DTs should be hospitalized for follow-up and referral, because the acute syndrome usually lasts several days, and long-term treatment is required to alleviate the underlying cause (See also pp. 539-542).

Disulfiram (Antabuse) reactions†

Disulfiram (Antabuse) is frequently prescribed to assist individuals during alcoholic treatment programs. The drug action primarily depends on its production of unpleasant side effects when combined with alcohol in any form (including alcohol-based cough syrups, fermented vinegar, and sauces or other food cooked or combined with alcohol).‡ Symptoms appear within 90 (usually 5 to 15) minutes after ingestion of alcohol. (It is important that recipients understand that disulfiram effects continue for as long as 6 to 12 days after ingestion.) Extrasensitive individuals may have a reaction even to external use of alcohol such as rubbing alcohol or shaving lotion.

Signs and symptoms include bright red flushing of the face, neck, and upper thorax; sweating; throbbing headache; hyperventilation; tachycardia; hypotension; nausea and vomiting; decreased level of consciousness or coma; and reddened conjunctiva.

---

*Phenytoin can be hazardous in large IV doses and should be reserved for situations in which the patient has an intolerance to other drugs or has chronic seizure disorders, or when serial neurological examinations are required for diagnosis and management.

†Mild reactions may be confused with other drug reactions. Look for an Antabuse card.

‡Metronidazole (Flagyl) and certain oral hypoglycemics can produce a similar response, although usually less severe.

Emergency management

1. Ask the patient to lie down and reassure him about what is happening. Position on the side if possible, since vomiting is likely. Determine how much alcohol has been ingested. (More than 2 to 3 ounces is cause for alarm, because shock and coma are likely.)
2. Elevate the legs.
3. Initiate an IV infusion of normal saline.
4. Administer (depending on local protocol):
   500 mg ascorbic acid
   12 mg chlorpheniramine (Chlor-Trimeton)
   50 mg diphenhydramine (Benadryl)
   25 mg Pyribenzamine
5. A nasogastric tube may be indicated if there is a decreased level of consciousness.
6. Oxygen by nasal catheter may be useful if acute respiratory distress is not relieved by antihistamines.
7. Continue to monitor the ECG and vital signs.
8. Report the incident to the alcohol treatment center or physician who dispensed the disulfiram.

DIABETES-RELATED EMERGENCIES
Ketoacidosis

Ketoacidosis is a metabolic disturbance caused primarily by insulin depletion. There may be a factor of noncompliance (that is, failure to inject insulin as required) or a situation in which the body's demand for insulin is greater than normal. Stresses of menstruation, pregnancy, surgery, trauma, infection, certain drugs, or even an emotional upheaval can precipitate ketoacidosis. It usually develops slowly over a period of 36 to 48 hours.

The early phenomenon in ketoacidosis pathogenesis is hyperglycemia. Since sugar acts like an osmotic diuretic, there is an excessive loss of water, sodium, and potassium. A hypovolemic state with severe electrolyte imbalance ensues. As metabolic aberrations continue, protein and fat are broken down to meet the body's energy requirements, yielding increased plasma

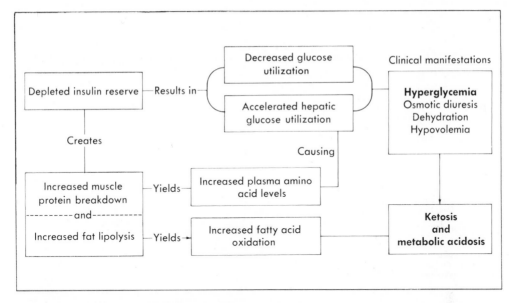

Fig. 24-1. Pathophysiology of diabetic ketoacidosis. (From Barber, J., and Budassi, S.: J.E.N. **3**:9-13, May-June, 1977.)

amino acid levels and fatty acid oxidation, respectively, which give rise to the acidotic state. To make matters worse, hepatic glucose production is triggered, which aggravates the preexisting hyperglycemic state (Fig. 24-1).

Initial assessments. Patients with a history of diabetes or who come to the emergency department in an altered state of consciousness should be screened for ketoacidosis (Fig. 24-2). In the meantime, continue with the initial historical data collection, beginning with the reason for coming to the hospital. Search for evidence of dehydration or gastrointestinal complaints (such as nausea, vomiting, diarrhea, abdominal pain or tenderness). Remember that diabetic ketoacidosis may mimic an acute abdomen (see Chapter 18).

Kussmaul-type respirations should be noted since they characterize acidosis. The rapid, deep, "air hunger" breathing helps get rid of excessive carbon dioxide, producing a respiratory alkalosis that helps balance the falling pH. Sniff the patient's breath too. It may be helpful in detecting acetone or ETOH intoxication.

Tachycardia and hypotension should be noted because they reflect hypovolemia.

The level of consciousness is an important parameter to monitor carefully throughout the emergency department encounter. Seizure activity may occur and should incite the investigation of a neurological basis for the current clinical problem, in addition to a metabolic one.

It is imperative to determine if the patient takes any medication on a regular basis, since certain agents affect insulin requirements (such as phenytoin, phenobarbital, and steroids).

Of course, miscellaneous data about allergies, previous illness or hospitalization, or the presence of unusual stress states that might alter insulin requirements should be noted.

Emergency management. After basic life support needs have been ensured, blood should be drawn for blood sugar, CBC, electrolytes, type and crossmatch, toxicology screening, and arterial blood gases. A Dextrostix (or similar device) may be employed for a rapid gross approximation of blood sugar levels. An IV of half-normal saline or normal saline should be

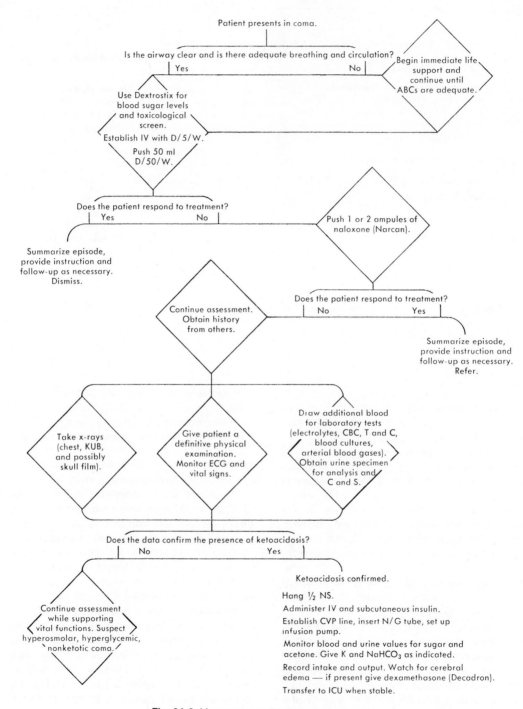

Fig. 24-2. Management of the comatose patient.

initiated. (Normal saline is preferred in instances of severe volume depletion.) Naloxone and 50% dextrose should be pushed for all unconscious patients (see p. 281). Since D/50/W is extremely sclerosing if it extravasates into subcutaneous tissue, be certain to aspirate before and at intervals during the push of dextrose. The use of D/50/W in diabetic coma, which is a hyperglycemic condition, is sometimes difficult for nurses to understand. However, the odds in diabetic-related coma are in the favor of hypoglycemia and the victim would dramatically improve. Since ketoacidosis already is accompanied by a very high blood sugar level, this bolus dose would have little effect on the outcome, and thus the risk is quite small. Essentially, the possible benefits far outweigh the risk of its use.

The physician may order a KUB or chest film to "rule out" infectious processes such as pneumonia or a wound abscess, or to detect other clues to the precipitation of ketoacidosis.

Urine is obtained for urinalysis, culture, and sensitivity as well as for sugar and acetone. Urinary tract infections are frequent causes of ketoacidosis. A fresh specimen is desirable, so the first emergency department voiding should be discarded. (Sugar concentrates in urine that is static in the bladder.) Catheterization should be avoided, since it risks infectious processes. Remember to use incandescent (rather than fluorescent) lighting to read color changes on chemical test strips for greater accuracy.

The emergency nurse may be asked to assist in detailed neurological testing of patients with ketoacidosis, especially those in coma, since reflexes help differentiate between metabolic and neurological phenomena.

FLUID MANAGEMENT. The early fluid management of ketoacidosis is directed toward correcting hypovolemia and hemoconcentration as well as dehydration of body tissue. The usual fluid deficit in ketoacidosis is 5 to 7 liters, and the sodium deficit, 300 to 500 mEq. Initially, 1 liter of normal saline is given over 30 to 60 minutes, followed by 500 mg/hour until hydration status is satisfactory. Occasionally plasma or other colloid volume expanders may be used

Table 24-3. Initial intravenous insulin therapy for ketoacidosis (in units of regular crystalline zinc insulin)*

If serum or plasma acetone is 4+	Adults	Children over 10 years	Children under 10 years
Undiluted specimen	100	50	25
1:2 dilution	200	100	50
1:4 dilution	300	150	75
1:8 dilution	400	200	100

*From Barber, J. M., and Budassi, S. A.: Mosby's manual of emergency care, St. Louis, 1979, The C. V. Mosby Co.

to combat severe hypovolemia. After the acute problems of hydration have been rectified, hypotonic fluids should be used (that is, 0.45% saline). The CVP should be carefully monitored.

INSULIN. The insulin dosage is calculated according to an established formula (which varies considerably from institution to institution); one half the requirement is given IV push, and the other half injected subcutaneously (Table 24-3). For a maintenance drip the following formula is recommended to achieve a rate of 1 unit/ml.

1 ml (unit 100) regular crystalline insulin

100 ml normal saline

4 ml serum albumin (as stabilizer)

(Use an infusion pump and regulate it at 0.1 unit/kg/hour.

There are several other modes of insulin therapy, including hourly IM and IV doses. Much experimentation is currently being done to circumvent the problem of insulin's short plasma half-life. Subcutaneous and intramuscular routes are unlikely to be satisfactory when used alone, especially if dehydration is severe.

ELECTROLYTES. Electrolyte determinations as well as blood sugar levels should be obtained at least every 2 hours. Potassium chloride (20 to 40 mEq/liter) may be added to the infusion after adequate renal function is assured. Sodium bicarbonate may also be indicated if the pH falls below 7.0. However, its use is controversial, with certain clinicians contending that it may contribute to both cerebral edema and hypokalemia. The ECG should be monitored judiciously during the administration of potassium chloride.

Glucose may be required when the blood level falls to 250 to 300 mg/100 ml to prevent precipitant hypoglycemia and to speed the clearance of ketone bodies. Five-percent or 10% dextrose can be given in saline by infusion, or 50 ml of D/50/W can be pushed.

OTHER CONSIDERATIONS. In the event that nausea and vomiting remain a problem during the management of ketoacidosis, a nasogastric tube should be anchored. Urine output should be measured at hourly intervals and specimens obtained for sugar and acetone levels. If infection is suspected as the cause of the problem, blood cultures may be requested. Continue to observe for complications of cerebral edema throughout the course of ketoacidosis, since they are commonly associated because of osmolality dynamics operant between the extracellular fluid and the central nervous system tissue.

Hyperosmolar hyperglycemic nonketotic coma

Hyperosmolar hyperglycemic nonketotic coma (HHNC) is a syndrome that includes marked hyperglycemia, dehydration, and coma; it is found in individuals with mild or unknown diabetes. The patient with HHNC is usually in the sixth or seventh decade of life. Significant acidosis and ketonemia do not occur. The primary difference between HHNC and ketoacidosis is that in the former there seems to be enough insulin in circulation to inhibit lipolysis (Fig. 24-3).

Signs and symptoms include coma, stupor, and focal grand mal seizures, all of which can be easily confused with a cerebrovascular accident. There may be a wide variety of bizarre behavioral manifestations. The history of illness may reveal important clues to HHNC. Commonly associated conditions include cardiovascular or renal disease, sepsis, pancreatitis, gastrointestinal hemorrhage, uremia, ingestion of certain drugs, and stress.

Certain laboratory values differ markedly between ketoacidosis and HHNC. For example, the serum glucose is usually much higher in HHNC, often reaching 2,800 mg/ml. Serum ketones are absent in HHNC.

The medical management of HHNC is similar to ketoacidosis, with much attention given to

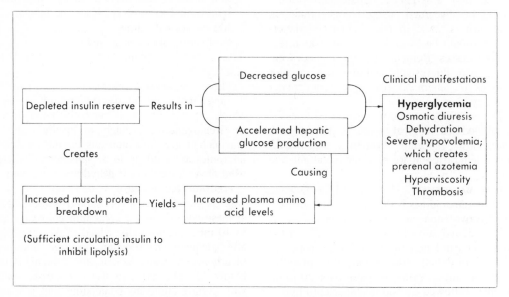

Fig. 24-3. Pathophysiology of hyperosmolar hyperglycemic nonketotic coma. (From Barber, J., and Budassi, S.: J.E.N.**3**[1]:16, 1977.)

Table 24-4. Insulins—administration and actions*

Type of insulin	Time and route of administration	Time of onset (hours after administration)	Peak action (hours after administration)	Duration of action (hours)
Crystalline zinc† (pH 3-3.5; Zn 0.02-0.04 mg/100 units) (regular)	IV (emergency), subcutaneously 15-20 min. before meals	Rapid, within 1 hour	2-4	6-8
Semilente† (amorphous zinc) pH 7.2; Zn 0.2-0.25 mg/100 units)	½ to ¾ hour before breakfast; deep subcutaneously; never IV	Rapid, within 1 hour	2-4	8-10
Globin zinc (pH 3.4-3.8; Zn 0.25-0.35 mg/ 100 units)	½ to 1 hour before breakfast; subcutaneously	Intermediate, rapidity of onset; increases with dose–within 1 to 2 hours	6-8	12-14; also increases with dose
Lente† (combination of 30% Semilente and 70% Ultralente) (pH 7.1-7.4; Zn 0.2-0.25 mg/100 units)	1 hour before breakfast; deep subcutaneously; never IV	Intermediate, within 1 to 2 hours	6-8	14-16
NPH (neutral-protamine-Hagedorn) (isophane) (pH 7.1-7.4; Zn 0.016-0.04 mg/ 100 units)	1 hour before breakfast; subcutaneously	Intermediate, within 1 to 2 hours	6-8	12-14
Protamine zinc (pH 7.4; Zn 0.2-0.25 mg/ units)	1 hour before breakfast; subcutaneously	Slow-acting, within 4 to 6 hours	16-20	36-72
Ultralente† (pH 4.8-5.7; Zn 0.2-0.25 mg/ 100 units)	1 hour before breakfast; deep subcutaneously; never IV	Slow-acting, within 4 to 6 hours	8-12	24-36

*From Barber, J. M., and Budassi, S. A.: Mosby's manual of emergency care, St. Louis, 1979, The C. V. Mosby Co.
†Contains no modifying protein (protamine or globin).

hydration and electrolyte balance. Intensive care nursing is required for this gravely ill individual. Complications to be watched for include cerebral edema, thrombophlebitis, acute pulmonary edema, cardiac dysrhythmias, electrolyte disturbances, and urinary tract infections. The mortality rate is 40% to 70% unless early management is aggressive and appropriate.

Hypoglycemia

Diabetics who take either insulin or oral hypoglycemic agents can develop hypoglycemia if there is too much of the agent present in the body for the amount of glucose. When an individual takes his insulin or hypoglycemic agent and does not ingest enough glucose or expends an abnormally high amount of energy, hypoglycemia can result. When the blood sugar falls, catecholamines are released to help cope with this stress. As a result, the individual feels hungry. Perspiration, anxiety, dilating pupils, headache, restlessness, and weakness may also occur. The energy-starved brain can become chemically toxic, thus triggering seizure activity. Unconsciousness will follow if glucose is not rapidly supplied.

Most hypoglycemic victims are managed by prehospital care paramedics before reaching the emergency department and have already recovered from the crisis as a result of a bolus of D/50/W in the field.

It is important for emergency personnel to know when various insulins "peak" in order to predict from the history when the blood sugar may reach its lowest point (Table 24-4). A baseline blood sugar should be drawn and a Dextrostix determination made promptly before administering the D/50/W. It is advisable to also obtain a heparinized blood sample for insulin assay and an additional one for cortisol assay. Alcoholics who appear hypoglycemic need both glucose and thiamine administered (see p. 553).

Other than drawing a blood sugar and administering D/50/W, the other major role of the emergency department nurse relates to instructions, follow-up care, and referrals as indicated to prevent subsequent hypoglycemic episodes.

ACUTE ADRENAL CRISIS (INSUFFICIENCY)

The adrenal cortex produces glucocorticoids, mineralocorticoids, and androgens. The deficiency of either glucocorticoids or mineralocorticoids can be life-threatening.

Cortisol is synthesized and released from the adrenal under the influence of the adrenocorticotropic hormone (ACTH), a pituitary hormone. It is responsible for sustaining the blood glucose level and has a part in sympathetic toning of arterial walls and thus the maintenance of blood pressure. Cortisol also has a role in energizing the body (that is, appetite, mental acuity, sense of well-being) and in stimulating the kidneys to excrete extra water. The most vital role of cortisol, however, relates to its role in the stress-adaptation response. It is capable of a tenfold production increase to sustain the body during stress. Aldosterone and desoxycorticosterone (another mineralocorticoid) act together to sustain blood volume by promoting sodium reabsorption in the distal renal tubules and by enhancing hydrogen ion and potassium secretion. (Aldosterone levels rise sharply in response to hyperkalemia.)

The patient who comes to the emergency department with adrenal insufficiency (Addison's disease) in crisis will relate a history of fatigue, nausea, vomiting, abdominal pain, anorexia, weight loss, weakness, and postural hypotension. Fever, tachycardia, and shock may be profound.

Patients with long-term Addison's disease may exhibit the classic mucocutaneous pigmentation on extensor surfaces such as the elbows, knees, and knuckles. These darkened areas may also be noted on the lips and buccal mucosa as well as on any surgical scars induced after the onset of the disease. Vitiligo (depigmented skin patches) are not uncommon.

The emergency care team should suspect adrenal crisis in all shocky patients whose hypotension cannot be explained, or who have been under stress, or have a history of infection, trauma, or surgery, or have suddenly ceased taking oral steroids. Patients known to have had hypophysectomy, adrenalectomy, or radiation therapy that would affect these areas are prime suspects for adrenal crisis manifestations.

An IV line should be established at once, and baseline blood studies drawn for cortisol levels, CBC, electrolytes, and blood sugar. The fluid of choice is saline with additives of dexamethasone phosphate and corticotropin or hydrocortisone sodium succinate. Desoxycorticosterone acetate (DOCA) and fludrocortisone acetate (Florinef) may be used for mineralocorticoid replacement if hypotension or hyperkalemia persists after initial fluid and drug therapy. Only glucocorticoid therapy is used for patients with hypopituitarism or ACTH suppression. The first liter is usually infused rapidly, within the first hour, followed by D/5/saline after another plasma cortisol assay has been drawn (10 ml venous blood). A urine collection (for 24-hour steroids) should be initiated shortly after the patient is admitted to the intensive care unit, where steroid and fluid therapy continues. Emphasis is on correcting sodium depletion, so up to 3 liters of saline may be given in a few hours. CVP and PWP monitoring are vital (see Chapter 12).

Therapy for Addison's disease requires admission to the hospital so that stabilization can be achieved while searching for the underlying cause of the crisis.

THYROID CRISES
Myxedema coma

The patient with myxedema in crisis usually comes to the emergency department in coma. The family may relate a history of recent apathy, lack of energy, and severe intolerance to cold. Frank psychosis sometimes is seen. There are usually longer-term signs such as dry skin, coarse hair, alopecia, periorbital edema, and abdominal distention and constipation. Ileus is sometimes noted. Body temperature may be subnormal (as low as 75° to 80° F), and tendon reflexes may be markedly hypoactive. The ECG exhibits low voltage with wide depressed or inverted T waves and a prolonged Q-T interval. Bradycardia is the predominant rhythm, and respiratory depression may be marked.

The causes of myxedema coma may include absent pituitary stimulation of the thyroid or possibly surgical absence of the gland. If hypofunction of the pituitary is the cause, facial, axillary, and pubic hair are absent and testes atrophic.

The laboratory results of blood analysis reveal a low level of serum thyroxine and serum sodium.

The coma of myxedema is triggered by a combined effect of poor ventilation, hyponatremia, and hypothermia. The management therefore includes attention to all these facets.

Airway. The airway is preferably maintained by tracheostomy if frank respiratory failure exists. (Patients usually relapse following routine extubations after 3 to 4 days. Achievement of results with thyroxine takes 7 to 10 days.) Respiratory assistance is provided with high-flow oxygen; arterial blood gases must be carefully monitored.

Thyroid and steroid replacement. An IV is initiated, and levothyroxine is administered, along with steroid replacement of cortisol. Careful ECG monitoring is done to detect cardiac ischemia secondary to the increase of tissue oxygen requirements as a result of thyroxine replacement.

Sodium replacement. If serum sodium levels fall below 115 mg/100 ml, hypertonic saline is given with extreme caution, along with a fluid restriction regimen in the intensive care unit.

Other management. Underlying causes of the crisis are searched for and any infection that is detected is treated specifically. The management of toxic states may contribute to a prompt reversal of the coma state. External rewarming *is not appropriate,* even though the core body temperature is low, because it would pull an already diminished vital organ blood flow and cardiac output to the periphery and thus invite profound cardiovascular collapse.

Thyrotoxic crisis (thyroid storm)

Most diseases of the thyroid progress slowly, but thyrotoxic crisis has a rapid onset and is life-threatening. It is triggered by conditions such as infections, sepsis, diabetes, or surgical stress.

The patient coming to the emergency department with thyroid storm is difficult to ignore in triage. Restlessness, nervousness, agitation, and a labile affect are noted. It is not uncommon that his inability to concentrate and constant movements make adequate history taking difficult. Fine tremors may be so profound that the individual can barely sign his admission forms or keep the thermometer in his mouth safely. Complaints of weakness, weight loss, excessive perspiration, shortness of breath, diarrhea, and heart palpitations are typical. Exophthalmos may be marked, with concurrent conjunctivitis, since the lid is no longer closely adequately to protect the eye. The thyroid gland may be noticeably enlarged, although this is not imperatively associated. Tachycardia and systolic hypertension are classic symptoms. It is important to also look for underlying pathologic conditions by linking symptoms of fever, abdominal pain, dysuria, and coughing with the classic thyroid storm indicators. It is easy to naively conclude that the individual is a "psych case" from his appearance, behavior, and admixture of complaints if you are not thinking critically about endocrine causes of such a presentation.

The initial diagnostic workup may include a 2-hour I-131 uptake since some other assay studies of value take several days to complete. Baseline serum thyroxine levels are also obtained, but therapy is usually instituted before the results are known because of the gravity of circumstances.

Emergency management. An IV is initiated with D/5/normal saline, and hydrocortisone (100 mg) and sodium iodide (1 to 2 gm) are infused. Propranolol, guanethidine, or reserpine is also given to block the adrenergic neurotransmitter that mediates the effects of excessive thyroid hormones. (The choice of agents depends on consideration of underlying disease such as asthma or congestive heart failure.) Propylthiouracil and methimazole (Tapazole) are initiated to block the synthesis of the thyroid hormone. These agents are given orally or by nasogastric tube, since parenteral preparations are not commercially available.

Sodium iodide (IV) or supersaturated solution of potassium iodide (SSKI) (orally) may be used to block the release of thyroid hormone. Generally they should be administered 1 hour after propylthiouracil or methimazole to prevent the iodide from being directed into new hormone stores. (Synthesis must be adequately blocked.*) Atrial fibrillition and congestive heart failure may require specific interventions (see p. 371).

Extreme cases of thyroid storm may be treated by exchange transfusions or peritoneal dialysis to remove excessive circulating thyroxine.

General measures useful in managing the patient with thyroid storm include rehydration, antipyretics (not aspirin) to reduce the fever, and possibly the use of a cooling blanket. Glucose and soluble B and C vitamin supplements are also advised to support the patient during the crisis.

The individual with thyroid storm is critically ill and should be managed in the intensive care unit. Nurses should be aware of the need for maximizing the resting state and care should be planned accordingly. Monitoring of ECG and careful supervision of medication and fluid therapy are paramount to detect impending complications related to the clinical management.

FLUID AND ELECTROLYTE DISTURBANCES: GUIDELINES FOR MANAGEMENT (TABLE 24-5)

1. Clinical assessments must correlate with laboratory findings. Remember that serum levels do not reflect the status of intracellular spaces.
2. Treat imbalances at the approximate rate of development.
3. Maintenance of airway, intravascular volume, and tissue perfusion are always the first priorities in treatment.

---

*Since the half-life of thyroxine in plasma is approximately 7 days, and that of triiodothyonine is 1 day, the effects of blockade are slow to appear.

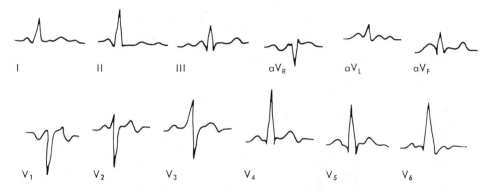

Fig. 24-4. Patient with serum potassium level of 2.7 mEq/liter. Hypokalemia is characterized by broadened T waves in limb leads with U waves most prominent in anterior precordial leads. (From Principles and techniques of critical care, Kalamazoo, Mich., 1976, The Upjohn Co.)

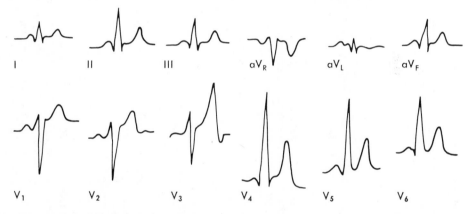

Fig. 24-5. Patient with serum potassium level of 7.5 mEq/liter. Hyperkalemia is characterized by tall, peaked T waves seen best in precordial leads. (From Principles and techniques of critical care, Kalamazoo, Mich., 1976, The Upjohn Co.)

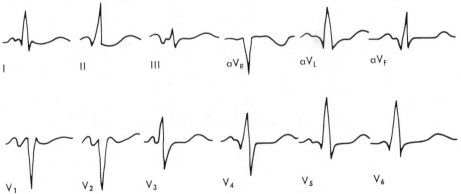

Fig. 24-6. Hypocalcemia. Note lengthened Q-T interval. (From Principles and techniques of critical care, Kalamazoo, Mich., 1976, The Upjohn Co.)

Table 24-5. Fluid and electrolyte imbalances*

Imbalance	Clinical signs and symptoms	Therapy	Anticipate in
Dehydration	Thirst, anxiety, weight loss, poor skin turgor, slow vein filling, elevated temperature, tachycardia, dry mucous membranes, decreased level of consciousness, increased hematocrit, increased BUN, increased RBC concentration	Volume replacement	Any condition in which water output exceeds intake; vomiting, diarrhea
Edema	Weight gain exceeding 5%; rales; dyspnea; puffy eyelids, swollen ankles, etc.; bounding pulse	Salt-poor albumin, exchange resins, diuretics	Protein deficiency, venous obstruction, heart failure, obstructed lymphatics, toxin ingestion, liver disease, renal disease
Third space syndrome	Hypotension, tachycardia, peripheral vasoconstriction, oliguria, no weight loss, increased hematocrit with no evidence of fluid loss	Plasma, salts, water replacement, diuretics, paracentesis, thoracentesis	Ascites, cellulitis, crush injuries, vascular occlusion, intestinal obstructions
Hypokalemia	Weakness, flaccidity; diminished reflexes; weak pulse, hypotension; ECG changes (Fig. 24-4)—increased P wave amplitude, flat or inverted T waves, ST segment depression, prominent U wave, prolonged PR interval; dyspnea; nausea, vomiting; mental depression	Oral or IV potassium therapy	Long-term diuresis (i.e., thiazides), vomiting, diarrhea, draining fistulas, heat stroke, diabetic acidosis, alcoholism, malnutrition
Hyperkalemia	Muscle cramps; nausea, diarrhea, vomiting; weakness; hyperactivity; dizziness; paresthesias; ECG changes (Fig. 24-5)—early, high-peaked T waves, ST segment depressed, P wave disappears, later—QRS widens, T waves taller, premature ectopic beat; escape beats, ventricular flutter, fibrillation, and standstill	NaHCO₃: mEq IV over 5 min; may repeat in 10 min NaCl: IV Calcium gluconate: 0.5 ml/kg of 10% solution over 2-4 min (do not give in central line) Infuse D/50 over 30-60 min with insulin Exchange resins: Kayexalate 20-50 gm in 100-200 ml of 20% sorbitol orally (repeat every 3-4 hr) or 50 mg with 50 gm sorbitol and 200 ml water as retention enema over 30-60 min Steroids Peritoneal dialysis or hemodialysis	Adrenal cortical insufficiency, acidosis, burns or other major tissue trauma, renal failure; overshooting IV or oral potassium

*Modified from Barber, J., Stokes, L., and Billings, D.: Adult and child care, ed. 2. St. Louis, 1977, The C. V. Mosby Co.

Continued.

Table 24-5. Fluid and electrolyte imbalances—cont'd

Imbalance	Clinical signs and symptoms	Therapy	Anticipate in
Hyperkalemia—cont'd		Glucose-insulin infusion: 2-4 gm glucose and 20-30 units insulin IV in 200-700 ml D/20/W over 30-60 min; or 1000 ml D/10/W with 90 mEq NaHCO₃ (infuse 300 ml over 30 min and remainder over 2-3 hr; give 25 units regular insulin SC at beginning of infusion)	
Hypocalcemia	Abdominal and muscle cramps, tetany, tingling of fingers and circumoral area, hyperactive reflexes, impaired mental functioning, laryngeal stridor, local or generalized seizures, ECG changes: prolonged QT interval due to lengthened ST segment (Fig. 24-6)	IV calcium: 20-30 ml of 10% calcium gluconate IV over 10-15 min	Infections, burns, diarrhea, excessive use of citrated blood, pancreatitis, parathyroid malfunction
Hypomagnesemia	Positive Chvostek's sign,* hyperactive reflexes, coarse tremors, seizures, disorientation, gait disturbances, chloreiform or athetoid movements, stupor	Magnesium sulfate: 2 mEq/kg body weight IV over 4 hr at rate not exceeding 150 mg/min	Vomiting, diarrhea, enterostomal drainage, cirrhosis, diuretic therapy, delirium tremens
Hyponatremia	Heat cramps; general weakness and fatigue; decreased cardiac output; hypotension; fainting; lip and nailbed cyanosis; cool, clammy skin; scant urine output; elevated intracranial pressure with headache, confusion, agitation, etc.; seizures; coma	Hypertonic saline (do not give more than 300 ml in 4 hr; monitor plasma chloride and bicarbonate levels cautiously)	Salt deficit, cirrhosis, diabetic ketoacidosis, heart failure, hormonal disturbances, (e.g., ADH, ACTH), poorly managed diuretic therapy; diarrhea, perspiration
Hypernatremia	Irritability, lethargy, coma, seizures, delirium, weakness, signs and symptoms of dehydration, high-pitched cry in infants	Balanced IV solution	Perspiration, fever, failure of thirst mechanism, inadequate water intake with high-protein feedings

*Unilateral contraction of facial muscle on facial nerve percussion (anterior to ear).

BIBLIOGRAPHY

Ansbaugh, P.: Emergency management of intoxicated patients with head injuries, J.E.N. **3:**9-12, May-June 1977.

Arieff, A. I., and Carroll, H. J.: Nonketotic hyperosmolar coma with hyperglycemia: clinical features, pathophysiology, renal function, acid-base balance, plasma cerebrospinal fluid equilibria and the effects of therapy in 37 cases, Medicine **51:**73-94, 1972.

Beeson, P. B., and McDermott, W.: Textbook of medicine, ed. 14, Philadelphia, 1975, W. B. Saunders Co.

Blum, M.: Myxedema coma, Am. J. Med. Sci. **264:**432-443, 1972.

Doromal, M., and Canter, J. W.: Hyperosmolar hyperglycemic nonketotic coma complicating intravenous hyperalimentation, Surg. Gynecol. Obstet. **136:**729-732, 1973.

Greenblatt, D. J., and Greenblatt, M.: Which drug for alcohol withdrawal? J. Clin. Pharmacol. **12:**429-431, 1972.

Greenblatt, D. J., and Shader, R. I.: Treatment of the alcohol withdrawal syndrome. In Shader, R. I., editor: Manual of psychiatric therapeutics: practical psychopharmacology and psychiatry, Boston, 1975, Little, Brown and Co.

Gross, M. M., Lewis, E., and Hastey, J.: Acute alcohol withdrawal syndrome. In Biology of alcoholism, Vol. 3, Clinical pathology, New York, 1974, Plenum Press.

Kalant, H.: Effects of ethanol on the nervous system. In Tremolieres, J., editor: Alcohols and derivatives, Sect. 20, Vol. 1, International encyclopedia of pharmacology and therapeutics, Oxford, 1970, Pergamon Press, Ltd.

Keyvan-Larijarni, H., and Tannenberg, A. M.: Methanol intoxication: comparison of peritoneal dialysis and hemodialysis treatment, Arch. Intern. Med. **134:**293-296, 1974.

Kolin, M.: A third diabetic shock syndrome, J.E.N. **3:**15-17, January-February 1977.

Lauler, D. P., Williams, G. H., and Thorn, G. W.: Diseases of the adrenal cortex. In Wintrobe, M. M., and others: Harrison's principles of internal medicine, ed. 6, New York, 1970, McGraw-Hill Book Co.

Macklin, J. F., Canary, J. J., and Pittman, C. S.: Thyroid storm and its management, N. Engl. J. Med. **291:**1396-1398, 1974.

Maling, H. M.: Toxicology of single doses of ethyl alcohol. In Tremolieres, J., editor: Alcohols and derivatives, Sect. 20, Vol. 11, International encyclopedia of pharmacology and therapeutics, Oxford, 1970, Pergamon Press, Ltd.

McCurdy, D. K.: Hyperosmolar hyperglycemic nonketotic diabetic coma, Med. Clin. North Am. **54:**683-699, 1970.

Plum, F., and Posner, J. B., editors: Diagnosis of stupor and coma, ed. 2, Philadelphia, 1975, F. A. Davis Co.

Sandler, J. A.: Endocrine emergencies. In Warner, C. G., editor: Emergency care: assessment and intervention, ed. 2, St. Louis, 1978, The C. V. Mosby Co.

Schwartz, G. R., and others: Principles and practice of emergency medicine, Philadelphia, 1978, W. B. Saunders Co., pp. 1061-1087.

Selenkow, H. A., and Ingbar, S. H.: Diseases of the thyroid. In Wintrobe, M. M., and others: Harrison's principles of internal medicine, ed. 6, New York, 1970, McGraw-Hill Book Co.

Thorn, G. W., and Lauler, D. P.: Clinical therapeutics of adrenal disorders, N. Engl. J. Med. **53:**673-684, 1972.

Urbanic, R. C., and Mazzaferri, E. L.: Thyrotoxic crisis and myxedema coma, Heart and Lung **7:**435-447, May/June 1978.

Toker, P.: Hyperosmolar hyperglycemic nonketotic coma: a cause of delayed recovery from anesthesia, Anesthesiology **41:**284-285, 1974.

Vinik, A., Seftel, H., and Joffe, B. I.: Metabolic findings in hyperosmolar nonketotic diabetic stupor, Lancet **2:**797-798, 1970.

Wilkins, E. W., editor, Dineen, J. J., and Moncure, A. C., Assoc. editors: MGH textbook of emergency medicine, Baltimore, 1978, The Williams and Wilkins Co., pp. 226-269.

Wulfson, H. D., and Dalton, B.: Hyperosmolar hyperglycemic nonketotic coma in a patient undergoing emergency cholecystectomy, Anesthesiology **41:**286-290, 1974.

CHAPTER **25**

Outdoor emergencies

Peter A. Dillman and Janet M. Barber

SNAKEBITE

There are approximately 3,000 species of snakes in the world, of which fewer than 200 actually pose a threat to humans. Evolutionary process has enabled different species of snakes to adapt and live in almost every type of environment. Snakes can be found in the water, ground, deserts, and trees from South America to the Arctic circle. In the United States it is estimated that there are 120 species of snakes, of which only about 20 are venomous. Only Maine, Alaska, and Hawaii are free from current ranges of poisonous snakes.

The snakes that are dangerous to humans in America and therefore concern us are divided into two different families and five species:

A. The pit vipers *(Viperidae)* contain the following species:
   1. Rattlesnakes *(Crotalus)*
   2. Moccasins *(Agkistrodon piscivorus)*
   3. Copperheads *(Agkistrodon contortrix)*
B. The coral snakes *(Elapidal)* contain the following species:
   1. Eastern coral *(Micrurus fulvius)*
   2. Texas coral *(Micrurus tenere)*

Approximately 7,000 venomous bites are incurred annually in the United States, of which fewer than 20 fatalities are reported. Pit vipers account for the majority of these injuries. This is because of their size, aggressiveness, and amount of venom that may be injected into their victims.

Characteristics of venomous snakes
(Fig. 25-1, *A*)

Pit vipers have such a name because of a facial pit located between their eye and nostril. This pit serves as a heat-sensing organ, allowing the reptile to locate warm-blooded prey. Also characteristic to the pit vipers are:
   1. A triangular head,
   2. Movable hollow upper jaw fangs,
   3. Vertical pupils,
   4. A single row of scales on the under surface of the tail.

Coral snakes are very colorful, and they vary considerably in color patterns. One should not rely on color markings alone to rule out whether or not these snakes are poisonous; coral snakes have the following characteristics:
   1. Relatively short fangs
   2. Colored rings of red and yellow that touch
   3. Black snout with yellow head ring
   4. Round pupils

Characteristics of nonvenomous
snakes (Fig. 25-1, *B*)
   1. Round pupils
   2. No facial pit
   3. Double row of scales on the under surface of the tail.

Venom

Poisonous snake venom is a complex mixture of enzymes, nonenzymatic proteins, and pep-

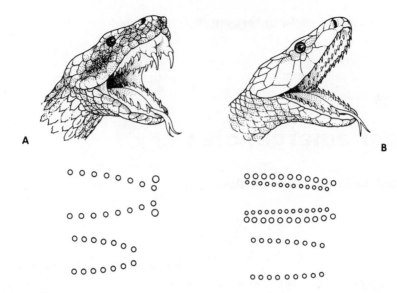

Fig. 25-1. A, Characteristics of venomous snake (pit viper). **B,** Characteristics of nonvenomous snakes.

tides, and other elements that have yet to be isolated and identified. Envenomation in humans causes a myriad of different effects in almost every body system because of the neurotoxic, hematoxic, and cardiotoxic properties the venom may possess, depending on the species. Some of the known enzyme constituents of snake venom include (Jiménez-Porras, 1970):

1. Hyaluronidase
2. Exopeptidase
3. Adenosine triphosphatase (ATPase)
4. Ribonuclease (RNase)
5. Deoxyribonuclease
6. Phospholipase
7. 5-Nucleotidase
8. Phosphodiesterase
9. Nucleotide pyrophosphatase
10. L-amino acid oxidase
11. Cholinesterase
12. Transaminase
13. Acid phosphatase
14. Alkaline phosphatase

Human pharmacological constituents that may be released and combine with the ensuing destructiveness of the venom once injected includes:

1. Histamine
2. Bradykinin
3. Adenosine

Signs, symptoms, assessment

Signs and symptoms of evenomation and the rapidity at which they appear depend on several factors:

1. The size and species of the snake
2. The location, depth, and number of bites
3. The amount of venom injected
4. Individual sensitivity to venom
5. The age and weight of the victim
6. General health of the victim
7. Microorganisms (type and number) in the oral cavity of the snake.

The immediate application of effective first aid measures and early medical care also affect the course of morbidity.

Early emergency assessment of any snake bite should be focused on the inflicted wound and condition of the patient.

Envenomation by a poisonous snake may or may not have taken place, so be skeptical and check quickly but thoroughly.* Although it

---

*In about one out of five or six poisonous snake bites, no envenomation takes place.

may seem logical to inspect for two fang marks, there may be only scratches or just one fang mark. One puncture wound may indicate that the other fang had been broken off in previous attack encounters. It is also possible that the snake may have more than two fangs. This is because every time a rattlesnake sheds its skin its fangs are shed too, and new ones are added.

Immediate and early responses

Besides the puncture wounds of the snakebite, other local tissue reactions include edema, vascular compromise, neuromuscular change with paresthesias, and possibly loss of function if the bite involves the feet, ankles, or hands. Burning pain is usually present. Hypotension and a resultant compromise of cardiac output are seen early. There is a decrease in circulating blood volume (largely because of an increase in vascular permeability similar to that phenomenon that accompanies anaphylaxis), and plasma proteins are substantially reduced. The red cell mass is depleted rapidly by bleeding and hemolysis.

Other changes and delayed responses

The nerve-muscle membranes are irritated by venom fractions, and resultant edema and hemorrhage may produce paresthesias, paralysis, and neuromuscular transmission disturbances.

Local and systemic hemostatic disturbances also develop after envenomation. Hemorrhage, petechiae, and ecchymosis are commonly observed. Four types of hemostatic-related phenomena occur.

1. Coagulant (clotting factors active, thrombinlike action of venom substance, or exposure of collagens to factor XII)
2. Anticoagulant (inactivation or destruction of clotting factors, or difibrination or defibrinogenation)
3. Hemolytic (direct lytic action in response to phospholipase A)
4. Platelet-related response

First aid measures

While assessing the victim, reassurance and immobilization are paramount. Apply a tourniquet to the extremity (almost all bites occur in the hands and lower legs) about 3 to 4 inches proximal to the bite. The purpose of this tourniquet is to obstruct lymphatic and venom flow to discourage systemic absorption of the venom.

Keep the wounded extremity at or below the level of the heart, and assess the distal pulses to ensure that arterial circulation has not been impaired. Remove as quickly as possible all jewelry to prevent tissue, nerve, and blood vessel damage that could result from edema. *Do not apply ice or any other coolant to the bite.*

Incision and suction.* If instituted within 5 to 10 minutes, suction can remove as much as 25% to 50% of the venom from an extremity. (If more than 30 to 40 minutes has elapsed, the technique is of little value, and could merely further traumatize the surrounding tissue.) Rinse the surface with an antiseptic if you have one available. Make a linear incision through each definite fang mark incising only as deep as the fangs had gone. (Usually this is very superficial, about ⅛ inch.) Do not criss-cross the incision or incise over the fang marks in a horizontal fashion. By not doing so, you minimize the risk of transecting nerves, blood vessels, ligaments, and so on.

Use suction for about 20 minutes. If the rescuer has any open wounds in or around the mouth the method should not be used. The wound fluid extracted with the mouth suction technique should be discarded regularly. However, if inadvertently swallowed, do not panic. The venom will be inactivated in the stomach.

Acquire an *accurate description of the snake* as best you can, but do not go out of your way to kill or capture it.

Rapidly transport the victim to an emergency facility. Never permit the victim to run.

Do not give any alcohol, stimulants, or depressants.

Record the time that progressive signs and symptoms develop and when you instituted your emergency treatment.

Emergency department care

Establish an IV of normal saline as soon as basic life support issues are resolved. Fluid

---

*This technique is recommended if there is rapid swelling around the bite, nausea, loss of consciousness, or the inability to reach a medical facility within 4 to 5 hours.

Table 25-1. Grading of envenomation*

Grade	Clinical findings	Amount of antivenin needed
0	History of suspected snake bite; presence of fang wound(s); no evidence of envenomation; minimal pain may be present; also minimal edema and erythema; no systemic manifestations during first 12 hours	None
I	Estimated minimal envenomation; history and signs of snake bite; moderate pain or throbbing localized at fang wound(s) surrounded by 2.5-12.5 cm of edema and erythema; no evidence of systemic involvement after 12 hours of observation	IM anterolateral should be given in thigh or buttocks; 1 vial
II	Moderate envenomation; symptoms and signs of grade I rapidly progress during first 12 hours; pain becomes more severe and widely distributed; edema spreads toward trunk; petechiae and ecchymoses limited to area of edema; systemically, nausea, vomiting, giddiness, and mild elevated temperature usually present	Part IV (50%), remainder IM; 2-4 vials
III	Severe envenomation; signs and symptoms begin like I and II but rapidly progress in severity; shock may ensue soon after the bite; within 12 hours edema spreads up extremity and may involve part of trunk; petechiae and ecchymoses may be generalized; systemic manifestations include rapid pulse, shocklike state, subnormal temperatures	All IV; 5 or more vials
IV	Very severe envenomation; seen especially after envenomation by a large rattlesnake; symptoms and signs of sudden pain, rapidly progressive swelling that may reach and involve trunk within a few hours with ecchymoses, bleb formation, and necrosis; systemic reactions often start early and usually include weakness, nausea and vomiting, tingling of lips and face; muscular fasciculation, painful muscular cramping, pallor, sweating, cold and clammy skin, rapid and weak pulse, incontinence, convulsions, and coma also may be observed; death may occur	All IV; 10 or more vials

*From Warner, C. G., editor: Emergency care, ed. 2, St. Louis, 1978, The C. V. Mosby Co.

volume replacement is essential in venom shock, preferably using colloidal substances. Specific intervention for hemostatic defects may include fresh frozen plasma, fresh blood, platelets, or fibrinogen.

Evaluation of the puncture wound. *Edema* begins at once after the bite and may involve the entire extremity in 1 hour. It continues for up to 36 hours after bites by certain poisonous snakes. *Ecchymosis* and general discoloration may also be noted in the first hour or two, with the subsequent formation of vesiculations, hemorrhage, and petechiae. Later (16 to 36 hours after the bite), superficial vessels may thrombose and injured tissue may slough. Coral snake bites usually are not accompanied by dramatic local tissue reactions. However, within 4 hours, blurred vision, increased salivation, difficulty in speaking, and ptosis may occur (Table 25-1).

General complaints. The victim may complain of pain, faintness, nausea, vomiting, sweating, tingling and numbness, and a metallic or rubberlike taste in the mouth. Muscle fasciculations may be noted in some instances. Hemorrhagic phenomena may be evident in hematemesis, melena, and hematuria. Shock, CNS dysfunction, and hematological abnormalities are indications of a serious envenomation.

The venom of the coral snake produces curarelike effects on the nervous system. Early symptoms include lethargy, euphoria, tremors, and excessive salivation. Soon after these phenomena are noted, slurred speech and double vision point to cranial nerve involvement. Fixed, constricted pupils, ptosis, dyspnea, seizures (especially in children), and paralysis of respiratory mechanisms follow if no treatment is given.

Laboratory data. Venous blood should be drawn for testing:

Hemoglobin

Hematocrit

CBC

BUN

Electrolytes

Typing and crossmatching

Serum protein

Coagulation studies (fibrinogen titer and partial thromboplastin time)

Elevated *hematocrit* (early) followed by a decrease in both hematocrit and hemoglobin accompany the classic poisonous snake bite. Bleeding and clotting times may be prolonged, with possible reduction in serum fibrinogen and lengthening of prothrombin and partial thromboplastin times.

Arterial blood gases are of little value except as a baseline study and to confirm acidemia, which sometimes accompanies venom shock.

An *ECG* may demonstrate ectopy.

Collect *urine* initially and on a daily basis thereafter for analysis. Renal functions may be affected by hemolysis, muscle necrosis, and shock. Monitor intake and output. Observe especially for microscopic hematuria.

Initial wound care and follow-up consideration

Culture and measure the circumference of the extremity at several points proximal to the wound to evaluate the degree of edema before thorough cleansing with a surgical soap solution. *Avoid any deliberate cooling* (even though cold applications might relieve pain), because it leads to unnecessary tissue destruction and even amputations in some instances.

Measure the circumference every 15 to 30 minutes. Note and record the presence of ecchymosis and bullae. Consider fasciotomy in any instance of intense swelling to relieve pressure and enhance circulation. An incision deep enough to enter the muscle compartment should be made. (Fasciotomy wounds are usually closed in 5 to 10 days).

Dress the wound, taking care to immobilize the extremity in functional position (for example, finger in flexion). Use a generous, bulky dressing because the drainage will be copious. Leave the tips of the fingers exposed so that circulatory status may be assessed regularly.

Plan for hospitalization. Write follow-up orders directing that the wound be immersed daily in 1:20 Burrow's solution with oxygen bubbled through the liquid, followed by application of a sterile, bulky dressing as before. Consider the inclusion of an active and passive exercise regimen to speed recovery, and alert personnel to observe for these complications: shock, pulmonary edema, serum sickness, wound infection, respiratory arrest, disseminating intravascular coagulation, coma, and contractures. Wound care suggestions for 3 to 5 days after the bite include the following:

- Continue Burrow's solution soaks but reduce time to 1 to 2 hours. After 3 to 5 days, debride vesicles and necrotic tissue. Follow debridement with hydrogen peroxide cleansing three times daily.
- Cover the wound with triple dye solution or another suitable agent.
- Dress the wound as previously instructed.
- *Ensure that all medical and nursing personnel assess the neurological and motor functions of the involved extremity on an hour-to-hour basis.*

Consider orthopedic consultation, especially when hands or feet are involved.

Consider administration of antibiotics to prevent secondary infection with gram-negative organisms, which comprise much of the normal flora of the snake's mouth.

Administer appropriate tetanus prophylaxis (see p. 233).

Antivenin therapy

Antivenin should be reserved for life-threatening envenomations since it carries the risks of serious sensitivity reactions, including anaphylaxis. *It should be administered in the first 4 hours after the bite if possible. It is of little or no value if venom shock has already occurred or if 12 or more hours have elapsed since the bite.* (See Table 25-1.)

Antivenin is not recommended for field usage because the risk of anaphylaxis is quite high. Intradermal skin or conjunctival testing must precede the administration of antivenin. See antivenin manufacturer's instructions, or follow these steps:

1. Have all equipment for resuscitation at hand, including epinephrine.
2. Obtain a complete allergy history.
3. Using a short 25- or 27-gauge needle and syringe, inject 0.1 ml of a 1:10 dilution intradermally. In the case of a history of sensitivity to horse serum, dilute the test material to 1:100. The wheal will be white at first; if the patient is sensitive to horse serum, it will become red in 10 to 15 minutes. Wait at least 20 minutes after the test, and if no local or systemic reactions are noted, proceed with the antivenin. *If there is a severe reaction to the test* (urticaria, wheezing, cyanosis, edema, and so on, indicative of anaphylaxis), give 0.3 to 0.5 ml of 1:1000 epinephrine subcutaneously, and be prepared to resuscitate the patient. (See p. 252 for management of anaphylaxis.)

An alternate test method is to drop 1 to 2 drops of a 1:10 solution of horse serum onto the conjunctiva. If the result is positive, the conjunctiva will redden. Following a positive test for sensitivity, a 1:1000 solution of epinephrine may be placed on the area to neutralize the horse serum effects.

Special notes on antivenin

1. The dose should be calculated to the *severity of reaction,* not weight, even in children (see Table 25-1).
2. The patient should be tested for horse serum sensitivity. (See antivenin package insert for this procedure.) *A negative sensitivity test is no real assurance that anaphylaxis will not occur. Have epinephrine and all other resuscitation support at hand.*
3. IV infusion of normal saline must be functional. Antivenin is usually given by IV piggy-back (diluted 1 unit of antivenin to 50 to 100 ml of normal saline). Of course, severe reactions may require a higher concentration. IM administration is also acceptable, but never inject anti-

venin into a finger or toe. Direct infiltration into a snakebite wound is probably ineffective. Intraarterial administration is acceptable using 1 vial of antivenin to 100 ml of normal saline.*

4. Monitor response to antivenin frequently —at least every hour.

GILA MONSTERS

A gila monster *(Heloderma suspectum)* is a lizard that has the capacity to milk venom into a victim by hanging on and chewing with its grooved teeth. Ordinarily, gripping the monster and forcibly jerking him off the body will extract the teeth and prevent envenomation.

Gila monster venom is essentially a neurotoxin and an anticoagulant. Resultant bites may bleed profusely, with edema and ecchymosis quite apparent. Death may be caused by cardiac and respiratory failure.

The management regimen for gila monster bites is the same as for pit viper bites.

STINGS, BITES, AND LOCAL IRRITATIONS FROM ARTHROPODS AND MARINE LIFE

Stings and bites from arthropods pose a more genuine threat to man than those of venomous snakes in the United States. About 45 to 50 fatalities are attributed to their inflictions each year in this country. Stings or bites from arthropods and marine life may become emergencies because of the victim's hypersensitivity or allergic response to the protein substance in the venom.

Stings

A sting is caused by the anatomical injection of a device known as the "stinger" into the flesh of a victim. For the most part a stinger is a defense weapon used as a vehicle for venom and differs in form and location from one animal species to another.

Hymenoptera: fire ants, bees, hornets, wasps, and yellow jackets. These insects have

---

*Corticosteroids have questionable value in the management of coagulation disturbances and tissue injuries and are of no value in venom shock reversal. However, they should be used when antivenin is administered intraarterially.

their stingers located in the terminal portion of the abdomen connected to a venom gland. About 50% of the deaths that occur from the stings of this group are attributed to the honeybee. The honeybee's stinger, unlike other insects in this group, is barbed. So once injected into the flesh of its victim, it becomes anchored. Therefore, when an attempt is made by the insect to fly away or when it is brushed off, it loses the posterior abdominal contents, including the venom sac, which is connected to the stinger. The bee then dies. It is important if stung by a honeybee that you brush or scrape the stinger away. If you pull the stinger off you are inadvertently squeezing more venom into the wound.

The remaining group of insects (fire ants, hornets, wasps, and yellow jackets) have the ability to sting their victim repeatedly because their stingers are not barbed, and therefore inject more venom. Hymenoptera tend to swarm the victim when they or their nesting quarters are disturbed, some species being more aggressive than others. Only the female Hymenoptera can sting, because the stinging apparatus is a modification of the ovipositor.

VENOM OF HYMENOPTERA. Each species from this order of insects has its own distinct toxins although there are some similarities.

BEE VENOM. Bee venom contains hyaluronidase and the polypeptides melittin and apamin, mastocytolytic (MCL) peptide, histamine, and phospholipase A and B.

WASP VENOM. Wasp venom contains serotonin, hyaluronidase, and wasp kinin; *hornet venom* contains serotonin, acetylcholine, and hornet kinin; *fire and velvet ant venom* has not been completely analyzed and isolated, but it is thought to contain histamine, phospholipase, and hyaluronidase.

Scorpions (Scorpinada). Scorpions are relatives of spiders and all are poisonous, some species more than others. Of approximately 40 species of scorpions in the United States only two are known to possess lethal venom, *Centruroides sculpturatus* and *Centruroides gertschi*. These deadly species are localized to Arizona and its neighboring states. Scorpions are a problem of considerable medical and public health importance in Arizona, since scorpions kill more people there than do poisonous snakes. Scorpions have their stinger on the terminal portion of their tails. Most stings occur to the hands or feet of the victim.

Bites

A bite from an arthropod is caused by vice-like jaws (chelicera) or beak that pierces the flesh of the victim.

Ticks. These creatures become attached to the body (usually in the head, neck, or groin) by burrowing their heads into the skin of the host to feed on blood. Once engorged, they detach and fall off the victim. The body of this insect relative is very flat when not engorged with blood and is difficult to locate once embedded in hairy areas of the host body. Care should be taken when in endemic areas by wearing proper field clothing. Some species carry the virus that causes Rocky Mountain spotted fever.

Spiders (Arachnida). Almost all spiders are poisonous but most are too small to do humans harm. Spiders have fangs associated with a venom gland connected to their jaws. Spiders use their fangs by injecting venom into their prey and anesthetizing them, then suck the insect body fluid for nourishment.

In the United States only two spiders are of medical significance, the black widow and the brown recluse. These spiders are poisonous and can cause medical grief when not identified by the victim as the cause of injury or illness.

Vesicating and urticating irritations

Many insects do not bite or sting their victims out of defense; some release a toxic substance (fluid or hair) when disturbed. The toxic substance affects the skin of humans by either causing hives or blistering. Insects in this category include blister beetles and certain species of caterpillars.

Summary

Bees and wasp stings account for the majority of all deaths caused by arthropods, probably because of an allergic response to the protein

Table 25-2. Bites and stings*

Type of Arthropod	Signs and symptoms	Management
Stinging		
Honeybee *(Apis mellificus)* Bumblebee *(Bombus)*	Painful injection wound with stinger often visibly protruding; edema and itching may be apparent.	Remove stinger by scraping with dull object. *Do not grasp and pull,* since this contracts the venom sac, releasing more toxin. Cleanse site and apply antiseptic. Apply ice and elevate part. Oral antihistamines and steroids may be indicated.
Yellow jacket *(Vespula maculifrons)* Wasp *(Chlorion ichneumonica)* Hornet *(Vespula maculata)*	Painful injection wound. Do not leave stinger behind. Stings repeatedly. Wheal formation, edema, itching may be present.	See bee sting. Watch for anaphylaxis. (See p. 251.)
Velvet ant *(Mutilla sacken)* Fire ant *(Solenopsis geminata)*	Painful injection wound with wheal, which expands into large vesicle; as purulence develops, reddening of area occurs; scarring and crusting follow reabsorption of pustule.	See bee sting. Watch for anaphylaxis. (See p. 251.)
Scorpions *(Centravoides vittatus* and *Centruroides gertschi)*	*Lethal:* No visible local effect. Sharp pain, hyperesthesia followed by hypoesthesia, itching, and speech disturbances are common. Jaw muscle spasms, nausea, vomiting, incontinence, and seizures follow. Death may occur from cardiovascular or respiratory failure.	Apply tourniquet as near to sting site as possible, and pack area in ice well beyond the tourniquet. After 5 minutes loosen tourniquet and reapply.
	Nonlethal: Sharp burning pain at sting site with edema and discoloration; anaphylaxis is rare.	*Caution:* Morphine and opiates are contraindicated, since they enhance toxic effects.
Biting and piercing		
Tick *(Dermacentor variabilis)*	Victim unaware of presence. Local irritation and possible injection when body is pulled off and head remains in tissue. Some species (which transmit Rocky Mountain spotted fever) cause flaccid paralysis from neurotoxin. Initial symptoms are paresthesias and pain in lower extremity. Respiratory failure results from bulbar paralysis.	Remove the offending ticks. Apply gasoline, ether, or a hot (not burning) match to the body. Wait 10 minutes for disengagement. Do not manually remove, for squeezing the body may inject more virus into the victim. The paralysis will dramatically subside.

*From Barber, J. M., and Budassi, S. A.: Mosby's Manual of emergency care, St. Louis, 1979, The C. V. Mosby Co.

Table 25-2. Bites and stings—cont'd

Type of Arthropod	Signs and symptoms	Management
Biting and piercing—cont'd		
Centipedes		
Eastern house centipede *(Scutigera cleoptratu)*	Wound site is red, edematous, and painful; sometimes tissue necrosis occurs.	Cleanse wound. Employ analgesics and antibiotics if indicated.
Wester house centipede *(Scolopendra heros)*		
Spiders		
Black widow *(Latrodectus mactans)* (Hourglass spider) (Female)	Pricking sensation is followed by dull, numbing pain. Edema and tiny red fang marks may become visible. Chest and abdomen pain may be evident adjacent to the site of the bite. Pain and rigidity of muscles subside after 48 hours. Blood pressure, temperature, and white blood count may be elevated. Hematuria rarely develops. Spinal fluid has been known to be under increased pressure.	Use ice locally to slow absorption of toxins. Employ muscle relaxants and 10% calcium gluconate IV to reduce spasms. Use antivenin *(Latrodectus mactans)*. Do skin test before administration of the horse serum. Symptoms subside 1-3 hours after antivenin administration.
Brown recluse *(Loxosceles reclusa)* (Fiddleback)	Local reactions begin 2-8 hours after bite with pain, edema, bleb formation, and ischema. On third or fourth day after bite, central area turns dark and is firm to touch. In the second week, the central area becomes depressed and demarcated with open ulceration formation. Healing may take place in about 3 weeks. Fever, chills, malaise, weakness, nausea, vomiting, joint pain, and petechiae may also be noted. Blood dyscrasias such as hemolytic anemia and thrombocytopenia rarely occur.	Immediate excision of wound with toxins may be useful. Steroids, antihistamines, and antibiotics are to be employed as indicated. Skin grafting may be necessary if healing does not take place.
True bugs		
Kissing bug *(Conenose triatoma)*	Mild or no pain at wound site. Redness, edema, itching, or nodular hemorrhagic lesions, depending on sensitivity.	Cleanse wound with soap and water. Oral antihistamines may be indicated. Anaphylaxis has been re-reported.
Assassin bug *(Arilus Christatus)* (Wheel bug)	Intense pain at wound site. Usually lasts 2-5 hours. Localized edema, itching and redness.	Cleanse wound with an antiseptic solution. Anaphylaxis rare.
Vesicating or urticating		
Blister beetles	A clean amber fluid (cantharidin) is released from the insects knee joints, prothorax, and genetalia. A mild burning sensation may become apparent due to fluid released at site.	Cleanse area with soap and water as soon as possible.

Continued.

Table 25-2. Bites and stings—cont'd

Type of Arthropod	Signs and symptoms	Management
Vesicating or urticating—cont'd		
Lepidoptera (larva)		
Io caterpillar *(Automeris io)* Puss caterpillar *(Mega-lopyge opercularis)* Saddle back caterpillar *(Sibine stimulea)* Range caterpillar *(Hemi-leuca oliviae)*	A distinct row of released spines may be seen at the site of intense pain. Nausea, vomiting, headache, and fever may be present.	Remove the spines with adhesive tape if possible. Apply ice to the wound; analgesics may be indicated. Unremoved spines could cause infection.
Aquatic organisms†		
Stingray	Wound contains venom sacs from furrowed spine of stingray tail. Fainting, nausea, vomiting, and diarrhea occur with occasional progression to muscle paralysis, respiratory distress, seizures, and even death.	Immediately irrigate wound to remove venom sacs (that is, flush with normal saline). Follow initial irrigation with immersion in hot water for 30 minutes (110°-114° F) to inactivate venom. Antibiotics are recommended; antihistamines and steroids may also be indicated. In severe cases have ventilatory support and resuscitation equipment at hand. Surgical closure of wounds may be necessary in some instances.
Catfish	Wound from dorsal spine causes pain and infection.	Use deep irrigations of hydrogen peroxide. Employ antibiotics as indicated.
Portuguese man-of-war *(Physalia physalis)*	Tentacles become embedded in skin. There may be welts, burned areas, or streaks. Pain may be intense enough to produce shock and collapse. Headache, cramps, and paralysis are also noted.	Tourniquet may be tried. Remove tentacles with alcohol and sodium bicarbonate scrub (prevents further stinging and neutralizes acid). Leave alcohol on for 6-8 min. Follow with sodium bicarbonate, allowing it to dry. Employ antihistamines and steroids locally and systemically. General anesthesia may be necessary to control pain.
Stings (cone shell snails, sea anemones, corals, and jellyfish)	Acid wound produced.	Cleanse wound with alkali (ammonia, sodium bicarbonate).
Bites (sea snake and octopus)	Wounds contain neurotoxin. Muscle stiffness, paralysis, myoglobinuria, and death from respiratory arrest can occur.	Apply tourniquet. Control shock; use indicated resuscitation measures.
Scorpionfish	Intense pain, edema, shock, and ECG changes.	See stingray injuries for wound cleansing and heat application. Give antivenin.
Sea urchins	Painful injection site with erythema, edema, numbness, and paralysis. Respiratory distress and death may occur.	Use heat as described under stingray. Do not attempt to remove spines initially but do attempt to locate them using x-ray films. Granulomatous lesions often develop from embedded spines.

†Antivenins for most aquatic bites and stings (stonefish, jellyfish, sea snake, and so on) are available from Commonwealth Serum Laboratories, Melbourne, Australia.

substance in the venom. Other arthropods also have the ability to create a medical concern but to a lesser degree, depending on the species. A person with a known hypersensitivity to any bite, sting, or other irritation from arthropods should acquire medical alert identification and carry it with him at all times. One should also consult a physician concerning the acquisition of an emergency anaphylactic kit when going afield.

Most insects and other arthropods go unnoticed until a sting or bite is incurred. Because there are just a few venomous or irritating arthropods in the United States, one should know and be able to identify those species indigenous to his geographical location.

Emergency nurses find it appropriate in their community to distribute information regarding venomous anthropods (Table 25-2). An example is this guide.

General guidelines to avoid venomous arthropods

1. Become familiar with the habitat and the identification of venomous arthropods.
2. Do not disturb insects or their nesting quarters.
3. Do not wear loose fitting clothing when afield.
4. Avoid the use fragrances such as colognes, after-shaves, and hair sprays.
5. Bright colored clothing attracts insects; dark colors repel.
6. Apply insect repellent to exposed area of the body when afield.
7. Never touch an insect unless positive identification has been established.
8. Examine the scalp, groin, and other body parts when coming in from afield for the possibility of ticks.
9. Check house pets for ticks and fleas if they are in and out of doors routinely.
10. Keep sheds, outbuildings, and privies as clean as possible to avert nest building.

LIGHTNING INJURIES

Injuries caused by lightning are not a common occurrence. It has been estimated that between 150 to 300 persons die each year in the U.S. from direct or indirect contact with lightning. Lightning occurs when ice particles collide in clouds being carried upward by warm air and downward by cooler air. Because of a large buildup of negative electrical charges in the bottom of the cloud and the positive charge of the earth, an attraction of negative and positive charges occurs, resulting in a bolt of lightning. It has been estimated that the current from such a bolt of lightning contains between 12,000 and 200,000 amperes and takes between $1/100$ and $1/1000$ of a second to hit the ground.

Patients with lightning injuries who are not responsive and in cardiac arrest should have CPR started immediately. Resuscitation efforts should continue for an extended period of time. Many cardiac arrest victims from lightning injuries have been resuscitated successfully and without sequelae; the 4- to 6-minute rule for cell death does not apparently apply. It is thought that cell degeneration is halted for an undeterminable period of time, because when lightning passes through the body all cell metabolism stops immediately, therefore requiring a longer period of time for the body cells to begin degeneration.

All patients who arrive in the emergency department with lightning injuries should have the following medical intervention.

Patent airway should be maintained with 4 to 6 liters of oxygen.

Continuous heart monitoring is essential. Usually these patients have elevated S-T segments and T wave inversion on their electrocardiogram. Recent literature also suggests that a delay in the effects of a damaged myocardium may not show up for 8 to 24 hours after the injury. Dysrhythmias should be treated with appropriate antidysrhythmic agents.

Fluid resuscitation should begin by utilizing a low molecular weight dextran and possible osmotic diuretic.

Baseline arterial blood gases should be obtained along with other routine blood values.

A CVP should be inserted to monitor the acuity of the pulmonary circuit.

Continuous monitoring of vital signs should take place, as in any other emergency.

Because of the nature of injury, tetanus prophylaxis should be administered.

The electrical burns should be treated with appropriate topical chemotherapy. (Be sure to inspect all areas of the body for entrance and exit points.)

Supportive measures and observation with monitoring equipment for at least 24 hours should be considered, regardless of the apparent condition of the patient.

Lightning is a natural occurrence that can threaten one's health and safety. Some tips on how to avoid its injuries during a thunderstorm include the following:

Stay out of water. (This includes the bathtub if indoors.)

Stay clear of any single tall object. They are prime targets for lightning.

Stay off the telephone (unless it's an emergency) because lightning may travel through the wires to you.

If in a car during a lightning storm, stay in it. It is well grounded because of the tires.

Discard all sporting equipment such as golf clubs, fishing rods, aluminum ball bats, and so on.

If afield with no apparent protection, head for dense woods; if you have rubber rain gear, lay on it.

Do not run.

If indoors, do not stand between an open door and open window, or lightning may strike in a linear fashion between the door and window along a current of hot or moist air.

FROSTBITE

Frostbite is a condition of trauma induced when ice crystals form and expand in extracellular spaces. The enlarging ice particles compress the cell, resulting in cell membrane rupture, thus interrupting enzymatic activity and basic metabolic processes. As histamine is then released, there is increased capillary permeability with red cell aggregation and microvascular occlusion similar to that common with burns. Frostbite is commonly accompanied by hypothermia (see p. 579).

Superficial frostbite involves the fingertips, ears, nose, or cheek. There is burning, tingling, and numbness, with failure of the part to recolor or pink up after blanching. The skin may take on a grayish cast with underlying tissue remaining soft. At this phase, warmth can be applied as long as friction is avoided. It is crucial not to allow cold exposure immediately after rewarming, however.

Deep frostbite is more serious and usually involves the hands or feet. The tissue appears white and is cold and solid to touch. After thawing, it changes its color to pink or purplish blue, with pain, blister formation, and even necrosis.

The triage nurse should elicit the nature of the individual's exposure (length of time, type of clothing worn, temperature, and wind chill). A history of other concurrent disease, especially disorders that affect circulation should be obtained, noting if there has been prior rewarming or refreezing, since these processes extraordinarily increase destruction of tissue. Clinicians, as well as patients, should realize that the length of exposure (once deep frostbite has occurred) does not affect the prognosis.

Emergency management

Emergency management involves rapid rewarming and water baths of 100° to 105° F (37.8° to 40.6 C). Water warmer than 106° F may cause excessive tissue destruction. The nurse should avoid any mechanical friction in the rewarming process, such as rubbing the area or allowing the part to touch the bottom of a basin or tub. Analgesics may need to be given to facilitate the rewarming process.

If there is deep extensive tissue destruction, the victim will have to be hospitalized. Subsequent management of the frostbitten part will include elevation on sterile sheets, using a foot cradle or other device to protect it from pressure friction and reduce the surrounding edema. If fingers or toes are involved, they should be separated with cotton balls or other dry dressing material. Large skin areas involved may require the patient to be isolated.

Tetanus prophylaxis should be provided as indicated by the patient's history. Ordinarily, antibiotics are not necessary. If blisters form related to the frostbitten area, they should be permitted to remain intact, because they will rupture spontaneously in 3 to 7 days. Occasionally, in rare circumstances a fasciotomy may be required to permit adequate circulation of a frostbitten extremity. Amputation is seldom necessitated, and should be avoided until it is well documented that no viable tissue is lying beneath the dead skin surface. Long-term effects of frostbitten areas include: cold sensitivity, excessive sweating, and paresthesias.

Teaching and follow-up advice for patients

Patients who have been seen in the emergency department and treated for frostbitten areas or who have required hospitalization for the treatment of such injuries should be given follow-up instructions in order to prevent the problems from occurring in the future.

Some rules that are helpful for people exposed to cold environments, particularly when the wind chill factor is high, include the following:

Use mittens rather than gloves, since the fingers each give off heat that keeps adjacent fingers warm.

Keep the feet dry, and wear two pairs of socks, one cotton (next to the skin) and one wool.

Avoid tight fitting shoes or boots, since they interfere with circulation and increase the effect of cold.

Do not use alcohol when exposed to extremely low temperatures; it has a vasodilating effect on the peripheral circulation, and thus adds to heat loss.

Keep active. Muscular activity generates heat.

Eat high caloric foods to supply heat.

Do not smoke in an extremely low temperature environment, since nicotine constricts blood vessels and reduces blood flow to the periphery.

Avoid high wind chill velocities in conjunction with low temperatures.

Wear several layers of clothing to trap air between them.

Wear hoods, hats, and scarfs.

Carry blankets and extra clothing in the car during cold episodes. An aluminum space-age blanket is ideal, since it is inexpensive and compact.

The follow-up care of frostbite may include range-of-motion exercises, whirlpool treatments, or other similar therapeutic modalities to enhance circulation. Wet dressings or petrolatum-impregnated gauze and ointments should be strictly avoided in conjunction with the skin lesions.

HYPOTHERMIA

Hypothermia is generally defined as a condition in which the core temperature of the body is less than 95° (35° C). However, adverse physiological circumstances do not occur until a 90° F (32.2° C) level is approached, when shivering stops and muscle rigidity sets in. Death usually occurs if the core temperature falls below 78° F (25.5° C). *It is imperative to attempt resuscitation of suspected hypothermia victims, despite apnea, pulselessness, dilated fixed pupils, a comatose state, and cold, rigid body*. It has been established that successful resuscitations have occurred after 2 or 3 hours of "clinical death," because the lowered body temperature protects the brain from the effects of anoxia associated with prolonged circulatory arrest. In order to assess core temperature, all emergency departments should possess a special rectal thermometer with a scale that extends down to 80° F (27° C) or a low scale esophageal thermometer.

When a victim of hypothermia has been received in the emergency department, initial life support measures should be taken at once if necessary. In the meantime, all wet clothing should be removed. Ordinarily, at least one, or preferably two, large IV lines for fluid and medication administration should be initiated. One line may be reserved for CVP monitoring. Venous blood should be drawn for the following tests: CBC, BUN, serum electrolytes, serum amylase, blood sugar, and coagulation studies. Some clinicians may also request an arterial blood gas sample. The nurse should prepare to monitor the ECG and to observe for conduction disturbances. Asystole occurs ordinarily at temperatures of 70° to 75° F (21.1° to 23.8° C).

Atrial fibrillation is the most common cold-related dysrhythmia. Look for a J, or Osborn, wave (positive deflection of the terminal 0.04-

second period of the QRS complex). Continue resuscitation despite a flat line ECG for up to 2½ to 3 hours. When the core temperature reaches 88° to 90° F either during cooling or rewarming, ventricular fibrillation may occur. If defibrillation is required, the operator should be especially cognizant of the hazards posed by the rewarming process, which usually involves using basins of warm water. The environment can become very precarious under such circumstances. Rubber boots and a 12-volt battery defibrillator unit are used in some institutions to minimize these risks. However, most departments do not have access to such devices unless previous experiences with hypothermia episodes have demonstrated their utility.

Active rewarming by core and external processes should follow initial resuscitation. *Ensure that the core temperature increases concurrently with the external temperature to prevent ventricular fibrillation.* When body surfaces are rewarmed, their initial demand for oxygen is quite high and the hypothermic heart is unable to meet this accelerated demand through increasing cardiac output. Hence, surface and myocardial hypoxia and acidosis are aggravated. Some of the following measures may be useful during the rewarming process:

A thermal blanket regulated at 98° to 100° F (36.6° to 37.7° C) can be incorporated into the plan to increase the body temperature at a rate of 1° to 2° per hour.

An immersion tub bath at a temperature of 104° F (40° C) can also be instituted. This will supplement other measures when life support electrical apparatus can be abandoned.

Core rewarming can involve several different procedures. Some of the ones most commonly used are the following:

Give IV fluids warmed with a blood-rewarming coil immersed in basins of warm water (99° F) 37° C. Be certain to maintain a constant temperature of the water by frequent changes and careful thermal monitoring.

Perform warm peritoneal lavage with normal saline heated to 98° to 100° F (36.6° to 37.7° C). (The bladder must be decompressed by a Foley catheter before the procedure to avoid accidental perforation of the bladder.) Dialysis solutions may be employed on the recommendation of a renal consultant. Constant electrolyte monitoring is imperative.

Nasogastric or rectal lavage with warm normal saline may be done to warm the gastrointestinal tract.

Thoracotomy with mediastinal lavage using heated fluids is another acceptable procedure.

Cardiopulmonary bypass with heat exchange may be done.

Ventilator managed respiration employing warm humidified air is also recommended.

Monitor laboratory values including electrolytes, hematocrit, blood sugar, BUN, and arterial blood gases. Record intake and output every 15 to 30 minutes. Assess the CVP and neurological status on at least an hourly basis. Monitor the heart rhythm constantly. Record a 6-second strip at least hourly to plot cardiovascular electrical trends. The nurse should also assess the external and core temperature at least hourly and constantly if electronic adjuncts are available. *Remember:* Do not rewarm the core faster than 1° or 2° per hour to prevent rewarming shock. Ensure that external rewarming does not occur at a faster pace than core rewarming to prevent the grave consequence of ventricular fibrillation.

HEAT SYNDROMES: CURRENT MANAGEMENT PRINCIPLES
Charles McElroy

Heat illness spans the spectrum from minor aberrations in physiology attended by minimal clinical symptoms to full-blown heat stroke accompanied by major clinical manifestations and occasional death of the victim. In this presentation, we will concentrate on individual syndromes that have widely accepted clinical and pathological substrates, and for which there is an evolving consensus on appropriate therapeutics.

Heat edema

Swelling of the feet and ankles is often reported by individuals, most especially the aged, upon visiting tropical and semitropical areas.

Most such individuals have no underlying cardiac, liver, venous, or lymphatic disease to explain this abnormality. The edema is usually minimal, is not accompanied by any significant impairment in function, and often resolves after several days of acclimatization. Since this entity is of inconsequential clinical import, accurate and detailed assessment of its pathophysiology is lacking. It is presumed that vasodilation of the cutaneous and muscular vessels, combined with venostasis, leads to vascular leak and accumulation of interstitial fluid in the lower extremities. The most important reason for being aware of this clinical presentation is to prevent overly vigorous diagnostic and therapeutic intervention in patients with this problem. Certainly, brief diagnostic evaluation is appropriate, but vigorous invasive diagnostic techniques and/or vigorous pharmacological therapy is clearly not indicated. There is no evidence for example, that diuretic therapy is appropriate in these individuals; rather, where possible, simple elevation or mechanical support hose can be employed. In the majority of individuals, benign neglect is the order of the day, and the problem will eliminate itself either through adequate acclimatization of the individual or with the individual's return to his or her place of origin.

Heat syncope

The next possible stage in the spectrum of heat illness is that of fainting in those exposed to and unaccustomed to the ambient heat. Although anyone may faint after prolonged standing because of peripheral pooling of blood in the lower extremities, this mild aberration in normal vasomotor regulatory control is exacerbated in hot climates. Since volume loss secondary to sweating, coupled with peripheral vasodilatation to lose body heat, in circumstances demanding prolonged standing, creates an ideal situation for inadequate blood return to the central circulation, individuals in these circumstances have an inordinately high incidence of syncope. Although it is mandatory to rule out other significant causes of syncope, most are suffering from simple postural syncope and can be adequately treated by postural adaptation. The patient should be orally volume re-

pleted and encouraged to avoid prolonged standing. Prophylactic instruction in the mechanism of the event may be helpful in preventing repeated episodes. Patients should be encouraged to assume a horizontal or head-between-knees position whenever postural syncope becomes imminent.

Heat exhaustion

This condition is a rather vague pathophysiological state that is one step further along the spectrum of heat illness. It clearly is of more consequence than the previously mentioned syndromes, but does not have the attendant morbidity and mortality of frank heat stroke. The temperature encountered in these patients is generally between 39° and 40° C, thus providing a useful objective measure to help the therapist discriminate between frank heat exhaustion and heat stroke. More important, the syndrome itself is one characterized by dizziness, nausea, headache, and low-grade temperature elevation.

Water deficiency is believed to contribute significantly to a portion of the patients complaining of heat exhaustion. Since 1 liter/hour is commonly lost during extremes of environmental heat stress, and 2 to 3 liters/hour have been reported, it is not unreasonable to expect that individuals could easily become water depleted. Each liter of sweat contains between 20 and 50 mEq sodium chloride, thus adding salt deficiency to the pathophysiological substrate. Hence, both water and salt deficiency, in variable proportions, combine to cause electrolyte, volume balance, and vasomotor regulatory disturbances, which contribute to inadequate peripheral and cerebral perfusion. These are mild, and the patient is usually easily treated by oral volume replacement. Quite obviously, this syndrome may blend inexorably and imperceptibly into heat stroke, but under ordinary circumstances, it is an easy differential diagnosis, since the symptoms are only minimally aberrant.

Muscle cramps. Muscle cramps may be a significant problem to patients suffering from heat exhaustion. The problem of muscle cramps is extremely common in hot climes and is felt to be primarily due to a rapid change in extracellular fluid osmolarity resulting from salt and water losses, which may occur rapidly under the circumstances described. Muscle cramps and the heat exhaustion syndrome in general are usually easily treated with appropriate salt and water replacement. Interestingly, agents such as Gatorade (a relatively balanced salt solution) and other similar fluid vehicles available for oral volume replacement are effective in both prevention and therapy of this problem.

Heat stroke
Etiology and predisposing factors

CLIMATE. Quite obviously, severely hot conditions, particularly those with simultaneous high humidity and without wind, optimally predispose to the development of heat stroke. It is most important, however, to consider the diagnosis at other times, as will become apparent when we consider other predisposing factors. Extremes of exercise, age, and underlying illness establish conditions wherein, even under the more mild of climatic conditions, patients can become extremely hyperthermic and suffer from the consequences of heat stroke.

EXERCISE. Extremes of exercise, including strenuous physical performance under hot environmental conditions, are notorious for establishing circumstances under which heat stroke will develop even in normal individuals. Unfortunately, however, even conditioned athletes may develop untoward consequences of heat retention when proper acclimatization has not been established before beginning vigorous physical activity. Football training programs are notorious for contributing an unreasonable share of heat stroke deaths to the annual morbidity and mortality statistics. In fact, heat illness as a consequence of football activities is second only to head injuries as a cause of death in American football. The ignorance that still surrounds organized and unorganized exercise activities, including football and a variety of other team sports, leads to the development of such heat-associated illness. Coaches who labor under the unfortunate misconceptions that water should not be provided during exercise and that young individuals can tolerate great excesses of physical exertion without undue

negative effects, along with clothing that retains any heat generated by the body, all contribute to this unfortunate circumstance. With proper acclimatization, conditioning, appropriate clothing, proper fluid replacement, and education of both supervisors and players, the majority of these problems could easily be avoided. Other precipitating activities include the armed services, where large numbers of unacclimatized and unconditioned individuals are pushed rapidly to or beyond their tolerance of physical activities and hence contribute to the medical literature relating to heat illness. The contemporary enthusiasm for jogging has produced another situation that generates large numbers of heat illness. In one recent morning of activities at UCLA, we received eight patients with heat illness, of whom three were suffering from frank heat stroke, one of whom remained hospitalized for approximately 10 days with major neurological, hepatic, renal, and muscle abnormalities. To detail all of the circumstances under which exercise is capable of producing heat illness is unproductive; it is enough to say that any unacclimatized, nonconditioned individual who suddenly undertakes excessive physical activity is at risk to develop heat stroke.

AGE. The aged are at great risk for developing heat illness under conditions that would ordinarily be safe. Underlying heart failure, minor neurological aberrations, the use of multiple drugs, and general frailty all contribute to the propensity for older individuals to suffer from heat stroke.

HEART FAILURE. Individuals suffering from myocardial dysfunction with inadequate ability to adapt to changes in environmental or physical stress, are clearly at increased risk of developing heat stroke under a variety of circumstances.

OBESITY. Whether obesity per se has a risk factor, or whether it is in fact the accompanying lack of physical conditioning that establishes this as a risk factor for developing heat stress is not clear from an evaluation of the available literature. Nonetheless, in most papers consulted, obesity has been referred to as a potential risk factor, though a minor one; hence, individuals with extremes of body weight should be viewed as being more at risk than otherwise normal individuals.

DRUGS. A variety of medications have been listed as being associated with the development of heat stroke and are presumed to be causal. Most of these drugs affect the ability to sweat, to peripherally vasodilate, or increase the basic metabolic activity of the individual. Some may have additional effects on central thermal regulatory activity, most notably the phenothiazines. The following drugs have been documented to have a putatively causal association with the development of hyperthermia: anticholinergics, phenothiazines, tricyclic depressants, monoaminoxidase inhibitors, glutethimide, LSD, and amphetamines. In addition, drugs restricted to hospital use, including nitrous oxide, halothane, ethylene, ethyl chloride, and succinyl choline have all been reported to be associated with the development of hyperthermia. It is important to note at this time that even though phenothiazines are listed as causally related to the development of heat stroke, there is no evidence to suggest that they should not be used in the full-blown case of heat stroke when the therapist needs to control shivering that may develop in the course of therapy. Though phenothiazines have been reported to alter the hypothalamic control of temperature regulation, when a patient is being cooled by artificial means and has been removed from ambient climatic conditions or circumstances under which physical exercise generated intolerable heat production, phenothiazines would not be expected to potentiate persistence or aggravation of hyperthermia. Phenothiazines have been repeatedly reported to block shivering and hence are listed as agents of choice for this special circumstance.

ALCOHOL. Alcohol, through a complex set of mechanisms, has been said to predispose towards heat illness. Interestingly, it also predisposes towards hypothermia. These reports are poorly documented, but appear often enough to require attention.

SPECIAL CLINICAL STATES. Excessive use of sauna baths, Turkish baths followed by exceptionally vigorous physical activity, incarceration in the Black Hole of Calcutta, and other similar unusual circumstances have all been reported to be remarkably effective in generating large numbers of heat casualties. In addition, patients suffering from mucoviscidosis, exfoliative dermatitides, Riley-Day syndrome, and a variety of other unusual illnesses have all been reportedly associated with an increased risk of developing heat illness.

Pathophysiology. The cause of heat stroke is clearly an accumulation of body heat because of failure or inadequacy of thermal regulatory mechanisms that, under ordinary circumstances, are sufficient to maintain core temperature at a level compatible with normal physiological activity. In humans, temperatures above 42° C appear to be routinely associated with marked resultant aberrations in the homeostasis of the individual. The figure 42° C is fairly well established, since large numbers of humans undergoing experimental temperature elevation in an attempt to control terminal cancer were demonstrated to tolerate temperatures up to 41.8° C. Nonetheless, occasional individuals will undergo full-blown heat stroke at lower temperatures. Above 42° C and certainly in the 44° C to 46° C range, enzymes denature, membranes liquefy, the mitochondria become nonfunctional, coding of proteins becomes disrupted, and the coordination of physiological processes ceases.

It appears that thermal regulation is controlled in hypothalamic thermal regulatory centers, which receive their information largely from the temperature of the blood circulating through the area. Skin sensors also receive and send information relating environmental temperature. In response to hypothalamic stimulation, respiratory rate increases to increase heat loss via exhaled air. Simultaneously, cardiac output increases in order to provide increased blood flow through skin and muscle. Blood flowing through the skin then allows for radiation of heat from the body. Simultaneously, sweat glands are activated, producing large quantities of sodium chloride and water, which then evaporate from the skin, adding to heat loss by evaporation. In acclimatized individuals, the concentration of sodium chloride in the sweat is lower than in nonacclimatized individuals. In the least trained subjects, sodium chloride levels are as high as 40 to 50 mEq/liter. With more training, the amount of sodium chloride falls so that a more dilute sweat is produced, thereby reducing the amount of salt loss.

In many discussions of heat illness, it has been stated that heat stroke occurs when either destruction of sweat glands occurs, or when the sweat glands undergo temporary dysfunction because of input overload. It is quite clear that this is an error and that continued sweating is quite possible even in a full-blown case of heat stroke. Similarly, although cardiovascular disease certainly predisposes to the development of heat stroke because of the inability of the cardiovascular system to maintain adequate blood flow through the periphery to maximize heat loss, heat stroke is nonetheless possible even with optimal cardiac function. Dehydration, often an accompanying parameter of heat stroke, is also not necessary for the patient to develop overt heat stroke.

The temperature achieved by the body is apparently the culprit in the destructive events that occur. Other proposed mechanisms include hypoxia, intravascular coagulation, electrolyte abnormalities, and severe acidosis. Although all of these physiological aberrations certainly accompany heat stroke, it is apparent that it is the temperature itself that is the primary pathological force.

Differential diagnosis. Although obvious cases of heat stroke are easy to diagnose, one must not be lulled into a false sense of security in making the diagnosis without ruling out other possible causes that might mimic heat stroke. Meningitis, encephalitis, malaria, typhoid fever, typhus, and hypothalamic hemorrhage have all been reported to cause syndrome complexes similar to heat stroke.

Clinical presentation

CENTRAL NERVOUS SYSTEM. Disturbances of the central nervous system often dominate the early course of heat stroke, with abrupt onset of confusion, irrational behavior, and sudden change or loss of consciousness. Convulsions are not uncommon and may appear early or be delayed. Early seizures may not be as ominous prognos-

tically as the late development of the same problem, perhaps because when seizure activity occurs at a later time, it often reflects an underlying structural abnormality such as in situ thrombosis, frank hemorrhage, or cytopathological changes resulting in loss of neuronal structure and function. Hemiplegia, ataxia, and permanent dementia have all been reported as residuals of heat stroke.

HYPOTENSION. Hypotension, leading into frank shock, is a common early manifestation of heat stroke. The mechanism of this aberration is complex. Volume depletion is certainly present, but has been repeatedly stated to be a minor component of hypotension. Since both water and sodium chloride are lost during sweating, with documented losses of 1 liter/hour being common, and with as much as 2 to 3 liters being documented under special circumstances, large amounts of water and sodium chloride may be lost from the body in short order. Sweat frequently contains 10 to 50 mEq/liter of sodium chloride. The less the conditioning of the individual, the higher the sodium chloride concentration. In one interesting case in the literature, a football player was reported to have lost 22 pounds during one early season game, with resultant confusion, hypotension, and signs of heat exhaustion. Thus, hypotension from water and electrolyte loss is to be expected if adequate replacement is not carried out prophylactically.

Peripheral vasodilatation with resultant *peripheral pooling* of intravascular contents is both a mechanism of heat loss and a contributor to hypotension. Furthermore, when lactic acidosis intervenes, peripheral pooling is enhanced, thereby augmenting any detriment in myocardial performance or hypovolemia that may simultaneously be present.

Myocardial dysfunction also plays a role in the development of hypotension and/or shock. Most especially noted in the elderly, pulmonary edema with high central venous pressure and wedge pressures between 25 and 40 mm Hg are frequently reported. Younger individuals, however, are not free of the spectre of heart failure. Myocardial infarction and death from heart failure or arrhythmias have been repeatedly reported in the setting of heat stroke. Interestingly, both at postmortem and in those cases where cardiac catheterization is done, coronary arteries are usually completely normal or have insignificant atherosclerotic change. Pathological section of the hearts of victims dying from heat stroke show mild to moderate hemorrhage into various areas of the myocardium, cellular degeneration, and spotty inflammatory infiltration of the heart muscle. Although these are frequently seen, the extent of the pathological change is not sufficient to explain the incidence or degree of cardiac dysfunction, and are even less sufficient to explain a cardiac cause of the death of the individual. Nonetheless, aberrations in myocardial performance are certainly frequent and can contribute to the development of hypotension and/or shock.

Disseminated intravascular coagulation or local areas of intravascular coagulation leading to in situ thrombosis further contributes to multiple organ dysfunction and pulmonary and cardiac insufficiency. These aberrations, and occasional episodes of massive gastrointestinal hemorrhage, all combine to present numerous causes for hypotension and shock.

RESPIRATORY FUNCTION. As mentioned, pulmonary edema is not uncommon, and is felt to be the result of both myocardial dysfunction with elevated pulmonary capillary wedge pressures and intravascular coagulation with resulting in situ vascular thrombosis. All of these, plus the systemic acidosis, generally lead to tachypnea, hypoxemia, and hypercarbia.

GASTROINTESTINAL FUNCTION. Gastrointestinal dysfunction is often present and is felt to reflect poor perfusion, electrolyte abnormalities, and intravascular coagulation, which may lead to frank gastrointestinal ulceration and massive gastrointestinal bleeding.

ADRENAL FUNCTION. Adrenal function appears to be well maintained during the course of heat stroke for reasons that are not clear, despite occasional pathological findings, including hemorrhage and inflammatory infiltrate. No cases have been reported of adrenal insufficiency under these circumstances.

RENAL FUNCTION. The renal system is reportedly one of the most commonly involved organ systems in the setting of heat stroke. The aberrations in renal function are felt to be secondary to hypovolemia and hypoperfusion because of all the conditions listed above. This may lead to only transient renal function embarassment, or to frank acute vasomotor nephropathy, which may require temporary dialysis for maintenance of the patient. The urine under these circumstances has occasionally been described to look like machine oil; it often shows a low specific gravity because of the inability of the kidneys to concentrate; red and white cells; white cell, hyaline, and granular casts; and mild to moderate protein. Ketone bodies are routinely found.

HEPATIC FUNCTION. The liver is frequently injured during the course of heat stroke. Frank jaundice may occur, either because of hepatocellular dysfunction or, presumably, edema of the head of the pancreas. Surprisingly, frank pancreatitis is only rarely reported, even though pathological sectioning routinely discloses local intravascular coagulation and cellular infiltrate, or hemorrhage into the substance of the pancreas. The liver itself is frequently enlarged and tender when examined, and laboratory evaluation often demonstrates elevation of SGOT, SGPT, minimal elevation of alkaline phosphatase, and mild to marked increases in bilirubin, lactic dehydrogenase, and gamma-glutamiletranscarbamylase. All these hepatocellular enzymes reflect hepatocellular death, which pathological evaluation reveals by occasional central lobular necrosis, dropping out of hepatocytes, and a diffuse monocellular infiltrate.

CLOTTING DISORDERS. Hemostasis is routinely abnormal during heat stroke. Clotting disturbances, believed to be mediated by a drop in platelet count, hypoprothrombinemia, hypofibrinogenemia, and increased capillary fragility are hallmarks of this disorder. Liver dysfunction certainly contributes to this picture, but diffuse intravascular coagulation is felt to similarly play a major role, as does thermal damage to cells and protein.

LABORATORY ABNORMALITIES.
- An ECG may show conduction disturbances and nonspecific ST and T wave changes. On occasion, changes compatible with true myocardial infarction are re-

ported. It is of interest that the cross-correlation with pathological findings compatible with coronary artery disease are not ordinarily found; in fact, in most cases, the arteries are normal or only minimally compromised by atherosclerotic change.

- The white cell count in these individuals is routinely elevated and may be between 20,000 and 30,000/cu mm. Indeed, white counts between 40,000 and 50,000/cu mm with a marked left shift are not uncommon with marked hyperthermia.

- Potassium values are routinely quite low. This is believed to be the result of renal loss incurred when renal regulatory mechanisms are shifted toward sodium retention by the renin-angiotension-aldosterone axis. Potassium is also lost through sweating, but the complete explanation remains in question.

Therapy. Immediate therapy of heat illness involves the usual ABCs of emergency management plus energetic and definitive control of body temperature.

THE ABCs. As is always the case, airway management is critical in the immediate resuscitation of seriously ill patients. Since pulmonary edema is commonly reported, oxygen is always provided, and intubation with positive pressure breathing is indicated for those patients with pulmonary edema. Pulmonary edema occurring in heart stroke may be the result of either the capillary leak syndrome and/or myocardial dysfunction. Because of this, a CVP or Swan-Ganz catheter is indicated to confirm the diagnostic category of pulmonary edema or heart failure, and to aid in patient management. In those individuals with a low CVP reading, cautious fluid administration averaging 1 to 1½ liters of Ringer's lactate or saline is appropriate to restore deficient intravascular volumes incurred during the stress that caused the heat stroke. It is surprising that volume deficits are frequently less than might be expected, and caution is indicated in avoiding overly vigorous volume replacement. In those individuals with a high CVP or a Swan-Ganz pressure reading in the pulmonary edema range, digitalization and isoproterenol (Isuprel) administration are indicated to improve cardiac output and tissue perfusion. If pulmonary edema is found with CVP or Swan-Ganz readings in the low-to-normal range, then the primary modality of choice is positive pressure ventilation.

Rhythm monitoring is routinely indicated, since these patients have been reported to incur ECG changes suggestive of myocardial infarction, ST and T wave aberrations suggestion of electrolyte abnormalities or ischemia, and dysrhythmias that may require urgent management.

COOLING. This therapeutic modality is of primary importance, and must be initiated as early as possible. The patient should be removed from the initiating environmental cause(s), clothing removed where appropriate, and any of a variety of cooling measures instituted. Modalities that have been reported to be effective include:

Alcohol sponge baths
Ice packs
Large circulating fans
Immersion in a tub of cold water
Cooling blankets

Aspirin is clearly contraindicated, since aspirin not only fails to correct the temperature aberration in these individuals, but has the added potential negative effect of aggravating the underlying abnormality of hemostasis. Most important, the temperature should be lowered as quickly as possible to 39° C as measured by a rectal thermometer. When the temperature reaches 39° C, the cooling measures should be stopped to avoid a hypothermic overshoot. Careful continued monitoring is then necessary to avoid rebound hyperthermia.

If shivering develops during the course of temperature lowering, then chlorpromazine (Thorazine) 10 to 25 mg by intravenous slow push has been recommended. The wisdom of utilizing chlorpromazine to block shivering has been questioned, but on grounds that seem unreasonable. Specifically, chlorpromazine has been implicated as a possible cause of heat stroke by interfering with normal regulatory mechanisms. Despite this, once a patient with heat stroke is in the hands of competent medical management utilizing external means of temperature lowering, there is no indication that phenothiazines would do harm. Since chlorpromazine has been demonstrated to effectively stop shivering, and hence block further heat production, there appears to be adequate scientific support for its cautious use. It should be noted that phenothiazines are alpha-blockers, and hence may potentiate hypotension when present; are cardiotoxic and have been reported to cause arrhythmias; and are known to lower the seizure threshold. For these reasons, the phenothiazines should probably be utilized only when effective temperature control cannot be obtained because of excessive shivering.

CENTRAL NERVOUS SYSTEM ABNORMALITIES. The level of consciousness is routinely depressed in victims of acute heat stroke. Although this is expected, it is important to carefully assess for the presence of cerebral edema, which would indicate the need for mannitol and steroid administration. If cerebral edema is found, 1 to 2 gm/kg mannitol should be given intravenously over 15 to 20 minutes. Dexamethasone 4 mg IV stat and 4 mg IV q6h are also indicated. If focal neurological deficits are found, then the patient should have an emergent EMI or other appropriate diagnostic scan to rule out the presence of an intracerebral hemorrhage, which might be amenable to neurosurgical decompression. Neurosurgical consultation is indicated.

Seizures should be treated with IV diazepam (Valium) or barbiturates in conventional dosages. Phenytoin (Dilantin), though effective, is more difficult to administer and probably should be reserved for those patients with a demonstrable intracranial pathological condition, which would then indicate the need for chronic medication for seizure control.

RENAL FUNCTION. Of all the organ systems involved in heat stroke, the kidneys represent a necessary focus of intense interest. Renal failure, both transient and permanent, is commonly reported. Victims of heat stroke almost always have demonstrable urinalysis abnormalities and routinely demonstrate a rise in BUN and creatinine. Management principles commonly reported to minimize the pathological condition in victims of heat stroke include the early and vigorous use of mannitol. In oliguric individuals who do not respond immediately to intravenous volume expansion, 0.25 gm/kg mannitol should be delivered intravenously. Furthermore, rhabdomyolysis leading to myoglobinuria is routinely reported and may be of paramount importance to the production and propagation of renal failure. For this reason, maintenance of a brisk urine output and alkalinization of the urine is indicated if myoglobinuria is documented or strongly suggested. Occasional patients require acute or chronic dialysis. This is obviously to be avoided, but when necessary may in fact render the patient capable of near full recovery.

MISCELLANEOUS THERAPEUTIC PRINCIPLES

NASOGASTRIC ASPIRATION. Nasogastric aspiration is routinely required to prevent regurgitation of gastric contents and concomitant pulmonary aspiration. Since hypokalemia is a common accompaniment of the heat stroke syndrome, ileus may be induced, leading to gastric atony and a high incidence of pulmonary aspiration. In addition, the gastric contents should be tested for the presence of blood, since GI bleeding has been reported to complicate the heat stroke syndrome.

STEROID USE. As is almost always the case in a serious illness, steroids have been used in the therapeutic management program but are of no proven benefit, and there is no documented evidence indicating their routine use. Specifically, Addisonian crisis, secondary to adrenal apoplexy, has not been reported in this syndrome.

ANTIBIOTIC ADMINISTRATION. There are no special circumstances in heat stroke that justify the routine prophylactic administration of antibiotics.

DISSEMINATED INTRAVASCULAR COAGULATION. This syndrome has been frequently reported to accompany the heat stroke rate. Heparin, as well as clotting factor replacement, has been reported to be effective management. It appears, however, that as is the case for disseminated intravascular coagulation in general, there is no evidence that the addition of heparin, or the replacement of clotting factors, is in fact therapeutically effective in improving morbidity and mortality. The standard management principles for eliminating the underlying cause for the intravascular coagulation should be followed.

HYPERKALEMIA. Although most heat stroke patients are hypokalemic, occasional patients are observed to rapidly develop hyperkalemia. This is believed to be caused by rhabdomyolysis with the release of potassium into the bloodstream, often coupled with renal insufficiency, thereby minimizing renal excretion. Such patients must be managed with great caution, and early dialysis is indicated.

SUGGESTED LABORATORY PARAMETERS

CBC

Urinalysis

BUN and creatinine

SGOT and bilirubin

Creatinine phosphokinase (MM and MB fractions)

Protime, PTT, platelet count, and fibrinogen levels

Serum and urinary amylase evaluation

Chest x-ray studies

ECG monitoring

Stool for guaiac

Lumbar puncture and EEG have not been routinely helpful and are not routinely indicated unless special circumstances dictate

DIVING EMERGENCIES

In diving, a person submits himself to pressures greater than those he is normally exposed to on land. As the gases in the lungs contract as a result of the increased atmospheric pressure, the diver must take in greater quantities of air from the SCUBA (self-contained underwater breathing apparatus) tank so that his lungs will not collapse. These greater atmospheric pressures bring with them a whole array of medical problems that are unique to underwater diving (or other situations that cause increased atmospheric pressures).

When a person is at sea level, the pressure exerted on his body is 1 atmosphere. At a water depth of 33 feet, the pressure exerted on the diver's body is 2 atmospheres. At a water depth of 66 feet, the pressure is 3 atmospheres.

Water depth (feet)	Pressure (atmospheres)
Sea level	1
33	2
66	3
100	4
133	5
166	6
200	7
300	10
400	13
500	16

Depth of dive and effect on gas volume

As Boyle's law states, the volume of a gas varies inversely with the absolute pressure. In other words, as pressure increases, gas volume decreases. For example, if a normal pair of lungs contains 2,000 cc of air at sea level, the volume of air decreases as the diver descends:

Depth	Air in each lung (cc)
Sea level	1000
33 feet	500
100 feet	250
233 feet	125

At a depth of 33 feet the total volume of air would be 1,000 cc (half of normal), at 100 feet it would be 500 cc (one fourth of normal), and at 233 feet, it would be 250 cc (one eighth of normal).

A SCUBA tank is added to the normal lungs at sea level. If the diver forcefully inhales supplemental air from the tank, his lungs will still contain 1,000 cc each:

Depth	Air in each lung (cc)
Sea level	1,000
33 feet	1,000
100 feet	1,000
233 feet	1,000

If the diver ascends but forgets to exhale on the way up, the pressure will decrease as he ascends, and the gas in the lungs will expand:

Depth	Air in each lung (cc)
233 feet	1,000
100 feet	2,000

Depth	Air in each lung (cc)
33 feet	4,000
Sea level	8,000

One can see what will happen; as the gas expands, the lungs expand, to a limit. Then the lungs rupture, a spontaneous pneumothorax results, and air escapes into the circulation, producing an air embolism. The mechanism of injury is breathholding on ascent.

Air embolism

Signs and symptoms
Tightness of chest
Shortness of breath
Pink frothy sputum from nose and mouth
Vertigo (loss of visual point of reference)
Limb paresthesias or vertical (one-sided) paralysis
Seizures
Loss of consciousness
Other signs and symptoms of pneumothorax (See Chapter 17.)

This is an extremely serious condition. If the diver does not die before reaching the surface, he must receive extremely prompt therapy.

Therapeutic intervention
1. Oxygen under positive pressure
2. If tension pneumothorax is present, needles inserted into anterior chest wall (See Chapter 17)
3. Trendelenburg position in left lateral decubitus position to avoid cerebral embolization
4. Prompt recompression

Preventive measures
The diver should exhale while ascending. Note that pneumothorax can occur in as little as 4 feet of water.

Nitrogen narcosis

Nitrogen narcosis is a condition in which, in accordance with Henry's law,* nitrogen (which is 79% of air) is dissolved in solution because the person is breathing nitrogen under greater

---

*At a constant temperature, the solubility of any gas in a liquid is almost directly proportional to the pressure of the liquid.

pressures than normal. Dissolved nitrogen produces effects similar to those of alcohol. The deeper one dives, the greater the narcosis. After 1 hour the effects of nitrogen at various depths are as follows:

Depth	Effects
125-150 feet	Narcosis begins
150-200 feet	Drowsiness, decreased mental functions
200-250 feet	Decreased strength, decreased coordination
300 feet	Diver becomes useless
350-400 feet	Unconsciousness, death

Therapeutic intervention consists of a gradual ascent to shallower water; symptoms of narcosis should disappear. Nitrogen narcosis can be prevented by avoiding dives to excess depths.

Decompression sickness

If a diver is at a depth long enough for nitrogen to be dissolved and then ascends rapidly, there is not enough time for the nitrogen to reabsorb, and nitrogen bubbles form, producing decompression sickness (the bends, dysbarism, caisson disease, diver's paralysis). Exercise (such as swimming toward the surface) causes a rapid release of nitrogen bubbles, similar to the effect of shaking a bottle of a carbonated beverage, causing gas to be released from solution.

Signs and symptoms
Itch
Rash
Fatigue
Dizziness
Paresthesias or paralysis
Seizures
Crepitus
Visual loss
Unconsciousness
Joint soreness
Shortness of breath

Factors increasing severity of signs and symptoms
Extremes of water temperature
Increasing age
Obesity
Fatigue
Poor physical condition

Alcohol consumption

Peripheral vascular disease

Heavy work while diving

Therapeutic intervention

1. Recompression
2. Oxygen at 10 liters/minute by mask
3. IV infusion
4. IV sodium bicarbonate
5. Transport in left lateral Trendelenburg position to decrease the possibility of air embolization.

Special notes

Any complaint of joint soreness 24 to 48 hours following a dive should be treated by decompression in a decompression chamber.

Bends can occur at depths less than 33 feet (1 atmosphere).

There are several common errors in treating decompression sickness:

Victim's failure to report his signs and symptoms

Failure to treat the patient in questionable cases

Failure to identify severe symptoms as a result of a dive accident

Prevention

Do not dive too deeply.

Do not stay down too long.

Follow the U.S. Navy's repetitive dive tables (Tables 25-3 to 25-6) recommendations within a safe range for repetitive dives.

Always carry a SCUBA identification card for at least 48 hours following a dive.

Use of decompression tables. Use of decompression tables allows for gradual ascent with delays at certain depths ("decompression stops") to allow nitrogen to be released by the lungs. Decompression tables are used to calculate the rate of nitrogen absorption by the body. Any dive within 12 hours of resurfacing is a repetitive dive, and the repetitive dive table should be used.

Other medical problems encountered in diving

The "squeeze" (Fig. 25-3). The squeeze results from a compression of air trapped in hollow chambers, producing severe, sharp pain, when outside pressure is greater than inside pressure. It may occur in these areas:

Ears

Sinuses

Lungs and airways

Gastrointestinal tract

Thoracic cavity

Teeth

Added air spaces (face mask or wet suit)

The signs and symptoms are as follows:

Pain

Edema

Capillary dilatation

Rupture

Bleeding

The mechanism by which this occurs is breath holding on descent or trapping of air in a hollow cavity.

Therepeutic intervention consists of gradual ascent to shallower depths to decrease the pressure and maintenance of airway, breathing, and circulation.

Ear squeeze or sinus squeeze. The cause of the ear squeeze or sinus squeeze is a blocked eustachian tube or paranasal sinus and an inability to equalize the pressures.

Therapeutic intervention consists of ascent to shallower water.

Hyperpnea exhaustion syndrome. Hyperpnea exhaustion syndrome usually results from diver fatigue. The signs and symptoms are as follows:

Tachypnea

Anxiety

Feeling of impending doom

Difficulty floating

Exhaustion

Therapeutic intervention consists of ascent to the surface and rest aboard a floatation device or boat.

General safety rules for SCUBA and snorkle divers*

1. Never dive alone.
2. Always wear an inflation vest.

---

*Adapted from class notes taken at Dworet Dive School in Boston, Mass.

Text continued on p. 597.

Table 25-3. U.S. Navy standard air decompression table*

Depth (feet)	Bottom time (min)	Time to first stop (min:sec)	Decompression stops (feet)					Total ascent (min:sec)	Repetitive group
			50	40	30	20	10		
40____	200	-----------	------	------	------	------	0	0:40	(*)
	210	0:30	------	------	------	------	2	2:40	N
	230	0:30	------	------	------	------	7	7:40	N
	250	0:30	------	------	------	------	11	11:40	O
	270	0:30	------	------	------	------	15	15:40	O
	300	0:30	------	------	------	------	19	19:40	Z
50____	100	-----------	------	------	------	------	0	0:50	(†)
	110	0:40	------	------	------	------	3	3:50	L
	120	0:40	------	------	------	------	5	5:50	M
	140	0:40	------	------	------	------	10	10:50	M
	160	0:40	------	------	------	------	21	21:50	N
	180	0:40	------	------	------	------	29	29:50	O
	200	0:40	------	------	------	------	35	35:50	O
	220	0:40	------	------	------	------	40	40:50	Z
	240	0:40	------	------	------	------	47	47:50	Z
60____	60	-----------	------	------	------	------	0	1:00	(†)
	70	0:50	------	------	------	------	2	3:00	K
	80	0:50	------	------	------	------	7	8:00	L
	100	0:50	------	------	------	------	14	15:00	M
	120	0:50	------	------	------	------	26	27:00	N
	140	0:50	------	------	------	------	39	40:00	O
	160	0:50	------	------	------	------	48	49:00	Z
	180	0:50	------	------	------	------	56	57:00	Z
	200	0:40	------	------	------	1	69	71:00	Z
70____	50	-----------	------	------	------	------	0	1:10	(†)
	60	1:00	------	------	------	------	8	9:10	K
	70	1:00	------	------	------	------	14	15:10	L
	80	1:00	------	------	------	------	18	19:10	M
	90	1:00	------	------	------	------	23	24:10	N
	100	1:00	------	------	------	------	33	34:10	N
	110	0:50	------	------	------	2	41	44:10	O
	120	0:50	------	------	------	4	47	52:10	O
	130	0:50	------	------	------	6	52	59:10	O
	140	0:50	------	------	------	8	56	65:10	Z
	150	0:50	------	------	------	9	61	71:10	Z
	160	0:50	------	------	------	13	72	86:10	Z
	170	0:50	------	------	------	19	79	99:10	Z

*Courtesy United States Navy.   *Continued.*
†See Table 25-4 for repetitive groups in no-decompression dives.

Table 25-3. U.S. Navy standard air decompression table—cont'd

Depth (feet)	Bottom time (min)	Time to first stop (min:sec)	Decompression stops (feet)					Total ascent (min:sec)	Repetitive group
			50	40	30	20	10		
80____	40	----------	------	------	------	------	0	1:20	(*)
	50	1:10	------	------	------	------	10	11:20	K
	60	1:10	------	------	------	------	17	18:20	L
	70	1:10	------	------	------	------	23	24:20	M
	80	1:00	------	------	------	2	31	34:20	N
	90	1:00	------	------	------	7	39	47:20	N
	100	1:00	------	------	------	11	46	58:20	O
	110	1:00	------	------	------	13	53	67:20	O
	120	1:00	------	------	------	17	56	74:20	Z
	130	1:00	------	------	------	19	63	83:20	Z
	140	1:00	------	------	------	26	69	96:20	Z
	150	1:00	------	------	------	32	77	110:20	Z
90____	30	----------	------	------	------	------	0	1:30	(*)
	40	1:20	------	------	------	------	7	8:30	J
	50	1:20	------	------	------	------	18	19:30	L
	60	1:20	------	------	------	------	25	26:30	M
	70	1:10	------	------	------	7	30	38:30	N
	80	1:10	------	------	------	13	40	54:30	N
	90	1:10	------	------	------	18	48	67:30	O
	100	1:10	------	------	------	21	54	76:30	Z
	110	1:10	------	------	------	24	61	86:30	Z
	120	1:10	------	------	------	32	68	101:30	Z
	130	1:00	------	------	5	36	74	116:30	Z
100____	25	----------	------	------	------	------	0	1:40	(*)
	30	1:30	------	------	------	------	3	4:40	I
	40	1:30	------	------	------	------	15	16:40	K
	50	1:20	------	------	------	2	24	27:40	L
	60	1:20	------	------	------	9	28	38:40	N
	70	1:20	------	------	------	17	39	57:40	O
	80	1:20	------	------	------	23	48	72:40	O
	90	1:10	------	------	3	23	57	84:40	Z
	100	1:10	------	------	7	23	66	97:40	Z
	110	1:10	------	------	10	34	72	117:40	Z
	120	1:10	------	------	12	41	78	132:40	Z
110____	20	----------	------	------	------	------	0	1:50	(*)
	25	1:40	------	------	------	------	3	4:50	H
	30	1:40	------	------	------	------	7	8:50	J
	40	1:30	------	------	------	2	21	24:50	L
	50	1:30	------	------	------	8	26	35:50	M
	60	1:30	------	------	------	18	36	55:50	N
	70	1:20	------	------	1	23	48	73:50	O
	80	1:20	------	------	7	23	57	88:50	Z
	90	1:20	------	------	12	30	64	107:50	Z
	100	1:20	------	------	15	37	72	125:50	Z

Table 25-3. U.S. Navy standard air decompression table—cont'd

Depth (feet)	Bottom time (min)	Time to first stop (min:sec)	Decompression stops (feet)					Total ascent (min:sec)	Repetitive group
			50	40	30	20	10		
120	15	----------					0	2:00	(*)
	20	1:50					2	4:00	H
	25	1:50					6	8:00	I
	30	1:50					14	16:00	J
	40	1:40				5	25	32:00	L
	50	1:40				15	31	48:00	N
	60	1:30			2	22	45	71:00	O
	70	1:30			9	23	55	89:00	O
	80	1:30			15	27	63	107:00	Z
	90	1:30			19	37	74	132:00	Z
	100	1:30			23	45	80	150:00	Z
130	10	----------					0	2:10	(*)
	15	2:00					1	3:10	F
	20	2:00					4	6:10	H
	25	2:00					10	12:10	J
	30	1:50				3	18	23:10	M
	40	1:50				10	25	37:10	N
	50	1:40			3	21	37	63:10	O
	60	1:40			9	23	52	86:10	Z
	70	1:40			16	24	61	103:10	Z
	80	1:30		3	19	35	72	131:10	Z
	90	1:30		8	19	45	80	154:10	Z
140	10	----------					0	2:20	(*)
	15	2:10					2	4:20	G
	20	2:10					6	8:20	I
	25	2:00				2	14	18:20	J
	30	2:00				5	21	28:20	K
	40	1:50			2	16	26	46:20	N
	50	1:50			6	24	44	76:20	O
	60	1:50			16	23	56	97:20	Z
	70	1:40		4	19	32	68	125:20	Z
	80	1:40		10	23	41	79	155:20	Z
150	5	----------					0	2:30	C
	10	2:20					1	3:30	E
	15	2:20					3	5:30	G
	20	2:10				2	7	11:30	H
	25	2:10				4	17	23:30	K
	30	2:10				8	24	34:30	L
	40	2:00			5	19	33	59:30	N
	50	2:00			12	23	51	88:30	O
	60	1:50		3	19	26	62	112:30	Z
	70	1:50		11	19	39	75	146:30	Z
	80	1:40	1	17	19	50	84	173:30	Z

Continued.

Table 25-3. U.S. Navy standard air decompression table—cont'd

Depth (feet)	Bottom time (min)	Time to first stop (min:sec)	Decompression stops (feet)					Total ascent (min:sec)	Repetitive group
			50	40	30	20	10		
160____	5	------------	------	------	------	------	0	2:40	D
	10	2:30	------	------	------	------	1	3:40	F
	15	2:20	------	------	------	1	4	7:40	H
	20	2:20	------	------	------	3	11	16:40	J
	25	2:20	------	------	------	7	20	29:40	K
	30	2:10	------	------	2	11	25	40:40	M
	40	2:10	------	------	7	23	39	71:40	N
	50	2:00	------	2	16	23	55	98:40	Z
	60	2:00	------	9	19	33	69	132:40	Z
	70	1:50	1	17	22	44	80	166:40	Z
170____	5	------------	------	------	------	------	0	2:50	D
	10	2:40	------	------	------	------	2	4:50	F
	15	2:30	------	------	------	2	5	9:50	H
	20	2:30	------	------	------	4	15	21:50	J
	25	2:20	------	------	2	7	23	34:50	L
	30	2:20	------	------	4	13	26	45:50	M
	40	2:10	------	1	10	23	45	81:50	O
	50	2:10	------	5	18	23	61	109:50	Z
	60	2:00	2	15	22	37	74	152:50	Z
	70	2:00	8	17	19	51	86	183:50	Z
180____	5	------------	------	------	------	------	0	3:00	D
	10	2:50	------	------	------	------	3	6:00	F
	15	2:40	------	------	------	3	6	12:00	I
	20	2:30	------	------	1	5	17	26:00	K
	25	2:30	------	------	3	10	24	40:00	L
	30	2:30	------	------	6	17	27	53:00	N
	40	2:20	------	3	14	23	50	93:00	O
	50	2:10	2	9	19	30	65	128:00	Z
	60	2:10	5	16	19	44	81	168:00	Z
190____	5	------------	------	------	------	------	0	3:10	D
	10	2:50	------	------	------	1	3	7:10	G
	15	2:50	------	------	------	4	7	14:10	I
	20	2:40	------	------	2	6	20	31:10	K
	25	2:40	------	------	5	11	25	44:10	M
	30	2:30	------	1	8	19	32	63:10	N
	40	2:30	------	8	14	23	55	103:10	O
	50	2:20	4	13	22	33	72	147:10	Z
	60	2:20	10	17	19	50	84	183:10	Z

Tables 25-4 to 25-6. THE "NU-WAY" REPETITIVE DIVE TABLES

TABLE 25-6 REPETITIVE DIVE TIMETABLE FOR AIR DIVES

Repet. group																
A	7	6	5	4	3	3	3	3	3	2	2	2	2	2	2	2
B	17	13	11	9	8	7	7	6	6	5	4	4	4	4	4	4
C	25	21	17	15	13	11	10	10	9	8	7	7	6	6	6	6
D	37	29	24	20	18	16	14	13	12	11	10	9	8	8	8	8
E	49	38	30	26	23	20	18	16	15	13	12	11	10	10	10	10
F	61	47	36	31	28	24	22	20	18	16	15	14	13	13	12	11
G	73	56	44	37	32	29	26	24	21	19	18	17	16	15	14	13
H	87	66	52	43	38	33	30	27	25	22	20	19	18	17	16	15
I	101	76	61	50	43	38	34	31	28	25	23	22	20	19	18	17
J	116	87	70	57	48	43	38	34	32	28	26	24	23	22	20	19
K	138	99	79	64	54	47	43	38	35	31	29	26	24	23	22	21
L	161	111	88	72	61	53	48	43	40	35	32	29	27	26	25	24
M	187	124	97	80	68	61	53	48	43	38	35	32	30	29	27	26
N	213	142	107	87	73	64	57	52	47	42	38	35	33	31	29	28
O	241	160	117	96	80	70	62	55	50	44	40	38	36	34	31	30
Z	257	169	122	100	84	73	64	57	52	46	42	40	37	35	32	31
RESIDUAL NITROGEN TIMES (MINUTES) FOR REPETITIVE DIVE DEPTH BELOW (FT)	40'	50'	60'	70'	80'	90'	100'	110'	120'	130'	140'	150'	160'	170'	180'	190'

TABLE 25-5 SURFACE INTERVAL CREDIT TABLE (TIMES IN HR:MIN)

Present repetitive group at left; select elapsed surface interval; new repetitive group given by the column. (All times hr:min; diagonal cell upper limit is 12:00 for group A.)

Group	New group : surface interval range
A	A 0:10–12:00
B	B 0:10–2:10 ; A 2:11–12:00
C	C 0:10–1:39 ; B 1:40–2:49 ; A 2:50–12:00
D	D 0:10–1:09 ; C 1:10–2:38 ; B 2:39–3:22 ; A 3:23–12:00
E	E 0:10–0:54 ; D 0:55–1:57 ; C 1:58–2:28 ; B 2:29–3:20 ; A 3:21–12:00
F	F 0:10–0:45 ; E 0:46–1:29 ; D 1:30–1:57 ; C 1:58–2:28 ; B 2:29–3:20 ; A 3:21–12:00
G	G 0:10–0:40 ; F 0:41–1:15 ; E 1:16–1:59 ; D 2:00–2:24 ; C 2:25–2:58 ; B 2:59–3:43 ; A 3:44–12:00
H	H 0:10–0:36 ; G 0:37–1:06 ; F 1:07–1:41 ; E 1:42–2:23 ; D 2:24–2:44 ; C 2:45–3:20 ; B 3:21–4:02 ; A 4:03–12:00
I	I 0:10–0:33 ; H 0:34–1:00 ; G 1:01–1:29 ; F 1:30–2:02 ; E 2:03–2:44 ; D 2:45–3:04 ; C 3:05–3:43 ; B 3:44–4:19 ; A 4:20–12:00
J	J 0:10–0:31 ; I 0:32–0:54 ; H 0:55–1:19 ; G 1:20–1:47 ; F 1:48–2:20 ; E 2:21–3:04 ; D 3:05–3:21 ; C 3:22–4:03 ; B 4:04–4:35 ; A 4:36–12:00
K	K 0:10–0:28 ; J 0:29–0:49 ; I 0:50–1:11 ; H 1:12–1:35 ; G 1:36–2:03 ; F 2:04–2:38 ; E 2:39–3:21 ; D 3:22–3:36 ; C 3:37–4:19 ; B 4:20–5:03 ; A 5:04–12:00
L	L 0:10–0:26 ; K 0:27–0:45 ; J 0:46–1:04 ; I 1:05–1:25 ; H 1:26–1:49 ; G 1:50–2:19 ; F 2:20–2:53 ; E 2:54–3:36 ; D 3:37–3:52 ; C 3:53–4:35 ; B 4:36–5:16 ; A 5:17–12:00
M	M 0:10–0:25 ; L 0:26–0:39 ; K 0:40–0:59 ; J 1:00–1:18 ; I 1:19–1:39 ; H 1:40–2:05 ; G 2:06–2:34 ; F 2:35–3:08 ; E 3:09–3:52 ; D 3:53–4:17 ; C 4:18–5:03 ; B 5:04–5:40 ; A 5:41–12:00
N	N 0:10–0:24 ; M 0:25–0:36 ; L 0:37–0:55 ; K 0:56–1:11 ; J 1:12–1:30 ; I 1:31–1:54 ; H 1:55–2:18 ; G 2:19–2:47 ; F 2:48–3:22 ; E 3:23–4:04 ; D 4:05–4:29 ; C 4:30–5:16 ; B 5:17–5:48 ; A 5:49–12:00
O	O 0:10–0:23 ; N 0:24–0:36 ; M 0:37–0:48 ; L 0:49–1:02 ; K 1:03–1:18 ; J 1:19–1:36 ; I 1:37–1:55 ; H 1:56–2:17 ; G 2:18–2:42 ; F 2:43–3:10 ; E 3:11–3:45 ; D 3:46–4:29 ; C 4:30–5:48 ; B 5:49–6:32 ; A 6:33–12:00
Z	Z 0:10–0:22 ; O 0:23–0:34 ; N 0:35–0:48 ; M 0:49–1:02 ; L 1:03–1:18 ; K 1:19–1:36 ; J 1:37–1:55 ; I 1:56–2:17 ; H 2:18–2:42 ; G 2:43–3:10 ; F 3:11–3:45 ; E 3:46–4:29 ; D 4:30–5:27 ; C 5:28–7:35 ; B 7:36–10:05 ; A 10:06–12:00

BOTTOM TIMES FOR AIR DIVES (MINUTES)

TABLE 25-4 "NO DECOMPRESSION" LIMITS AND REPETITIVE GROUP DESIGNATION TABLE FOR NO DECOMPRESSION AIR DIVES

DEPTH (FT)	NO DECOMPRESSION LIMITS	A	B	C	D	E	F	G	H	I	J	K	L	M	N	O
10	—	60	120	210	300											
15	—	35	70	110	160	225	350									
20	—	25	50	75	100	135	180	240	325							
25	—	20	35	55	75	100	125	160	195	245	315					
30	—	15	30	45	60	75	95	120	145	170	205	250	310			
35	310	5	15	25	40	50	60	80	100	120	140	160	190	220	270	310
40	200	5	15	25	30	40	50	70	80	100	110	130	150	170	200	
50	100	—	10	15	25	30	40	50	60	70	80	90	100			
60	60	—	10	15	20	25	30	40	50	55	60					
70	50	—	5	10	15	20	30	35	40	45	50					
80	40	—	5	10	15	20	25	30	35	40						
90	30	—	5	10	12	15	20	25	30							
100	25	—	5	7	10	15	20	22	25							
110	20	—	—	5	10	13	15	20								
120	15	—	—	5	10	12	15									
130	10	—	5	8	10											
140	10	—	5	7	10											
150	5	—	5													
160	5	—	—	5												
170	5	—	—	5												
190	5	—	—	5												

CAUTION

THESE "RESIDUAL NITROGEN TIMES" ARE THE TIMES A DIVER MUST ASSUME HE HAS ALREADY SPENT ON THE BOTTOM BEFORE HE STARTS A REPETITIVE DIVE TO A SPECIFIC DEPTH.

ALL TABULATED BOTTOM TIMES (MINUTES), AND ALL TABULATED DEPTHS (FEET) HAVE BEEN TAKEN FROM THE U.S. NAVY DIVING MANUAL OF MARCH 1970.

—— INSTRUCTIONS ——

1. TO CALCULATE A REPETITIVE DIVE INVOLVING EXPOSURES UP TO AND INCLUDING THE "NO DECOMPRESSION LIMITS" ENTER TABLE 25-4 ON THE EXACT OR NEXT GREATER DEPTH THAN THAT TO WHICH EXPOSED, AND SELECT THE LISTED EXPOSURE TIME EXACT OR NEXT GREATER THAN THE ACTUAL EXPOSURE TIME. THE REPETITIVE GROUP DESIGNATION IS INDICATED BY THE LETTER AT THE HEAD OF THE VERTICAL COLUMN WHERE THE SELECTED EXPOSURE TIME IS LISTED.

2. CONTINUE THE VERTICAL MOTION ALONG THE STRAIGHT LINES JOINING TABLE 25-4 TO TABLE 25-5 ENTER THE TABLE VERTICALLY TO SELECT THE ELAPSED SURFACE INTERVAL TIME. THE NEW REPETITIVE GROUP DESIGNATION FOR THE ELAPSED SURFACE INTERVAL IS TO THE RIGHT OF THE HORIZONTAL COLUMN WHERE THE ELAPSED SURFACE INTERVAL TIME IS LISTED.

3. CONTINUE THE RIGHTHANDED MOTION TO ENTER 25-6 ON THE HORIZONTAL COLUMN TO THE RIGHT OF THE NEW REPETITIVE GROUP DESIGNATION. THE TIME IN EACH VERTICAL COLUMN IS THE RESIDUAL NITROGEN TIME. IT IS A PENALTY TIME, ie. THE TIME A DIVER MUST ASSUME HE HAS ALREADY SPENT ON THE BOTTOM BEFORE HE STARTS A REPETITIVE DIVE TO THE DEPTH SPECIFIED AT THE BOTTOM OF THE COLUMN.

Reprinted courtesy of Ralph M Maruscak

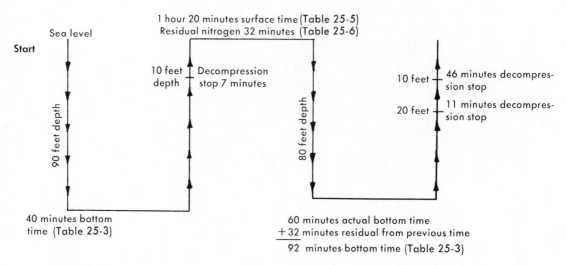

Fig. 25-2. Sample dive plan with use of U.S. Navy repetitive dive tables. (From Barber, J. M., and Budassi. S. A.: Mosby's manual of emergency care, St. Louis, 1979, The C. V. Mosby Co.)

Table 25-7. Gas toxicities in diving*

Gas	Signs and symptoms	Therapeutic interventions
Oxygen (from breathing 100% oxygen)	Twitching, nausea, dizziness, tunnel vision, restlessness, paresthesias, seizures, confusion, pulmonary edema, atelectasis, shock lung	ABCs, intubation, controlled ventilation to reduce FIO_2, decompression, PEEP
Carbon dioxide (from inhaling expired air; 8%-10% causes toxicity)	Dizziness, lethargy, heavy labored breathing, unconsciousness	Ascent to surface, ABCs, 100% oxygen
Carbon monoxide (from contaminated tank—filled too close to internal combustion engine)	Dizziness, pink or red lips and mouth, euphoria	Ascent to surface, ABCs (CPR if necessary), 100% oxygen in hyperbaric chamber at 3 atmospheres for 1 hour

*From Barber, J. M., and Budassi, S. A.: Mosby's manual of emergency care, St. Louis, 1979, The C. V. Mosby Co.

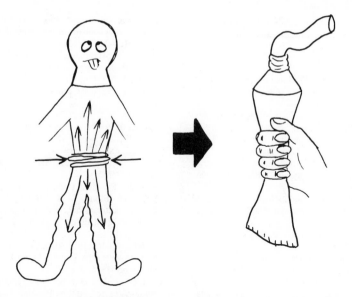

Fig. 25-3. The squeeze. (From Barber, J. M., and Budassi, S. A.: Mosby's manual of emergency care, St. Louis, 1979, The C. V. Mosby Co.)

3. Tow a surface float with a diver's flag.
4. Do *not* use ear plugs while diving.
5. Do *not* use nose clips while diving.
6. Do *not* dive with an upper respiratory infection.
7. Check your equipment prior to diving. Regulators should be overhauled every year, and tanks should be hydrostatically tested every 5 years.
8. In SCUBA, *always* exhale on ascent.
9. In SCUBA, do *not* hold your breath.
10. Do not consume alcohol or drugs prior to diving.
11. Observe the "decompression limits" chart.
12. Do not remain at depth when the tank is on reserve.
13. Have an annual physical checkup.
14. Be physically fit; do not dive if you do not feel well.
15. Know the area where you are diving.
16. Avoid dangerous places and poor conditions.
17. Plan your dive.
18. Be ready for emergencies; be certified in lifesaving, first aid, and CPR; have first aid equipment.
19. Carry a diver's identification card for 48 hours following a dive.
20. Seek medical attention if problems occur following a dive.

Reasons for not diving to great depths

Water temperature much colder
Visibility poor/darker
Less color/less animation
Less tank time/air used faster
Extra equipment required
Need for "decompression stops"
Drug and alcohol effect greater
Emergency ascent difficult

Emergency information

The following information should be kept readily available when diving:
Coast Guard telephone number and radio frequency
Police telephone number and radio frequency
Paramedic telephone number and radio frequency
Decompression chamber location and telephone number*

---

*If this information is unavailable, call the U.S. Navy Experimental Diving Unit in Washington, D.C. (202-433-2790, 24 hours a day/7 days a week) and ask for the duty officer, who will give you the name, location, and telephone number of the nearest decompression chamber.

Name and telephone number (24-hour number) of a physician trained in underwater emergencies

BIBLIOGRAPHY

Biery, J.: Venomous Arthropod Handbook, Washington, D.C., 1976, U.S. Govt. printing office, p. 42, 46, 47, No. 008-070-00397-0.

Clowes, G. H. A., and Donnell, T. F.: Heat stroke, New Engl. J. Med. **291**(11):564-567, September 12, 1974.

Collins, K. J.: Heat illness: diagnosis, treatment and prevention, Practitioner **219**:193-198, August 1977.

Ellis, F. P.: Heat illness. III. Acclimatization, Trans. Royal Society of Trop. Med. and Hygiene **70**(5/6):419-425, 1976.

Ellis, F. P.: Heat illness. I. Epidemiology, Trans. Royal Society of Trop. Med. and Hygiene **70**(5/6):402-411, 1976.

Gephart, D.: Anaphylaxis from insect stings, J.E.N. **4**:19-20, May-June 1978.

Hamilton, D.: The immediate treatment of heatstroke, Anaesthesia **31**:270-272, 1976.

Hoagland, R. J., and Bishop, R. H., Jr.: A physiologic treatment of heat stroke, Am. J. Med. Science **241**:415-422, 1961.

Horen, P.: Insect and scorpion sting, J.A.M.A., **221**:894, August 21, 1972.

IDEM: Scorpions, Tempe, Ariz., 1956, Poisonous Animals Research Laboratory, Arizona State College.

Jiménez-Porras, J. M.: Biochemistry of snake venoms, Clin. Toxicol. **3**:389, September 1970.

Kew, M. C.: Effects of heatstroke on the function and structure of the kidney. Quarterly J. Med. **36**(143):277-300, July 1967.

Kew, M. C., Bersohn, I., and Seftel, H.: The diagnostic and prognostic significance of the serum enzyme changes in heat stroke, Trans. Royal Society of Trop. Med. and Hygiene **65**(3):325-330, 1971.

Knochel, J. P.: The renal, cardiovascular, hematologic and serum electrolyte abnormalities of heat stroke, Am. J. Med. **30**(2):299-309, February 1961.

Knochel, J. P., Dotin, I. N., and Hamburger, R. J.: Patho-physiology of intense physical conditioning in a hot climate. I. Mechanisms of potassium depletion, J. Clin. Invest. **51**:242-255, 1972.

Malamud, N., Haymaker, W., Custer, R. P.: Heat stroke—A clinicopathologic study of 125 fatal cases, Milit. Surg. **99**:397-449, November 1946.

Murphy, R. J.: Heat illness, J. Sports Med. **1**(4):26-29, 1973.

O'Donnell, T. F., and Clowes, G. H. A.: Circulatory abnormalities of heat stroke, New Engl. J. Med. **287**(15):734-737, October 12, 1972.

Pal, A. K., and Chopra, S. K.: Cardiopathology of heatstroke, Indian J. Med. Sciences **29**(12):299-301, December 1975.

Proulx, R. P.: Heat stress disease. In Schwartz, G. R., Safar, P., Stone, J. H., Storey, P. B., and Wagner, D. K., editors: Principles and practice of emergency medicine, Philadelphia, 1978, W. B. Saunders Company, p. 815.

Schwartz, G. R.: Phenothiazines and anticholinergics in heat stroke (Letter to the Editor), J.A.C.E.P. **5**(12):995, December 1976.

Schwartz, G. R., Safar, P., Stone, J. H., Storey, P. B., and Wagner, D. K., editors: Principles and practice of emergency medicine, Vol. I, Philadelphia, 1978, W. B. Saunders Co., p. 823.

Shibolet, S.: Fibrinolysis and hemorrhages in fatal heatstroke, New Engl. J. Med. **266**(4):169-173, January 25, 1962.

Shibolet, S., Lancaster, M. C., and Danon, Y.: Heat stroke: a review. Aviat. Space Environ. Med. **47**(3):280-301, March 1976.

Stahnke, H. L., and Stahnke, J.: Treatment of scorpion sting, Ariz. Med. **14**:576, 1957.

Vertel, R. M., and Knochel, J. P.: Acute renal failure due to heat injury—an analysis of ten cases associated with a high incidence of myoglobinuria. Am. J. Med. **43**:435-451, September 1967.

Watt, C. H.: Poisonous snakebite treatment in the U.S., J.A.M.A. **240**:655, August 18, 1978.

Wheeler, M.: Heat stroke in the elderly, Med. Clin. North Am. **60**(6):1289-1296, November 1976.

CHAPTER 26

Burns

Burns are one of the most dread emergencies that nurses encounter and require a systematic, thorough approach. The psychological as well as physiological factors that attend these injuries produce a problematic clinical situation that requires the attention of an entire team of caregivers. This chapter, in addition to discussing the immediate management of burns, will consider early efforts that can positively influence the total rehabilitation of the victim.

Pathophysiology

The severity of a burn depends largely on the intensity and duration of the thermal insult and on the unique characteristics of the tissue area involved. Density, water content, vascularity, subcutaneous fat, and content of the tissue affect the degree of burn damage and influence the response to healing. For example, tissue with little or no subcutaneous fat is more prone to contractures and scarring than is tissue with a substantial layer of fat, and well-vascularized tissue dissipates heat more readily.

Immediately after a burn there is a generalized vasoconstrictor response; later, dilatation is prominent, and plasma is permitted to extravasate into the tissue. Ischemia is pronounced because of aggregation of platelets and leukocytes in the underlying capillaries, resulting in thrombosis. Leukocytes cannot migrate easily in the thrombosed capillary bed; thus, the infection potential is increased. Therefore, it may be 4 or 5 days after a burn until the severity of the burn can be realized fully. Water and heat are lost from the involved area; if the area is large, severe hypothermia can result.

In the first hours after the burn, water and electrolytes are shunted into the skeletal muscles, and shock can result. Cardiac output may fall because of the hypovolemia, and a decrease in myocardial contractility may be demonstrated. This compromise may not always respond to volume administration. In later hours, this process reverses itself and stabilizes by the end of the first day after the burn.

Hematopoietic effects

Anemia after burns is caused by several factors, including erythrocyte hemolysis from direct heat damage, a decreased half-life of damaged red cells, a loss of red blood cell mass, and a shortened half-life of transfused red cells. Platelet function and half-life are decreased, and leukocyte counts may fall. Several days (even up to 2 weeks) may be required to restore normal blood counts after a major burn.

Classification

Burns are tissue injuries caused by thermal (liquid or flame), chemical, or electrical stimuli. Radiant energy and friction may also create tissue burns, but they account for only a small percentage of burns encountered in the emergency department. Therefore, the majority of this discussion will relate to thermal, chemical, and electrical burns.

The severity of burns is determined primarily by the amount of body surface area (BSA) involved, the depth (degree) of the burn, and to some extent by other factors, such as age, the presence of concurrent medical or surgical

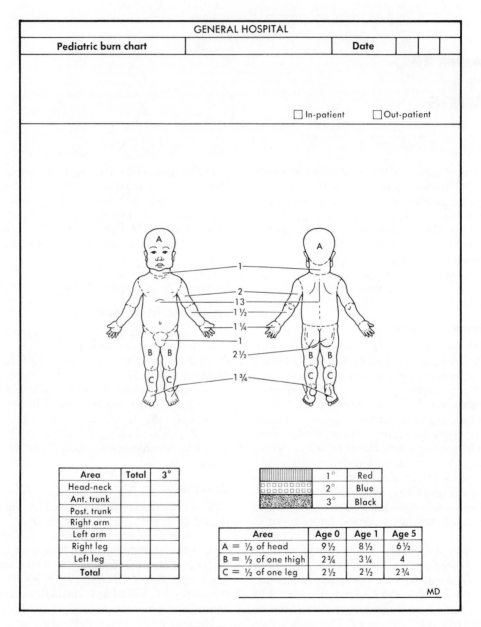

Fig. 26-1. Pediatric burn chart.

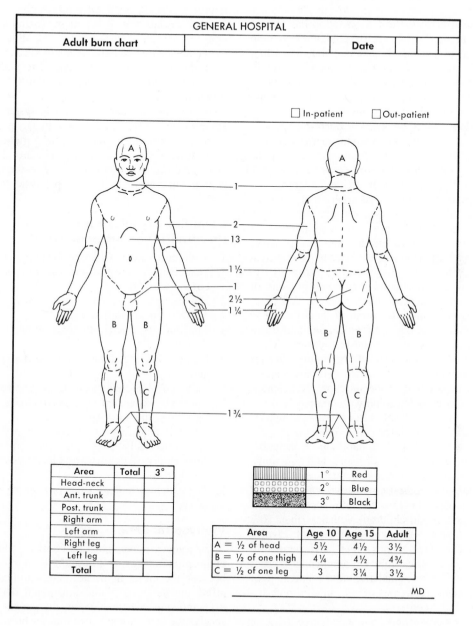

Fig. 26-2. Adult burn chart.

problems, and complications that attend certain types of body burns such as those of the face, hands, and genitalia (Figs. 26-1 to 26-3).

The American Burn Association has formulated the following set of guidelines to help emergency personnel make decisions regarding which burned patients can be managed safely on an outpatient basis, which ones should be hospitalized, and which ones should be transferred to a major burn center.

Categories of severity of burn injury*

MAJOR BURN INJURY. Second degree burns of greater than 25% of the body surface in adults (20% in children); all third degree burns of 10% of body surface area or greater; all burns involving hands, face, eyes, ear, feet, or perineum; all inhalation injuries; electrical burns; complicated burn injuries involving fractures or other major trauma; and all poor risk patients. Such patients would normally enter the system at the site of the injury and be transported to a hospital with optimal facilities (burn unit or burn center) dependent on distance and time, burn complications (respiratory shock), and bed availability. Direct communications and transfer agreements in this regard are extremely important. If seriousness of the injury dictates transportation to the closest effective emergency department or special expertise hospital, then transfer to a hospital with optimal facilities should be arranged after cardiopulmonary stabilization and intravenous fluid therapy for shock are established. Rehabilitation, including corrective surgery for cosmetic and functional deficiencies, completes the therapeutic circle.

MODERATE UNCOMPLICATED BURN INJURY. Second degree burns of 15% to 25% BSA in adults (10% to 20% in children) with less than 10% third degree burns and that do not involve eyes, ear, face, hands, feet, and perineum. Excludes electrical injury, complicated injuries such as fractures, inhalation injury, and all poor risk patients (extremes of age, intercurrent diseases, and so on).

MINOR BURN INJURY. Second degree burn of less than 15% BSA in adults (10% in children)

---

*From Dimick, A. R.: ABA—striving to improve burn care, Emerg. Product News **9**(4), 1977.

with less than 2% third degree burn, not involving eyes, ears, face, hands, feet, and perineum. Excludes electrical injury, complicated injuries and all poor risk patients (extremes of age, intercurrent disease, and so on). Such patients may be treated at the scene of the accident by EMT personnel and transported to hospital emergency department, where definitive care is initiated, including follow-up to complete recovery and discharge from the system. A similar course would be followed by any patient admitting himself to the hospital emergency department for treatment. Primary care physicians may function either in the emergency department role or as follow-up physician, or both.

Definition of major burns (hospitalization recommended)

1. Total burns exceed 10% of the body surface area, or there are unequivocal third degree burns over 2%.
2. Hands, feet, or genitalia are involved.
3. The burn is circumferential.
4. The burn is electrically or chemically induced.
5. Burns are concomitant to suspected child abuse.
6. Infection of the wound is already apparent.
7. There are associated injuries (fractures, dislocations, and so on).
8. There is a history of illness or injury that could adversely affect prognosis (diabetic peripheral vascular disease, blood dyscrasia, and so on).
9. The patient is under 2 years or over 40 years of age.

Prehospital care

Emergency nurses must be familiar with the prehospital management of major burn injuries, because the initial field care may significantly affect the outcome of the injury and perhaps even influence whether or not the patient will survive the first critical hours after the burn.

Extinguishing the fire. If the victim is still on fire, since flames rise upward, get him supine to protect the face and upper airways. Do not throw sand or dirt on the fire since such

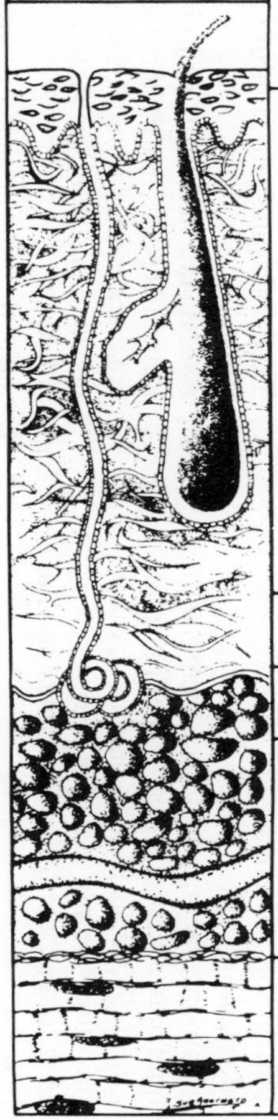

	Depth of burn (Detailed classification)	Pain and pinprick sensitivity	Appearance	Healing time	End result of healing	Treatment
1° Partial skin loss	Erythema only, no loss of epidermis	Hyperalgesia	Erythema		Normal skin	Allow to heal by natural processes Protect from further injury and infection
2° Partial skin loss	Superficial, no loss of dermis	Hyperalgesia or normal		6-10 days	Normal skin	Allow to heal by natural processes Protect from further injury and infection
2° Partial skin loss	Intermediate, healing from hair follicles	Normal to hypoalgesia	Erythema to opaque, white blisters are characteristic	7-14 days	Normal to slightly pitted and/or poorly pigmented	Allow to heal by natural processes Protect from further injury and infection
2° Partial skin loss	Deep, healing from sweat glands	Hypoalgesia to analgesia		14-21 days	Hairless and depigmented Texture normal to pitted or flat and shiny	Elective skin grafting may save time and give better end result
3° Whole skin loss	Deep dermal, occasionally heal from scattered epithelium	Analgesia	White opaque to charred, coagulated; subcutaneous veins may be visible	More than 21 days	Poor texture Hypertrophic Scar frequent	Elective skin grafting may save time and give better end result
3° Whole skin loss	Whole skin loss, healing from edges only			Never if area is large	Hypertrophic scar and chronic granulations unless grafted	Skin grafting mandatory
4° Deep tissue loss	Deep structure loss	May be some algesia				Skin grafting mandatory

Fig. 26-3. Classification of burns according to depth of burn. (From Warner, C. G., editor: Emergency care: assessment and intevention, ed. 2, St. Louis, 1978, The C. V. Mosby Co.)

agents contaminate the wounds and interfere with a satisfactory evaluation. It may be helpful to smother flames with a blanket or garment or by rolling the individual. Remove smoldering clothing at once, leaving only tightly adhering items that cannot easily be taken off. Remove all jewelry or belts that could interfere with circulation when edema formation begins. (See special notations regarding chemical burns on p. 615 and electrical burns on p. 613).

History and assessment. The initial assessment of the burned individual should be similar to the approach used for any trauma patient, with primary attention first directed toward the airway, breathing, and circulation. In the meantime, attempts should be made to learn the nature of the injury. What was the thermal source, or other stimuli? If there is evidence of smoke or fire, determine whether or not the burned victim was in a closed space. Was there an explosion? Are any noxious chemical or other subtances thought to have been involved? Were there any related accidents, such as jumping from a window, falling, or colliding? Consider child abuse and/or criminal intent (see p. 41). Remember that the burn might be the most obvious injury but other serious and even life-threatening crises might be lurking, such as cervical injury, serious chest or intraabdominal trauma, or airway obstruction in an early phase, such as from edema. Assess the level of consciousness. Burns do not create unconsciousness, so CNS injuries should be considered. Look for hemorrhage. Since burns do not hemorrhage, in the event of severe bleeding, other injuries are present. Splint any obvious fractures, and take measures to control shock (see Chapter 12). Evaluate the burn as the last factor in the multiple trauma exam and be prepared to describe it in terms of depth, extent, type, exact body parts and areas involved, age of victim, history of concurrent disease, and other attendant injuries.

For transport, the burn may be covered with a dry (preferably sterile) sheet. If the transport time is short (less than 15 to 20 minutes), other care procedures are not essential. However, if the time is longer, the following points should be considered.

An IV line should be initiated using Ringer's lactate. A peripheral vein such as the antecubital vein is desirable. Although it is not desirable to cannulate through the burn wound, it is appropriate in some instances when other suitable veins are inaccessible. If shock is profound from multiple injuries (such as abdominal bleeding and large bone fractures), antishock trousers may be used, but their use should be limited if there are lower extremity burns, since the counterpressure may increase ischemia in those areas.

Repeated airway assessments must be made throughout transport, and all major burn patients should be given high-flow oxygen.

It is important that the prehospital care team alert the receiving hospital, giving a succinct but thorough summary of the patient's condition in order that the emergency department can be properly prepared when the patient arrives. Be certain to elevate burned extremities en route to minimize edema formation.

Prehospital care of major burns
1. Consider environmental hazards to the rescuer before approaching the victim, such as poisonous fumes (especially from plastics containing polyvinylchloride), flames, or explosions.
2. When the rescuer and the victim are in a relatively safe environment (away from immediate danger), evaluate the airway, breathing, and circulation. Establish and maintain the airway (see p. 132). Use caution with persons who could have spinal injury or fractures, for example, victims of auto accidents, falls, and explosions.
3. a. Control any hemorrhage. Burn wounds do not hemorrhage; if severe bleeding is present, look for other injuries.
   b. Splint fractures.
   c. Take measures to control shock if apparent.
   d. Assess the level of consciousness. Remember that burns themselves do not create unconsciousness, so other nonapparent injuries should be considered.
4. Evaluate the burn, quickly estimating the body surface area involved and depth of

injury. (Refer to Figs. 26-1 and 26-2). *Do not break blisters. Do not apply anything to the burn!*

a. If extremities are involved, elevate them to minimize edema formation.
b. Remove clothing that is smoldering or damp, but *do not* tear away clothing adherent to the skin.
c. Remove constricting jewelry if possible.
d. Place the individual in a clean (preferably sterile) sheet and keep him warm and dry for transport.

Avoid using iced saline-soaked dressings or cool compresses (even though they help alleviate pain of superficial burns) since they unnecessarily lower body temperature. If the burned area requires rinsing to remove a substance or considerable surface debris, use saline and rinse the wound with copious amounts of water. Cover with a dry, sterile dressing and sheets before transport.

5. Obtain baseline vital signs and continue to monitor. The blood pressure cuff, electrodes for the ECG, and so on may be placed safely over the burned area if necessary.
6. Initiate IV Ringer's lactate on all major burns (as defined on p. 602).* Use a large percutaneous plastic catheter for delivery. Avoid sites with circumferential burns (of the extremities), since developing edema could impede the flow. A venesection through burned skin is better than placing an IV line in an extremity with a tiny scalp vein needle! Establish the flow rate and monitor cautiously.
7. Administer oxygen during transport, and be prepared to suction the airway and support ventilation mechanically if necessary.
8. When long-distance transfer (over 1 hour) is necessary:
   a. If time and conditions permit, insert a No. 18 nasogastric tube (see p. 608), because major burns are frequently accompanied by paralytic ileus and vomiting.
   b. Place a Foley catheter.
   c. Consider administration of an analgesic. Morphine sulfate or other narcotic agents may be indicated for the extreme pain that is associated with first degree (and some second degree) burns. Monitor the respiratory status cautiously.
   d. Assess extremity pulses regularly throughout the transfer. (Escharotomy may be necessary in very long transfers if peripheral arterial blood flow is obliterated by impinging edema (see p. 610).
9. Reassure and comfort the victim as much as possible. Explain the procedures and rationale. Relate what events will take place at the hospital.

EMERGENCY MANAGEMENT

The receiving room in the emergency department should be readied with sterile sheets, dressings, debridement trays, and other supplies essential for resuscitation, initial wound care, and management of concomitant injuries, such as lacerations and fractures. Assigned personnel, whose activities should be strictly confined to the trauma room, should don surgical attire; only sterile linen should be used.

Anticipation of any decontamination needs is an important early consideration in certain burn injuries, especially chemical burns. Any remaining burned or damp clothing should be cut away or otherwise removed. A 1:1 solution of saline and hydrogen peroxide is recommended to facilitate removal. A ring cutter should be at hand to remove constricting jewelry.

The hospital medical photographer or other assigned individual should be summoned to take initial and postdebridement burn wound photos for medical documentation.

As fluid therapy is begun, venous blood samples should be obtained for bilirubin, phosphorus, clotting studies, alkaline phosphatase, complete blood count, hemoglobin and hematocrit, electrolytes (including calcium and mag-

---

*Some authorities suggest that IV fluid administration is not necessary unless the victim is "shocky" or the unit is more than 30 minutes from the nearest hospital.

nesium), BUN, blood sugar, total protein, and creatinine. Obtain a toxicology screen for selected situations (burns of criminal intent, suspected foul play, and so on). Consider typing and cross-matching. An arterial carboxy-hemoglobin level is desirable for guiding therapy, too, particularly in inhalation injuries.

A urine specimen should be sent to the laboratory for baseline values.

Soon after the care of the patient is well underway, validate the details of the accident and search for concomitant injuries and clues to chronic illness. Ascertain any history of allergies, and provide appropriate tetanus prophylaxis (see p. 613).

Airway considerations

About 30% of major burn injuries involve some smoke inhalation. Carbon monoxide, chemical pneumonitis, and airway obstruction can occur in relation to the inhalation insult, and its damaging effects are proportional to the length of exposure as well as the temperature and nature of the offending substance.

Carbon monoxide and other inhalations may be detected easily by emergency personnel who are alert to their potential.* Look for singed nasal hairs, a rasping cough, hoarseness, soot in the sputum, hemoptysis, respiratory stridor, and bronchospasm as factors that strongly point to inhalation complications.

The characteristics of the patient's ventilatory effort are far more important than the rate of respirations. Many noxious inhaled substances depress the vital centers, so care should be taken to scrutinize tidal volume and to assist with bag-valve-mask when indicated.

A baseline chest x-ray film should be obtained promptly.

The face, chest, and neck should be inspected for edema formation and escharotomy con-

sidered (see p. 610). If the patient is in the emergency department for more than 30 minutes, every 20 to 30 minutes he should be turned and asked to cough and breathe deeply to enhance respiratory functioning.

An arterial blood gas should be obtained early in the management of the patient with inhalation injuries, and serial determinations made throughout the initial hours after the injury. An arterial pO_2 less than 50 mm Hg is an indication for endotracheal intubation and respiratory assistance by mechanical devices. Humidified oxygen should be administered and the airway suctioned as necessary. The patient may prefer to sit upright to relieve dyspnea. (Table 26-1).

The treatment of inhalation varies according to clinical signs and symptoms and the results of arterial blood gas monitoring. It may include bronchodilators, mechanical respiratory support, intubation, epinephrine, steroids, and cricothyrotomy, depending upon the nature and severity of the problem as well as local protocol. All patients (without exception) with inhalation injury, however, should receive high-flow oxygen.

A gastric tube (No. 18) should be used to decompress the stomach, since major burn patients tend to develop abdominal distention and paralytic ileus. The tube should be connected to 40 mm Hg suction.

Resuscitation and shock management

One and preferably two large-bore IV lines should be established for fluid administration and to facilitate CVP monitoring (preferably by a subclavian route). A venesection may be necessary for burns exceeding 20% of the body surface or if a large line cannot be placed percutaneously.

Fluid replacement should be calculated and replaced accordingly. A Foley catheter should be placed early to monitor urinary output and to observe for myoglobinuria or hemoglobinuria. An initial sample should be sent to the laboratory for baseline urinalysis and osmolality and electrolyte determination. Do urinometer output readings at 15-minute intervals,

---

*Carbon monoxide at levels of 20% concentration of carboxyhemoglobin produces only a mild, throbbing headache. At 30% to 50% carboxyhemoglobin levels there is irritability, confusion, visual disturbances, dizziness, nausea, vomiting, dyspnea, and syncope. At levels of 50% to 80%, coma, seizures, respiratory failure and death occur. The patient may not appear cyanotic or flushed, even though significant hypoxemia is present.

Table 26-1. Noxious gases*

Type of product	Commercial use	Toxic combustion product	Toxicity—clinical symptoms	Remarks
Plastics				
1. Polyvinyl chloride	Unbreakable bottles, electrical insulation, wall coverings, car and airplane interiors	a. HCl b. CO	a. Dyspnea, burning mucous membranes, chest pain, ectopy, lightheadedness, laryngeal and pulmonary edema b. Lightheadedness, nausea, dyspnea, chest pain, seizures, coma	a. Toxic levels appear before significant amounts of smoke and persist up to 1 hour after fire is extinguished b. Symptoms depend on CO concentration and reflect tissue hypoxia
2. Polyurethane	Thermal insulation wall coverings, seat cushions, carpets, mattresses	a. CO b. Toluene 2 4-Diisocyanate, hydrocyanic acid	a. See 1b above b. Lightheadedness, nausea, dyspnea, chest pain, syncope	a. See 1b above b. Binds Fe^{3+} ions, interrupts cellular electrolyte transport Rx: sodium nitrite and sodium thiosulfate
3. Styrene	Piping, wall covering, luggage, appliances, food and drink containers	a. CO b. Styrene	a. See 1b above b. Conjunctivitis, rhinorrhea, mucous membrane burning	a. See 1b above b. Less toxic than other noxious gases
4. Acrylics	Aircraft windows, textiles, wood finishes, wall coverings, furniture, piping	a. CO b. Acrolein	a. See 1b above b. Burning mucous membranes, lightheadedness, dyspnea	a. See 1b above b. Toxicity results from denaturing proteins
Nylon	Carpeting, clothes upholstery	a. Ammonia b. Hydrocyanic acid	a. Conjunctivitis, burning mucous membranes, laryngeal and pulmonary edema b. See 2b above	a. Binds with cells and produces liquefaction necrosis b. See 2b above

*From Fitzgerald, R. T.: Prehospital care of burned patients. Crit. Care Q. **1**(3):21, 1978.

maintaining the output at 30 to 75 ml/hour for adults. Hourly specimens should be sent to the laboratory on a regular basis for repeat analysis and determination of specific gravity and myoglobin levels. Baseline vital signs (temperature, pulse, respirations, CVP, and blood pressure) must be obtained and monitored subsequently at 15-minute intervals. Consideration should be given to employing arterial pressure line monitoring when the distribution of the burn precludes regular assessment of cuff blood pressure readings. Obtain a 12-lead ECG to assess the cardiac status, and monitor cardiac rhythm to detect hyperkalemic dysrhythmias, which can result from tissue and red cell destruction.

Weigh the patient as soon as feasible for a baseline value.

Some clinicians feel that central venous lines are unnecessary in the emergency department management of burns and should be avoided unless no other IV route can be achieved, leaving the central veins undisturbed for later use in hyperalimentation.

Fluid formulas

There are several formulas widely used for calculating fluid replacement in the burn victim. They are designed to replace sodium and plasma proteins in a controlled manner during the first 24 to 48 hours after the injury.

The Baxter formula is designed to administer crystalloids based on the percent of burned surface (4 ml of Ringer's lactate per kilogram of body weight per percent of body surface area burned). The fluid is administered by delivering one half in the first 8 hours after the injury, and one fourth of the amount in each of the second and third 8-hour periods. Note that additional water is not provided, since the slightly hypotonic Ringer's solution provides approximately 120 ml of excess water per liter. Sugar is not administered in the first 24 hours because of the risk of stress-induced pseudodiabetes seen in conjunction with massive burns.

The second day provides dextrose, potassium supplement, and colloids (plasma proteins, albumin, and so on) to correct other tissue and plasma volume deficits. Adjustments are made based on a monitoring of vital signs, CVP or PCWP, urinary output, and general status, such as sensorium and gastrointestinal activity.

Fluid administration is monitored and adjusted in relation to cardiovascular status. Special care should be exercised in regard to the elderly with compromised myocardial reserve because of a high mortality associated with fluid volume excess. An adequate blood pressure, a slowing pulse, and normal cerebration indicate a positive response to fluid therapy.

Nasogastric intubation

Burn patients are prone to gastric dilatation and paralytic ileus; therefore, gastric decompression is desirable to prevent vomiting and aspiration. The tube may also be used to administer antacids to reduce gastric irritation and the potential for ulceration. Thirty milliliters of a suitable antacid are administered, and suction is interrupted for 10 minutes (by clamping the tube). This procedure may be repeated hourly.

Pain relief

Until the patient's postburn shock status is fairly well stabilized, IV narcotics should be avoided, especially if there are concomitant injuries that could require early surgery. When fluid resuscitation has brought shock under control, small doses of meperidine (Demerol) (20 to 25 mg for adults; 0.2 mg/pound for children) can be given IV while the cardiorespiratory status is cautiously monitored.

Since the need for analgesia is inversely proportional to the depth of the burn, patients with first and mixed second degree (partial-thickness) burns may benefit from analgesia. Full-thickness burns are essentially painless because of the destruction of sensory nerve endings.

Sterile saline compresses (towels dipped in solution cooled to 55° to 60° F) may be applied to wounds to reduce pain. Do not, however place any ice directly on the burn, because frostbite can result, as well as a serious drop in body temperature. Small surface areas may be cooled; however, cooling of body surfaces

Baxter formula for resuscitation

First 24 hours

Ringer's lactate 4 ml/kg of body weight X% of body
  surface burn
No plasma or plasma substitutes.
No dextrose-containing solutions.
Administered:
  One half of 24-hour in first 8 hours
  One fourth of 24-hour total in second 8 hours
  One fourth of 24-hour total in third 8 hours

Second 24 hours

Dextrose in water sufficient to maintain serum sodium level at 140 mEq/liter.
Potassium chloride supplements to maintain serum
  potassium within normal limits.
Plasma or plasma substitutes to return plasma volume
  to normal.

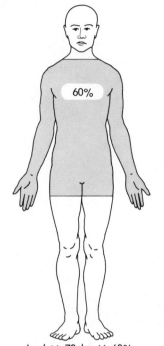

60%

4 ml × 70 kg × 60%
16,800 ml Ringer's lactate solution for first 24 hours

(over 10% to 20%) must be avoided to prevent hypothermia. An antiseptic soap may be added to the compresses; however, avoid hexachlorophene-based agents because of their potential neurotoxicity, which can cause seizures when they are rapidly absorbed through exposed body surfaces.

All burn wounds should be kept covered, because circulating air, especially drafts, seems to cause increased pain in certain partial-thickness injuries.

In some major burn cases it may be necessary to warm patients with sterile blankets. In any event, do not permit the unclothed victim to lie for a lengthy period unprotected in an air-conditioned room.

Care of the burn wound

The burn wound is usually not attended until all initial stabilization procedures have been accomplished. Before initiating wound care, ensure that the wound is photographed. Scrupulous surgical asepsis should be employed, and the area involved must be protected from sources of contamination. The first step involves cleaning the burned surfaces with half-strength iodine-containing solution, such as diluted povidone iodine (Betadine).

Loose tissue and foreign material such as sand, glass, or dirt should be removed, and a careful inspection then made to determine the depth and extent of the injury. Do not use brushes or scrubbing to remove debris or car-

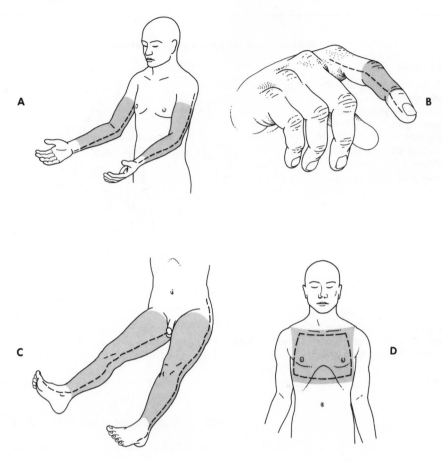

Fig. 26-4. Proper sites for escharotomy. **A,** Arms; **B,** fingers; **C,** legs; **D,** anterior thorax.

bon since they may further injure tissue. Shave the hair in and adjacent to the burned area, but avoid shaving eyebrows, because they may not grow back. Excise skin fragments and blister debris, but *do not* disturb intact blisters. Reevaluate the burn wound after initial cleaning and debridement, and rephotograph. Culture each major area for baseline values.

Throughout the early care phase, the nurse should be alert to circumferential burns that could create constricting edema, thus impairing circulation. (Ensure that the IVs, for example, are not infusing into an arm with the potential of extensive edema.) Perform escharot-

omies as necessary to relieve compression from circumferential wounds (Fig. 26-4). Continue to protect the wound from contaminants until it can be properly dressed or covered with a biological dressing, such as a homograft or heterograft. As much as feasible, keep the involved extremities or other body parts elevated to minimize edema.

There are two popular topical agents for burn therapy: mafenide (Sulfamylon) and silver sulfadiazine (Silvadene). Silver nitrate is also used, but its disadvantages include skin discoloration and pain on application to second degree burns; thus, it has largely been replaced by mafenide and silver sulfadiazine.

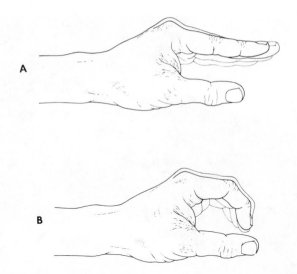

Fig. 26-5. Positioning hand in dressing. **A,** "Duck-bill" position. **B,** Functional position.

Mafenide is a bacteriostatic, broad-spectrum agent. It penetrates the wounds with ease and is rapidly oxidized, absorbed, and excreted. It is used as a 10% cream in twice daily applications along with daily washing and debridement of the wound. Mafenide is not inactivated by pus or body fluids, but it is painful on application and tends to macerate the skin when used under a dressing. Close monitoring of renal function is essential when using this agent, since it can contribute to metabolic acidosis, especially in the presence of impaired renal activity.

Silver sulfadiazine is bacteriostatic, bacteriocidal, and broad spectrum. It is used as a 1% cream applied three times daily or every 48 hours (in dressing). It can be washed away without debriding the area. Despite its advantage, it is not as effective as mafenide in management of burns with established wound infection.

Sulfa sensitivities must be ascertained before using either agent.

There are several methods of dressing burn wounds. Here are three examples.

1. Cover wound with 4½ burn gauze (knitted mesh roller gauze) impregnated with silver sulfadiazine cream. Use spiral wrap or cut in strips of appropriate length and layer onto the wound. Be sure to wrap fingers and toes separately. If the eyelids are involved, the cut gauze is smoothed over the closed lids. All face burns should be covered, except for the nose and the mouth. Protect dressed ears with individual dressings and paddings. Perineal and genitalia burns are left exposed by placing the patient on a pad of polyurethane foam lathered with silver sulfadiazine.

   Cover impregnated gauze dressings with six turns of similar nonimpregnated gauze. Put hands and fingers in the position of function, or use the alternate "duck-bill" position (Fig. 26-5). Sterile burn pads may be appropriate: 32-ply cheesecloth for large areas, especially in the adult.

   Enclose the dressing in bias-cut stockinette, and secure with tape. A burn dressing should always extend well beyond the wound.

2. Hydron burn dressings* may be sprayed directly on the wound to produce a bacterial barrier effect (Fig. 26-6).

---

*Hydrophilic polymer, poly(2-hydroxyethyl methacrylate) and polyethylene glycol 400.

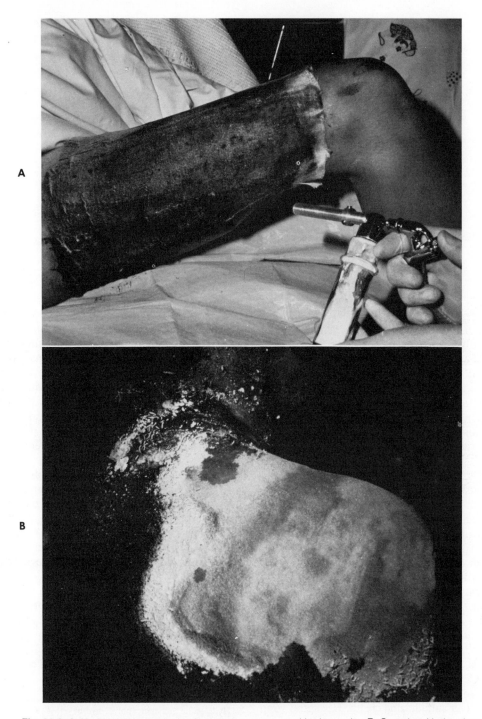

Fig. 26-6. A, Hydron being applied to fine mesh gauze over skin donor site. **B,** Complete Hydron burn bandage over partial-thickness burn wound. (Courtesy Abbott Laboratories, Chicago.)

Table 26-2. Guide to tetanus prophylaxis in burn patients*

History of tetanus immunization (doses)	Tetanus and diphtheria toxoid ("Td") (adult type)	Tetanus immune globulin (human)†
Uncertain	Yes	Yes
0-1	Yes	Yes
2	Yes	No‡
3 or more	No§	No

*From Edlich, R. F.: J.A.C.E.P. **7**(4):152, 1978.
†When tetanus toxoid and globulin are given concurrently, separate syringes and separate sites should be used.
‡Unless burn more than 24 hours old.
§Unless more than 5 years since last dose.

3. Allografts (cadaver skin) or xenografts (pigskin) may be used if available in emergency department.

NOTE: If the patient is to be transferred to a burn unit or regional burn center, the wound may be merely cleansed, grossly debrided, and wrapped in sterile sheets if the transfer time is within 1 or 2 hours.

Tetanus prophylaxis

Tetanus prophylaxis should be assessed and agents appropriately administered (Table 26-2). Antibiotics such as aqueous penicillin, 50,000 units/kg/day, should be initiated. It is further advocated that gamma globulin be given for infants and small children to ensure maximum protection from infectious complications. Nystatin (oral and vaginal) should be considered for all those with burns that exceed 20% of the body surface area.

Care of minor burn wounds

- Evaluate the extent and depth of injury.
- Remove clothing; if it is adherent to the wound, soak as previously described. Remove jewelry.
- Relieve pain by applying cool compresses or immersing the part in cool tap water (55° F) for 1 to 2 hours.
- Cleanse the wound gently with a mild detergent soap. Shave the surrounding hair.
- Debride as necessary.
- Dress the wound with an antimicrobial agent and apply a bulky protective dressing (see p. 609). (Always place fine mesh gauze directly over the wound.) If a responsible individual is available, demonstrate the dressing technique, and provide instructions for daily soaks and dressings. Explain how elevation may be useful in controlling edema. Provide descriptions for all dressing items.
- Provide tetanus prophylaxis (Table 26-2).
- Consider an antibiotic regimen.
- Plan follow-up care at 48- and 72-hour intervals in the outpatient department or physician's office.
- Provide written instructions for the burn wound regimen, and ensure that they are understood.

ELECTRICAL INJURIES

Electrical injuries, especially burns, create some unusual and challenging problems for emergency personnel. If the current passes through vital organs, death can be immediate from ventricular fibrillation or respiratory arrest; other delayed complications include nervous system damage, severe tissue destruction, and vascular injury, as well as renal failure. Renal complications are common, because myoglobin from damaged muscle cells induces acidosis and interferes with renal tubular function, effecting shutdown.

Electrical burns can be quite deceiving, since a small surface wound can be underladen with widespread destruction of muscle, nerves, and blood vessels. When electricity passes through living organisms, intensive heat (up to 20,000° C) is produced, which devitalizes the tissue along the pathway of the current.

Electrical flash or arc injuries are usually industrially related, and the intense heat in-

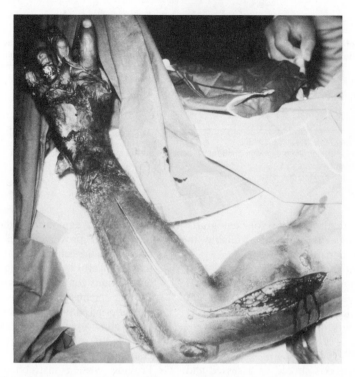

Fig. 26-7. High voltage electrical injury. Obvious charring of hand and wrist. Incision through skin caused bleeding only in mid-arm. Muscle in both arm and forearm was necrotic; shoulder disarticulation was necessary. (From Hartford, C. E., and Boyd, W. C.: In Liechty, R. D., and Soper, R. T.: Synopsis of surgery, ed. 4, St. Louis, 1980, The C. V. Mosby Co.)

volved may generate temperatures of 4,000° C or more, producing larger thermal burns. Since the current in these injuries does not transverse the body, internal organ damage is unlikely.

Electrical burns are classified into three types:

Type I electrical burns are characterized by tissue damage along the conduction route. Thrombosis and blood vessel damage may be concealed by a small surface erosion burn.

Type II electrical burns are the result of flash or arching incidents from high-tension sources. External skin damage may range from a small entrance wound to a huge, exploded exit wound. Extensive skin discoloration, edema, charring, and deformity may accompany this burn (Fig. 26-7).

Type III burns are electrical current injuries accompanied by an ignition of clothing, producing an added insult to body tissue.

Emergency management

As soon as the victim has been disengaged from the source of electricity, the ABCs of basic life support should be checked at once, and cardiopulmonary resuscitation initiated as needed. (Since there are numerous reports of an arrested individual recovering without sequelae after 6 or 8 hours of resuscitation efforts after electrocution, it is appropriate to continue CPR for an extended period of time before abandoning hope.) Defibrillation may be required repeatedly. It is crucial to monitor any heart rhythm constantly, since serious dysrhythmias may appear after satisfactory cardiac activity seems certain. Respiratory arrest may demand intubation and the delivery of high-flow oxygen.

An IV should be established promptly using Ringer's lactate to combat shock. No formula for fluid administration is used, however, since the surface area involved is deceivingly small compared to the hidden tissue damage. Large quantities of fluid may be required to maintain the urinary output at the level of 100 ml/hour for adults, the desirable quantity for adult victims of electrical injuries. Mannitol may be ordered to ensure renal filtration and prevent acute tubular necrosis. Sodium bicarbonate alkalinization therapy may also be tried to prevent precipitation of myoglobin in the renal tubules. The output should be carefully monitored using a Foley catheter with specimens sent to the laboratory at 2-hour intervals for myoglobin content analysis.

When the victim has been stabilized, analgesia may be considered before wound cleansing and debridement. The entrance and exit sites for current should be located to predict the pathway of current through the body and thus anticipate the internal organ damage. Hidden areas such as the groin, rectum, axilla, and mouth should not be overlooked in the search for surface wounds of exit.

All individuals with electrical burns should be hospitalized (even if the wounds seem minor) if either unconsciousness or cardiac dysrhythmias are noted at *any time* after the injury.

The sequelae of electrical injuries are multiple. Later complications include those related to deep muscle, fascia, nerve, and blood vessel destruction. There may be delayed wound sloughing, neurological impairment, gangrene, infection, septicemia, and hemorrhage, which could lead to amputation of body parts and even death. There are also chances for other delayed complications, including cardiac arrest, respiratory paralysis, and renal shutdown up to several weeks after the injury, so follow-up is critical.

CHEMICAL BURNS

Chemical burns may be induced by surface contact, ingestion, inhalation, and even injection. Most chemicals ''burn'' by a process other than the usual thermal mode. Tissue is damaged and destroyed by chemical coagulation of protein, precipitation of cellular substances, dehydration, protoplasmic poisoning, or tissue proteins being dissolved by their action. (See p. 325 for chemical burns of the eye.)

Most chemicals should be immediately flushed from the body surface by copious amounts of water. A shower, if available, is ideal for areas involving much body surface area. Exceptions are sulfuric acid, hydrochloric acid, and muriatic acid. Weak bases tend to be more helpful in managing these latter substances, since water alone creates a heat-producing chemical reaction. Mustard gas, sodium metal, phenol, and white phosporous are best handled initially by covering with oil. Gasoline should be washed quickly from the skin using a soap solution, since prolonged contact can foster cutaneous absorption with resultant respiratory damage and destruction of vascular endothelium involving the liver, spleen, and kidneys. Sodium metal, white phosphorus, and alkyl mercuric agents may require surgical excision. Dry chemicals should be brushed from skin surfaces before flushing the skin with water to reduce the amount of heat generated in the resultant chemical reaction.

Hydrofluoric acid burns

Hydrofluoric acid burns should be washed with copious amounts of water to decrease the rate of inflammatory and chemical reaction, minimize the hygroscopic effects, and restore the normal pH. A calcium hydroxide solution should be used in cleansing any wound surface. Skin areas penetrated by the agent require infiltration of calcium gluconate into the skin edges and subcutaneous layers. Antibiotic ointment and dressings typical for a second degree thermal burn may be then applied. Third degree hydrofluoric acid burns are likely to require skin grafting.

TAR BURNS

Tar should be cooled with cold water and peeled away. If it is difficult to remove, it can be dissolved with mineral oil. The resultant burns should be dressed with polymyxin B sulfate (Neosporin) and redressed every 12 hours until healed.

SUNBURN

Severe sunburn should be carefully evaluated as any burn according to the degree and percentage of surface area involved. Any sunburn is serious if the body temperature exceeds 101° F (38° C) or if blistering is apparent over broad areas. Evaporative cooling is useful, so the nurse should apply a wet cloth or dressing over the burn and expose the involved area to air. A wet tee-shirt works well for large surface and trunk burns. A bland sunburn lotion with an anesthetic agent, topical steroids, or other preparations may be useful. Infrared radiation, if available, can be helpful in reducing erythema.

FRICTION BURNS (ABRASIONS, "FLOOR BURNS," OR "STREET BURNS")

These injuries involve both mechanical friction and heat trauma. Since they are frequently contaminated with surface debris (from gymnasium floors, tennis courts, or pavements), particulate matter should be carefully removed after cleansing and before dressing. A local anesthetic agent may be necessary for accomplishing this feat. Hydrogen peroxide and vigorous scrubbing may be useful in ridding the wound of debris. Particles left in the wound may create permanent changes in the skin appearance, that is, a "tattooing" effect.

SUMMARY

The major burns seen in the hospital emergency department represent a challenge to the personnel in terms of physical care and emotional support to the victim and his significant others.

In communities that have a well-developed prehospital care system, the severely burned individual is often provided the critical "edge" of a difference in treatment that makes survival possible. Early attention to airway management, concomitant injuries, fluid resuscitation, and transport without delay to a burn center has benefited hundreds of victims. Despite these improvements in the delivery of emergency care, the morbidity and mortality of full-thickness, extensive burns is high, especially in the very young and the elderly.

Emergency care in the hospital consists of airway management, resuscitation and shock management, pain relief, and early care and protection of the burn itself. An important nursing responsibility is monitoring the critical cardiovascular parameters in the early postburn hours by careful attention to blood gases, central venous pressure, urine output, and other vital signs. Preventing secondary complications of infection, circulatory impairment, renal failure, and respiratory complications deserves the attention of all emergency personnel.

Special burns, chemical or electrical, have unique hazards that must be considered in the early hours after the accident.

The knowledge of the pathophysiological responses to the burn wound provides a fundamental basis for understanding the rationale for the sequence of events in the medical management of this injury.

BIBLIOGRAPHY

Allyn, P.: Inhalation injuries, Crit. Care Q. **1**(3):37-42, 1978.

Braen, G. R.: Emergency management of major thermal burns, Monograph, Kansas City, Mo., 1977, Marion Laboratories.

Crews, E. R.: The practical manual for the treatment of burns, Springfield, Ill., 1967, Charles C Thomas, Publisher.

Edlich, R. F., and others: Emergency department treatment, triage, and transfer protocols for the burn patient, J.A.C.E.P. **7**:152-158, 1978.

Emergency Product News, **9**(4), June 1977 (entire issue).

Feller, I., and Jones, C. A.: Nursing the burned patient, Ann Arbor, Mich., 1973, Institute for Burn Medicine.

Fisher, J. C.: Immediate care of the burn victim, Emerg. Prod. New **9**(4):58-59, 1977.

Fitzgerald, R. T.: Prehospital care of burned patients, Crit. Care Q. **1**(3):13-24, 1978.

Gursel, E., and Tintinalli, J. E.: Emergency burn management, J.A.C.E.P. **7**:209-212, 1978.

Harding, J., and Walraven, G.: Prehospital management of burn injuries: a case study, Emerg. Prod. News **9**(4): 34-37, 1977.

Hersperger, J. E., and Dahl, L. M.: Electrical and chemical injuries, Crit. Care Q. **1**(3):43-49, 1978.

Jacoby, F. G.: Nursing care of the patient with burns, ed. 2, St. Louis, 1976, The C. V. Mosby Co.

Marvin, J.: Acute care for the burn patient, Crit. Care Q. **1**(3)25-35, 1978.

McGranahan, B. G.: Nursing care of the burn patient, A.O.R.N.J. **20**:787-793, November 1974.

Simmons, R.: Emergency management of electrical burns, J.E.N. **3**:14, 1977.

CHAPTER 27

Poisons and toxicology

The individual with a reported or suspected overdose requires prompt management and should never be relegated to a waiting area in the emergency department. If the victim is unconscious or has a depressed level of consciousness (either accidental or intentional) or if there is local evidence of contact with a toxic agent, serious poisoning should be suspected.

BASIC LIFE SUPPORT
Airway

The management of cardiopulmonary arrest should always be paramount in the minds of emergency personnel, even though the victim of poisoning or overdose may be cardiovascularly stable upon arrival at the hospital. Apneic patients should be intubated and ventilations assisted mechanically. (Do not use an esophageal obturator if corrosive substances have been ingested, because perforation could be induced.) Provide supplemental oxygen to *all* overdose victims. Use 100% oxygen for inhalation injuries (see Table 26-1). The individual should be placed in a semiprone, side-lying position (head down, feet elevated 10° to 15°) to minimize the risk of aspiration. If the individual is not intubated, oral airways and oropharyngeal suctioning should be employed as necessary. Auscultate the lungs frequently to ensure adequacy of ventilations and to detect the onset of pulmonary edema.

Cardiovascular status

Since many toxic agents affect cardiac rhythm, the ECG should be monitored continuously. The nurse should be prepared to defibrillate or initiate CPR if indicated. After baseline blood samples are obtained for sugar, CBC, BUN, electrolytes, and toxicology screens, an IV of saline or D/5/W should be initiated to serve as a line for drug administration. Baseline ABGs should be obtained periodically, and sodium bicarbonate administered as needed to correct acidosis.

All unconscious patients should have a bolus or two of D/5/W and naloxone (Narcan) to rule out hypoglycemia or narcotic-related causes of coma. Otherwise, valuable time should not be spent searching for an antidote. The ones that exist for a specific poisoning however, should be well known (Table 27-1).

Hypotension should be initially managed by infusing 200 ml of IV fluid every 5 minutes three times for a total of 600 ml or until a normotensive state is reached. For residual hypotension, add dopamine at 5 to 20 μg/kg/minute. (Lower doses may aggravate hypotension.) A CVP line may be a useful adjunct for monitoring fluid therapy in individuals who have a history of heart, renal, or respiratory disease. A Foley catheter is an important element of management of poisonings and overdoses for assessing qualitative and quantitative renal function.

Seizures

Almost all patients in a toxic condition have the potential for seizures and thus should be observed for seizure activity. Anticonvulsants may be required in certain instances, but they

Assessment guide and possible considerations for patient who has ingested poisons*

Assessments	Possible considerations
1. Respiratory assessment	
a. Are respirations depressed?	Barbiturates, sedatives, hypnotics
b. Is the patient experiencing dyspnea? Hyperpnea?	Salicylates
c. Is the patient coughing?	Indication that patient possibly aspirated
d. Is cyanosis present?	Kerosene, cyanide, nitrites, aniline compounds
e. What signs of hypoxia are evident? Restlessness? Confusion?	Barbiturates, sedatives, hypnotics
2. Circulatory assessments	
a. What are the vital signs?	
b. Is the blood pressure decreased?	Barbiturates, sedatives, hypnotics
c. Is bradycardia present?	Organic phosphorus
3. Central nervous system assessments	
a. Is the patient confused?	Organic phosphorus, PCP, LSD, marijuana
b. Is the patient comatose?	Organic phosphorus, central nervous system depressants
c. Is the patient having seizures?	Organic phosphorus, central nervous system stimulants, strychnine, camphor
4. Assessments related to sensory function	
a. Eyes: What is the condition of the pupils? Are they dilated? Are they pinpoint?	Cocaine, atropine, amphetamines, antihistamines, nicotine (late effect) Nicotine (early effect), opiates, physostigmine
b. Integument: Is the skin flushed or pink?	Carbon monoxide, cholinergic drugs
5. Gastrointestinal assessments	
a. Is the patient vomiting?	Acids, alkalis, metallic compounds, organic phosphorus
b. Is the patient having diarrhea?	Same as above
c. Is abdominal pain a presenting symptom?	Acids alkalis, metallic compounds
d. Are there burns about the mouth?	Caustic alkalis
e. Is there a characteristic breath odor?	Turpentine, arsenic, cyanide, wintergreen, phosphorus
6. Urinary assessments	
a. Are changes noted in urine?	
b. Presence of albuminuria?	Mercury
7. Musculoskeletal assessments	
a. Is trismus being experienced?	Phenothiazides
b. Is opisthotonus present?	Phenothiazides

*Modified from Barber, J. M., Stokes, L. G., and Billings, D. M.: Adult and child care, a client approach to nursing, ed. 2, St. Louis, 1977, The C. V. Mosby Co.

Table 27-1. Specific antidotes*

Poison or agent	Antidote
Narcotics, dextropropoxy-phene (Darvon), pentazo-cine lactate (Talwin), and diphenoxylate (Lomotil)	Naloxone (Narcan)
Mercury, arsenic, lead, copper, cobalt	Dimercaprol (BAL [British anti-lewisite])
Iron	Deferoxamine
Cyanide	Nitrate thioscilfate
Organic phosphates (insecti-cides) such as para-thion, malathion	Atropine Pralidoxime (2-PAM)
Lead	Versene Penicillamine
Carbon monoxide	Oxygen
Anticoagulants	Vitamin K
Tricyclics (scopolamine, belladonna, alkaloids, diphenhydramine [Bena-dryl]), jimsonweed	Physostigmine
Acetaminophen	N-Acetylcysteine

*Specific antidotes are usually not available for most poisons. However, a few important ones should be known to the emergency nurse because their prompt use could be lifesaving; therefore, their availability in the department is vital.

must be carefully used if the respiratory status is already depressed due to overdose.

Vomiting

Vomiting may be appropriate as a mode to empty the stomach of an ingested substance, but its use is limited to conscious patients who do not have a deteriorating level of consciousness. It is also not recommended for ingestions of strong acid, alkali, or possibly petroleum products. In general, emesis is not useful if the ingestion occurred 4 hours or more before emergency intervention, because systemic absorption would already have taken place. (Aspirin is an exception; see p. 624.)

Ipecac syrup is administered in doses of 30 ml for the adult and 15 ml for the child orally. (It may be repeated once if no results are noted.) Ipecac should be followed with one or two glasses of water. Larger amounts of water may result in a reflex emptying of the stomach into the small intestine, thus defeating the intent of the emetic. If feasible, ambulate the patient, because it hastens the effect of the emetic agent. Vomiting usually is induced within 15 to 20 minutes for children and within 30 to 60 minutes for adults. *Save all emesis.* The initial emesis should be isolated from the total specimen if possible for qualitative analysis. If emesis is not produced for any reason after the initial and repeated dose of ipecac, the drug should be lavaged from the stomach since it is a myocardial irritant if systemically absorbed.

Apomorphine is a potent emetic, but is seldom used because ipecac is effective and much safer. Apomorphine may be given safely only to adults. The dose is usually 0.1 mg/kg IV or subcutaneously followed by a generous amount of oral fluids (two glasses) to hasten vomiting. Emesis should ensue in 5 to 15 minutes. However, if the drug is ineffective, do not repeat the dose. Reverse the effects of the drug with naloxone (see p. 731) as soon as effects have been obtained or after 20 minutes without desired results.

Lavage

Lavage is often used to recover ingested substances if there are contraindications for emetic use. Emergency nurses will find that all their skill, ingenuity, and physical stamina are required to accomplish this feat in an uncooperative child or adult. Explanations of the rationale and efficacy of lavage are generally worthless, because the child who has accidentally ingested a toxic substance is too young to comprehend and the adult who has ingested a toxic substance is likely to be suicidal and thus initially wants to die rather than being helped by well-meaning emergency personnel. A guideline for the lavage procedure follows.

Lavage procedure

1. Protect the airway with endotracheal intubation in an unconscious patient or by using a head-down, left side-lying position in an alert patient. Have suctioning at hand. Remember that strong vagal stimulation can also induce cardiac dysrhythmias and cardiopulmonary ar-

rest. Be prepared for all phases of resuscitation. *If you must partially restrain a combative patient, do not hold him down on his back so forcefully that he could not turn or be turned in the event of vomiting.*

2. Select a lavage tube. A 28 (Fr) Ewald tube is the smallest tube acceptable for lavage. A 36 (Fr) Ewald tube is preferred. (A 16 to 18 [Fr] nasogastric tube is inadequate for lavaging any substance other than liquids.)

3. Lubricate the tube with a water-soluble lubricant if it is to pass through the nose; with cold water if it is to be passed orally.

4. If the patient is able to cooperate, have him sit up and swallow or take sips of water, which will close the epiglottis and prevent accidental passage into the trachea.

5. Before lavage, aspirate to ascertain that the tube is in the stomach or listen with a stethoscope over the stomach as air is introduced via a syringe. A third test for proper placement of the tube involves placing the free end in a glass of water to check for fluctuations that correspond to respirations. Do not proceed with lavage if there are fluctuations corresponding to inspiration and expiration or if there are other signs of respiratory distress.

6. Secure the tube with tape to avoid dislodgement.

7. Place the patient in the head-down, left side-lying position.

8. Lavage with normal saline in a tidal volume of no less than 50 to 300 ml for adults and 10 ml/kg per wash in children. Larger tidal volumes may cause reflex emptying of the stomach into the small bowel, defeating the purpose of the procedure. Warm the normal saline after the initial liter is used to prevent a lowering of the body temperature. Lavage until the return is clear by instilling the saline and either siphoning or aspirating the return. Charcoal may be used after collection of the initial aspirate and then *repeated* after lavage. Remember that the aspirate may be of limited value to the laboratory, however, once the charcoal has been given. Administration of citrate of magnesium, magnesium sulfate, sodium sulfate, or another saline cathartic may be given after the charcoal to hasten elimination of the remaining substance.

9. Remove the tube quickly. (Anticipate gagging and possible aspiration.) Provide oral hygiene care as indicated.

10. Permit the individual to sit up after lavage.

ACUTE IRON POISONING

Acute iron poisoning is essentially a toddler's disease resulting from ingestion of iron tablets. The toxic and potentially lethal dose is approximately 60 mg/kg or 1 tablet/kg (since ferrous sulfate tablets are characteristically 60 mg each). Iron-fortified vitamins and other similar preparations usually contain less per unit, often as little as 15 mg.

The signs and symptoms that should alert the emergency nurse to the problem are related to the substance's effects on the gastric mucosa. There may be brisk gastric or lower gastrointestinal bleeding occurring an hour or two after ingestion. Within 4 to 6 hours, there may be a rapid development of shock, acidosis, and/or coagulopathy. Delayed effects include hepatic necrosis, pyloric stenosis, and other strictures of the gastrointestinal tract.

If acute iron poisoning is suspected, emesis and lavage with 5% sodium bicarbonate (or Fleet's enema solution diluted 1:4 with water), which acts as an iron-trapping solution, are recommended. Follow emesis or lavage with catharsis. An IV of D/5/W may be required to manage the shock caused by the relaxation of capacitance vessels, venous pooling, decreased CVP, and reduced cardiac output. Volume infusion is usually sufficient to alleviate this problem.

Venous blood samples should be drawn for testing serum iron and iron-binding capacity levels, prothrombin time and partial thromboplastin time, and type and cross-match. An arterial blood gas may also be desired to assist in the clinical management of the acidosis. Since iron tablets are radiopaque, the extent of a recent poisoning may be evaluated on x-ray films.

Deferoxamine is the specific chelation therapy for binding iron at a weight ratio of 100:9. Deferoxamine is given IV (15 mg/kg/hour) or IM (90 mg/kg every 8 hours). The nurses should be aware of the potential for anaphylaxis, noted initially by urticaria and hypotension. Since the anaphylaxis may be histamine-mediated, the administration of an antihistamine may be useful prophylactically. Since iron complexes resulting from binding are filtered into the urine, the urine will be reddish pink. Exchange transfusion may be useful in selected cases. All victims of acute iron poisoning should be admitted to the hospital for follow-up therapy.

PETROLEUM DISTILLATE (HYDROCARBON) INGESTION

One of the most dread ingestions is a petroleum distillate (or hydrocarbon). The most common substances (in rank order) that are ingested are kerosene, charcoal lighter fluid, mineral seal oil, furniture polish, turpentine, gasoline, lighter fluid, and insecticides in a petroleum-distillate base. The lethal dose of most of these substances is 3 to 4 ounces for an adult and considerably less for a child. (Exact amounts have not been documented.)

In order to assess how much was ingested, it is useful to know the contents of the container (before and after ingestion) or at least the number of swallows that were taken if the ingestion was witnessed. (A child ingests about 2 ml per swallow.) It is usually difficult to assess from the history how much was taken, because gagging, coughing, spitting, and aspiration can affect the amount actually ingested. Always determine if vomiting has occurred, and if so, evaluate the airway with added caution since aspiration could have occurred, too.

NOTE: Do not spend precious time determining the exact nature of the petroleum distillate or the amount ingested. Proceed with emergency management if there is a strong suspicion or if the history seems reliable. In the meantime, decontaminate the skin with soap and warm water if surface contamination is evident, noting skin color and temperature.

Airway

The child should be assessed thoroughly in regard to the airway. Look for redness, blisters, or other irritation in the mouth and pharynx. Suspect aspiration, and listen for rales, rhonchi, dullness, diminished breath sounds at the bases, and note any dyspnea. Smell the breath for the presence of a volatile petroleum distillate. Most smell the way they do in containers, except turpentine, which gives off an odor resembling violets. Coughing may be a sign that aspiration has already occurred. Obtain a chest film and have it checked thoroughly for infiltrate, edema, and atelectasis. Pulmonary compromise can be ascertained partially by ABGs. An increased pCO_2, hypoxia, and the clinical indices of respiratory compromise may signal the need for intubation and ventilatory support. Supplemental oxygen is a necessity if there is evidence of cyanosis. Position to prevent aspiration.

Other aspects of emergency management

Obtain baseline laboratory data. Take the temperature, and record it. Weigh the child, because therapy will depend partially on the amount of ingested substance per kilogram of body weight. Draw blood for arterial blood gas measurement, obtain a chest film, and draw venous blood for routine complete blood count, toxicology screening, and liver function studies. Monitor the ECG for dysrhythmias. Obtain a baseline urinalysis. (Later a bone marrow analysis may be made to reveal hypoplasia.) Determine the need for emetics or lavage. (A few milliliters are unlikely to cause systemic toxicity, and the major risk of aspiration has already occurred.) Spontaneous vomiting occurs in 50% of petroleum distillate ingestions. If a potentially toxic dose has been ingested and the patient has an intact gag reflex and is breathing normally, ipecac-induced emesis is recommended to remove the substance before the onset of central nervous system, respiratory, and cardiac depression. Most aspiration occurs on ingestion—not during vomiting. Save all vomitus. Isolate the initial specimen. Send it and the remainder of vomitus to the laboratory in separate containers labeled appropriately for qualitative and quantitative analysis. Note on the chart if prehospital emesis occurred. If the patient has a depressed level of consciousness or is having seizures indicating systemic involvement (either of which would make vomiting dangerous), gastric lavage may be used to remove the stomach contents. Protection of the airway by nasotracheal or endotracheal intubation, however, must precede the procedure. Half-normal saline is used to prevent water intoxication from excess absorption. When less than 0.5 ml/kg of a hydrocarbon (nonchlorinated or non–metal containing) has been ingested, catharsis may be helpful. However, do not give any oil-based cathartic. Several hours after ingestion there may be diarrhea with blood-tinged stools with the characteristic hydrocarbon odor.

The victim of hydrocarbon ingestion should be admitted. The white blood count and temperature should be monitored at frequent intervals because an elevation in either is a good indicator of the development of pneumatoceles. IV antibiotics and steroids are used by some clinicians to thwart the progression of pneumonitis, but their efficacy has not been proved thus far. Follow-up chest films are essential, with the second one scheduled 6 to 8 hours after ingestion.

The neurological status deserves ongoing concern, especially if the ingestion is thought to be greater than 1 ml/kg. Seizure precautions are indicated.

The ingestion of petroleum distillates (hydrocarbons) is a critical circumstance, and emergency nurses should take every opportunity to do preventive guidance within their community in regard to the problem.

DIGITALIS TOXICITY

The major effects of digitalis include the following: increasing the contractility of the heart, prolonging atrioventricular node conduction, prolonging the atrioventricular refractory period, and shortening action potential of the Purkinje fibers and ventricular muscle.

Its overall mechanisms enhance cardiac output and reduce the cardiac rate. Digitalis is widely used to treat congestive heart failure, atrial fibrillation and flutter, and occasionally paroxysmal atrial tachycardia. It is important to note, however, that therapeutic doses of the agent exert little or no effect on a normal functioning heart.

Digitalis in its several forms is the fourth most commonly prescribed drug, although it has a small margin of safety. The therapeutic dose is approximately 50% to 60% of the toxic dose. Digitalis toxicity is statistically the most common adverse drug reaction, in part because it has a long half-life (approximately 36 hours for digoxin and 5.7 days for digitoxin [Crystodigin]). It is therefore extremely important for emergency personnel to know signs, symptoms, and dangers inherent in digitalis intoxication.

Symptoms of mild intoxication include: anorexia, ventricular ectopic beats, bradycardia, nausea and vomiting, headache, malaise, and ventricular premature beats, bigeminy.

Symptoms of severe intoxication include: blurring of vision, disorientation, diarrhea, ventricular tachycardia, sinoatrial and atrioventricular block, ventricular fibrillation, and color (yellow) disturbances in visual perception.

Digitalis intoxication should be suspected when these symptoms are evident, especially in the elderly or in a person with a history of the following, since each contributes to toxicity.

Hypopotassemia (hypokalemia) is especially likely in those who concurrently take thiazide diuretics. Prolonged vomiting or the use of insulin, amphotericin B (Fungizone), ethacrynic acid (Edecrin), furosemide (Lasix), chlorthalidone (Hygroton), and corticosteroids also contributes to hypopotassemia. This low potassium state causes weakness, diminished reflexes, low blood pressure, weak pulse, and a characteristic ECG. There is usually an elevated P wave amplitude, prolonged PR interval, ST depression, flat or inverted T waves, and a prominent U wave.

Concurrent use of calcium (parenteral) (stimulates ectopic pacemakers); catecholamines or sympathomimetics (stimulate ectopic pacemakers); barbiturates (accelerate metabolism by reducing half-life by 50%); or reserpine (parenteral) (causes dysrhythmias from sudden catecholamine release)

Accompanying physical conditions that increase sensitivity to digitalis or retard its renal elimination

Hypoxia

Emergency management consists initially of discontinuing all digitalis and diuretics, which contribute to hypokalemia. Venous blood samples for digitalis level and electrolyte determination should be drawn, and any electrolyte imbalances noted should be corrected during the course of therapy. Antidysrhythmics are sometimes used to treat selected cases.

JIMSONWEED

Jimsonweed is a psychedelic agent that produces atropinelike effects, hallucinations, and disturbances of thought processes. It is essential that this agent's effects be differentiated from those of LSD and that the presentation not be confused with schizophrenia. Leaves may be used as a tea drink or smoked, and seeds may be chewed and swallowed (Fig. 27-1). If death occurs, it is usually from cardiac and respiratory arrest.

Signs and symptoms include dryness of the mouth and intense thirst; dilated pupils; blurred vision; photophobia; warm, flushed skin; fever; difficulty in swallowing, talking, and urinating; palpitations and tachycardia; possibly hyperactivity; disorientation (unlike that of LSD); central nervous system depression—even seizures and coma have been noted after large dose ingestions.

Emergency management

The patient should be placed in a quiet room with low lighting to reduce stimulation. Emesis or lavage is useful, even if the ingestion

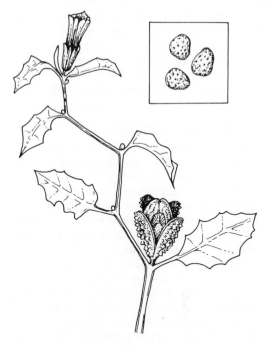

Fig. 27-1. Jimsonweed.

has occurred several hours previously, since jimsonweed delays emptying of the stomach.

Vital signs and the ECG should be carefully monitored to detect cardiac irritability or cardiovascular decompensation. If fever is present, antipyretics may be used.

Physostigmine is administered as follows:*

Adult: 2 mg diluted to 10 ml IV over 2 minutes. Repeat every 5 minutes up to a 6-mg maximum dose.

Child: 0.5 mg diluted to 10 ml IV over 2 minutes. Repeat every 5 minutes up to a 2-mg maximum dose.

Physostigmine may need to be repeated in 30 to 60 minutes (because of its short half-life) if toxic signs and symptoms reappear. Side effects of physostigmine include excessive peristalsis with cramping and diarrhea, acceler-

---

*Neostigmine bromide and pyridostigmine bromide do not enter the central nervous system and are not useful in treatment of jimsonweed poisoning.

ated salivation, and urinary urgency. It should be used with caution in patients with asthma, cardiovascular disease, or gastrointestinal or urinary obstruction. Reverse severe side effects with atropine (see p. 715).

The most sensitive index to successful therapy is the slowing of a rapid pulse.

SALICYLATE POISONING

It is most important for emergency personnel to be familiar with salicylate poisoning, because it is frequently responsible for death in accidental or intentional overdosage. Most salicylate poisoning involves aspirin; however, methyl salicylate (oil of wintergreen), even when applied topically in certain situations, also may provoke a crisis.

The most crucial initial task of emergency personnel is to determine if the amount of aspirin ingested is serious enough to indicate the need for definitive clinical management.

Any ingestion of methyl salicylate is dangerous, however. (The potentially lethal dose for a 2-year-old child is approximately 1 teaspoon.)

Calculate the salicylate ingestion from aspirin (acetylsalicylic acid; ASA) using either of the following formulas (1 gr = 65 mg):

$$\frac{\text{Number of tablets ingested} \times \text{gr ASA tablet}}{\text{Weight of patient in pounds}} =$$

$$\text{Dose in gr/pound}$$

$$\frac{\text{Number of tablets ingested} \times \text{mg ASA/tablet}}{\text{Weight of patient in kg}} =$$

$$\text{Dose in mg/kg}$$

If the dose is less than 1 gr/pound, or less than 150 mg/kg, no further treatment is needed unless there is concurrent febrile illness, dehydration, or renal dysfunction, which would contribute to serious toxicity, even at lower doses.

Treatment is needed if the ingestion exceeds 3.0 gr/pound, or 400 mg/kg, or if any signs or symptoms of salicylate intoxication appear: unexplained hyperpnea, especially accompanied by vomiting, tinnitus, fever, confusion, lethargy, seizures, and coma.

Induce emesis with syrup of ipecac even if

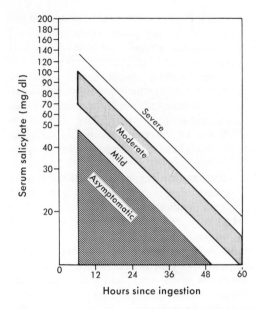

Fig. 27-2. Nomogram for estimating the severity of poison from the serum salicylate level at varying intervals after ingestion of a single dose. This nomogram is only useful if the ingestion has occurred in a single dose. If symptoms have developed over an extended period of time, other clinical criteria must be used to estimate potential severity. (From Barber, J. M., and Budassi, S. A.: Mosby's manual of emergency care, St. Louis, 1979, The C. V. Mosby Co.)

the patient has previously vomited. Emesis may be valuable up to 24 hours after ingestion to evacuate salicylate concretions. (Some clinicians also administer a cathartic to hasten the drug through the intestine.)

Obtain laboratory specimens for testing of blood pH, serum CO_2, sodium and potassium, BUN or creatinine, and glucose; urine is obtained for specific gravity determination. (Urine pH is of no value for evaluating acid-base disturbances.) A blood salicylate level should be determined approximately 6 hours after ingestion to give the peak blood level concentration and to estimate the severity of the poisoning, which may have been seriously underestimated (Fig. 27-2).

Treat accompanying phenomena according to clinical manifestations:

Fever: Tepid sponging

Dehydration: Oral or parenteral fluids

Acid-base disturbances: Do not use oral sodium bicarbonate; it enhances the absorption of salicylates

Seizures (with or without tetany): Diazepam or barbiturates IV; calcium IV to rule out hypocalcemia as a cause for seizures

Cerebral edema: See p. 289

Pulmonary edema: See p. 367

Hemorrhage: Vitamin K or its oxide (25 to 50 mg) may be justified prophylactically

Renal failure: Alkalinizing urine to hasten excretion of drug is futile, because it cannot be accomplished if there is a potassium deficit. Correction of the latter could not be accomplished rapidly enough for practicality. Tromethamine (Tham) or acetazolamide (Diamox) may be tried to alkalinize urine; osmotic diuresis with mannitol may have a slight effect in accelerating elimination. Peritoneal dialysis or hemodialysis may be valuable in augmenting elimination

Hyperpnea: Do not treat. This is essential for providing sufficient oxygen to meet tissue demands created by accelerated metabolic rate

Respiratory depression: Artificial ventilation with supplemental oxygen

PHENOTHIAZINE AND BUTYROPHENONE REACTIONS

Extrapyramidal side effects may occur as a characteristic reaction after only a single dose of any one of the phenothiazine drug group (see p. 547) or after administration of butyrophenone agents including haloperiodol (Haldol).

There are three motor disorders commonly included:

1. Parkinsonism: Depression, masklike facies, motor retardation, pill-rolling tremor, rigidity, excessive salivation, and a shuffling gait
2. Akathisia*: Motor restlessness, a strong urge to move about, and a near inability to sit down
3. Dystonia and dyskinesias: Torticollis, tics, abnormal eye movements, facial grimacing, and involuntary muscle activity
   a. Oculogyric crisis: Upward gaze, eye rotations, tics, and lid contractions
   b. Torticollic crisis: Labored breathing, severe contractions of neck muscles, and torticollic or retrocollic manifestations (most common, usually occur together)
   c. Buccolingual crisis: Dysarthria, dysphagia, mutism, protrusion retraction of the tongue, facial grimacing, and distortion
   d. Opisthotonic crisis: Scoliosis, lordosis, or opisthotonus
   e. Tortipelvic crisis: Abdominal wall spasms, bizarre gait, inguinal pain, and slumping to the ground

Accompanying clinical findings may be atropinelike symptoms, postural hypotension, and fever.

Adverse reactions can occur 4 to 5 days after ingestion. Always inquire if any drugs were taken in the past week to avoid overlooking a causative agent.

Signs and symptoms of reactions can be reversed by diphenhydramine (Benadryl) 25 to 50 mg by IV push over 1 to 4 minutes followed by a prescription for oral diphenhydramine to cover 2 to 3 days, since the half-life of phenothiazines is 24 hours.

Dyskinesias can be life threatening if they involve throat muscles and interfere with breathing.

Extrapyramidal reactions are not necessarily associated with drug abuse or illicit drug use. They may occur after a single dose of a prescribed agent.

Reassure the patient that he is not allergic to the medication. The emergency physician should consider providing a prescription for an antiparkinsonian agent, such as trihexyphenidyl (Artane) (2 mg twice a day) or benztropine (Cogentin) (2 mg twice a day). A week's supply should be given with instructions to contact

---

*These reactions usually occur only after several doses or long-term use. They seldom are acute manifestations likely to be seen by emergency personnel as a primary problem.

the physician who prescribed the phenothiazine drug. See p. 547 for more information on these agents.

ACETAMINOPHEN OVERDOSE

Acetaminophen, a metabolite of phenacetin, is widely used as an aspirin substitute and is commonly found in miscellaneous remedies for colds, coughs, and fever. In adults, toxicity is rarely seen in overdoses of less than 10 grams (30 regular strength or 20 extrastrength tablets or capsules), and fatalities are rare under 15 grams (45 regular strength or 30 extrastrength tablets or capsules). Overdoses in children are not typically a crisis with children under 5, possibly due to their unique way of metabolizing the substance. However, treatment is recommended anyway.

The half-life of acetaminophen is 2 to 4 hours in healthy adults. Peak plasma levels for tablets are reached within the first hour, slightly sooner for liquid preparations. Peak levels may be delayed if acetaminophen is taken with food or other substances that could retard absorption. Alcohol tends to accelerate absorption. Baseline acetaminophen and liver enzyme levels should be drawn before initiating further management. Other baseline laboratory tests to be obtained are SGOT, SGPT, prothrombin time, bilirubin, glucose, sodium, potassium, chlorides, carbon dioxide, and creatinine.

Emergency personnel should be alert to signs and symptoms of all three stages of toxicity.

Emergency management

After estimating the quantity of acetaminophen ingested and the time of the ingestion, proceed with gastric emptying. (If bowel

---

Clinical course of acetaminophen overdose*

The clinical course of acetaminophen overdose occurs in a three-phase sequential pattern. Remember that the patient may be asymptomatic during the early phases. Therefore, in cases of suspected acetaminophen overdose, begin specific antidotal therapy as soon as possible.

Phase I: The first phase begins shortly after ingestion of a potentially toxic overdose and lasts for 12 to 24 hours. The patient may manifest signs of gastrointestinal irritability, nausea, vomiting, anorexia, diaphoresis and pallor. Coma or other evidence of central nervous system depression is not present unless, as may be the case in suicide attempts, the patient has also ingested toxic doses of barbiturates, tranquilizers, alcohol or other central nervous system depressants. For many patients, symptoms of acetaminophen toxicity never progress beyond this phase.

Phase II: If toxicity ensues, there is a latent phase of 24 to 48 hours but it may last as long as four days. The earlier symptoms abate and the patient may feel well. During this interval, hepatic enzymes, serum bilirubin and prothrombin time begin to rise as hepatic necrosis progresses. Right upper quadrant pain may develop as the liver becomes enlarged and tender. The vast majority of cases do not progress beyond this phase and their subsequent clinical course is characterized by a gradual return of liver function tests to normal.

Phase III: For the relatively few patients who develop significant hepatic necrosis, the signs and symptoms of the third phase of the clinical course depend on the severity of hepatic damage, and usually occur from three to five days following ingestion. Symptoms may be limited to anorexia, nausea, general malaise and abdominal pain in less severe cases or may progress to confusion, stupor and hepatic necrotic sequelae including jaundice, coagulation defects, hypoglycemia and encephalopathy as well as renal failure and myocardiopathy. Death, when it occurs, is due to hepatic failure.

*Developed by McNeil Consumer Products Co., for use in the brochure Management of Acetaminophen Overdose with N-Acetylcysteine. Fort Washington, Pa.

sounds are not evident, use emetic and lavage even if the ingestion has occurred up to 12 hours ago. See p. 619 for procedures.) Do not administer activated charcoal, however, unless its use is essential for a mixed ingestion of toxic agents. It will interfere with the absorption of the antidote to be given later. If it is administered for other agents, lavage should be done before initiating antidotal therapy.

The antidote for acetaminophen is acetylcysteine, commercially available as Mucomyst. Regardless of the quantity reportedly ingested (as long as it occurred within 24 hours or less), an initial loading dose of 140 mg/kg acetylcysteine should be given. It should be diluted with cola, grapefruit juice, orange juice, or water to achieve a 5% solution. (Do not store this mixture longer than 1 hour.) If the patient vomits the dose within 1 hour, it should be repeated. (The dose may be better tolerated and retained when administered via a nasoduodenal tube.)

When the patient is stabilized after initial therapy, he should be transferred to the intensive care unit where further acetylcysteine therapy is done. The maintenance dose is 70 mg/kg of body weight every 4 hours for 17 doses. Acetaminophen assays should be repeated every 4 hours; liver function studies should be done every 24 hours for at least 4 days after ingestion while the patient's general status is observed and supportive therapy is continued.

FOOD POISONING

Food poisoning occurs in two forms: *food infection* and *food intoxication*. Food infection involves the ingestion of substances that contain bacteria that produce illness after their multiplication in the intestinal tract. Food intoxication indicates that the food ingested contained toxins from a previous multiplication of bacteria, resulting in poisoning from toxin release into the body system.

Symptoms occur within 1 to 5 hours after ingestion of contaminated food. The onset is abrupt, with nausea, vomiting, diarrhea, and abdominal cramping. A history of the food intake should be obtained. Ascertain if other individuals who ate the same foods are similarly affected.

Obtain blood samples for electrolyte and osmolarity studies, and initiate IV therapy if dehydration is severe or if signs of shock are present. Electrolyte imbalances should be corrected as they are detected.

Monitor the temperature throughout therapy to detect elevations. Characteristically, the temperature is subnormal in acute food poisoning.

Botulism

Suspect botulism in the presence of any neurological signs and symptoms that mimic a cerebrovascular occlusive disease, Guillain-Barré syndrome, myasthenia gravis, or arsenic intoxication.

Botulism is a relativley rare condition, but occurs typically in a sporadic family or other group outbreak. The usual exotoxins causing poisoning are A, B, and E (E is commonly from fish); rarely toxins C and F are encountered. Botulism is the most serious type of food poisoning, with a mortality of 60% for persons poisoned by botulism spores. (Botulism can also occur following wound contamination with *Clostridium botulinum*.)

The typical cause of botulism is poorly processed or "spoiled" home-canned vegetables, especially nonacid types such as green beans. Bulging cans or lids (resulting from expanding gases as the organisms grow) are often implicated in the history.

Symptoms develop generally 12 to 36 hours after ingestion of contaminated food but may be delayed for as long as 4 days. The presenting symptoms are often vague and may consist of lethargy, constipation, visual disturbances, and a dry, sore throat with hoarseness. Weakness, paralysis, eye movement limitations, dilated pupils, decreased tendon reflexes, and impaired speech may also be noted or reported. Headache is a common associated finding. There is no fever in early botulism; in fact, the temperature may be subnormal.

Emergency management. If the patient is asymptomatic or the exposure is questionable, emesis may be induced, particularly in recent consumptions. If several hours have elapsed after the ingestion, cathartics may be useful, since the toxin is slowly absorbed. Sodium sulfate (250 mg/kg orally) or magnesium (250 mg/kg orally) are likely choices of the physician.

The victim of suspected botulism should be hospitalized and subsequently treated with antitoxin if symptoms develop.

For patients who initially have clinical and neurological symptoms, induce emesis if there is no depression in the level of consciousness or evidence of seizure activity. Report the case at once to the Center for Communicable Disease in Atlanta (404-633-2176), and determine the location of the nearest laboratory for toxin analysis and antitoxin administration. In the meantime, draw 30 ml of venous blood for toxin assay.

If the antitoxin is recommended to be given, a skin test for horse serum sensitivity should be done. If there is sensitivity, the instructions for desensitization on the package insert are to be followed before IM or IV antitoxin administration is accomplished.

All patients being treated with antitoxin should be admitted to the intensive care unit or other area where mechanical respiratory support is available.

Guanidine hydrochloride (15 to 50 mg/kg per NG tube) in divided doses may be administered to assist in the blockade of the toxin. Excess dosage of this agent may result in tremors and muscle twitching.

Infant botulism. This rather rare clinical condition occurs secondary to an infant's producing *Clostridium botulinum* toxin within his small intestine. Signs and symptoms include constipation, poor feeding, decreased activity, hypotonia, generalized weakness, ophthalmoplegias, and, in severe cases, respiratory paralysis.

It is important that emergency personnel detect the signs and symptoms and differentiate them from failure to thrive, Guillain-Barré syndrome, myasthenia gravis, or CNS disease. A stool sample should be obtained for toxin studies. The ill infant is admitted for stabilization of fluid and nutritional status and further studies.

Mushroom poisoning

The acute onset of nausea, vomiting, and diarrhea—especially in the spring, late summer, and early fall—should alert emergency personnel to the consideration of mushroom poisoning.

Determine if any "wild" mushrooms were consumed within the last 24 hours, and obtain a specimen of the mushroom if possible for mycological examination.

If sample mushrooms cannot be obtained, elicit where they were harvested.

Induced emesis or gastric lavage is of little value unless the ingestion occurred within the past 1 or 2 hours. It may be useful, however, if the patient has not vomited. Catharsis may be attempted to hasten passage of the mushrooms through the gastrointestinal tract. Save the stool specimen for toxin verification.

Atropine is usually given for muscarinic poisoning symptoms (0.5 to 1.0 mg) subcutaneously every 30 minutes until symptoms cease. Fluid and electrolyte imbalances should be treated as usual, and hallucinogenic and intoxication reactions should be managed with phenothiazine drugs.

The patient must be hospitalized for delayed mushroom reactions. Hemodialysis is often helpful in managing renal failure.

Thiotic acid is thought to be of some value in coping with hepatocellular damage if it is administered within the first 3 days after poisoning. Thiotic acid is given IV by slow drip (100 to 300 mg/day) concurrently with dextrose in saline for control of resultant hypoglycemia, a side effect of thiotic acid.

Helvella esculanta poisoning can occur by ingestion or inhalation of a volatile toxin (gyromitrin) from certain varieties (see p. 631). Blood transfusion is recommended along with dialysis and a rigorous protocol to monitor and maintain fluid and electrolyte balance. A disulfiram-type reaction can occur as a secondary intoxication response to the mushroom *Cop-*

Text continued on p. 638

Table 27-2. Food toxins—differential findings*

Usual source	Incuba-tion period	Nausea and vomiting	Diarrhea	Neurological findings	Other common characteristics	Comments
Fish						
Grouper, amberjack, po'ou' (ciguatoxin)	30 min-30 hours	X	X			Fish tastes normal; toxin not inactivated by heat
Puffer (tetrodotoxin)	10 min-4 hours	X	X	Paresthesias, numbness, floating feeling, respiratory paralysis		
Tuna, bonito, dolphin or mahi-mahi (scombrotoxin)	5 min-2 hours	X	X		Flushing, headache, urticaria, dizziness	
Shellfish (paralytic and neurotoxin poisoning from dinoflagellate)	10 min-1 hour	X	X	Facial paresthesias, especially respiratory		20% mortality
Uncooked (*Vibrio parahemolyticus*)	12-24 hours	X	X			
Heavy metals (beverages)	Minutes–3-4 hours	X			Metallic taste	
Reheated meats (*Clostridium*)	8-12 hours	X				
Confections, meat, milk (*Staphylococcus*)	1-6 hours	X				
Poultry, turtles, human carriers (*Salmonella*)	8-48 hours	X	X		Fever	
Food, water, human contact (*Shigella*)	1-7 days	X	X			
Water, fresh vegetables (cholera)	1-5 days	X	X			
Amoeba	Days to weeks	X	X			
Monosodium glutamate (Chinese food)	5-30 min				Burning sensation of chest, neck, abdomen and extremities; feeling of pressure over face and chest	

*From Barber, J. M., and Budassi, S. A.: Mosby's manual of emergency care, St. Louis, 1979, The C. V. Mosby Co.

Continued.

Table 27-2. Food toxins—differential findings—cont'd

Usual source	Incubation period	Nausea and vomiting	Diarrhea	Neurologic findings	Other common characteristics	Comments
Mushrooms—rapid onset						
Group I: Rhodphyllus sinuatus; Agaricus arvensis, A. hondensis, A. placemyces; Boletus miniatodivaceus, B. luridus, B. satanas; Cantharellus floccopus; Chlorophyllum molydites; Lactarius glaucescens, L. rufus, L. torminosus; Naematoloma fasciculare; Paxillus involutus; Phaeolepiata aurea; Russula emetica; Scleroderma aurantium; Tricholoma pardinum, T. venenatum	½-2 hours	X	X			
Group II: Clitocybe dealbata; Inocybe napyses, I. mixtilis, I. griseolilacina, I. lacera, I. decipientoides; Omphalotus olearius	15 min-3 hours	X	X	Seizures	Visual disturbances, sweating, excessive salivation, muscular weakness, tearing, bradycardia, dysrhythmias	Low mortality

		X	X		
Group III: Amanita muscaria, A. pantherina, A. flavivala, A. cothurrata	15-30 min	X	X	Hallucinations, intoxication	Muscular weakness, visual and auditory disturbances
Group IV: Conocybe cyanopus, C. smithii; Psilocybe caerulescens, P. mexicana, P. pelliculosa, P. cyanesches, P. baeocystis, P. cubensis	1-3 hours			Drowsiness, dizziness, ataxia	
Mushrooms—delayed onset Group I: Amanita phalloides, A. virosa, A. bisporigera, A. verna; Galerina marginata, G. autumnalis, G. venenata	6-24 hours	X	X	Abdominal pain, bloody stool, malaise Remission after 2-3 days followed by Paralysis and other variable neurologic disturbances and coma	Hematuria, albuminuria, anuria, peripheral vascular collapse, and hepatic failure 30-50% mortality
Group II: Helvella esculenta	6-12 hours	X	X	Vertigo, confusion	Symptoms essentially same as above, less severe
Mushrooms—secondary intoxication Coprinus atramentarius	12-24 hours until sensitization to alcohol begins	X	X	Tachycardia, flushing, hyperventilation, palpitations, hypotension, weakness, blurred vision	

Table 27-3. Poisonous house plants*

Plant	Toxic parts	Symptoms	Treatment
Bird-of-paradise *(Poinciana gilliesi)*	Pods and seeds	Vomiting, diarrhea, dizziness, vertigo, drowsiness	Gastric lavage or emesis, symptomatic treatment, demulcents, replace fluids
Dumb cane *(Dieffenbachia)* and philodendron	All parts, especially stem and leaves	Instantaneous swelling of tongue and throat with difficult swallowing, blisters, paralysis of vocal cords	Gastric lavage or emesis (if no blisters present), cold pack to lips and mouth, demulcents, antihistamines, especially epinephrine
Elephant ear *(Colocasia)*	Same as above	Same as above	Same as above

*Modified from Turk, S.: J.E.N. **5**(2):9, 1979.

Table 27-3. Poisonous house plants—cont'd

Plant	Toxic parts	Symptoms	Treatment
English ivy (Hedera helix)	All parts, especially leaves and berries	Skin irritation, nausea, vomiting, severe diarrhea, increased thirst, increased salivation, abdominal pain, difficulty breathing; can lead to coma	Gastric lavage, symptomatically supportive treatment—paraldehyde (2-10 ml) IM, O_2, sometimes artificial respiration
Holly (Ilex sp.)	Berries and leaves	Vomiting, diarrhea, stupor, narcosis	Gastric lavage or emesis, symptomatic treatment
Hunter's robe (Rhaphidophora aurea)	Sap	Irritation of skin, lips, tongue; can lead to diarrhea	
Jack-in-the-pulpit (Arusrema triphyllum)	Leaves	Irritation of gastrointestinal tract, swelling of tongue, lips, and palate	Gastric lavage, symptomatic treatment, demulcents, cold packs to lips and mouth, antihistamine (epinephrine), aluminum hydroxide (neutralizer)

Continued.

Table 27-3. Poisonous house plants—cont'd

Plant	Toxic parts	Symptoms	Treatment
Jerusalem cherry *(Solanum pseudocapsium)*	All parts	Stomach pain, low temp, paralysis, dilated pupils, vomiting, diarrhea, circulation, respiratory depression, loss of sensation, death	Gastric lavage or emesis, support respirations, paraldehyde (2-10 ml) IM
Mistletoe *(Phoradendron serotinum)*	Berries	Stomach and intestinal irritation, diarrhea, bradycardia	Gastric lavage or emesis, supportive potassium, procainamide and quinidine sulfate have been effective (treatment as for digitalis intoxication)
Pencil tree *(Euphorbia tirucalli)*	Spurges, milky sap	Severe irritation of mouth, throat, and stomach	Gastric lavage, symptomatic treatment

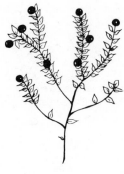

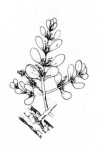

Table 27-3. Poisonous house plants—cont'd

Plant	Toxic parts	Symptoms	Treatment
Poinsettia (*Euphorbia pulcherima*)	Milky sap, stem, leaves, flowerbud	Irritation of mouth, throat, stomach, skin, dangerous to eyes	Gastric lavage or emesis, symptomatic treatment
Star of Bethlehem (*Ornithgalum umbellatum*)	All parts—bulbs and leaves (both fresh and dried)	Nausea, intestinal disorders	Gastric lavage or emesis, symptomatic treatment
English yew (*Taxacere*)	All parts, especially leaves and seeds	Diarrhea, vomiting, trembling, pupil dilation, difficulty breathing, muscular weakness, coma, convulsions, dysrhythmias, death	Gastric lavage or emesis, control pain with meperidine, symptomatic treatment

Continued.

Table 27-3. Poisonous house plants—cont'd

Plant	Toxic parts	Symptoms	Treatment
Rhubarb (Rheum rhaponticum)	Leaf blades	Stomach pains, nausea, vomiting, weakness, difficulty breathing, burning of mouth and throat, internal bleeding, coma, death	Gastric lavage or emesis with lime water, chalk, or calcium salts; calcium gluconate, parenterally forced fluids; supportive treatment
Peach	Pits	Breathing difficulty, vocal paralysis, weakness, coma, convulsions	Gastric lavage, emesis
Mushrooms (fly agaric, false morel, death cap)	All parts	Respiratory distress, central nervous system disturbances, stomach pains, parasympathomimetic effects, coma, death	Lavage with potassium permanganate, atropine

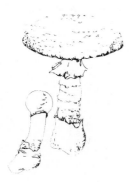
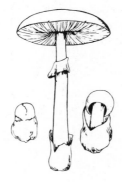
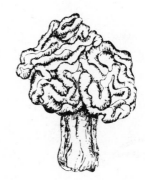

Plant	Toxic parts	Symptoms	Treatment
Cherry	Pits	Shortness of breath, vocal paralysis, convulsions, coma	Gastric lavage or emesis

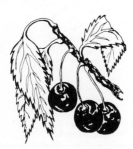

Table 27-3. Poisonous house plants—cont'd

Plant	Toxic parts	Symptoms	Treatment
Lily of the valley	All parts	Gastrointestinal distress, dysrhythmias	Gastric lavage or emesis, potassium, sodium
Castor bean	Leaves, pods (beans)	Gastrointestinal distress, convulsions	Gastric lavage or emesis, sodium bicarbonate

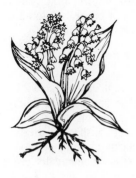

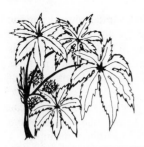

rinus atramentarius if it is consumed along with alcohol. No specific treatment is necessary. (See Table 27-2 for a comparative description of mushroom poisonings.)

Table 27-3 includes descriptions of poisonous house plants.

POISON CONTROL SYSTEMS

The emergency nurse may be called upon to answer poison control calls on a community action line phone, often located in the emergency department of the hospital. The caller may be a frantic parent, concerned friend, neighbor, or the actual victim of an acute ingestion, accidental overdose, or contact with a toxic agent. It is important for the nurse to gather important reference data systematically during the call in the event that an ambulance needs to be subsequently dispatched and to ensure adequate follow-up. A form for this data gathering should contain these initial items: name of caller and relationship to victim; address and phone number of caller and victim; age and weight of victim; nature of ingestion (name of substance, type, ingredients, amount); and the caller's evaluation of the severity of the problem. If the patient's life is in immediate or potential danger, an ambulance should be dispatched, rather than risking private transportation to the hospital. The toxic substance, the containers, and any environmental clues to an unknown overdose should be gathered, and, if feasible, transported to the hospital with the patient.

There are situations in which the toxic substance has come into contact with the skin where it can be inhaled, absorbed, or cause chemical injury (see p. 615). In such instances, surface decontamination should be begun at once. The poison control phone call may provide the opportunity for the nurse to instruct the caller about the modes of decontamination appropriate to the offending substance.

The poison control nurse may also instruct the caller in techniques of emesis using ipecac, because many parents of young children have the agent in their home as a result of a pediatrician's advice. If vomiting does occur, the parent or significant other should save all emesis and bring it to the hospital. If there is no ipecac in the home, milk may be advisable as a method of diluting the agent and as a mode to slow down the emptying of the stomach. Obviously, any oral intake is contraindicated in the presence of a depressed level of consciousness, seizures, or the loss of a gag reflex.

Most emergency departments that have a poison control line will have a systematic drug/toxicology reference program with a teletype, a computer, card file, or Microfiche index. A popular program is Poisindex, published by Micromedex, Inc. in association with the National Center for Poison Information, 2645 South Santa Fe Drive, Denver, Colorado, 80223; Barry H. Rumack is the editor.

Poisindex system for poison control information

The Poisindex is a computer-generated Microfiche system of specific and detailed emergency poison treatment protocols. The entire product information is republished quarterly, integrating any new data or revising previous management regimens. It is automatically provided to users of the Poisindex system on a regular basis so that only the most recent information will be at hand for emergency care.

Topics in management of specific product poisonings include available forms, pharmacology, clinical effects, range of toxicity, laboratory considerations, treatment regimens, and major references.

Entries are found under trade names, generic names, chemical names, slang terms, or imprint code designations. For a few items (such as snakes, plants, and mushrooms) color pictures are provided to assist in rapid identification of the offending item.

Access to poison control information can be accomplished within less than a minute and necessary management instituted promptly if indicated.

Prevention of poisoning

Any phone contact or emergency department contact provides an opportunity to quickly discuss the storage spaces in the home where hazardous materials are commonly found, especially under the sink, in the bathroom, and in the basement or garage. It should be pointed out that drain cleaning crystals or liquid, automatic dishwater detergents, paints and thinners, insecticides, pest control devices (rat or mice bait) and automotive products (lubricants, transmission fluid, antifreeze) are dangerous and could be lethal. Of course, medicines should be kept out of the casual reach of everyone but the user, because even some vitamins and iron supplements pose serious threats to life when ingested in large amounts. Even adults, on occasion, accidentally ingest someone else's drug as a result of poor labeling, improper storage, or mixing of several types of substances within one container. Such careless practices as keeping ''old'' medicine around for a future bout of the same illness are dangerous habits in relation to health maintenance; they also pose a risk for accidental or intentional multidrug toxicity, which is difficult to diagnose and treat because of interrelated responses of the agents involved.

A community health nurse referral may be indicated in selected instances of repeated ingestions among children within the same household. Such multiple ingestions may be a form of child battering (see p. 41).

All poisoning involving young children should prompt the emergency nurse to provide the mother or father with ipecac (along with instructions regarding its use) for further emergencies of toxic ingestions.

BIBLIOGRAPHY

Ambre, J., and Alexander, M.: Liver toxicity after acetaminophen ingestion: inadequacy of the dose estimate as an index of risk, J.A.M.A. **238**:500-501, 1977.

Arena, J. M.: Poisoning—toxicology, symptoms, treatment, Springfield, Ill. 1974, Charles C Thomas, Publisher.

Barber, J. M., Stokes, L. G., and Billings, D. M.: Adult and child care: a client approach to nursing, ed. 2, St. Louis, 1977, The C. V. Mosby Co.

Beamon, Richard F., and others: Hydrocarbon ingestions in children: a six-year retrospective study, J.A.C.E.P. **5**:771-775, October 1976.

Becker, C. E., and others: Diagnosis and treatment of *Amanita phalloids*—type mushroom poisoning: use of thiotic acid, West. J. Med. **125**:100-109, 1976.

Burks, J. S., and others: Tricyclic antidepressant poisoning: reversal of coma, choreoathetosis, and myoclonus by physostigmine, J.A.M.A. **230**:1405-1407, 1974.

Done, A. K., and others: Treatment of salicylate poisoning, Mod. Treat. **8**:528-551, 1971.

Dreisbach, R. H.: Handbook of poisoning, Los Altos, Calif., 1969, Lange Medical Publications.

Eastman, J. W., and others: Hypertensive crisis and death associated with phencyclidine poisoning, J.A.M.A. **231**:1270-1271, 1975.

Fauman, B., and others: Psychosis induced by phencyclidine, J.A.C.E.P. **4**:223-225, 1975.

Fenichel, R. R.: Iron poisoning, Acute Care Bull. **1**: 23-28, November, 1977.

Hamlyn, A. N., and others: Liver function and structure in survivors of acetaminophen poisoning—a follow-up study of serum bile acids and liver histology, Am. J. Dig. Dis. **22**:605-610, 1977.

Hansen, A. R., and others: Glutethimide poisoning, a metabolite contributes to morbidity and mortality, N. Engl. J. Med. **292**:250-252, 1975.

Hrnicek, G., and others: Pulmonary edema and salicylate intoxication, J.A.M.A. **230**:866-867, 1974.

Is danger growing in your house? Am. Baby **39**:24-26, May 1977. J. Am. Pharm. Assoc. **NS17**:517-521, 1977.

Jollow, D. H., and others: Acetaminophen induced hepatic necrosis. II. Role of convalent binding in vivo, J. Pharmacol. Exp. Ther. **187**:195-202, 1973.

Kingsbury, J. M.: Poisonous plants of the U.S. and Canada, Englewood Cliffs, N.J., 1964, Prentice-Hall, Inc.

Landecker, E. M.: Fundamentals of the fungi, Englewood Cliffs, N.J., 1972, Prentice-Hall, Inc., p. 414.

Litten, W.: The most poisonous mushrooms, Sci. Am. **232**: 90-101, March 1975.

Little, T. L., and Moniz, D. M.: Toxicity associated with acetaminophen overdose, Nurse Pract. **2**:31-32, 1977.

Management of Acetaminophen Overdose with N-Acetylcysteine (Monograph): Fort Washington, Pa., January 1979, McNeil Consumer Products Company.

McJunkin, B., and others: Fatal massive hepatic necrosis following acetaminophen overdose, J.A.M.A. **236**: 1874-1875, 1976.

Mahler, D. A.: Anticholinergic poisoning from jimson weed, J.A.C.E.P. **5**:440-442, 1976.

Mann, J. B., and others: Therapy of sedative overdosage, Pediatr. Clin. North Am. **17**:617-628, 1970.

National Clearinghouse for Poison Control Centers Bulletin, Bethesda, Md., February 1977, U.S. Department of Health, Education, and Welfare.

National Clearinghouse for Poison Control Centers Bulletin, Bethesda, Md., April 1977, U.S. Department of Health, Education, and Welfare.

Pierce, A. W.: Salicylate intoxication, Postgrad. Med. **48**: 243-249, September 1970.

Prescott, L. F., and others: Treatment of paracetamol (acetaminophen) poisoning with N-acetylcysteine, Lancet **2**:432-434, 1977.

Pretty poison . . . plant poison, Family Health **9**:29-32, July 1977.

Ray, O.: Drugs, society, and human behavior, ed. 2, St. Louis, 1978, The C. V. Mosby Co., pp. 230-231.

Rumack, B. H., and others: Lomotil poisoning, Pediatrics **53**:495-500, 1974.

Rumack, B. H., and Matthew, H.: Acetaminophen poisoning and toxicity, Pediatrics **55:**871-876, 1975.

Rumack, B. H.: Hydrocarbon ingestion in perspective, J.A.C.E.P. **6:**172-173, April 1977.

Russman, B. S: Convulsive seizures in infancy and childhood, Pediatr. Ann. **5:**39-45, May 1976.

Shirkey, H. C.: Treatment of petroleum distillate ingestion, Mod. Treat. **8:**580-592, 1971.

Turk, S.: Houseplant poisoning in children, J.E.N. **5:**9-13, March/April 1979.

Walker, W. E., and others: Physostigimine—its use and abuse, J.A.C.E.P. **5:**436-439, 1976.

Williams, R., and Davis, M.: Therapeutic aspects of paracetamol overdose including management of acute liver failure, Acta Pharmacol. Toxicol. **41**(suppl.):300-310, 1977.

CHAPTER 28

Disaster aspects in emergency nursing

Joan Kelley Simoneau

Not very long ago the principles of disaster casualty management were only briefly discussed in schools of nursing around the country. Lack of in-depth nursing focus on potentials for catastrophic events was but a microcosm of a similar lack of awareness and concern about planning that existed in the populace at large. People are generally not comfortable in preplanning for a true catastrophe. It is difficult to believe that such a situation really could occur, or if it did, that it might affect us. Contemplating a mass disaster is overwhelming, yet no community is safe from the potential. It is difficult to protect citizens from disasters unless disaster-related adaptive behavior is second nature. When such behavior is not second nature, the potential for chaos and uncoordinated response is extremely likely. Because death and disability are fearsome, many people dislike discussing community disaster programs. People simply do not willingly involve themselves in planning and in practicing for the possibility—indeed, most "drills" are looked upon and treated as though they are games. Because of their integral involvement in community health and emergency operations, emergency nurses are in a unique position to encourage the development of in-hospital and community disaster plans and to educate one another, other health professionals, and the lay public in prevention of and survival in disasters.

It is an indisputable fact that our losses after disaster events would be far less if people were prepared to meet the emergency, knew what actions to take, and took them. This chapter is dedicated to the presentation of vital elements in the development of effective disaster plans and behavior for families, communities, and emergency facilities.

DEFINITION OF A DISASTER

Definitions of disasters are as numerous as the ideas people may have of what disasters involve. Practically every journal article or textbook chapter dealing with the issue promotes a different definition. Regardless of the words used, each community and medical facility must determine what a disaster is to them. In simple terms, a disaster is any patient-generating incident that results in overload either of existing personnel or of supplies and equipment, or a patient-generating incident that occurs in a situation wherein resources for backup of staff and equipment are not readily available in a reasonable amount of time. One could say "that about covers it," yet a more precise breakdown may help in planning for specific situations in terms of expected patient volume.

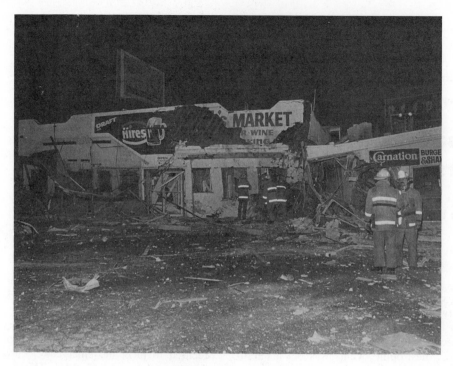

Photo courtesy *Los Angeles Times.*

Multiple patient incident

A multiple patient incident may generate fewer than 10 casualties, who may or may not arrive at the same facility for treatment. Typical kinds of disasters are bomb explosions, multiple vehicle collisions (perhaps even a single vehicle such as a bus carrying several passengers), and apartment fires. Generally, local community resources (ground rescue vehicles, manpower, and local medical facilities) can handle this situation effectively in a minimal period of time without requiring mutual aid from outside the community. These incidents also tend to be limited in terms of the generation of victims; the patients initially injured are the only victims involved that the medical resources can expect to handle. Because of the minimal numbers of patients, it is possible to provide on-scene stabilization and identification, with an organized dispersal of victims to several facilities instead of overloading one or two. Therefore, a reasonable time

delay between occurrence of the incident and the initial hospital receipt of patients can be expected. Under these circumstances, although a disaster indeed exists, effective planning and response can prevent it from being transferred into one hospital, thereby causing a disaster situation in the emergency department.

These "disasters" are fairly common. Those of us who work in emergency department certainly appreciate that day-to-day patient volumes fluctuate in irregular patterns, and staffing may not be adequate to meet the load at all times. According to the definition of a disaster presented here, 10 seriously ill or injured patients at one time constitute a disaster in the ED. Emergency department personnel often handle situations that may be termed "mini-disasters," yet implementation of a fixed disaster plan is not necessary. Most departments have staff call-back plans as a contingency in these circumstances that are usually sufficient to meet the need. However, true disasters re-

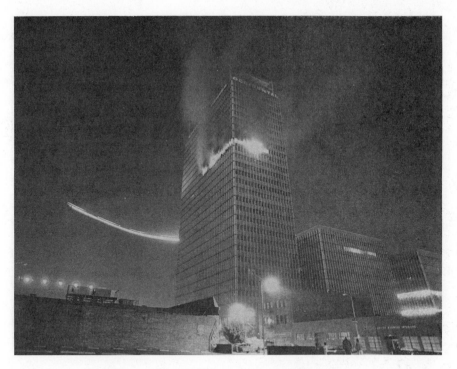

Photo courtesy *Los Angeles Times.*

quire an entirely different response than a sudden increase in volume does. A disaster that results in many victims usually generates casualties with severe trauma as opposed to slight increases in volume, which may yield only 3% to 4% critical or potentially critical patients.

Multiple casualty incident

A multiple casualty incident necessitates multiple field unit response with the initiation of a medical communications command post where responsibility for triage and disposition of casualties to appropriate facilities is centered. This incident generates 100 or fewer casualties with a fairly reliable time lag between occurrence of the incident and initial hospital receipt of victims. The local hospital emergency administrative radio (HEAR) network is activated if the community has such a system, making possible the coordination of field dispatch, dispersal of victims to hospitals depending on the status of each facility, the num-

bers of victims they can handle, and movement of supplies and equipment. Such a disaster situation involving 100 or fewer victims occurs in air collisions or crashes, dam breaks, riots, snowstorms, floods, tornadoes, hurricanes, and minor earthquakes.

Mass casualty incident

A mass casualty disaster overwhelms existing community resources, necessitating mutual aid, either from adjacent communities or from other states. Because such a circumstance will significantly overtax the existing medical response system locally, implementation of an organized response (consisting of complete field triage operations, HEAR network coordination of the event, and coordination of incoming medical teams, supplies, and equipment from outside the region involved) will be necessary. The state and possibly federal disaster plans may be implemented. At the very least state disaster officials become integrally

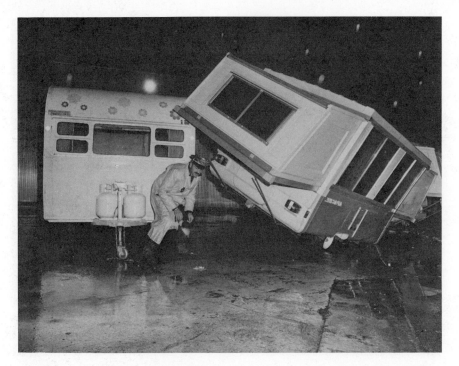

Photo courtesy *Los Angeles Times*.

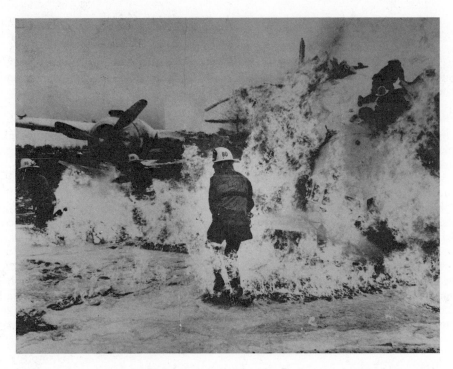

Photo courtesy *Los Angeles Times*.

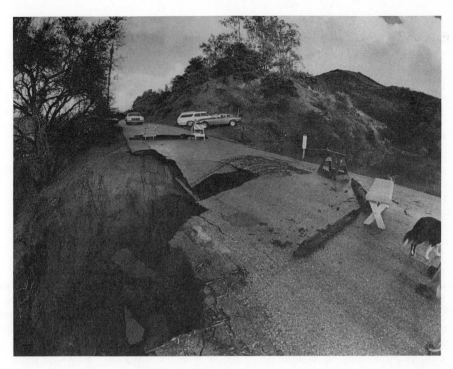

Photo courtesy *Los Angeles Times*.

involved to help maintain extensive communications and to respond when exhaustion of internal and external resources occurs. The patient load in this case may be anywhere from hundreds to thousands of casualties often in a continuous generation of casualties over a prolonged period of time. The time lag between occurrence and initial hospital receipt of victims may vary from little advance warning to an inordinate time between notification and receipt. There also may be disruption of local communication capability, including the HEAR network, and if so, the hospitals may receive little to no adequate information about the status of the disaster site or the numbers of casualties that may be expected. Often the duration and extent of the incident require continuous manpower and provisions for food, shelter, clothing, and medical care for the survivors and their families.

There have been very few true incidents of this nature and extent, but it is to this potential that planning of disaster programs and plans of operation must be directed. It makes little difference whether a disaster is man-made or natural; response must be predicated on the extent of the incident as defined by the numbers of casualties actually or potentially generated by the disaster.

There are as many different "types" of disasters as there are communities in which they might occur. Yet not to be forgotten in any planning on the part of emergency facilities are those disasters that might conceivably occur *inside* the facility itself, necessitating a completely different response relative to the location and type of the incident (consider a bomb explosion destroying the *emergency department*). Each hospital must not only be prepared to meet the needs of the community, but also to meet its own needs should a disaster occur that disrupts its own normal operations.

In all cases, one must bear in mind that each disaster will vary from any other experience in terms of degree, onset, duration, and amount of time available to initiate mechanisms for response. Because of this variance, it is helpful for organized plans to include contingencies for step-wise mobilization and implementation of response. Such methodology will be discussed later in this chapter.

PLANS FOR SELF AND FAMILY

Because a disaster can occur at any time anywhere, without regard for any individual or his family, a considerable amount of peace of mind can be obtained in the chaos of the moment if you and your family develop a plan for survival. Evaluate your particular locale to determine what type of natural disasters your area is likely to experience. Develop a plan of action relative to the possibilities, before a disaster occurs!

Before a disaster

- Predetermine a location where your family and you can contact one another in the event of a disaster prewarning by community officials, or in the event a disaster strikes.
- Learn how your community disaster plan will function. Contact either your local health department, or your state's office of emergency services.
- Inquire how the school or industry with which your family members are affiliated will respond. Knowing what can be expected of others in the protection of your family if you are not together when a disaster occurs will help free you to function in your own survival and for the protection of others in your neighborhood.
- *Always* carry your nursing license and any other appropriate nursing identification. If you have this information available, you will be able to gain access to police lines to present yourself either to an emergency facility or to an organized medical response team in the field. Some states have initiated a program of issuing disaster cards to emergency personnel to promote more effective utilization of their services in the event of a disaster.
- Predetermine possible access routes to your hospital and *all* hospitals close to your home.

- One or more of your family members should have the ability to initiate first aid procedures in the event that medical facilities cannot be reached, are damaged, or you are either injured or not with them.
- Learn how to turn off electricity, gas, and water, and teach your family members. Locate and practice disengaging all main switches.
- In earthquake country, remove or correct all earthquake hazards, such as fastening heavy pictures or bookcases to the wall, and placing heavy objects low on shelves. Bolt water heaters to the floor (in addition to heavy appliances), and use flexible connections wherever possible.
- Keep on hand supplies of food and water, a flashlight with new batteries (replace them every 3 months if you are storing this flashlight), a first aid kit, a battery-operated radio, and some candles for use in an emergency.
- Cooperate to the fullest extent in the planning of your hospital and/or community disaster response program. Actively participate in drills for the purpose of evaluating the efficiency and effectiveness of the plan.

After a disaster

- Report the disaster, if appropriate.
- Check for injuries in your family, and in your neighborhood. Attempt to help people avoid panic and unsafe behavior. Use common sense when presented with the need to enter buildings that may be unsafe. If you are uninjured, do not place yourself, as a rescuer, in jeopardy.
- When rendering aid, evaluate the extent of the disaster before deciding to perform CPR. Stop bleeding, immobilize fractures if necessary, but keep in mind that becoming involved with essentially morbid injuries will reduce your effectiveness as a rescuer.
- Check for fires or fire hazards. Check utility lines for damage and if there are gas leaks, turn off the main valve, which is usually near the meter. Clean up spilled flammable liquids as soon as you can. Turn off the main electrical power; the switch is usually located in or near the main fuse box.

- Do not use the telephone. Turn on the battery-operated radio for information and specific instructions.
- In the case of earthquakes, prepare for aftershocks of various intensity; be certain that young children are not left alone.
- Consider reporting to your hospital if appropriate and possible. If not, you might report to the nearest *accessible* hospital, based on radio reports or as instructed by police or fire personnel. *Do not mobilize if roadways adjacent to your location are dangerous to travel.*
- Community plans will affect how you can best become involved in postdisaster operations. If you are unable to report to your facility, or to any other facility because of impairment or obstruction of roadways, make reasonable attempts to present yourself to organized medical teams if concurrent with your local disaster plan. Identify yourself and your specialty, advising the team commander of your particular skills. Obey the directions given you, and ask for an assignment. *If you are not an emergency nurse, do not attempt to interfere with organized field medical operations.* It will be necessary for you to evaluate your own abilities and use common sense regarding where you could best be utilized after a disaster strikes.

COMMUNITY PLANNING

Community planning is essential for an organized, methodical response to a sudden and possibly unforeseen situation that imperils the safety of persons and property within individual communities. Yet this planning must not exist in a vacuum; it must be in concert with regional or state and federal models.

Federal plan

A plan currently exists for the federal government to aid a state that has exhausted its resources during or after a disaster. The Federal Disaster Relief Act is administered by the President of the United States when, in his determination, a disaster has resulted in damage and injury of sufficient severity and magnitude to warrant major assistance beyond the scope

of the state or states involved. Military aid and medical assistance are also available as emergency services through the federal government to help alleviate the burden on the area involved when the area is clearly overwhelmed by the magnitude of the event. Such support is requested by the governor of the state in concert with local medical disaster coordinators.

State plan

State plans may vary in some technical points; however, most plans involve similar concepts.
- Initial response is a local responsibility.
- Mutual aid will become available to support local efforts when such aid becomes an identified need by local disaster officials.
- All local, regional, and state plans should be integrated for maximum efficiency in an emergency situation.
- The state government must establish a mechanism for priority allocation of resources that may have multiple claims. In many areas the state office of emergency services is the coordinator of these requests during disaster situations.
- There must be uniform procedures for response at the regional and state levels in the event of mass casualty disasters beyond the scope and capability of a county or the region.

Fig. 28-1 illustrates level II and level III disasters in terms of response by the region (two or more counties) and the state of California, according to that state's plan, which is currently being updated. The California plan is consistent with the federal model and is similar to the plans of other states. A level I disaster is one in which adequate local medical resources are available to provide for on-scene triage and stabilization, movement of casualties to local facilities, and management of those casualties in the facilities to which they are taken. Level II disasters are those in which the large number of casualties and/or lack of local medical facilities require multicounty medical mutual aid. A level III disaster is one in which medical resources in and near the disaster area are in-

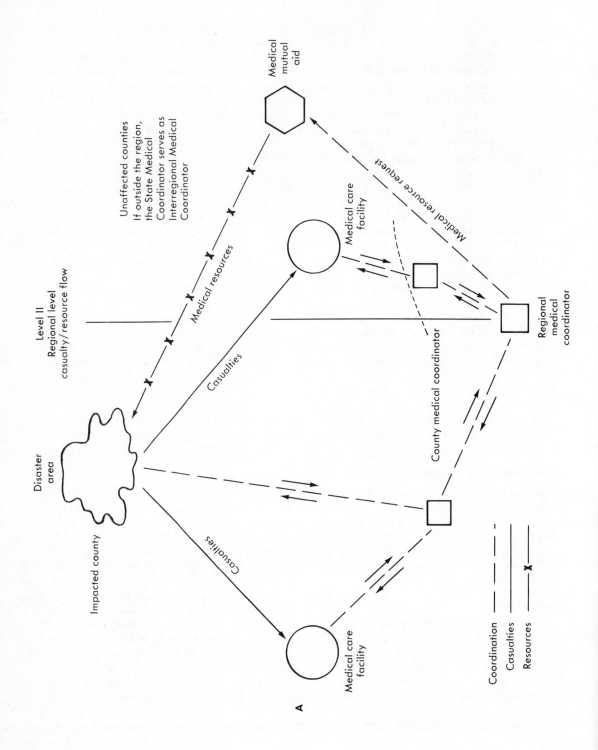

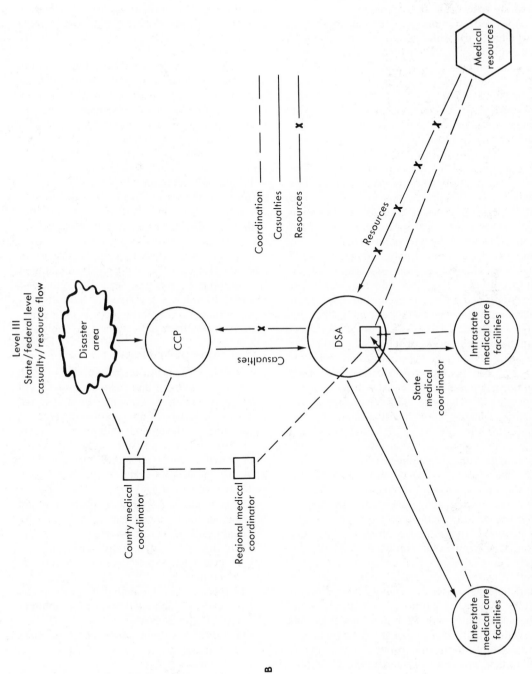

Fig. 28-1. A, Level II: Regional level casualty/resource flow. **B,** Level III: State/federal level casualty/resource flow.

undated and require the assistance of state and possibly federal medical resources.

A level III example is an earthquake of great magnitude, particularly near a densely populated urban area. Such an event requires a substantial temporary reorganization of governmental and agency structure and function, permeating all the way to the rescue operation, where the necessity to revert to a military-type triage would be indicated to save the most lives and relieve the most suffering.

A level III disaster requires multipurpose staging areas (MSA) to be established. These areas stage equipment and personnel as they arrive from outlying regions or states. The MSA also serves as a base for coordination and direction of localized emergency operations. Casualty collection points (CCP) are also initiated for the assembly, triage, medical stabilization, and evacuation of casualties. Both the location of the MSA and the CCP must be established before the event, through careful planning, with consideration given to access by land, air, or sea. Disaster support areas (DSA) are established on the periphery of the disaster to serve as an area where disaster relief resources can be received, stocked, allocated, and dispatched into the disaster area. In addition, the DSA can be used for receipt of casualty evacuees or for their evacuation by aircraft. Multiple MSAs, CCPs, and DSAs are necessary in a large-scale disaster. In addition, ground ambulances might be used as satellite first aid stations in the impacted area. Those medical personnel who survive the initial event but who cannot get to their medical facility because of either damage to the facility or impairment of roadways are utilized at casualty collection points. Of particular value in the first hours of a major disaster are personnel with expertise in emergency care who can support field personnel in triaging and setting up CCPs. Medical facilities on the periphery of the disaster area will likely be inundated with casualties and cannot be counted on for medical resources to the area or for general support of further casualty evacuation. The CCPs are the essential delay factor in preventing further overload of these medical facilities by triaging and stabilizing victims, subsequently evacu-

ating them to facilities at some distance from the site. Evacuation might be accomplished by air and sea if destruction of the disaster area is extensive enough to prevent safe and timely ground transport.

In the event the disaster is of long duration and requires a level III response, state and local plans must have a process for managing disaster-related factors in the aftermath of the impact: vector-borne disease control, sanitation, psychological management of survivors, survivor relocation with family, and establishment of shelters for the noninjured.

Further considerations in state planning are effective responses to hazardous material accidents and acts of terrorism. Each of these potentials for disaster exists in our modern society, and each requires vastly different knowledge and response than do natural disasters. In addition, there must be mutual understanding of responsibilities, abilities, and limitations of military, local law enforcement, and health disciplines, in managing these types of civil emergencies to maximize protection of the public.

Local community plans

Local plans for disaster response, although in concert with state and federal models, will often vary, relative to local resources and needs. Such variations may involve the areas of prewarning methods and timing, evacuation predisaster, initial local notification of officials, field activities and communications, interhospital communications, and methods for dispersement of casualties.

The hierarchy involved in the planning might best include the following categories of people.

Local health officer or designee

Local medical disaster coordinator

Chairperson, local medical association disaster committee

Chairperson, local emergency professional specialty organization disaster committees (ACEP and EDNA)

Local director of emergency servies (county or region)

Local chief of police

Local fire chiefs (city and county or region)

Director of communication systems for the area

Local chief, highway patrol or state police

Representative, hospital council

Director, advanced life support field personnel

Chairman, county ambulance association

Director, local department of transportation

Commanding officer, local National Guard unit

Chairman, local American Red Cross disaster committee

Chairman, local Civil Defense and Disaster Corps

Other categories of persons might be included in the committee's efforts if, in the determination of the committee, such persons should be included for appropriate planning. Such people as shown in the foregoing list will lend a team approach to the planning of a realistic response to any type of disaster that the area might reasonably expect.

Important elements of the plan that should be addressed by this body of experts include:

- Establishment of guidelines for the declaration of a disaster (prewarning, evacuation, notification of personnel, type of data to be reported, and channels to be used)
- Communication link development
  a. Dispatch of ground, air resources
  b. Field to emergency operations center (EOC) or disaster coordinating center
  c. EOC to hospitals in the area
  d. EOC to field units
  e. EOC to mutual aid resources
- Record keeping and storage procedures
- Identification of the disaster coordinating center (DCC) and development of an organizational chart
- Process for mutual aid by the community to another inundated area in need of resources
- Utilization and coordination of rescue units
- Establishment of triage teams and field command post operational plan
- Identification of the type of triage that will be used in each level disaster (that is, two tier, three tier, four tier)
- Procedure for identifying medical personnel from different agencies and/or those out of uniform

- Process for maximizing use of ground transportation besides those regularly used in patient transport (other available resources are florist vans, milk trucks, hearses)
- Establishment of coordination for maintenance, repair, and restoration of damaged utilities and essential structures
- Establishment of procedures for procurement of medical equipment and supply back-up
- Identification of responsibilities and duties of key agencies and medical personnel
- Provisions for periodic review and updating of plan
- Exercise and testing of plan on a periodic basis

There are many other possible elements that might be evaluated and discussed; this list is therefore by no means all inclusive. Comprehensive planning will be necessary to develop a realistic community response, and persons involved in such planning must represent a united effort to identify their own community needs and to address a mechanism for optimal disaster operations. On a day-to-day basis, many groups work closely together to deliver emergency medical services and transportation to the citizens of the community. Representatives of these groups must work closely to plan for any changes in operations that may become necessary in a time of disaster. However, each community should identify what works well daily, and to plan on maintaining normal operational procedures during a major disaster. To change this system during a time of extreme stress may disrupt and confuse those performing emergency services. Smoothness in implementing and conducting disaster responses is essential in preventing chaos and disorganization. Although preplanning is an important part of disaster response, maintaining simplicity and adhering as closely as possible to routine may solidify a total response operation.

FIELD OPERATIONS

There are a few considerations that should be discussed as they relate to the impact of a disaster upon field rescue procedures. These considerations include prewarning, evacuation, communications, triage, and transport.

Prewarning and evacuation

There are many occasions wherein officials of a community or state are aware that a disaster is imminent before the citizens are aware. The question thus raised is "Should the citizenry be notified, and when they are, can we control panic?" Just as the ranking administrator and the emergency department medical director of a medical facility declare a disaster alert within the hospital, so must the ranking officials in the community and/or state determine the efficacy of prewarning or declaration. This decision must be made in concert with high ranking law enforcement officials and the EMS director. In many communities this is the responsibility of the mayor in concert with the disaster medical coordinator and the area police chief. Regardless of where the responsibility will rest, the decision to prewarn a community of an impending disaster is a crucial one that carries a heavy consequence. Panic may be a significant danger but generally depends on the type of disaster that is being prewarned. Some disasters, such as major earthquakes, are difficult to predict with any degree of accuracy, whereas others such as tornadoes or hurricanes are more accurately prejudged. Fear of generating panic may cause those in positions of authority to hesitate to evacuate—particularly when natural disasters threaten. Yet evacuation *before* a disaster can result in preservation of life, reduction in personal injury, and protection of property.

Evacuation behavior among the population may vary. Under some circumstances people may refuse to leave their homes, preferring instead to take the gamble while staying on to mitigate the negative consequence to their property. Others may refuse because they do not believe the event will take place. Unless a person is convinced that the impact is certain and that he is within the danger area, there is a general reluctance to cooperate with emergency evacuation plans. Further, those who are not certain where other family members are, or are otherwise not with their family members

at the time of the evacuation, often will not comply with evacuation orders.

Through several studies that have been conducted on the process of evacuation, there are some data to suggest that there are at least four factors that play a part in the individual's decision to participate in an evacuation process, or to respond to a warning (Glass, 1970):

- The individual's assessment of personal threat
- The reality of the disaster threat
- The content of the warning message
- The number of times the warning message was received

According to this same resource, in order to clear an area effectively, residents must either have prior knowledge of an existing evacuation plan or be informed of the procedure when warned. Safe routes must be identified for exit from the area, and appropriate destinations must be defined for the public. This information is a minimum of what must be transmitted to the public in order to achieve the intended response, which is to have the population leave the area! Drabeck and Baggs reported that in a study of flood warning response "families were warned through three distinct processes: (1) authorities, (2) peers, (3) mass media. Those warned by an authority (such as a roving police car with a loudspeaker emitting the warning) were less likely to be skeptical about the warning." It is reasonable to conclude from the foregoing information, that a community plan for warning and evacuation should incorporate the following points:

1. The warning message should be as detailed as possible, including information regarding the location of expected impact, how severe the impact is expected to be, how evacuation will be conducted, and when, and if necessary, safe routes for exit, and appropriate destinations.
2. The warning message must be repeated as urgently and often as possible.
3. The warning message must come from authorities in the community.

Once the decision to warn and/or evacuate is made by the official hierarchy of the community, it is essential to increase the level of perceived personal risk in order to obtain co-operation by the public. These simple steps listed above will promote such behavior.

Communications

If there is one most essential component to an organized disaster response, it is that an effective communication system exists and is supported by back-up systems capable of continuing communications in the event that the primary system fails. There is no one right way to develop and establish such a system; how-ever, major necessary elements include:

1. The major coordination center must be capable of communicating with each medical facility that participates in receiv-ing victims. This center also must have the equipment to communicate with local law enforcement, all rescue units includ-ing those dispatched through mutual aid, fire officials, and any other support agen-cy.
2. Each rescue unit should have the radio frequencies on which to communicate with one another, with local law enforce-ment, and with the medical facilities that they will transport to.
3. Any roving disaster coordinating vehicle must have radio frequencies on which to communicate with each rescue unit and local law enforcement.
4. A contingency capability should exist that will allow all the above to communicate with National Guard and state police.
5. Hand-held walkie-talkie radios must be available for the field triage operation. These radios must be capable of com-municating with the coordination center, all rescue units, and every other walkie-talkie being used in the field triage area.
6. A mechanism must exist for reasonable documentation of crucial communications transmitted and received by the major coordination center.

There are a variety of modalities that can provide the capabilities described above. Each community must decide which one will meet its specific needs. Many communities currently use a HEAR network (*h*ospital *e*mergency *a*dministration *r*adio), which links hospitals together for communication purposes. This net-work has served effectively in multiple casualty incidents in the past but does require central coordination to reduce transmission difficulties that develop when multiple hospitals use the same frequency. Every hospital that supports an emergency department and that potentially would receive casualties in the event of a disas-ter should have the capability of receiving and transmitting radio signals as opposed to relying on telephone systems, which might not be functional after a disaster.

Field triage

The term "triage" derives from the French word meaning "to sort." The triage process involves a sorting of patients based on the need to assign medical priorities and to provide the best care for the greatest number. Civilian tri-age is predominant in situations in which there is enough manpower to provide treatment, stabilization, and evacuation of all patients in a reasonable and timely manner. This type of triage is designed to save lives and limbs while less urgent problems await management, thus maximizing the health care system. Such triage is common to everyday emergency medicine.

Military triage differs in a significant way from civilian triage. Military triage is designed to provide the "best for the most with the least by the fewest" in situations where the numbers of casualties overwhelm by a great majority the numbers of medical personnel available to treat and stabilize them. In such a situation priorities are assigned to casualties based on the initial medical interpretation of presenting signs and symptoms. As more medical resources and the ability to evacuate cases become available, priorities must be reevaluated. *Triage of any type is not a one-time assessment and priority assignment;* rather, it is a continuum of reas-sessment and reassignment of priority relative to the dynamic changes experienced either by the patient or by the situation. Once a military triage is initiated, it may revert to civilian triage *only* after all triage personnel have received communication to that effect! Such decisions are the responsibility of the disaster medical coordinator or, in the absence of such a person, the triage medical coordinator at the scene.

Civilian triage is often possible even in multiple casualty situations if enough rescuers are available. Coordination of this activity *must* exist, because the tendency in many instances is to "load and go" as opposed to providing a primary (ABCs) survey and a secondary survey (2-minute head-to-toe evaluation for existing injuries) before assigning a triage priority. Again, in civilian triage, patients with major injuries and even cardiopulmonary arrest might receive immediate treatment and stabilization, whereas patients with minor wounds or fractures would await care and evacuation.

In situations in which mass casualties exist, or where the numbers of cases otherwise overload the available medical personnel, the decision to institute military triage must come from the medical coordinator at the scene. It is often a difficult decision; many patients who might be managed successfully in a nondisaster situation will likely not survive if military triage is instituted. The decision to utilize this more severe type of triage must be made relative to the magnitude of the disaster as determined by numbers of casualties, types of injuries, and the extent to which the disaster may be generating casualties (that is, finite and infinite), and also to the type and extent of resources available. Total patient care will be impossible in any disaster setting, particularly at or near the site. The type of triage used will depend on the setting itself and on the medical personnel available to provide the most optimal of care possible under the circumstances. In any event, such a process will never equate with the treatment possible in an emergency department in nondisaster settings. It *will*, however, provide for an orderly and progressive evaluation and evacuation of those injured in a disaster situation.

Those components necessary for an organized triage process at the disaster site include:
- Adequate communications to determine where, when, and how to evacuate sorted cases. Adequate communication includes utilizing a system to tag and mark all casualties with their initial triage priority and with subsequent changes in that priority if changes occur.
- A triage "team" of taggers and evaluators.
- A triage "officer" to coordinate type of triage and decisions relative to the process.
- Referral points as patient destinations, which must be accessible from the site of the disaster (in mass casualty situations, the referral point may be a casualty collection point). Such referral points may be first at the site, then to an ambulance or other vehicle for transportation to a medical facility. In small-scale disasters, a triage and evacuation process is usually simultaneous, and casualties are not sorted into sections to await evacuation. In larger disasters where casualties must await transport, designation of holding areas based on priority is necessary.
- A rating system—such a system may be two tier, three tier, four tier, or five tier (see boxed material, Triage Rating Systems). It must be kept in mind that the type of triage (military or civilian) is not the same as the rating used. The chart describing immediate and delayed cases on pp. 655-656 presents a two-tier system, and Fig. 28-2 depicts activity flow when a two-tier system is being used.

The tagging and record-keeping activities in the triage areas are vital ones that must be instituted at the very start of triage. Different systems use different forms; therefore, consideration of how the differences will effect mutual aid support is crucial. Everyone using the forms must be aware of how to complete and use them, or the recording and tagging systems (the crux of patient identification and priority assignment) will be useless. More important, these communication tools will be potentially dangerous. The ideal situation is for all components of the disaster response, retrieval, and receipt teams to use the same forms; however, such an ideal does not exist at this time.

The primary forms for effective field triage are the patient identification tag, which serves as a tool to record patient data and treatment in the first hour after the event occurs, and

Triage rating systems

Five-tier system (used in military triage)
Dead or will die
Life-threatening—readily correctable
Urgent—must be treated within 1 to 2 hours
Delayed—noncritical or ambulatory
No injury—no treatment necessary

Four-tier system
Immediate—seriously injured, reasonable chance of survival
Delayed—can wait for care after simple first aid
Expectant—extremely critical, moribund
Minimal—no impairment of function, can either treat self or be treated by a nonprofessional

Three-tier system
Life-threatening—readily correctable
Urgent—must be treated within 1 to 2 hours
Delayed—no injury, noncritical, or ambulatory

Two-tier system
Immediate versus delayed
Immediate—life-threatening injuries that are readily correctable on scene, and those that are urgent
Delayed—no injury, noncritical injuries, ambulatory victims, moribund, and dead

Description of immediate and delayed cases in simple triage during multiple casualty incidents, and in military triage during mass casualty incidents*

Simple triage

Immediate (Priority I)
1. Asphyxia
2. Respiratory obstruction from mechanical causes
3. Sucking chest wounds
4. Tension pneumothorax
5. Maxillofacial wounds in which asphyxia exists or is likely to develop
6. Shock caused by major external hemorrhage
7. Major internal hemorrhage
8. Visceral injuries or evisceration
9. Cardiopericardial injuries
10. Massive muscle damage
11. Severe burns *over* 25% BSA
12. Dislocations
13. Major fractures

*Courtesy, Office of Emergency Services, State of California

Continued.

Description of immediate and delayed cases
in simple triage during multiple casualty incidents,
and in military triage during mass casualty incidents—cont'd

Simple triage—cont'd

Immediate (Priority I)
14. Major medical problems readily correctible
15. Closed cerebral injuries with increasing loss of consciousness

Delayed (Priority II)
1. Vascular injuries requiring repair
2. Wounds of the genitourinary tract
3. Thoracic wounds without asphyxia
4. Severe burns *under* 25% BSA
5. Spinal cord injuries requiring decompression
6. Suspected spinal cord injuries without neurological signs
7. Lesser fractures
8. Injuries of the eye
9. Maxillofacial injuries without asphyxia
10. Minor medical problems
11. Victims with little hope of survival under the best of circumstances of medical care

Mass casualty triage with an overwhelming number of injuries

Immediate (Priority I)
1. Asphyxia
2. Respiratory obstruction from mechanical causes
3. Sucking chest wounds
4. Tension pneumothorax
5. Maxillofacial wounds in which asphyxia exists or is likely to develop
6. Shock caused by major external hemorrhage
7. Dislocations
8. Severe burns *under* 25% BSA†
9. Lesser fractures†
10. Major medical problems that can be handled readily

Delayed (Priority II)
1. Major fractures (if able to stabilize)†
2. Visceral injuries or evisceration†
3. Cardiopericardial injuries†
4. Massive muscle damage†
5. Severe burns *over* 25% BSA†
6. Vascular injuries requiring repair
7. Wounds of the genitourinary tract
8. Thoracic wounds without asphyxia
9. Closed cerebral injuries with increasing loss of consciousness†
10. Spinal cord injuries requiring decompression†
11. Suspected spinal cord injuries without neurological signs
12. Injuries of the eye
13. Maxillofacial injuries without asphyxia
14. Complicated major medical problems†
15. Minor medical problems
16. Victims with little hope of survival under the best of circumstances of medical care

---

†Conditions that have changed categories

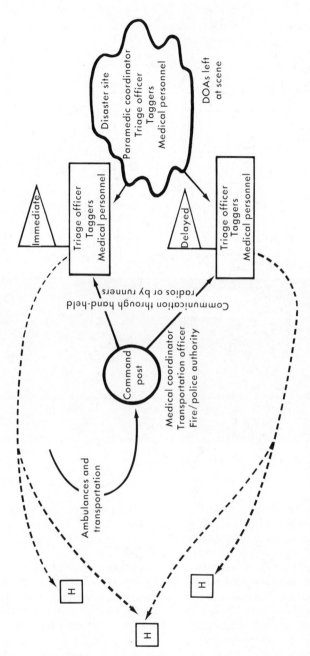

Fig. 28-2. Activity-flow ambulances and victims. Communications between all points of contact imperative to effort. (Adapted from Long Beach Disaster Plan, courtesy J. MacDonald, MD.)

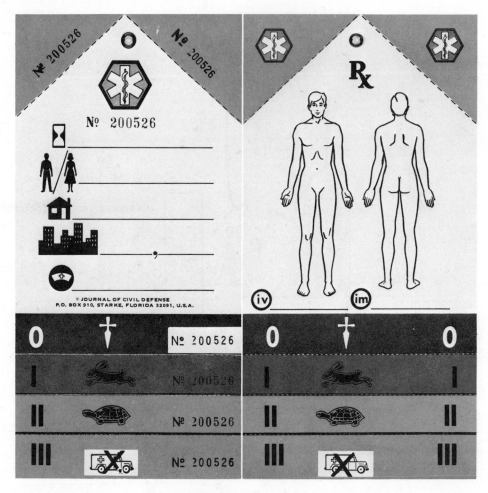

Fig. 28-3. Triage tag.

the casualty distribution log, which identifies the receiving facilities, numbers of casualties dispatched to each, and the time each casualty left the field triage area. Such a log will help prevent inadvertent overload of one or two facilities while others are available and ready. This log is most appropriately maintained by someone specifically assigned to ambulance/transportation coordination at each triage and/or holding area in order for the information to be continuously documented at the same time that evacuation is coordinated with the triage teams.

Examples of disaster tags and a casualty distribution log can be seen in Figs. 28-3 and 28-4.

Transport

Transport of casualties out of a disaster site requires great skill and caution in many instances. In large-scale disasters damaged buildings, vehicles, and roadways may seriously hamper rescue and evacuation efforts, and may present a danger to the rescuers themselves. The main concern under these circumstances must be that the rescuers avoid precarious and dangerous situations; they must discard samaritan heroics and keep themselves from harm in

Hospital	Location	Beds available

Tag No.	Destination	Ambulance name and Unit No.	Time out

Fig. 28-4. Casualty distribution log.

order to continue with rescue efforts. This is not to say that they must avoid any risk, but they should be careful not to take those risks that in all likelihood will cause their own injury or death. In smaller-scale situations in which many rescuers are available, a great deal more risk might be entertained on an individual basis, but retrieving and evacuating casualties in major disasters require much the same judgment as initiating military triage: some casualties who are still alive might have to be left to die so that more can be saved.

Retrieval from damaged buildings, destroyed commercial aircraft, fire ravaged areas, and so on requires consideration of correct technique for stabilization and extrication of patients with vertebral injuries or extremity fractures. Yet often perils exist that demand that more attention be directed at removing the victim from further harm, and the rescuers from potential harm, as rapidly as possible. There may not be enough spinal boards or extremity splints to use on everyone. In fact, depending on the extent of the disaster and the numbers of casualties, there may not be enough of any major equipment item. Decisions regarding the most expedient method to extricate each victim will have to be made on a case-by-case basis. There are no golden rules or absolutes to rely upon. Once the victims have been removed from danger and assigned a triage priority, the question becomes one of evacuation of victims from the scene to either casualty collection points, disaster service areas, or medical facilities—any of which are utilized relative to the level of the disaster. Such evacuation can be conducted on several levels, including ground transport, helicopter or airplane, or ship.

Ground transport does not have to be limited to ambulances, although most often this is so when multiple casualty incidents occur. Any community planning in regard to ground transport should include alternative means as a contingency for lack of sufficient regulation ambulances. Alternatives may include milk trucks, flower trucks, telephone company trucks, and hearses. No doubt there are few who are as aware of fast routes into every hospital in the area as flower delivery men! Whenever alternatives to ambulances are included in a community disaster plan, extensive education and coordination must take place in order for everyone involved in a disaster to be aware of how to use these resources. With some forethought, these alternative vehicles can be equipped with citizens band or comparable radio equipment when they are called into service during a disaster.

THE HOSPITAL PLAN

Much as community, state and federal plans are vital to effective response to disasters, so are intelligently developed plans for both the inpatient areas of a hospital and the emergency department—the hub of disaster activity in the hospital. The Joint Commission on Accreditation of Hospitals (JCAH) requires that every hospital develop, maintain, and practice (at least two times a year) a disaster plan. These drills are vital to the planning and training process, because inexperience and lack of understanding of the plan contribute to the very behaviors that a good plan should prevent: indecision and anxiety. What is needed is a brief, concise plan of action developed with input from those people who will be using it. Both during and after development, the plan must be tested, evaluated, and modified as necessary on a routine basis.

The emergency department plan

Plans specific to the ED are crucial to efficient and effective response to external *and* internal disasters. External disasters include earthquakes, floods, tornadoes, and acts of war. Internal disasters include fire in the hospital, bomb threats, water spills, and radiation accidents. The ED is the hub of response; hospital operations during a disaster are essentially an expansion of the ED and primarily there only for back-up to ED operations. Because of this, each area—inpatient and ED—must have individualized plans for disaster response. However, these plans cannot exist in a vacuum. The ED plan must be integrated into the hospital inpatient plans and coordinated with the patient services such as pharmacy, central supply, and dietetics. The graded responses of a step-wise implementation of the entire hospital plan might follow the guidelines below, depending on the size of the hospital and the ED:

Phase I (fewer than 15 patients received)—Management of all cases in the ED if possible, without disrupting normal hospital functions. If impossible to manage all the cases in the ED (because of existing patient load, lack of staff, and so on), proceed to phase II.

Phase II (15 to 40 patients received)—Management of all patients in the ED and adjacent areas if possible; cancellation of elective surgeries and admissions; allocation of more space for emergency management of immediate and delayed cases according to the plan.

Phase III (over 40 patients received)—Implementation of the entire hospital plan with total revision of hospital activities as necessary.

Disaster plans are an integral part of any emergency department operational plan, but the focus of these plans is generally on mass casualty disaster response, without a mechanism for step-wise implementation less disruptive to the facility. It is important that a working plan allow for implementation not only for large-scale disasters, but for the 5- to 50-patient incidents that occur more frequently in any community. The graded response of the emergency department plan will follow different criteria for step-wise implementation than the inpatient plans.

If the prevailing philosophy is to develop a plan flexible enough to meet the needs of varying situations, then criteria must be developed whereby the nurse and physician in charge at the time the incident occurs may make reasonably appropriate decisions on how to meet those needs. There is no fail-safe mechanism that will guarantee correct decisions. The nature of disasters is such that they are spontaneous, unpredictable, and contribute to initial confusion and uncertainty. The most critical information necessary for making appropriate decisions on how to mobilize the department and when to mobilize the entire facility follows.

1. What is the nature of the incident?
   a. Which category of disaster does the incident most readily fit into?

b. Is the number of casualties controlled (known fairly accurately) or uncontrolled (only a rough estimate)?

c. What type of injuries are prevailing (for example, burns, multiple trauma, respiratory)?

d. What is the expected severity of the majority of injuries (that is, many critical cases, minimal minor injuries)?

e. How much time exists between the initial notification of the facility and the expected receipt of the first patients?

2. What is the status of the department at the time of the initial awareness that a disaster exists that will affect the ability of the ED to respond?

a. How many nurses and physicians are on duty right now?

b. What is the relationship to hour of day, volume of patients already existing in the department, and availability of back-up staff?

c. How many beds within the department are available immediately? In 30 minutes? In 60 minutes?

d. What is the relative departmental supply status?

In order to collect information that will provide this data, the nurse receiving notification (whether given by layperson, outside agency, or the area disaster coordinating center (DCC) might complete an emergency situation report form (Fig. 28-5), which records verification of the caller and the incident. This form will document characteristics of the situation by which decisions can be made.

The variables are so vast that more thorough

```
┌─────────────────────────────────────────────────────────────────────────┐
│ Drill:    □Yes  No□      Notified by:                                      │
│ Date:                    Agency:                                          │
│ Time:                    Phone No.          Verified  □Yes    No□          │
├─────────────────────────────────────────────────────────────────────────┤
│ Situation, time of onset, location:                                       │
│                                                                           │
│                                                                           │
│                                                                           │
├─────────────────────────────────────────────────────────────────────────┤
│ Extent:                  □Multiple patient                                │
│                          □Multiple casualty                               │
│                          □Mass casualty                                   │
├─────────────────────────────────────────────────────────────────────────┤
│ Type of injuries predominating (chemical, thermal burns, radiation, head, │
│ neck, chest, abdomen wounds, and so on):                                  │
│                                                                           │
│                                                                           │
├─────────────────────────────────────────────────────────────────────────┤
│ Disaster coordinating center communications:                             │
│                                                                           │
│                                                                           │
│                                                                           │
│                                                                           │
├─────────────────────────────────────────────────────────────────────────┤
│ No. of casualties to be received:                                         │
│                                                                           │
│ _____Immediate        _____delayed                              │
│                                                                           │
│ No. actually received at triage area:                                     │
│                                                                           │
├─────────────────────────────────────────────────────────────────────────┤
│ Pink copy:   post in ED by assignment sheet                               │
│ Yellow copy: send to ED command post                                      │
│ White copy:  send to hospital administration                             │
└─────────────────────────────────────────────────────────────────────────┘
```

Fig. 28-5. Emergency situation report for hospital.

definition of initial action to take would be exhaustive. Essentially, the following steps for implementation might be considered:

1. Multiple patient incident with *no prior notification* (sudden arrival)
   a. Call for nursing house supervisor to proceed to the ED to assist with unexpected complications.
   b. Notify ranking hospital administrator that a potential ED overload situation exists.
   c. Discharge any existing patient who might be expedited.
   d. Request staff assistance from nursing office (critical care nurses).
   e. Review need for ED staff call-in on an as-needed basis.
2. Multiple patient incident with prior notification
   a. Complete emergency situation report, and notify the nursing supervisor and the ranking hospital administrator in the house to respond to the ED to assist with decision making.
   b. Take a quick overview of the department, evaluating whether current staffing and supplies will be able to handle incoming patients.
   c. Respond to the local DCC if contacted, stating the numbers of immediate patients that can be handled and the number of delayed cases that can be handled. Have an RN continue to monitor the communication system until or unless the ED command post is opened.
   d. Determine if the need can be met by the department only, by the department with staff call-in only, or by mobilizing the hospital and opening the clinic for added space.
   e. Assign a staff member (clerk) to call staff in and notify administrative personnel from the ED, unless the command post can assume responsibility.
   f. Prepare to, at a minimum, staff the triage area and a section of the ED for disaster patient care.
3. Multiple casualty incident with prior notification.
   a. Follow the preceding steps.
   b. Prepare to implement the ED command post regardless of whether the decision is made to mobilize the hospital or not.
   c. Open triage immediately.
   d. The decision to mobilize the entire hospital will depend on how many casualties the hospital can reasonably expect to receive. The community disaster plan will be in effect, and ideally casualties will be distributed in a manner that will prevent overload of any one facility. If the local DCC has been activated, the ED must ensure accurate communication relative to the department status at the time of the event and at the time of initial receipt of casualties. The ED might expect to have to tolerate short-term management of multiple casualties until effective control is generated by the DCC. From multiple field triage experiences, it is safe to predict that the majority of cases generated from a disaster will be of the salvageable delayed category.
   e. The following hospital departments must be notified:

X-ray	Central service
Laboratory	Security
Surgery	Housekeeping
Pharmacy	

   Accelerated in-patient discharges or evacuation of in-patient areas to accommodate multiple new admissions *may not* be necessary. Step-wise implementation will allow for each of these last two activities when the need becomes apparent. However, the decision may be to gather ED staff and supplies first, and accelerate to the full plan only as necessary.
4. Mass casualty incident with prior notification
   a. Complete the emergency situation report.
   b. Notify the ranking hospital administrator.
   c. Implement the disaster plan to mobilize the entire hospital.

These are the types of responses that may be utilized. The decision regarding which response to use should rest with the emergency physician on duty and the nurse in charge *at the time* of the incident. Hospital and nursing administrators present and accountable for hospital operations at the time may assist in the decision-making process but should not unnecessarily pursue hospital-wide mobilization. If the situation can be handled with the clearing of only a small number of operating suites or intensive care beds, perhaps that should be the primary action. Judgment regarding intelligent step-wise implementation can only be developed through familiarity with the disaster plan and the capability of the emergency department on the part of all decision makers.

Components of an emergency department plan

1. A description of the purpose and function of the plan
2. Definition of authority roles (remember that specific people may not be present, so do not list authorities by name, only by title)
3. Location and function of the command post
4. Provisions for staff call-in (including medical staff)
5. Personnel identification provisions
6. Personnel disaster action cards
7. Triage area activities, supplies, patient flow
8. Patient records and flow logs
9. Communications
   a. Intradepartment
   b. Interdepartment
   c. Hospital/community/rescue vehicles
10. Interface with hospital back-up services
    a. X-ray, lab, central service, pharmacy
    b. Admission, surgery, special care units
    c. Public relations, security, housekeeping, dietetics

An ED disaster planning committee should include representatives from all involved services and be conducted by a designated disaster officer for the ED.

Because many people will be involved in this planning, effective leadership will be crucial to avoiding such difficulties as difference of opinion, loss of motivation, and development of unrealistic goals. Most importantly, the completed plan must be simple and easy for the average employee to understand. The important points of some of the elements on the list will be discussed to promote an understanding of their application to effective disaster response.

LOCATION AND FUNCTION OF EMERGENCY DEPARTMENT COMMAND POST. The ED command post may, in many facilities, be a combined hospital and ED command post. Such an area has primary responsibility for coordination of the disaster effort within the hospital. It must be located central to the "action," with the capability of communication to all areas as well as outside the hospital. The interhospital communication radio should be moved into this area to be monitored by experienced personnel integrally involved in coordinating activities. The command post can significantly relieve the professionals in the ED from the responsibility to maintain central communications. The command post personnel can also accommodate other administrative functions, such as:

1. Staff call-back and documentation
2. Obtaining needed supplies and equipment
3. Distributing information to the press and to concerned citizens seeking information about family members
4. Delegating social services, language interpreters, transporters, volunteers, and so on into appropriate areas
5. Arranging for patient admissions

PERSONNEL CONSIDERATIONS

STAFF CALL-IN. Implementation of staff call-in should be initiated as soon as the ED nurse in charge determines that a need exists. A roster must be readily available that identifies each staff member alphabetically and by title and lists the current telephone number. It is helpful to shade the names of those ED staff members who live less than 15 minutes from the facility. Staff members should be aware that they should try to get to their hospital in the event of a major disaster, if there is any possible way to do so. But they should be asked to stay by their telephone in a lesser disaster to enable the hospital to reach them if they are needed.

Name	Telephone No.	Time called	Response WBI	No	No ans.	ETA	Time arrived	Comments
Sample, Joe	323-1111	10:40				5 min	10:53	
Jones, John	874-8833	10:42						Road inaccessible; he will come in when situation changes.
Smith, Jane	342-8351	10:45						Mother states she is out of town.
Lindsey, Roberta	395-6458	10:46				15 min		

Fig. 28-6. Staff call roster for disaster.

Name	Category	Area/duty	Changes	Time off duty
Jones, Cathy	RN	Treatment area Disaster coordinator		
Smith, Clark	MD	Treatment area Disaster officer		
Lindsey, Jack	MD	Triage physician		
Macy, Lynn	RN	Treatment area Team I		
Reynolds, Tracy	RN	Triage nurse		
Lane, Roger	EMT	Treatment area Team I		
Roy, Gary	EMT	Clinic	Treatment area Team 3 1040	
Michael, Nancy	RN	Clinic		

Fig. 28-7. Assignment sheet for disaster.

A flow sheet is necessary in order for those who are attempting to contact staff members to be aware of who has been called and what the result was. Fig. 28-6 is an example of such a list.

STAFF ASSIGNMENT. Once staff has been called in, it will be necessary to assign them to specific responsibilities and areas such as triage, treatment, or delayed treatment. When changes in assignments are made, such changes must be noted on the assignment sheet (Fig. 28-7). Many hospitals use a blackboard that is automatically hung on the wall for the sole purpose of identifying which staff members are in the area and where they have been assigned. This blackboard might be in addition to the working call-in and assignment sheets that are in the command post. Assignments of nursing personnel must be at the direction of the nursing coordinator in the ED, and assignment of physician personnel should be at the direction of the disaster medical officer. Ancillary staff, such as x-ray technicians, laboratory technicians, and IV nurses, should be requested by the ED nurse in charge to perform specific functions only, and then to return to their own areas to await further instructions.

STAFF IDENTIFICATION. It is imperative that adequate identification be employed to reduce unnecessary and dangerous traffic on the part of sightseers. Public members such as press people have been known to penetrate emergency facilities when specific methods for identifying personnel authorized to be in the area are not employed. Such identification may be in the form of color-coded arm bands or bibs with titles clearly marked on the front and back (RN, MD, triage officer, LPN, clerk). The security force in the hospital, who control traffic flow, must be instructed not to allow anyone without proper identification into the ED. Initial access can be accomplished more easily if wallet-sized disaster cards are given to employees of the ED. These should be photo cards and should have the employee ID number affixed. It is possible that the display of such a card will also help the employee through police or fire lines on the way to the hospital.

STAFF DUTY CARDS. Because true disasters are unpredictable and extremely variable, all the drills in the world might not enable everyone to function optimally in each specific circumstance. Staff turnover, excitement, and anxiety, and a feeling of urgency or haste may promote lack of understanding or recall of job functions. Disaster action cards are a simple method of assigning and identifying jobs and job responsibilities, by role description and shifts, to physicians, nurses, clerks, and technicians in the ED. Such cards can be employed in any area, but prove particularly beneficial in the ED. No one in an actual disaster has the time to read through a disaster manual; the need to do this is precluded by a card that, point by point, defines the necessary action for each person to take *in order of priority*. Fig. 28-8 is an example of the specific responsibilities of the nurse in charge of the ED at the time a disaster occurs. Following are also examples of the specific responsibilities for an ED clerk and an ED physician. Once the cards are handed out, everyone must undertake the specific tasks on his or her card immediately. *No one* should require further information about what to do as listed on the card.

ROLE OF THE TRIAGE AREA AND PERSONNEL

FUNCTION AND LOCATION. A triage area is essential in all emergency departments when a disaster strikes that generates 10 or more casualties with a time lag between occurrence, notification of hospitals, and receipt of victims. External triage at the scene, with disaster tags affixed to each patient, generally occurs in situations involving multiple casualties of more than 10 victims. Mass casualty situations, particularly those involving large-scale disasters may generate so many casualties that sorting and tagging in the field is hasty, sporadic, and may have a high classification error rate. The most critical function of the triage area is that of providing a rapid reassessment of all casualties and distribution of each victim to the appropriate treatment location. In addition, the triage area also serves as a physical barrier to unauthorized traffic and to friends, relatives, reporters, and noninjured. For this reason, all other accesses into the hospital must be closed and locked or guarded to avoid access of walk-

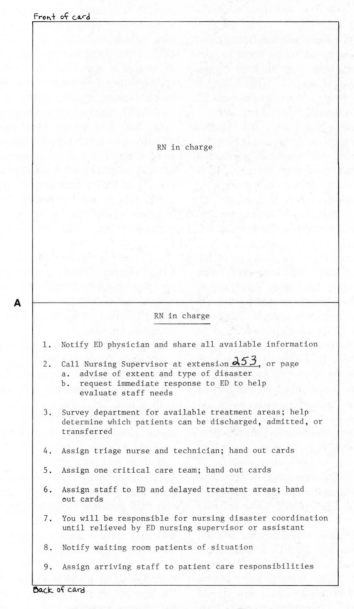

Front of card

RN in charge

A

Back of card

RN in charge

1. Notify ED physician and share all available information

2. Call Nursing Supervisor at extension 253, or page
   a. advise of extent and type of disaster
   b. request immediate response to ED to help
      evaluate staff needs

3. Survey department for available treatment areas; help
   determine which patients can be discharged, admitted, or
   transferred

4. Assign triage nurse and technician; hand out cards

5. Assign one critical care team; hand out cards

6. Assign staff to ED and delayed treatment areas; hand
   out cards

7. You will be responsible for nursing disaster coordination
   until relieved by ED nursing supervisor or assistant

8. Notify waiting room patients of situation

9. Assign arriving staff to patient care responsibilities

Fig. 28-8. Disaster action cards. **A,** RN in charge.

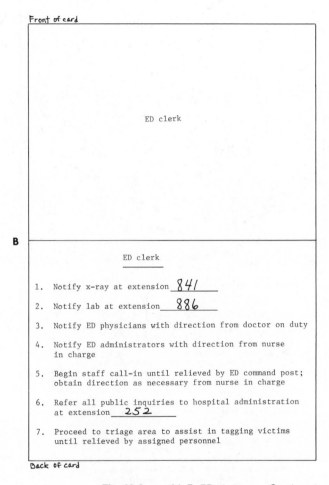

Front of card

ED clerk

B

ED clerk

1. Notify x-ray at extension _841_

2. Notify lab at extension _886_

3. Notify ED physicians with direction from doctor on duty

4. Notify ED administrators with direction from nurse in charge

5. Begin staff call-in until relieved by ED command post; obtain direction as necessary from nurse in charge

6. Refer all public inquiries to hospital administration at extension _252_

7. Proceed to triage area to assist in tagging victims until relieved by assigned personnel

Back of card

Fig. 28-8, cont'd. B, ED clerk.   *Continued.*

Front of card

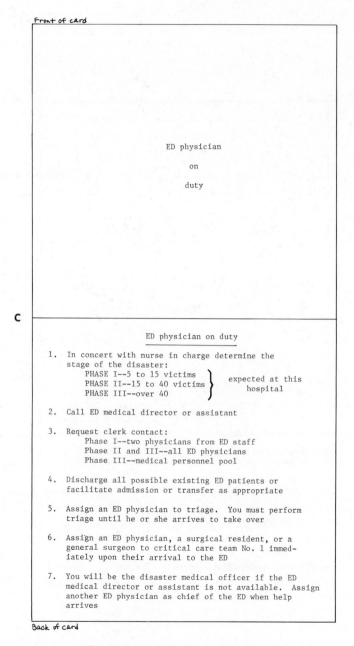

C

ED physician

on

duty

ED physician on duty

1. In concert with nurse in charge determine the stage of the disaster:
   PHASE I--5 to 15 victims
   PHASE II--15 to 40 victims ⎫ expected at this
   PHASE III--over 40 ⎭ hospital

2. Call ED medical director or assistant

3. Request clerk contact:
   Phase I--two physicians from ED staff
   Phase II and III--all ED physicians
   Phase III--medical personnel pool

4. Discharge all possible existing ED patients or facilitate admission or transfer as appropriate

5. Assign an ED physician to triage. You must perform triage until he or she arrives to take over

6. Assign an ED physician, a surgical resident, or a general surgeon to critical care team No. 1 immediately upon their arrival to the ED

7. You will be the disaster medical officer if the ED medical director or assistant is not available. Assign another ED physician as chief of the ED when help arrives

Back of card

Fig. 28-8, cont'd. C, ED physician on duty.

in victims into the wrong areas, or to avoid penetration of the facility by sightseers. Hospital personnel responding to the disaster may be directed into the facility through alternate doors identified to them as access routes for staff before the disaster. Emergency personnel, however, must be able to go directly into the ED through the triage area. The triage area itself must be located at the front entrance to the ED, ideally under a protective canopy to shield victims and triage personnel from adverse weather. Unfortunately, some of the physical problems encountered in this area are poor lighting, lack of major equipment, and lack of privacy. Other factors affecting the function of the triage area include heavy patient flow that overloads triage staff, an unbalanced patient flow perhaps with many immediate cases arriving at one time, and disorganization on the part of the triage personnel.

PERSONNEL. The personnel involved in the triage area should include message runners, transporters, clerical personnel, nurses, and physicians. The extent of the system will vary depending on the size of the ED and numbers of casualties expected. Minimal personnel would be:

One physician skilled in triage
One RN skilled in triage
One LPN or EMT
One clerk
Two transporters
Two message runners

If a physician is not available, a registered nurse with training in the concepts of multiple and mass casualty triage should be designated as the triage officer. *Anyone* assigned to this role must be able to perform rapid physical evaluations, make rapid triage decisions that are correct the majority of the time, and to remain calm for the duration of the activity. The effectiveness of nurse triage is commonly recognized in everyday emergency operations, with 80% or more accuracy. The remaining 20% are triaged to a higher category than necessary. Under disaster circumstances, however, it is crucial that an RN who is assigned as triage officer understand civilian and military triage concepts. Any triage officer must be able to

abandon traditional concepts of total patient care and instead to accept the clinical concept that the triage area must provide simple first aid and rapid distribution of patients who will benefit most by timely intervention.

A rule of thumb that has proved helpful in assigning sufficient triage personnel is the following: one triage officer can see one to two patients per minute for bursts of patient influx; the occasional patient may take 3 to 5 minutes; and more than 30 patients per hour will require a second triage officer and sufficient taggers to prevent unnecessary delay in the triage of victims. All the personnel assigned to triage must remain there until the disaster is officially over in terms of hospital receipt of casualties. Provisions must be made to allow sufficient rest breaks with the assistance of relief personnel if the disaster is long.

The triage officer will need to be able to evaluate patients according to how they were classified initially in the field and to whether they have changed in priority. To do this, the officer will need to have a good command of the criteria for classifying patients in order not to overload the treatment area or ambulatory care disaster staff. Correct classification on the part of triage officers and assistants will depend on their knowledge of the following areas (Richman, 1977):

1. Salvageable life-threatening situations
2. Nonsalvageable life-threatening situations
3. Immediate non-life-threatening situations
4. Burns and communicable diseases
5. Psychiatric/emotional problems
6. Minor lacerations (minor surgery)
7. Orthopedic problems
8. Obstetrical problems
9. Delayed problems such as sprains and minor eye injuries
10. Criteria for patient discharge from triage

In addition everyone at triage, particularly the transporters, should understand not only the classification (rating) system being used in that area but also the patient flow pattern and locations for distribution (clinic, morgue, recovery room, critical care unit, ED, decontamination

```
                        Triage officer

1.  Put on identification bib

2.  Obtain paperwork from triage cart (technician will bring
    cart to triage area)

3.  Ensure procurement of wheelchairs and stretchers by
    housekeeping

4.  Ensure sufficient personnel to assist you in evaluating,
    tagging, and documenting log sheet.  Nursing disaster
    coordinator will assign staff to triage

5.  DO NOT LEAVE YOUR AREA UNTIL RELIEVED BY DISASTER
    MEDICAL COORDINATOR

6.  Record information on tags and on the log accurately; do
    not "rush" victims out of triage without proper information

7.  These areas will receive the following categories of patients:
          ED................. Burns, multiple trauma, major wounds
          Clinic............. Minor wounds
          X-ray............. Simple fractures, no other injury
          Recovery room...... Major head injuries
          Coronary care...... Chest pain, no injuries
          Morgue............. Dead on arrival
          Obstetrics........ Term and high-risk OB
          Chapel............. Families, friends of victims
          Social services.... Hysteria, no injury
          Pathology......... Radiation contamination
          Administration..... Press
```

Fig. 28-9. Disaster action card for triage officer.

area). Signs should be posted to designate each of these areas. A location board that identifies access routes to each area designated as a receiving unit for casualties often proves helpful when many transporters are used or when volunteers are used who may not be familiar with the locations. It is very important to do whatever need be done to avoid dispersal of patients to incorrect locations, because such a situation can result in "lost casualties" for prolonged periods of time with obvious detriment to the patient. In addition, all triage personnel must be aware of where to send families, sightseers, press, blood donors, and any other category of person who may accidentally end up at the triage area.

Triage should occur at each level of treatment in whatever clinical areas are being utilized for patient receipt. Remember, triage is not a one time only function. Any patient triaged to a delayed treatment area, for instance, may develop complications that require im-

mediate attention and, depending on the capability of the delayed area, triage back to the ED or to any designated immediate care area. A sample triage officer disaster action card can be seen in Fig. 28-9.

PAPERWORK. Disaster tags must be used if the number of casualties exceeds 10. Any number less than 10 generally allows for initiation and utilization of the standard ED treatment record. Numbers over 10 (this figure is relative to the capability of each individual ED) require tagging, if field tags were not applied, or retagging if initial field triage classification has changed or the tag is unreadable. In large-scale disasters the standard emergency records are impractical and time consuming. The triage tags should be sufficient to include necessary patient data and space for recording treatment and disposition. Additionally, the tag must be *tied* onto the patient and not taped. No one should record essential treatment data on foreheads once the patient is in the hospital, *unless*

ATTACH SECURELY TO PATIENT

| Pink copy: administration |
| White copy: admitting |
| Hard copy: patient record |

NO. 524873

A

Hospital: St. Josephina

| Patient name   (Last) | (First) | (Middle) |
| Smith | Donald | K. |

Address
1252 N. 11th St.

| Date | Time | Age | Sex | Religion |
| 10/5/64 | 1015 | 32 | M | Cath. |

Description of patient: (Ht, Wt, Eyes, Hair, Compl, Marks, Clothing)
6ft. brn/green 180# Cauc.
torn blue shirt, brn trousers, blk shoes/socks

ALLERGIES:
Horse Serum

Next of kin:
(name)   (address)
Alice Smith   1252 N 11th St.   Wife

INITIAL ASSESSMENT:
2° burns face/hands
Open chest wound ® chest
Rigid belly, responds purposefully to voice

INITIAL TREATMENT:
- ☐ Airway
- ☑ Bleeding control
- ☐ Tourniquet
- ☐ Splint
- ☑ OTHER: Vaseline gauze dressing, occlusive bandage

- ☑ IV Rlc 1000 cc
- ☑ Oxygen @ 8L/min mask
- ☐ Medication:

INITIAL ROUTING AT HOSPITAL TRIAGE POINT:
- ☑ Surgery
- ☐ X-ray
- ☐ First aid
- ☐ Emergency Department
- ☐ ICU
- ☐ CCU
- ☐ Observation area
- ☐ Morgue

OTHER:

PRIORITY DESIGNATION
- ☑ Immediate
- ☐ Delayed
- ☐ Dead

RED

If immediate care affix
RED LABEL
If delayed care affix
BLACK LABEL

DO NOT DETACH TAG FROM PATIENT UNTIL INCORPORATED IN PATIENT RECORD
SEE REVERSE SIDE FOR TREATMENT, DISPOSITION, AND INSTRUCTIONS

Fig. 28-10. A, Completed disaster tag.   *Continued.*

a tourniquet is in place. In this case a marking pen should be used to mark "TK" on the patient's forehead as a warning alert to everyone treating him. When time permits, regular emergency or inpatient charts can be generated, in which case the tag will become part of the official treatment record. An example of a tag completed at the triage point and of a disaster patient flow log can be seen in Fig. 28-10. As each casualty enters the triage point, the tag

number assigned to him is recorded on the log, along with time to triage, priority, name (if possible), and initial disposition. The log is completed as information is received from the treatment areas via the command post, and during and after the disaster operation it can be utilized as a patient location and information log in answer to questions received from the press and from the local DCC.

SUPPLIES. Those supplies necessary to the tri-

Time to triage	Tag No.	Name	Priority	Initial disposition	Time out	Final disposition	Diagnosis

Fig. 28-10, cont'd. B, Hospital triage patient flow log.

age area will depend on what the situation is; however, a triage cart with the following basic minimum supplies should be kept stocked and stored near the site designated as the triage point.

Sterile gauze pads
Sterile kling bandage
Sterile kerlix
Splinting material
Irrigating sterile normal saline
Bag/valve/mask resuscitator
Rubber oral airways—all sizes
Assorted adhesive tape
Plastic IV solutions
Penlights
Delivery packs
Plastic bags—large and small
Blankets
Oxygen equipment and tanks
Disaster tags
Disaster patient flow log
Clipboards and pencils
Marking pens
Bullhorn
Walkie-talkie radios
Prepackaged supplies for rescue vehicles

In addition, provisions should be made for immediate delivery of sufficient numbers of wheelchairs, gurneys, sheets, and IV poles upon opening of the triage area in an actual disaster.

One of the supply needs frequently overlooked by facilities is that of the incoming ambulances. Prepacked supplies should be ready at the triage area for issuance to rescue vehicles; as they deliver a patient the rescue personnel will be able to accomplish a rapid, minimum restock of such items as sterile dressings and bandages, splinting materials, plastic IV solution bags, emesis basins, and airway equipment. The precise compilation of these ready-to-go supplies is best determined by the hospital and the rescue operations people before a disaster occurs.

Finally, a plan must be coordinated whereby central service is prepared to replace used triage supplies immediately; perhaps this can be accomplished by stationing a central service employee in the area with a simply inventory, such person to contact CS for runner service when supplies must be replaced. Treatment in the triage area must necessarily be minimal, but the area should be prepared to maintain or initiate simple first aid during the few moments that each victim is being triaged into the facility.

CRITICAL CARE TEAMS. The emergency department will generally handle multiple patient incidents with either existing staff or with supplements obtained from the nursing office or by staff call-in. However, in multiple casualty incidents with prior notification of facilities by the local DCC, the ED will more often than not be requested to identify how many "immediate" and how many "delayed" cases can be handled. In mass casualty situations, the ED should mobilize the entire hospital, and may have very little to say about how many casualties they may handle or even how much time exists before receipt of the casualties.

The concept of critical care teams developed out of a need to provide continuity of care under department overload conditions for those patients categorized as "immediate."

The teams functions very well under multiple casualty circumstances, and may provide more focused and efficient care during times when fragmentation of that care is highly likely and may prove disastrous for the patients.

In order to understand how the teams may work, one must be aware that, although triage is a continuous process during disasters, initially patients will be received in the triage area with a disaster tag affixed to one limb displaying their priority. These are field categories of relative priority when the patient is initially triaged at the scene. A patient may either improve or deteriorate; thus, on follow-up triage at the facility, recategorization may be necessary. One can assume that patients categorized as "immediate" will require one-to-one nursing care and efficient, continuous, medical and nursing intervention. In multiple casualty incidents with DCC notification of receiving facilities, the ED will often be able to limit the number of "immediate" priority cases that can be safely managed. Under these circumstances, one critical care team per "immediate" patient should be established.

STAFFING THE TEAMS. Each critical care team should consist of the following members:

Physician in charge of the team, experienced in emergency care
Emergency nurse
Emergency technician
Clerk
Transporter

Upon notification of a disaster, the nurse in charge of the department determines how many "immediate" cases may be safely handled in the 30 to 60 minutes after the disaster. The nurse in charge also determines how much staffing will be necessary to meet the need immediately, in 30 minutes, and in 60 minutes after the disaster. At least one critical care team (team No. 1) should be assigned *immediately* from the following:

1. One of the emergency department physicians on duty, *or* one of the third or fourth year surgical residents, *or* a general surgeon from the attending staff
2. One of the emergency department nurses on duty at the time of the disaster
3. One of the emergency technicians
4. Clerks and transporters may be assigned to team No. 1 as they become available

Teams 2, 3, 4, and so on should be established as soon as appropriate staff arrive from home, from the residency staff, and from the attending medical staff. It would not be appropriate to assign nurses who are floated to the emergency department, or to assign medical residents, as the theory and practice of disaster medicine are largely foreign to them. These people might be more effectively utilized to manage the existing patient load (nondisaster patients) in the department.

As specialists in neurosurgery and general surgery arrive from the attending staff, they may be assigned as physicians in charge of a team; however, they will need to be told exactly what is required of them by being given a disaster action card. Assigning these specialists is risky because they may have to leave the team abruptly to operate on a patient; therefore, if used, they should be replaced immediately upon arrival of more emergency department physicians.

FUNCTION OF A CRITICAL CARE TEAM. Disaster action cards must be available for each member of a team. Success of the operation depends upon how quickly the teams are established, how well they understand what their role should be, and how effectively they remain together and work as a team.

The objective of the team is to accept *one*

patient at a time, and to treat and transport their patient to the appropriate in-hospital area. If this concept is to function effectively, the ED cannot expect to handle more "immediate" cases than there are teams available. However, the idea is that each team accepts a patient, performs appropriate and *reasonable* life-saving intervention, and admits the patient either to an operating room or to a critical care unit for further stabilization. The time a patient remains in the ED should be relatively brief, and as soon as disposition is accomplished, the team should return for immediate reassignment to another patient. In mass casualty situations where sufficient teams cannot be generated, each team may need to modify the concept by accepting two patients. The process will remain the same but the team will have to coordinate the care of two patients instead of one. Managing more than two cases would be counter-productive to the purpose of the teams. Under these circumstances, more teams (as many as necessary) should be assembled; staffing needs are obvious, because the teams have a constant staff requirement.

Critical care teams should function according to the points below:

1. A critical care team must remain together until the disaster is resolved and there is no further receipt of patients at the department. Therefore, teams should not disband until the disaster coordinator is advised by the command post that the DCC has declared the disaster operation over and the triage officer has advised the coordinator that no further patients are being processed at the triage area.

2. A team should manage their patient as quickly as possible by evaluating priorities of treatment and accomplishing them as a unit, going as a team with the patient as he is admitted. They will be responsible for all aspects of that patient's care as a team, until after a complete report is given to the physician and nurse receiving the patient in the inpatient area.

3. A team should reassemble *together* for reassignment to another case as quickly as possible.

4. A team should be identified by number, and each member should wear an armband stating *team* and *number*.

5. The physician member will generate the medical treatment orders and serve as principal clinician. The RN or LPN will administer medications, provide critical care nursing, and document. The emergency technicians will provide equipment and supplies and assist the nurse and physician. The clerk will prepare clothing lists and bag clothes and valuables, make certain that laboratory and x-ray requisitions are complete, and make certain that the patient is listed on the disposition log. The transporter will serve as messenger between the disaster coordinator and the team, and in addition will provide safe transport when the patient is admitted. The transporter also delivers specimens and paperwork that the team generates.

Again, in order to function effectively, the ED cannot consider itself as a definitive care unit.

EMERGENCY DEPARTMENT SUPPLIES. Emergency department and hospital supplies could become a major problem in mass casualty events unless provisions are made for access to more than a 30-day supply of materials. Backup for disasters will require sufficient major tray supplies for both the ED and the operating rooms. If supply sources are interrupted between supply house and hospital, the hospital must be able to function for a reasonable period of isolation. Many hospitals maintain sterile supplies, instruments, beds, and so forth in the warehouse to accommodate the additional patient load. Arrangements should be made with local medical supply houses to respond to increased needs in the event that hospital supplies become exhausted. In addition, a simple and rapid inventory system should be utilized by a central supply/service administrator during the entire event to pinpoint dwindling supplies and arrange for procurement before the need is severe or before resupply is impossible. Food and water can become another major consideration, particularly if the disaster condition persists over a period of days, weeks, or months, with hospital staff and patients unable to leave the premises. Contingency plans for food and water priority use may be helpful in extensive disasters.

EMERGENCY DEPARTMENT ANCILLARY SERVICES. Ancillary services vital to the ED during a disaster include laboratory and x-ray, social services, chaplain services, security, dietetics, housekeeping, and public relations. ED personnel will be so thoroughly involved clinically that time will not exist for many of the humanistic concerns of a population struck by disaster. The American Red Cross, who may be strategically involved in both field casualty triage and relocation, in-hospital victim location, and postdisaster ''clean-up'' work involving shelters, epidemic control, immunization services, and psychological support, will require patient updates from the hospital. Press and families will also be concerned about survivors. ED personnel will have little patience and time for these questions and will rely heavily on the social services, chaplain, and public relations people to provide advocacy.

Laboratory and x-ray personnel, who routinely work closely with the ED, will be required to maintain their supplies and staffing, and to make decisions relative to equipment and process that will not compromise the ability of the ED to handle the caseload efficiently. The security force will be vital to containment of treatment areas, direction of the curious and uninjured, protection of staff entrances, and patrol of all unneeded entrances and exits. These officers must be required to *demand* proper identification, or to refuse entry and direct unidentified people to appropriate screening areas. Under disaster circumstances, security officers in uniform are more effective than those in plain clothing.

Finally, sufficient personnel from housekeeping should be assigned to procure extra wheelchairs and gurneys, to patrol the ED to identify potential safety hazards, and to provide a clean environment after each patient is seen.

Careful planning, training, and practice will enable all of these vital service personnel to assist the ED cooperatively and efficiently. Including these services in the development and coordination of the plan will promote and facilitate interdepartmental rapport during a major event.

TRAINING AND DRILLS. Any disaster plan, whether under development or under revision, requires careful training and testing of *everyone* who will be involved. Although the JCAH requries only two drills per year, the actual need for training may far exceed that number. Attitude is extremely important, particularly when interest wanes or when nonchalance occurs. Training (which may not always include actual staged drills) must be constant and include such items as:

1. How and when to activate the plan
2. Where triage and backup supplies, ID bibs, and paperwork are located
3. Locations that will be utilized for patient receipt; what type of patients can be treated in those areas; how to get to those areas.
4. Methods for communication, communication process, and communication documentation
5. Implementation of staff call-in
6. Use of the disaster action cards

Because there is generally very little time between occurrence and receipt of casualties at the hospital, and because communications are so crucial to the response and follow-through, these two areas—implementing the plan and communications—must be stressed to all staff members consistently. Once a month is not too often: disaster response can be integrated into new employee orientation and staff in-services. The idea is to avoid complacency. Many ED experts agree that having a plan is not enough; continual testing and evaluation will point out deficiencies time and time again. The plan must be tested and revised as often as deficiencies are obvious, and upon revision, retesting of the changes should be conducted. A well-known learning maxim is ''When I hear it I forget it, when I'm shown it I will remember 50% of the time, but when I do it I never forget.'' Thus, the staff should have frequent opportunities to perform as though a disaster has occurred, with process recorders in the background doing nothing other than taking notes about the proceedings for discussion and evaluation in the postdrill critique. The goal in any drill must be that all personnel learn to function as effectively as possible in disasters both internal and external to the hospital. Drills that incorporate "scenarios" and mulaged "patients" may be helpful once or twice a year, but may be counterproductive when a plan has just been developed or is newly revised. There is some argument for realism, but realism for the sake of catching people unaware will negate any careful evaluation or training relative to a plan that is newly developed or revised. Further, realistic drills in which casualties are mulaged to reveal injuries tend to develop a circus air and are unfortunately prone to fragmentation of care for the true ED patients. If the purpose of the drill is to educate staff, test plans, and identify areas for improvement, it should not attempt absolute realism. On the other hand, once the plan is fully developed and staff members know how to function within it, realistic drills ensure comprehensive rehearsals. Any risk to the public during realistic drills must be minimized, with safety procedures clearly delineated. After every drill and true disaster there will always be a need for the personnel involved to give their input regarding the experience. It is through continual critique that needs are identified and resolutions to problems developed. From that critique, establish a program to address the problem areas and set a timetable; otherwise another incident might occur before changes have been made and tested. Any time that changes are made, the staff must be retrained and other departments must be advised. Once retraining is accomplished, the staff should be redrilled step by step.

In all, this process requires a significant investment of time and resources. Even so, it cannot be overlooked or ignored, for not being prepared when a disaster strikes is a disaster in itself, and contrary to the hospital's philosophy of responsiveness to the needs of the local community.

POSTDISASTER CONSIDERATIONS

The aftermath of a disaster will depend on the extent and duration of the disaster itself.

In major events in which hundreds or thousands of survivors are homeless and there has been extensive damage to cities, the immediate aftermath period will entail survivor relocation in shelters, emergency sanitation, and procurement of sufficient food and water. The American Red Cross and Civil Defense will be integrally involved in providing these elements. All citizens, however, should know how to prepare water that may be contaminated and convert it into drinkable fluid. Many people might have to await rescue for several days or even weeks, and this knowledge will help them survive until they are located and evacuated. (See boxed material on p. 677.)

Natural or nuclear disaster preplanning for the householder*

1. *Have a 2-week supply of stored water* (7 gallons per person). Do not forget the water in an undamaged water heater, storage tanks of the toilet, ice cubes in the refrigerator, and so on.
2. Have a 2-week supply of food—preferably food stored in cans that requires little water for preparation, or heating, or refrigeration. (Most canned items have greater than a 12-month safe shelf life).
3. Have a portable radio, and contact your local emergency services or disaster office now for the dial location of the Emergency Broadcasting Station in your area.
4. *Have two working flashlights and extra batteries* stored in refrigerator to prolong use.
5. *Have at least a quart of household clothes bleach such as Clorox (5.25% sodium hypochlorite) for purifying drinking water.*
6. *Know the location of the gas shut-off, water shut-off, and electrical power shut-off and how to shut down these utilities if necessary.* Have the proper tools available to accomplish these tasks. Candles should be used with caution.
7. *Have an extra supply of special foods and medications if such items are needed by a member of the household.*
8. *Have a 2-week supply of paper plates, cups, towels, and plastic utensils to conserve what water is available for drinking.* And don't forget to have a can-opener available that does not require electricity to operate.
9. *Have one metal waste can with a tight-fitting*

---

*Prepared by California Medical Association Committee on Disaster Medical Care, December 1978, San Francisco.

cover to store human waste until sewage facilities are restored. Keep a supply of plastic bag liners and ties to fit the waste can.

10. *Do not use your telephone immediately after the disaster unless absolutely necessary.*
11. *Have an adequate basic first-aid kid and a Red Cross first-aid handbook available.* Take training now in first aid.
12. *Know the location of your nearest hospital and nuclear attack shelter.*
13. *Preplan how to reunite the family after a major disaster.*
14. *Contact your local disaster office for more specific literature on earthquakes, floods, landslides, fires, air pollution, and nuclear attacks or accidents.*
15. Where it would prove useful, keep a shovel, axe, and matches.

Obtaining safe drinking water.* Public water supplies, protected for everyday use, may be unavailable in a disaster. If the supplies are shut off, water may become contaminated with typhoid, desentery, or infectious hepatitis.

EMERGENCY SOURCES. At home, limited supplies may be obtained from ice trays, toilets, hot water tank (toilet water must be purified). Outdoors, avoid surface sources such as ponds and lakes. Avoid water with dark color, odor, or floating materials. If surface water is used, obtain it from upstream source, dipped below surface, and purified. Try to use underground

---

*From the United States Department of Health, Education, and Welfare.

To purify water*

Heat
Strain water to remove debris.
Boil vigorously 1 full minute.
Cool.
Pinch of salt may help improve taste.

Chemicals
Strain water to remove debris.
Use liquid chlorine bleach or tincture of iodine as directed below.

	Drops per quart	
Available amount	Clean water	Cloudy water
Chlorine*		
1%	10	20
4% to 6% (common household bleach)	2	4
7% to 10%	1	2
If not known	10	20
Tincture of iodine†		
2%	5	10

*Let stand for 30 minutes. A slight chlorine odor should be detectable; if not repeat dosage and let stand 15 minutes more.
†Let stand 30 minutes.

Keep all purified water in clean, closed containers that are noncorrodible. With careful rationing, 7 gallons of water per person for drinking and food preparation can last 2 weeks. This amount will *not* allow for hygienic use.

---

*Adapted from a United States Department of Health, Education, and Welfare bulletin.

source if possible (well or spring); if not, look next for a creek or running stream instead of stagnant water.

Hazards

Postdisaster hazards that must be addressed include the spread of infectious disease, danger from hazardous chemicals and materials, starvation, and psychological crises. Mass immunization may become a necessity, and hospitals that develop disaster plans should identify a mechanism for mobilizing such supplies in the event that they are needed. Hospital epidemiology teams should also have plans for assisting the community if epidemic control becomes necessary. Finally, mental health services in every community should be aware of the psychological consequences of disasters, and be prepared to assist in meeting the needs of the victims and survivors in coping with the catastrophe and with the disruption of reality as they knew it.

Nurses who are involved in the management of casualties or in the management of survivors who are relocated into shelters will find that a redefinition of health care roles will occur. There will be a need to attend to sudden large numbers of people with multiple demands and needs, and a resulting expansion of the nursing role will develop. Physicians and nurses will rely on each other to address the medical, psychological, and welfare needs of the survivors and to evaluate the plan while engaged in action. Much of the actual nursing care will have to be delegated to less skilled and less knowledgeable persons, while nurses supervise their actions and teach them proper methods. Improvisation will require imagination and ingenuity, because supplies and resources will be limited. There is no question that a major reorganization and restructuring of the generally acceptable health manpower chain would become a necessity if the overpowering needs of the population affected by a major, large-scale disaster are to be addressed. Volunteers can be a major asset, and if they have had prior training in the principles and concepts of disaster plans, it will be much easier to allocate them to areas where they are needed. Indeed, survivors who are not physically disabled can effectively give assistance under supervision of health professionals. Often this activity will provide for a validation of the one thing that is left—self-respect—and will help prevent personal panic. The hard truth is that the aftermath of a disaster can be filled with difficult trials. It is a stressful time in which health professionals will need to intensify their leadership abilities while remaining as calm as they can.

SUMMARY

Disaster aspects of nursing involve a great number of considerations, including preplanning, immediate survival, management of great numbers of victims, and the potential problems in the days and weeks following a major catastrophe. The intricacies are very exciting to anyone who is willing to take the time to become involved in planning for an effective response, but these same intricacies predispose to alarm, confusion, and chaos unless there is intelligent and thoughtful direction during actual situations. Knowing what to expect is half the battle, because even though each disaster situation contains inherent differences, an awareness of the plan for action lends a great deal of stability to one's behavior. Disaster preparedness will vary depending on the population, geographic area, and culture, but the needs of the victims and survivors are basically the same, namely, first aid and evacuation, medical and nursing attention, psychological support, and shelter, food, and water.

Both the citizenry and the health profession must have plans for action, which can only be developed after accepting the possibility and anticipating the response. Public education is vital to developing public awareness and subsequently developing adaptive behavior. Nursing and medical disaster awareness can begin in the basic training curricula. The health profession has an obligation to psychologically and professionally prepare themselves for the potential of a disaster incident, and to become involved in the development and implementation of effective disaster plans.

BIBLIOGRAPHY

Department of Health, Education, and Welfare report, unpublished 1978.

Draback, and Baggs. In Perry, R.: Evacuation decision-making in natural disasters, Mass Emergencies **4:**25-37, March 1979.

Glass, A.: The psychological aspects of emergency situations. In Psychological aspects of stress, Springfield, Ill. 1970, pp. 64-7.

Guiffrida, L.: Training for trouble, Emergency **11:**41-48, October 1979.

MacDonald, J.: Principles of field triage, Disaster seminar, 1978, Long Beach, Calif.

Perry, R.: Evacuation decision-making in natural disasters, Mass Emergencies **4:**25-37, March 1979.

Richman, L.: Procedural guidelines for a triage officer, Los Angeles County Medical Association Bulletin December 1977.

State of California, Office of Emergency Services, Disaster Medical Procedures, unpublished draft, 1979.

Whitcraft, D.: A new system for hospital disaster assignments, Memorial Hospital of Long Beach, Calif., 1977, Unpublished paper.

ADDITIONAL READINGS

Accreditation Manual for Hospitals, Joint Commission on Accreditation for Hospitals.

ANA Committee on Nursing in National Defense: Nursing in disasters, Am. J. Nurs. **60**(8):1130-1133, 1960.

Austin, M.: Disaster management—coping with a catastrophe, Nurs. Times **70:**1880-1883, December 1974.

Bradley, J.: Nurse management during the bombing crisis in Birmingham, Nurs. Times July 1975, pp. 1186-1188.

Charlesworth, D.: Rescue, South African Nurs. J. **40:**24, 1973.

Cross, R.: The team approach to disaster care, J.E.N. **3:** 17-19, Nov/Dec 1977.

DeDominicis, C.: Crisis on the island, Emerg. Prod. News November 1977, pp. 41-43.

Fisher, C.: Mobile triage team in a community disaster plan, J.A.C.E.P.**6:**21-23, 1977.

Frederick, C.: Psychological first aid: emergency mental health and disaster assistance, Invited paper, National Institute of Health, unknown origin.

Gierson, E., and Richman, L.: Valley triage: an approach to mass casualty care, J. Trauma **15:**193-196, March 1975.

Harvey, E.: Disaster at moorgate, Nurs. Times **11:**1226-1227, July 1975.

Herst, W.: Disaster planning, Nurs. Times **70:**186-189, February 1974.

Holdman, P.: Nuclear accident, Newsweek April 9, 1979, pp. 24-36.

Hoyle, J.: The Beverly Hills Club disaster, Emerg. Med. Serv. **6**(4):50-56, 1977.

Hudson, L.: Heroes of the Johnstown Flood, Family Weekly September 1977, pp. 12-14.

In Time of an Emergency, Department of Defense bulletin, March 1968.

Mahoney, R.: Emergency disaster nursing, New York, 1967, MacMillan Publishing Co., Inc.

Neal, M.: Disaster and mass casualty nursing, Nurs. Outlook **8:**225, April 1960.

Newell, P.: Nurses at work, Aust. Nurs. J. **3**(16):16, 1974.

Patterson, C.: Explosion! A case study in disaster drills, J.E.N. **3:**9-16, Nov/Dec 1977.

Quake Guidelines for MD's: Los Angeles County Medical Association Bulletin, January, 1977.

Rosenblum, E.: What would you do in a disaster? Nurs. Times **6:**72-73, 1976.

Schulberg, H.: Picking up the pieces. . . intervening in disaster situations, Nurs. Dig. **3:**50-52, July/August 1975.

Simoneau, J.: Quake guidelines for RNs, Calif. Nurse July/August 1978.

Simoneau, J.: Role of the nurse in disasters, California Medical Association workshop on disasters, 1978.

Soffer, A.: War in Sinai—nursing care of the critically wounded, Heart Lung 3(3):385-389, 1974.

Theoret, J.: How a community hospital emergency department copes with a massive blizzard, Mass Emerg. **14:** 1-9, March 1979.

What to do in a disaster, Los Angeles County Medical Association Bulletin December, 1977.

Wiener, P.: Setting up an external disaster procedure, Hosp. Topics **54:**22-25, 1976.

Wilkins, E. W.: Massachusetts General Hospital textbook of emergency medicine, Baltimore, 1978, Williams and Wilkins, Co., p. 745.

Zschoche, D.: Radiological accidents, Crit. Care Update! April 1975.

APPENDICES

APPENDICES

Joint Commission on Accreditation of Hospitals requirements for emergency services*

Principle: Any individual who comes to the hospital for emergency medical evaluation or initial treatment shall be properly assessed by qualified individuals, and appropriate services shall be rendered within the defined capability of the hospital.

STANDARD I

A well-defined plan for emergency care, based on community need and on the capability of the hospital, shall be implemented by every hospital.

Interpretation

The hospital and its medical staff shall promote, help to develop, and implement a community-based emergency plan. Whenever feasible, all hospitals in a community that offer emergency medical services should make a joint effort to identify the readiness of each hospital and its staff to receive and treat emergency patients effectively. From such community planning, emergency medical service resources may be classified by capability. In any case, each hospital shall evaluate and classify itself to indicate its capability in providing emergency medical services to the community served. Classification shall be based on the overall capability of the hospital and its medical staff to meet the needs of the community.

The hospital must have some procedure

*From Joint Commission on Accreditation of Hospitals, Accreditation manual for hospitals, Chicago, The Commission.

whereby the ill or injured person can be assessed and either treated or referred to an appropriate facility, as indicated. A hospital's emergency service shall be classified according to the level of the services provided. Regardless of the nomenclature assigned, the levels vary from emergency services that are comprehensive to those of a first aid/referral level. The requisite staffing, facilities, and services shall be provided as delineated in this section of the *Manual.*

Specific and general requirements are established for four levels of emergency services. Other comparable classifications, such as state or regional, shall be considered acceptable, and the hospital shall be evaluated for compliance at the appropriate level.

It is recognized that hospitals may offer critical therapeutic services in specialized clinical areas such as spinal cord injury, burns, trauma, and so forth. Such hospitals shall be considered as providing comprehensive (Level I) services for the specific clinical focus of care, while the emergency services otherwise provided shall be evaluated at the appropriate level.

Level I. A Level I emergency service offers

comprehensive emergency care 24 hours a day, with at least one physician experienced in emergency care on duty in the emergency care area. There shall be in-hospital physician coverage for at least medical, surgical, orthopedic, obstetrical/gynecological, pediatric, and anesthesiology services by members of the medical staff or by senior-level residents, with other specialty consultation available within 30 minutes, as needed. The hospital's scope of services shall include in-house capabilities for managing physical and related emotional problems on a definitive basis. The above requirements apply to a comprehensive-level emergency service provided by a hospital offering care only to a limited group of patients, such as pediatric, obstetrical, ophthalmological, and orthopedic.

Level II. A Level II emergency service offers emergency care 24 hours a day, with at least one physician experienced in emergency care on duty in the emergency care area, and specialty consultation available within 30 minutes by members of the medical staff or by senior-level residents. The hospital's scope of services shall include in-house capabilities for managing physical and related emotional problems, with provision for patient transfer to another facility when needed.

Level III. A Level III emergency service offers emergency care 24 hours a day, with at least one physician available to the emergency care area within 30 minutes through a medical staff call roster. Specialty consultation shall be available by request of the attending medical staff member or by transfer to a designated hospital where definitive care can be provided.

Level IV. A Level IV emergency service offers reasonable care in determining whether an emergency exists, renders lifesaving first aid, and makes appropriate referral to the nearest facilities that have the capability of providing needed services. The mechanism for providing physician coverage at all times shall be defined by the medical staff.

Patient transfer. Transfer of patients shall be made in accordance with the community-based hospital emergency plan. A hospital providing emergency care shall be capable of instituting essential lifesaving measures and implementing emergency procedures that will minimize further compromise of the condition of any infant, child, or adult being transported.

When a patient is transferred, all pertinent medical information shall accompany the patient. Unless extenuating circumstances are documented in the patient's record, no patient shall be arbitrarily transferred to another hospital if the hospital where he is initially seen has the means for providing adequate care. The patient shall not be transferred until the receiving hospital or facility has consented to accept the patient, and the patient is considered sufficiently stabilized for transport. Responsibility for the patient during transfer shall be established.

Identifying signs. Appropriate signs, consistent with applicable law, shall indicate the direction of the hospital from major thoroughfares, and whether it is designated as a specialized emergency care center. The location of the emergency access area shall also be identified by clearly visible signs.

Disaster plans. The role of the emergency service in the hospital's internal and external disaster plans shall be consistent with the capabilities of the hospital and community served. For requirements of the hospital's disaster plans, refer to the Functional Safety and Sanitation section of this *Manual*.

External communication. There shall be a communication system, such as radio-telephone or other appropriate means, that permits instant contact with law enforcement agencies, rescue squads, and other emergency services within the community, to provide advance information concerning critically ill or injured patients.

Where required frequently in the emergency care area, there should be a means of communicating in the language of the predominant population groups served by the hospital emergency service.

STANDARD II

The emergency service shall be well organized, properly directed, and staffed according to the nature and extent of health care needs anticipated and the scope of services offered.

Interpretation

The relationship of the emergency service to other units and departments/services of the hospital shall be specified within the overall hospital organizational plan. The responsibility and accountability of the emergency service to the medical staff and hospital administration shall be defined in writing.

Direction. The emergency service shall be directed by a physician member of the active medical staff. A deputy director or other qualified physician member of the medical staff shall be designated and authorized to perform the functions of the director when he is unavailable. The director, the deputy director, or other qualified physician in charge of a Level I or Level II emergency service shall have at least three years of training and/or experience in a specialty appropriate (as determined by the medical staff) to the care and treatment of emergency patients. The director shall have the authority and responsibility for carrying out established policies, and for providing overall direction in the continuing operation of the service. The director shall assure that the quality, safety, and appropriateness of emergency patient care are evaluated, and the appropriate action based on the findings of review activities is taken. The credentials files of the director, deputy director, and all other practitioners with emergency service privileges shall reflect their training and experience, as well as evidence of current competence. The director of a Level I emergency service or his deputy or qualified physician designee shall be readily available. Except under unusual circumstances, the position of the director shall be held on a full-time basis.

Direction of a Level III emergency service may be provided by a physician member of the medical staff or through a multidisciplinary medical staff committee, with the chairman of the committee serving as director of the emergency service.

Medical staff coverage. The method of providing medical staff coverage shall be defined. Acceptable methods include the use of house staff under adequate medical staff supervision; the use of contract groups whose members must be members of the medical staff, unless otherwise provided by law; or assumption of such coverage by medical staff members. When the medical staff has assumed the responsibility, its members shall have an obligation for emergency room coverage as determined by the medical staff, each in accordance with his clinical competence and privileges. Specialists in limited practice shall be available on an established schedule for consultation and special services in response to the needs of the emergency patient. When physicians are employed for only brief periods of time, such as evenings, weekends, or holidays, their professional and personal qualifications shall be evaluated through the established medical staff credentialing mechanism to assure appropriate licensure, privilege delineation, staff categorization, and approval by the governing body. For medical staff membership requirements, refer to Standard I of the Medical Staff section of this *Manual*.

The degree of evaluation and treatment rendered to any patient who presents himself or is brought to the emergency care area shall be the responsibility of a physician. The priority with which persons seeking emergency care will be seen by a physician may be determined by specially trained personnel using guidelines established by the emergency service director and approved by the medical staff. Rosters designating medical staff members on duty or on call for primary coverage and specialty consultation shall be posted in the emergency care area.

Nursing service coverage. A designated registered nurse who is qualified by relevant training, experience, and current competence in emergency care shall supervise the care provided by all nursing service personnel within the emergency service. Level I and Level II emergency services shall have at least one registered nurse and a sufficient number of other nursing service personnel permanently assigned and on duty within the emergency service area at all times. The number of nursing service personnel shall be sufficient for the types and volume of patients served. A Level III emergency service shall have a registered nurse available at least on an on-call, in-house basis at all times. The emergency nurse supervisor or head nurse shall participate in committee activities concerned with the emergency service.

Other staff coverage. When emergency medical technicians or other allied health personnel are used, their duties and their responsibilities to physicians and nurses providing care within the emergency service area shall be defined in writing. Other staff disciplines shall be available as required.

STANDARD III

The emergency service shall be appropriately integrated with other units and departments of the hospital.

Interpretation

Laboratory services. Level I, Level II, and Level III emergency services shall have readily available at all times clinical laboratory services with the capability of performing all routine studies and standard analyses of blood, urine, and other body fluids. In addition laboratory services supporting Level I and Level II emergency services shall provide arterial blood gas and pH determinations, coagulation studies, serum and urine osmolality, microbiological studies, and, as required, toxicological studies. An adequate supply of blood shall be available at all times, either in-hospital or from an outside source approved by the medical staff. The hospital must provide for blood typing and cross-matching capability, and for blood storage facilities that are readily available to the emergency service.

Radiology services. Diagnostic radiology services shall be readily available at all times to provide routine studies using both fixed and mobile equipment. For Level I and Level II emergency services, angiography of all types, sonography, and nuclear scanning shall be readily available, as needed.

Operating suite special requirements. Level I emergency services shall have prompt access, as needed, to operating suites that have the following capabilities: cardiopulmonary bypass pump oxygenator; operating micro-

scope; thermal control equipment for the patient and for blood; fracture table; roentgenographic equipment, including image intensifier: endoscopes, all varieties; craniotomy equipment; electrocardiograph-oscilloscope-defibrillator; pacemaker insertion capability; mechanical ventilator; and equipment for monitoring direct blood pressure, temperature, blood flow rate, and respirations. It is essential that appropriate surgical specialists and anesthesiology and operating room personnel be in-house and available within a few minutes.

Level II emergency services shall have prompt access to operating suites with the following capabilities: thermal control equipment for the patient and for blood, fracture table, appropriate endoscopic equipment, electrocardiograph-oscilloscope-defibrillator, mechanical ventilator, and temperature-monitoring equipment. Roentgenographic equipment shall be readily available.

Other services. Depending on the level of emergency service provided, there shall be access to the obstetrical suite and special care units.

Other manual references. For other requirements related to emergency services, refer to the following section of this *Manual:* Anesthesia Services, Building and Grounds Safety, Functional Safety and Sanitation, Infection Control, Medical Record Services, Medical Staff, Nuclear Medicine Services, Nursing Services, Pathology and Medical Laboratory Services, Pharmaceutical Services, Radiology Services, and Social Work Services.

STANDARD IV

All personnel shall be prepared for their emergency care responsibilities through appropriate training and education programs.

Interpretation

Orientation program. A planned, formal training program shall be required for all registered and licensed nurses, and for specified professional personnel who provide patient care in the emergency service. When there is no in-house capability of providing this training, a qualified outside source of instruction shall be substituted. The program shall be acceptable to the physician director of the emergency service, or to the committee of the medical staff when there is no director, and to the director of the nursing service. The orientation program shall be of sufficient duration and substance to cover all patient care responsibilities related to each individual's level of participation in the emergency service. The program shall include training in:

- Recognition, interpretation, and recording of patient's signs and symptoms, particularly those that require notification of a physician;
- Initiation of cardiopulmonary resuscitation and other related life-support procedures;
- Parenteral administration of electrolytes, fluids, blood and blood components;
- Wound care and management of sepsis;
- Initial burn care;
- Initial management of injuries to the extremities and central nervous system;
- Effective and safe use of electrical and electronic life-support and other equipment used in the emergency service;
- Prevention of contamination and cross infection; and
- Recognition of and attention to the psychological and social needs of patients and their families.

Continuing education program. All emergency service personnel shall participate in relevant in-service education programs. The director or his qualified designees shall contribute to the in-service education of emergency service personnel. In-service education shall include safety and infection control requirements as described in this *Manual.* Cardiopulmonary resuscitation training shall be conducted as often as necessary for all physicians, nurses, and specified professional personnel who work in the emergency care area.

The hospital administration shall assure that there are opportunities for physicians, nurses, and, as required, other personnel to participate in emergency service continuing education programs outside the hospital, as needed. Education programs for emergency service personnel

shall be based at least in part on the results of emergency care evaluation studies. The extent of participation shall be documented, and shall be realistically related to the size of the staff and to the scope and complexity of the emergency care services provided.

STANDARD V

Emergency patient care shall be guided by written policies and procedures.

Interpretation

There shall be written policies and procedures specifying the scope and conduct of patient care to be rendered in the emergency service. Such policies and procedures must be approved by the medical staff and hospital administration, and shall be reviewed at least annually, revised as necessary, dated to indicate time of the last review, and enforced. The policies and procedures in Level I, Level II, and Level III emergency services and, as appropriate, in Level IV emergency services, shall relate to at least the following:

- Location, storage, and procurement of medications, blood, supplies, and equipment at all times.
- Provision of care to an unemancipated minor not accompanied by parent or guardian, or to an unaccompanied unconscious patient.
- Circumstances under which the patient's personal physician is to be notified or given reports.
- Confidentiality of patient information and the safeguarding of records.
- Release of authorized information and materials to police or health authorities.
- Transfer and discharge of patients.
- The emergency medical record, including any consent for treatment.
- Infection control measures, including procedures for eliminating the possibility of contamination and cross infection.
- Procedures to be followed in the event of equipment failure.
- Pertinent safety practices.
- Control of traffic, including visitors.
- Dispensing of medications in accordance

with the requirements of the Pharmaceutical Services section of this *Manual*.

- The handling and safekeeping of patients' valuables.
- The role of the emergency service in the hospital disaster plans.
- Specification of the scope of treatment allowed, including general and specific procedures that may not be performed by medical staff members in the emergency service, and the use of anesthesia.
- Who, other than physicians, may perform special procedures, under what circumstances, and under what degree of supervision. Such procedures include, but are not limited to, cardiopulmonary resuscitation, including cardiac defibrillation; endotracheal intubation; tracheostomy or cricothyrotomy; respiratory care, including assisted ventilation and humidification; the administration of parenteral antiarrhythmic and other specified medications; and the obtaining of arterial and venous blood samples and other laboratory specimens.
- The use of standing orders.
- The property exchange system, when necessitated by the transportation and transfer of patients.
- Circumstances that require the patient to return to the emegency service for treatment.
- The emergency management of individuals who have actual or suspected exposure to radiation or who are radioactively contaminated. Such action may include radioactivity monitoring and measurement; designation and any required preparation of space for evaluation of the patient, including, as required, discontinuation of the air circulation system to prevent the spread of contamination; decontamination of the patient through an appropriate cleansing mechanism; and containment, labeling, and disposition of contaminated materials. The individual responsible for radiation safety should be notified.
- Alleged or suspected rape, or sexual molestation. Criteria for an adequate medicolegal evaluation should include examination and treatment; required patient consent; collection, retention, and safeguarding of specimens, photographs, and other evidentiary material, maintaining a detailed receipt for all material released; and, as legally required, notification of, and release of information to, the proper authorities. Examination of and consultation with the patient shall take place only when visual and auditory privacy are assured.
- Alleged or suspected child abuse. Criteria for alerting emergency service personnel to the possibility of child abuse should be developed. Pertinent information may be obtained from the history, physical examination, laboratory and radiological tests, photographs, and observations of parent/child interactions. In addition to such information, the medical record should document the treatment given, and any required reporting to the proper authorities.
- The management of pediatric emergencies.
- Individuals dead on arrival, and any legally required collection and preservation of evidence, and reporting to the proper authorities.
- The management of patients who are under the influence of drugs or alcohol, or who are emotionally ill or become difficult to manage.
- The initial management of patients with burns, hand injuries, head injuries, fractures, multiple injuries, poisoning, animal bites, gunshot and stab wounds, and other acute problems.
- Precautions to be taken in preventing the occurrence of accidents to unconscious or irrational patients.
- Tetanus and rabies prevention/prophylaxis.

Current toxicologic reference materials and antidote information shall be readily available within the emergency service, along with the telephone number of the regional poison control information center. A list of referral and consultation services shall be prominently displayed and shall include, as appropriate, the regional coordinating office for radiological emergency assistance, antivenin service, county coroner or medical examiner, police department state and local health departments, ambulance transport and rescue services, tissue donation centers, and special care services not provided by the hospital.

STANDARD VI

The emergency service shall be designed and equipped to facilitate the safe and effective care of patients.

Interpretation

The emergency care area shall be easily accessible from within the hospital to permit rapid admission of patients treated initially in the emergency service. The emergency service should be in proximity to the emergency entrance, on the same level at which patients are transported to the area. The entrance shall be clearly identified externally, and shall be accessible to emergency vehicles and pedestrian traffic. If a separate approach is provided for ambulatory patients, any differences in levels shall be bridged by a ramp rather than by steps. All emergency service entrance doors shall be well lighted and protected from the weather. Entrance doors shall be wide enough to accommodate patients, attendants, and equipment. Stretchers and wheelchairs should be stored immediately adjacent to the emergency service entrance and should not obstruct entry. A waiting area, telephone, and lavatory facilities should be available to patients seeking emergency medical care and to individuals accompanying them. Unauthorized individuals shall be prohibited from entering the treatment and work areas of the emergency service.

The design of the emergency service area shall facilitate the visual and auditory privacy of the patients, without compromising patient care. Sufficient space shall be provided for the examination and treatment of patients seeking emergency care, particularly for the management of patients with life-threatening conditions.

Observation beds. When observation beds are permitted, there shall be guidelines for the type of patient use, the maximum time period of use, the mechanism for providing constant surveillance, and the type of nurse/patient call system. Use of an observation bed should ordinarily be limited to less than twelve hours for any one patient.

Internal communication. When warranted by the size and sophistication of the emergency care area, an intercommunication/alarm system shall be provided between the nurses' station and any examination, treatment, or other areas from which additional personnel may need to be summoned in an emergency. Rapid communications with other departments in the hospital must be assured.

Special provisions. When indicated, examination rooms, such as rooms for gynecological, ophthalmologic, orthopedic, or pediatric patients, should be provided. When general anesthesia is administered in the emergency service, the anesthesia area shall meet the requirements of the National Fire Protection Association standards (NFPA publication 56A, 1973) and the Anesthesia Services section of this *Manual*. Protective security may be requried in the care of combative or emotionally disturbed patients.

Equipment and supplies. Equipment and supplies used in the emergency service shall be of the same quality as those used throughout the hospital and shall be suitable for all sizes of patients treated. Equipment shall be checked on a scheduled basis in accordance with the hospital preventive maintenance program and the requirements of the Functional Safety and Sanitation section of this *Manual*.

At least the following shall be readily available for use within Level I and Level II emergency services and, as appropriate, Level III and Level IV emergency services:
- Oxygen and the means of administration;
- Mechanical ventilatory assistance equipment, including airways, manual breathing bag, and ventilator;
- Cardiac defibrillator with synchronization capability;
- Respiratory and cardiac monitoring equipment;
- Thoracentesis and closed thoracostomy sets;
- Tracheostomy set;
- Tourniquets;
- Vascular cutdown sets;

- Laryngoscopes and endotracheal tubes;
- Tracheobronchial and gastric suction equipment;
- Urinary catheters with closed volume urinary systems;
- Pleural and pericardial drainage set;
- Minor surgical instruments;
- Splinting devices; and
- Emergency obstetrical pack.

Standard drugs, antivenin (in geographic areas as indicated), common poison antidotes, syringes and needles, parenteral fluids and infusion sets, plasma substitutes and blood administration sets, and surgical supplies must be available for immediate use. Emergency drug carts or emergency drug storage areas shall be checked by an appropriate individual at least once per shift and after each use to assure that all items required for immediate availability are actually contained in the cart and are in usable condition. This requirement may be met by a system designed to assure continued integrity of the contents between periods of use. Uniformity in the arrangement of supplies is recommended to facilitate rapid implementation of emergency care. There shall be refrigerated storage for biologicals and all other supplies requiring such storage within the emergency service.

Examination tables shall be stable, should lock, and should be adjustable to required positions. Stretchers and examination tables that can be penetrated by X rays are recommended. Side rails and safety straps should be available.

STANDARD VII

A medical record shall be maintained on every patient seeking emergency care and shall be incorporated into the patient's permanent hospital record. A control register shall adequately identify all persons seeking emergency care.

Interpretation

Emergency medical record. All prior pertinent inpatient and outpatient medical record documentation, including previous visits to the emergency service, shall, whenever possible, be made available when requested by the attending physician or other authorized individuals. For each visit to the emergency service, the medical record shall contain documentation relating to the following:

- Patient identification. When not obtainable, the reason shall be entered in the medical record.
- Time and means of arrival.
- Pertinent history of the illness or injury, and physical findings, including the patient's vital signs.
- Emergency care given to the patient prior to arrival.
- Diagnostic and therapeutic orders.
- Clinical observations, including results of treatment.
- Reports of procedures, tests, and results.
- Diagnostic impression.
- Conclusion at the termination of evaluation/treatment, including final disposition, the patient's condition on discharge or transfer, and any instructions given to the patient and/or family for follow-up care.
- A patient's leaving aginst medical advice.

The medical record shall be authenticated by the practitioner who is responsible for its clinical accuracy.

It is recommended that the ambulance record of the patient be available to the practitioner providing emergency care and that it be filed with, but not necessarily as part of, the patient's record.

Control register. A control register shall be continuously maintained, and shall include at least the following information for every individual seeking care: identification, such as name, age, sex; date, time, and means of arrival; nature of the complaint; disposition; and time of departure. The names of individuals dead on arrival shall also be entered in the register. Information obtained from the register may aid in planning staffing for the emergency service, and can be used as a guide in selecting records for the evaluation of the quality and appropriateness of services provided. Information obtained from the register may also be used in appropriate institutional planning of health care services based on community need.

STANDARD VIII

The quality and appropriateness of patient care provided in the emergency service shall be continuously reviewed, evaluated, and assured through establishment of quality control mechanisms.

Interpretation

The director of the emergency service or the chairman of the emergency care committee shall be responsible for assuring that a timely review of emergency patient care is performed and documented. The review shall be performed at least monthly, and shall involve the use of the medical record and preestablished criteria. When there is rapid turnover of physician personnel, as in the case of medical staff rotation or the use of part-time physician coverage, it is recommended that a review be performed more frequently. Particular attention shall be given to the review of individuals who are dead on arrival and those who die in the emergency service area or within 24 hours of admission from the emergency service. Periodic conferences on the management of trauma and other aspects of emergency care are recommended for pertinent medical staff and nursing service personnel to identify and review any areas that require strengthening in the emergency team effort.

At least the following quality control mechanisms shall be established:

- When authorized, a copy of the record of emergency services rendered shall be available to the private practitioner or medical facility responsible for follow-up care.
- There shall be a timely review of X rays, with the official interpretation available to the private practitioner and to the practitioner providing emergency care. There shall be a mechanism for notifying and recalling patients who require additional radiologic studies or for whom a more definitive radiologic interpretaiton has been made.
- Reports of laboratory test results shall be available in a timely manner to the private practitioner and to the practitioner providing emergency care. There shall be a mechanism for notifying and recalling patients who require additional or repeat laboratory studies.
- Interpretation of electrocardiograms by physicians with such privileges shall be available to the private practitioner and to the practitioner providing emergency care. There shall be a mechanism for notifying and recalling patients who require additional electrocardiographic studies.
- Patient transfer shall be carried out safely and in accordance with written transfer protocol.
- Emergency service patients who receive blood transfusions shall be included in the medical staff's review of blood utilization.
- Emergency service patients who receive antibiotics shall be included in the medical staff's review of the clinical use of antibiotics.
- Emergency medical records of the previous 24 hours should, when possible, be reviewed daily on at least a representative sample basis by the medical director or his designee to assess the adequacy of the services rendered and of the documentation.
- Surgical specimens removed from patients in the emergency care area shall be sent to the pathologist for examination, except for those specimens that for legal reasons are given directly in the chain of custody to law enforcement representatives.

Normal laboratory values*

Many of the normal values are based on the experience in the Department of Pathology, Mount Sinai Hospital, Chicago, Illinois, and the Division of Clinical Pathology, State University Hospital, State University of New York, Syracuse, New York. Actual values may vary with different techniques or in different laboratories. Although only the more common tests are discussed in the text, others are included here for completeness.

Abbreviations used in tables

<	= less then	mIU	= milliInternational Unit
>	= greater than	mOsm	= milliosmole
dl	= 100 ml	mμ	= millimicron
gm	= gram	ng	= nanogram
IU	= International Unit	pg	= picogram
kg	= kilogram	μEq	= microequivalent
mEq	= milliequivalent	μg	= microgram
ml	= milliliter	μIU	= microInternational Unit
mM	= millimole	μl	= microliter
mm Hg	= millimeters of mercury	μU	= microunit

---

*Reproduced with permission from Davidsohn, I., and Henry, J. B., editors: Todd-Sanford Clinical diagnosis by laboratory methods, ed. 15, Philadelphia, 1974, W. B. Saunders Co.

Table B-1. Whole blood, serum, and plasma (chemistry)

Test	Material	Normal value	Special instructions
Acetoacetic acid			
Qualitative	Serum	Negative	
Quantitative	Serum	0.2-1.0 mg/dl	
Acetone			
Qualitative	Serum	Negative	
Quantitative	Serum	0.3-2.0 mg/dl	
Albumin, quantitative	Serum	3.2-4.5 gm/dl (salt fractionation)	
		3.2-5.6 gm/dl by electrophoresis	
		3.8-5.0 gm/dl by dye binding	
Alcohol	Serum or whole blood	Negative	
Aldolase	Serum	Adults: 3-8 Sibley-Lehninger U/dl at 37° C	
		Children: Approximately 2 times adult levels	
		Newborn: Approximately 4 times adult levels	
Alpha-amino acid nitrogen	Serum	3-6 mg/dl	
δ-Aminolevulinic acid	Serum	0.01-0.03 mg/dl	
Ammonia	Plasma	20-150 μg/dl (diffusion)	Collect with sodium heparinate; specimen must analyzed immediately
		40-80 μg/dl (enzymatic method)	
		12-48 μg/dl (resin method)	
Amylase	Serum	60-160 Somogyi units/dl	
Argininosuccinic lyase	Serum	0-4 U/dl	
Arsenic	Whole blood	$<3 \mu$g/dl	
Ascorbic acid (vitamin C)	Plasma	0.6-1.6 mg/dl	Analyze immediately
	Whole blood	0.7-2.0 mg/dl	
Barbiturates	Serum, plasma, or whole blood	Negative	
Base excess	Whole blood	Male: −3.3 to +1.2	
		Female: −2.4 to +2.3	
Base, total	Serum	145-160 mEq/L	
Bicarbonate	Plasma	21-28 mM/L	
Bile acids	Serum	0.3-3.0 mg/dl	
Bilirubin	Serum	Up to 0.3 mg/dl (direct or conjugated)	
		0.1-1.0 mg/dl (indirect or unconjugated)	
		Total: 0.1-1.2 mg/dl	
		Newborns total: 1-12 mg/dl	
Blood gases			
pH		7.38-7.44 arterial	
		7.36-7.41 venous	
P_{CO_2}		35-40 mm Hg arterial	
		40-45 mm Hg venous	
P_{O_2}		95-100 mm Hg arterial	
Bromide	Serum	0-5 mg/dl	

Continued.

Table B-1. Whole blood, serum, and plasma (chemistry)—cont'd

Test	Material	Normal value	Special instructions
BSP (bromsulfonphthalein) (5 mg/kg)	Serum	<6% retention after 45 min	
Calcium	Serum	Ionized: 4.2-5.2 mg/dl 2.1-2.6 mEq/L or 50-58% of total Total: 9.0-10.6 mg/dl 4.5-5.3 mEq/L Infants: 11-13 mg/dl	
Carbon dioxide (CO_2 content)	Whole blood, arterial	19-24 mM/L	
	Plasma or serum, arterial	21-28 mM/L	
	Whole blood, venous	22-26 mM/L	
	Plasma or serum, venous	24-30 mM/L	
CO_2 combining power	Plasma or serum, venous	24-30 mM/L	
CO_2 partial pressure (P_{CO_2})	Whole blood, arterial	35-40 mm Hg	
	Whole blood, venous	40-45 mm Hg	
Carbonic acid	Whole blood, arterial	1.05-1.45 mM/L	
	Whole blood, venous	1.15-1.50 mM/L	
	Plasma, venous	1.02-1.38 mM/L	
Carboxyhemoglobin (carbon monoxide hemoglobin)	Whole blood	Suburban nonsmokers: <1.5% saturation of hemoglobin Smokers: 1.5-5.0% saturation Heavy smokers: 5.0-9.0% saturation	
Carotene, beta	Serum	40-200 μg/dl	
Cephalin cholesterol flocculation	Serum	Negative to 1+ after 24 hours 2+ or less after 48 hours	
Ceruloplasmin	Serum	23-50 mg/dl	
Chloride	Serum	95-103 mEq/L	
Cholesterol, total	Serum	150-250 mg/dl (varies with diet and age)	
Cholesterol, esters	Serum	65-75% of total cholesterol	
Cholinesterase Pseudocholinesterase	Erythrocytes Plasma	0.65-1.00 pH units 0.5-1.3 pH units 8-18 IU/L at 37° C	
Citric acid	Serum or plasma	1.7-3.0 mg/dl	
Congo red test	Serum or plasma	>60% after 1 hour	Severe reactions may occur if dye is injected twice; check patient's record

Table B-1. Whole blood, serum, and plasma (chemistry)—cont'd

Test	Material	Normal value	Special instructions
Copper	Serum or plasma	Male: 70-140 μg/dl	
		Female: 85-155 μg/dl	
Cortisol	Plasma	8 A.M.-10 A.M.: 5-25 μg/dl	
		4 P.M.-6 P.M.: 2-18 μg/dl	
Creatine	Serum or plasma	Males: 0.2-0.6 mg/dl	
		Females: 0.6-1.0 mg/dl	
Creatine phosphokinase (CPK)	Serum	Males: 55-170 U/L at 37° C	See Chapter 4
		Females: 30-135 U/L at 37° C	
Creatinine	Serum or plasma	0.6-1.2 mg/dl	
Creatinine clearance (endogenous)	Serum or plasma and urine	Male: 123 ± 16 ml/min	
		Female: 97 ± 10 ml/min	
Cryoglobulins	Serum	Negative	Keep specimen at 37° C

Electrophoresis, protein	Serum		*percent*	*gm/dl*	
		Albumin	52-65	3.2-5.6	
		Alpha-1	2.5-5.0	0.1-0.4	
		Alpha-2	7.0-13.0	0.4-1.2	
		Beta	8.0-14.0	0.5-1.1	
		Gamma	12.0-22.0	0.5-1.6	

Test	Material	Normal value	Special instructions
Fats, neutral	Serum or plasma	0-200 mg/dl	
Fatty acids			
Total	Serum	9-15 mM/L	
Free	Plasma	300-480 μEq/L	
Fibrinogen	Plasma	200-400 mg/dl	
Fluoride	Whole blood	<0.05 mg/dl	
Folate	Serum	5-25 ng/ml (bioassay)	
	Erythrocytes	166-640 ng/ml (bioassay)	
Galactose	Whole blood	Adults: none	
		Children: <20 mg/dl	
Gammaglobulin	Serum	0.5-1.6 gm/dl	
Globulins, total	Serum	2.3-3.5 gm/dl	
Glucose, fasting	Serum or plasma	70-110 mg/dl	Collect with heparin-fluoride mixture
	Whole blood	60-110 mg/dl	
Glucose tolerance, oral	Serum or plasma	Fasting: 70-110 mg/dl	Collect with heparin-fluoride mixture
		30 min: 30-60 mg/dl above fasting	
		60 min: 20-50 mg/dl above fasting	
		120 min: 5-15 mg/dl above fasting	
		180 min: fasting level or below	
Glucose tolerance, IV	Serum or plasma	Fasting: 70-110 mg/dl	Collect with heparin-fluoride mixture
		5 min: Maximum of 250 mg/dl	
		60 min: Significant decrease	
		120 min: Below 120 mg/dl	
		180 min: Fasting level	
Glucose-6-phosphate dehydrogenase (G-6-PD)	Erythrocytes	250-500 units/10^9 cells	
		1200-2000 mIU/ml of packed erythrocytes	
γ-Glutamyl transpeptidase	Serum	2-39 U/L	
Glutathione	Whole blood	24-37 mg/dl	

Continued.

Table B-1. Whole blood, serum, and plasma (chemistry)—cont'd

Test	Material	Normal value	Special instructions
Growth hormone	Serum	$<$10 ng/ml	
Guanase	Serum	$<$3 nM/ml/min	
Haptoglobin	Serum	100-200 mg/dl as hemoglobin bind capacity	
Hemoglobin	Serum or plasma	Qualitative: Negative	
		Quantitative: 0.5-5.0 mg/dl	
Hemoglobin	Whole blood	Female: 12.0-16.0 gm/dl	
		Male: 13.5-18.0 gm/dl	
Hemoglobin A_2	Whole blood	1.5-3.5% of total hemoglobin	
α-Hydroxybutyric dehydrogenase	Serum	140-350 U/ml	
17-Hydroxycorticosteroids	Plasma	Male: 7-19 μg/dl	Perform test immediately or freeze plasma
		Female: 9-21 μg/dl	
		After 25 USP units of ACTH IM: 35-55 μg/dl	
Immunoglobulins	Serum		
IgG		800-1600 mg/dl	
IgA		50-250 mg/dl	
IgM		40-120 mg/dl	
IgD		0.5-3.0 mg/dl	
IgE		0.01-0.04 mg/dl	
Insulin	Plasma	11-240 μIU/ml (bioassay)	
		4-24 μU/ml (radioimmunoassay)	
Insulin tolerance	Serum	Fasting: Glucose of 70-110 mg/dl	Collect with heparin-fluoride mixture
		30 min: Fall to 50% of fasting level	
		90 min: Fasting level	
Iodine			
Butanol extraction (BEI)	Serum	3.5-6.5 μg/dl	Test not reliable if iodine-containing drugs or radiographic contrast media were given prior to test
Protein bound (PBI)	Serum	4.0-8.0 μg/dl	
Iron, total	Serum	50-150 μg/dl	Hemolysis must be avoided
Iron-binding capacity	Serum	250-450 μg/dl	
Iron saturation, percent	Serum	20-55%	
Isocitric dehydrogenase	Serum	50-250 U/ml	
Ketone bodies	Serum	Negative	
17-Ketosteroids	Plasma	25-125 μg/dl	
Lactic acid	Whole blood, venous	5-20 mg/dl	Draw without stasis
	Whole blood, arterial	3-7 mg/dl	
Lactate dehydrogenase (LDH)	Serum	80-120 Wacker units	See Chapter 4
		150-450 Wroblewski units	
		71-207 IU/L	

Table B-1. Whole blood, serum, and plasma (chemistry)—cont'd

Test	Material	Normal value	Special instructions
Lactate dehydrogenase isoenzymes	Serum	Anode: LDH$_1$ 17-27% LDH$_2$ 27-37% LDH$_3$ 18-25% LDH$_4$ 3-8% Cathode: LDH$_5$ 0-5%	
Lactate dehydrogenase (heat stable)	Serum	30-60% of total	
Lactose tolerance	Serum	Serum glucose changes are similar to those seen in a glucose tolerance test	
Lead	Whole blood	0-50 μg/dl	
Leucine aminopeptidase (LAP)	Serum	Male: 80-200 Goldbarg-Rutenburg units/ml Female: 75-185 Goldbarg-Rutenburg units/ml	
Lipase	Serum	0-1.5 Cherry-Crandall U/ml 14-280 mIU/ml	
Lipids	Serum		
Total		400-800 mg/dl	
Cholesterol		150-250 mg/dl	
Triglycerides		10-190 mg/dl	
Phospholipids		150-380 mg/dl	
Fatty acids		9.0-15.0 mM/L	
Neutral fat		0-200 mg/dl	
Phospholipid phosphorus		8.0-11.0 mg/dl	
Lithium	Serum	Negative Therapeutic level: 0.5-1.5 mEq/L	
Long-acting thyroid-stimulating hormone (LATS)	Serum	None	
Luteinizing hormone (LH)	Plasma	Male: <11mIU/ml Female: midcycle peak >3 times baseline value Premenopausal; <25 mIU/ml Postmenopausal: >25 mIU/ml	
Macroglobulins, total	Serum	70-430 mg/dl	
Magnesium	Serum	1.5-2.5 mEq/L 1.8-3.0 mg/dl	
Methemoglobin	Whole blood	0-0.24 gm/dl 0.4-1.5% of total hemoglobin	
Mucoprotein	Serum	80-200 mg/dl	
Nonprotein nitrogen (NPN)	Serum or plasma Whole blood	20-35 mg/dl 25-50 mg/dl	
5' Nucleotidase	Serum	0-1.6 units	
Ornithine carbamyl transferase (OCT)	Serum	8-20 mIU/ml	
Osmolality	Serum	280-295 mOsm/L	

Continued.

Table B-1. Whole blood, serum, and plasma (chemistry)—cont'd

Test	Material	Normal value	Special instructions
Oxygen			
Pressure (Po₂)	Whole blood, arterial	95-100 mm Hg	
Content	Whole blood, arterial	15-23 vol%	
Saturation	Whole blood, arterial	94-100%	
pH	Whole blood, arterial	7.38-7.44	
	Whole blood, venous	7.36-7.41	
	Serum or plasma, venous	7.35-7.45	
Phenylalanine	Serum	Adults: <3.0 mg/dl Newborns (term): 1.2-3.5 mg/dl	
Phosphatase, acid, total	Serum	0-1.1 U/ml (Bodansky) 1-4 U/ml (King-Armstrong) 0.13-0.63 U/ml (Bessey-Lowry) 1.4-5.5 U/ml (Gutman-Gutman) 0-0.56 U/ml (Roy) 0-6.0 U/ml (Shinowara-Jones-Reinhart)	Hemolysis must be avoided; perform test without delay or freeze specimen
Phosphatase, alkaline, total	Serum	Adults: 1.5-4.5 U/dl (Bodansky) 4-13 U/dl (King-Armstrong) 0.8-2.3 U/ml (Bessey-Lowry) 15-35 U/ml (Shinowara-Jones-Reinhart) Children: 5.0-14.0 U/dl (Bodansky) 3.4-9.0 U/ml (Bessey-Lowry) 15-30 U/dl (King-Armstrong)	
Phospholipid phosphorus	Serum	8-11 mg/dl	
Phospholipids	Serum	150-380 mg/dl	
Phosphorus, inorganic	Serum	Adults: 1.8-2.6 mEq/L 3.0-4.5 mg/dl Children: 2.3-4.1 mEq/L 4.0-7.0 mg/dl	Separate cells from serum promptly
Potassium	Plasma	3.8-5.0 mEq/L	
Proteins	Serum		
Total		6.0-7.8 gm/dl	
Albumin		3.2-4.5 gm/dl	
Globulin		2.3-3.5 gm/dl	
Protein fractionation	Serum		
Protoporphyrin	Erythrocytes	15-50 μg/dl	
Pyruvate	Whole blood	0.3-0.9 mg/dl	
Salicylates	Serum	Negative Therapeutic level: 20-25 mg/dl	
Sodium	Plasma	136-142 mEq/L	

Table B-1. Whole blood, serum, and plasma (chemistry)—cont'd

Test	Material	Normal value		Special instructions
Sulfate, inorganic	Serum	0.2-1.3 mEq/L 0.9-6.0 mg/dl as SO₄		Hemolysis must be avoided
Sulfhemoglobin	Whole blood	Negative		
Sulfonamides	Serum or whole blood	Negative		
Testosterone	Serum or plasma	Male: 400-1200 ng/dl Female: 30-120 ng/dl		
Thiocyanate	Serum	Negative		
Thymol flocculation	Serum	0-5 units		
Thyroid hormone tests	Serum	*Expressed as thyroxine*	*Expressed as iodine*	
T₄ (by column)		5.0-11.0 μg/dl	3.2-7.2 μg/dl	
T₄ (by competitive binding Murphy-Pattee)		6.0-11.8 μg/dl	3.9-7.7 μg/dl	
Free T₄	0.9-2.3 ng/dl	0.6-1.5 ng/dl		
T₃ (resin uptake)		25-38 relative % uptake		
Thyroxine-binding globulin (TBG)		10-26 μg/dl (expressed as T₄ uptake)		
Transaminases				
GOT	Serum	8-33 U/ml		
GPT	Serum	1-36 U/ml		
Triglycerides	Serum	10-190 mg/dl		
Urea nitrogen	Serum	8-18 mg/dl		
Urea clearance	Serum and urine	Maximum clearance: 64-99 ml/min Standard clearance: 41-65 ml/min or more than 75% of normal clearance		
Uric acid	Serum	Male: 2.1-7.8 mg/dl Female: 2.0-6.4 mg/dl		
Vitamin A	Serum	15-60 μg/dl		
Vitamin A tolerance	Serum	Fasting: 15-60 μg/dl 3 hr. or 6 hr. after 5000 units vitamin A/kg; 200-600 μg/dl 24 hr: fasting values or slightly above		Administer 5000 units vitamin A in oil per kg body weight
Vitamin B₁₂	Serum	Male: 200-800 pg/ml Female: 100-650 pg/ml		
Unsaturated vitamin B₁₂ binding capacity	Serum	1000-2000 pg/ml		
Vitamin C	Plasma	0.6-1.6 mg/dl		Collect with oxalate and analyze within 20 minutes
Xylose absorption	Serum	25-40 mg/dl between 1 and 2 hr; in malabsorption, maximum approximately 10 mg/dl Dose Adult: 25 gm D-xylose Children: 0.5 gm/kg D-xylose		For children administer 10 ml of a 5% solution of D-xylose per kg of body weight
Zinc	Serum	50-150 μg/dl		
Zinc sulfate turbidity	Serum	< 12 units		

Table B-2. Urine

Test	Type of specimen	Normal value	Special instructions
Acetoacetic acid	Random	Negative	
Acetone	Random	Negative	
Addis count	12-hr collection	WBC and epithelial cells: 1,800,000/ 12 hr RBC: 500,000/12 hr Hyaline casts: 0-5,000/12 hr	Rinse bottle with some neutral formalin; discard excess
Albumin			
Qualitative	Random	Negative	
Quantitative	24 hr	10-100 mg/24 hr	
Aldosterone	24 hr	2-26 μg/24 hr	Keep refrigerated
Alkapton bodies	Random	Negative	
Alpha-amino acid nitrogen	24 hr	100-290 mg/24 hr	
δ-Aminolevulinic acid	Random	Adult: 0.1-0.6 mg/dl Children: <0.5 mg/dl	
	24 hr	1.5-7.5 mg/24 hr	
Ammonia nitrogen	24 hr	20-70 mEq/24 hr 500-1200 mg/24 hr	Keep refrigerated
Amylase	2 hr	35-260 Somogyi units per hour	
Arsenic	24 hr	<50 μg/L	
Ascorbic acid	Random	1-7 mg/dl	
	24 hr	>50 mg/24 hr	
Bence Jones protein	Random	Negative	
Beryllium	24 hr	<0.05 μg/24 hr	
Bilirubin, qualitative	Random	Negative	
Blood, occult	Random	Negative	
Borate	24 hr	<2 mg/L	
Calcium			
Qualitative (Sulkowitch)	Random	1+ turbidity	Compared with standard
Quantitative	24 hr	Average diet: 100-250 mg/24 hr Low calcium diet: <150 mg/24 hr High calcium diet: 250-300 mg/24 hr	
Catecholamines	Random	0-14 μg/dl	
	24 hr	<100 μg/24 hr (varies with activity)	
Chloride	24 hr	110-250 mEq/24 hr	
Concentration test (Fishberg)	Random after fluid restriction	Specific gravity: >1.025 Osmolality: >850 mOsm/L	
Copper	24 hr	0-30 μg/24 hr	
Coproporphyrin	Random	Adult: 3-20 μg/dl	Use fresh specimen and do not expose to direct light; preserve 24-hr urine with 5 gm Na_2CO_3
	24 hr	50-160 μg/24 hr Children: 0-80 μg/24 hr	
Creatine	24 hr	Male: 0-40 mg/24 hr Female: 0-100 mg/24 hr Higher in children and during pregnancy	

Table B-2. Urine—cont'd

Test	Type of specimen	Normal value	Special instructions
Creatinine	24 hr	Male: 20-26 mg/kg/24 hr 1.0-2.0 gm/24 hr Female: 14-22 mg/kg/24 hr 0.8-1.8 gm/24 hr	
Cystine, qualitative	Random	Negative	
Cystine and cysteine	24 hr	10-100 mg/24 hr	
Diacetic acid	Random	Negative	
Epinephrine	24 hr	0-20 μg/24 hr	

Estrogens, total	24 hr	Male: 5-18 μg/24 hr
		Female
		    Ovulation: 28-100 μg/24 hr
		    Luteal peak: 22-105 μg/24 hr
		    At menses: 4-25 μg/24 hr
		    Pregnancy: up to 45,000 μg/24 hr
		    Postmenopausal: 14-20 μg/24 hr
			Keep refrigerated

Estrogens, Fractionated	24 hr	Non-pregnant, mid-cycle	
Estrone (E1)		2-25 μg/24 hr	
Estradiol (E2)		0-10 μg/24 hr	
Estriol (E3)		2-30 μg/24 hr	
Fat, qualitative	Random	Negative	
FIGLU (N-formi- minoglutamic acid)	24 hr	<3 mg/24 hr After 15 gm of L-histidine: 4 mg/8 hr	
Fluoride	24 hr	<1 mg/24 hr	
Follicle-stimulating hormone (FSH)	24 hr	Adult: 6-50 mouse uterine units/24 hr Prepubertal: <MUU/24 hr Post-menopausal: >MUU/24 hr	
Fructose	24 hr	30-65 mg/24 hr	
Glucose			
Qualitative	Random	Negative	
Quantitative	24 hr		
Copper-reducing substances		0.5-1.5 gm/24 hr	
Total sugars		Average: 250 mg/24 hr	
Glucose		Average: 130 mg/24 hr	
Gonadotropins, Pituitary (FSH and LH)	24 hr	10-50 MUU/24 hr	
Hemoglobin	Random	Negative	
Homogentisic acid	Random	Negative	
Homovanillic acid (HVA)	24 hr	<15 mg/24 hr	
17-Hydroxycortico- steroids	24 hr	Male: 5.5-14.5 mg/24 hr Female: 4.9-12.9 mg/24 hr Lower in children After 25 USP units ACTH, IM: a 2- to 4-fold increase	Keep refrigerated

Continued.

Table B-2. Urine—cont'd

Test	Type of specimen	Normal value	Special instructions
5-Hydroxyindole-acetic acid, qualitative	Random	Negative	Some muscle relaxants and tranquilizers interfere with test
5-HIAA, quantitative	24 hr	<9 mg/24 hr	
Indican	24 hr	10-20 mg/24 hr	
Ketone bodies	Random	Negative	Fresh, keep cool
17-Ketosteroids	24 hr	Male: 8-15 mg/24 hr	Keep refrigerated
		Female: 6-11.5 mg/24 hr	
		Children: 12-15 hr, 5-12 mg/24 hr; <12 yr, <5 mg/24 hr	
		After 25 USP units ACTH, IM: 50-100% increase	
Androsterone		Male: 2.0-5.0 mg/24 hr	
		Female: 0.8-3.0 mg/24 hr	
Etiocholanolone		Male: 1.4-5.0 mg/24 hr	
		Female: 0.8-4.0 mg/24 hr	
Dehydroepiandrosterone		Male: 0.2-2.0 mg/24 hr	
		Female: 0.2-1.8 mg/24 hr	
11-Ketoandrosterone		Male: 0.2-1.0 mg/24 hr	
		Female: 0.2-0.8 mg/24 hr	
11-Ketoetiocholanolone		Male: 0.2-1.0 mg/24 hr	
		Female: 0.2-0.8 mg/24 hr	
11-Hydroxyandrosterone		Male: 0.1-0.8 mg/24 hr	
		Female: 0.0-0.5 mg/24 hr	
11-Hydroxyetiocholanolone		Male: 0.2-0.6 mg/24 hr	
		Female: 0.1-1.1 mg/24 hr	
Lactose	24 hr	12-40 mg/24 hr	
Lead	24 hr	<100 µg/24 hr	
Magnesium	24 hr	6.0-8.5 mEq/24 hr	
Melanin, qualitative	Random	Negative	
3-Methoxy-4-hydroxy-mandelic acid (VMA)	24 hr	1.5-7.5 mg/24 hr (adults) 83 µg/kg/24 hr (infants)	No coffee or fruit two days prior to test
Mucin	24 hr	100-150 mg/24 hr	
Myoglobin			
Qualitative	Random	Negative	
Quantitative	24 hr	<1.5 mg/L	
Osmolality	Random	500-800 mOsm/L	May be lower or higher, depending on state of hydration
Pentoses	24 hr	2-5 mg/kg/24 hr	
pH	Random	4.6-8.0	
Phenolsulfonphthalein (PSP)	Urine, timed after 6 mg PSP IV		
	15 min	20-50% dye excreted	
	30 min	16-24% dye excreted	
	60 min	9-17% dye excreted	
	120 min	3-10% dye excreted	

Table B-2. Urine—cont'd

Test	Type of specimen	Normal value	Special instructions
Phenylpyruvic acid, qualitative	Random	Negative	
Phosphorus	Random	0.9-1.3 gm/24 hr	Varies with intake
Porphobilinogen			
Qualitative	Random	Negative	
Quantitative	24 hr	0-2.0 mg/24 hr	
Potassium	24 hr	40-80 mEq/24 hr	Varies with diet
Pregnancy tests	Concentrated morning specimen	Positive in normal pregnancies or with tumors producing chorionic gonadotropin	
Pregnanediol	24 hr	Male: 0-1 mg/24 hr Female: 1-8 mg/24 hr Peak: 1 week after ovulation Pregnancy: 60-100 mg/24 hr Children: Negative	Keep refrigerated
Pregnanetriol	24 hr	Male: 1.0-2.0 mg/24 hr Female: 0.5-2.0 mg/24 hr Children: <0.5 mg/24 hr	Keep refrigerated
Protein			
Qualitative	Random	Negative	
Quantitative	24 hr	10-100 mg/24 hr	
Reducing substances, total	24 hr	0.5-1.5 mg/24 hr	
Sodium	24 hr	80-180 mEq/24 hr	Varies with dietary ingestion of salt
Solids, total	24 hr	55-70 gm/24 hr Decreases with age to 30 gm/24 hr	
Specific gravity	Random	1.016-1.022 (normal fluid intake) 1.001-1.035 (range)	
Sugars (excluding glucose)	Random	Negative	
Titrable acidity	24 hr	20-50 mEq/24 hr	Collect with toluene
Urea nitrogen	24 hr	6-17 gm/24 hr	
Uric acid	24 hr	250-750 mg/24 hr	Varies with diet
Urobilinogen	2 hr	0.3-1.0 Ehrlich units	
	24 hr	0.05-2.5 mg/24 hr or 0.5-4.0 Ehrlich units/24 hr	
Uropepsin	Random	15-45 units/hr	
	24 hr	1500-5000 units/24 hr	
Uroporphyrins			
Qualitative	Random	Negative	
Quantitative	24 hr	10-30 μg/24 hr	
Vanillylmandelic acid (VMA)	24 hr	1.5-7.5 mg/24 hr	
Volume, total	24 hr	600-1600 mg/24 hr	
Zinc	24 hr	0.15-1.2 mg/24 hr	

Table B-3. Gastric fluid

Test	Normal value
Fasting residual volume	20-100 ml
pH	<2.0
Basal acid output (BAO)	0-6 mEq/hr
Maximal acid output (MAO) after histamine stimulation	5-40 mEq/h4
BAO/MAO ratio	<0.4

Table B-4. Cerebrospinal fluid

Test or constituent	Normal value	Special instructions
Albumin	10-30 mg/dl	
Albumin/globulin ratio	1.6-2.2	
Calcium	2.1-2.9 mEq/L	
Cell count	0-8 cells/μl	
Chloride	Adult: 118-132 mEq/L	These values are invalidated by
	Children: 120-128 mEq/L	admixture of blood
Colloidal gold curve	0001111000	
Globulins		
Qualitative (Pandy)	Negative	
Quantitative	6-16 mg/dl	
Glucose	45-75 mg/dl	
Lactate dehydrogenase (LDH)	Approximately $\frac{1}{10}$ of serum level	
Protein		
Total CSF	15-45 mg/dl	
Ventricular fluid	8-15 mg/dl	
Protein electrophoresis		
Pre-albumin	4.1 ± 1.2%	
Albumin	62.4 ± 5.6%	
Alpha-1 globulin	5.3 ± 1.2%	
Alpha-2 globulin	8.2 ± 2.0%	
Beta globulin	12.8 ± 2.0%	
Gamma globulin	7.2 ± 1.1%	
Xanthochromia	Negative	

Conversions and equivalencies

Measurements and temperature conversions*

Measurements

Oral temperature range	36.4°-37.2° C. (97.6°-99° F.)
Rectal temperature range	37.0°-37.8° C. (98.6°-100° F.)
Axillary temperature range	35.8°-36.6° C. (96.6°-98° F.)
"Average" pulse rate	70 beats/min.
Pulse rate range at rest	60-90 beats/min.
Pulse rate range for everyday activities	Women, 72-80 beats/min; men, slightly lower
Respiratory rate range	14-20 respirations/min.
Normal central venous pressure (CVP) range	2-10 cm H_2O or up to 20 cm H_2O
Normal fetal heart rate (FHR) range	125-155 beats/min. or 120-160 beats/min.
Average blood pressure (BP)	$\dfrac{120 \text{ mm Hg}}{80 \text{ mm Hg}}$
Tidal volume of air (tidal air)	500 ml (cc)
Inspiratory capacity	3500 ml (cc)
Inspiratory reserve volume (complemental air)	3000 ml (cc)
Expiratory reserve volume (supplemental air)	1200 ml (cc)
Vital capacity	4700 ml (cc)

Temperature conversions

$$C = \frac{5}{9}(\text{Fahrenheit reading} - 32) \qquad F = \left(\frac{9}{5} \times \text{centigrade reading}\right) + 32$$

*From McInnes, B.: The vital signs, with related clinical measurements: a programmed presentation, ed. 3, St. Louis, 1979, The C. V. Mosby Co.

Weight equivalencies*

Pounds	Kilograms	Pounds	Kilograms	Pounds	Kilograms
1	0.45	50	22.7	180	81.7
2	0.9	60	27.2	190	86.3
3	1.4	70	31.8	200	90.8
4	1.8	80	36.3	210	95.3
5	2.3	90	40.9	220	100.0
6	2.7	100	45.4	230	104.4
7	3.2	110	50.0	240	109.0
8	3.6	120	54.5	250	113.5
9	4.1	130	59.0	260	118.0
10	4.5	140	63.6	270	122.6
20	9.0	150	68.1	280	127.1
30	13.6	160	72.6	290	131.7
40	18.2	170	77.2	300	136.2

*From Barber, J. M.: Handbook of emergency pharmacology, St. Louis, 1978, The C. V. Mosby Co.

Aftercare suggestions*

BLAND DIET

The value of a bland diet is a matter of medical controversy. However, all physicians agree that caffeine, aspirin, any medicine containing aspirin (please read labels), and alcoholic beverages should be strictly avoided. Also don't eat any food that causes you discomfort. The following diet is a bland diet that you may find useful. It is limited in roughage and low in stimulating factors (concentrated sweets, extractives, acids, and condiments). It is adequate in all food essentials except Vitamin C. Chew all foods thoroughly before swallowing.

Foods allowed

Beverages. Milk, cream, eggnog, malted milk, vanilla milkshake, DeCafe, Sanka, skim milk where fat is limited; *avoid* buttermilk and chocolate milk.

Meat, fish, and poultry. Broiled, baked or roasted lean tender beef, veal, lamb, turkey, or chicken (white meat), broiled or baked fish, lean steak, lamb chop; *avoid* boiled meats and stew, fried meats, all smoked or cured meats and fish (such as sausage, corned beef, smoked fish, and so on).

Vegetables. Cooked carrots, beets, asparagus, spinach, squash, tender wax beans; *avoid* raw vegetables, vegetables in the cabbage family such as broccoli, brussel sprouts, cauliflower, vegetables with skins such as peas.

Fruits. Cooked or canned fruit without skins, ripe banana, applesauce, baked apple without skin; *avoid* raw fruit, citrus fruit.

Juices. Bland juices *only* such as pear nectar, apricot nectar, peach nectar, pineapple juice; *avoid* citrus juices, tomato juice.

Soups. Strained cream soups, strained vegetable soup, no seasoning; *avoid* meat soups, tomato soup, seasoned soup, bean soup.

Desserts. Jello, custard, junket, vanilla ice cream, simple puddings such as vanilla pudding, plain bread pudding, tapioca, plain rice pudding, angel food cake, sponge cake, lady fingers, plain vanilla cookies, fruit whip; *avoid* chocolate, nuts, raisins.

Cereals. Refined cereals such as Farina, Cream of Wheat, Cream of Rice, strained Corn Flakes, Rice Krispies, Special K, Puffed Rice, noodles, rice, plain spaghetti, plain macaroni, and cheese; *avoid* coarse, whole grain cereals.

Bread. Day-old white bread or white toast, Zwieback, white crackers, melba toast; *avoid* whole wheat bread, rye bread, bread with seeds and raisin bread.

Sweets. Sugar, jelly, honey in moderation; *avoid* concentrated sweets such as pie, pastry, rich cakes, and chocolate candy.

Fats. Butter, fortified margarine, cream.

Eggs. Any kind except fried.

---

*Courtesy Brotman Medical Center, Department of Emergency Medicine, Culver City, Calif.

Cheese. Cottage cheese, cream cheese, mild jack cheese, mild American cheese; *avoid* all others.

CLEAR LIQUID DIET

This diet is used in the treatment of vomiting and diarrhea. Clear liquids are very easy to digest and tend to reduce these problems. This diet will also help you maintain normal body fluid balance.

The diet explains itself. Any liquid that you can see through (excluding alcoholic beverages of course) is allowable. Examples are soft drinks, water, tea, bouillon, broth, Jello, honey, etc. Examples of excluded items are: milk, most soups, and all solid foods.

Start with small amounts. For example, 4 to 6 tablespoons each half hour. If this amount is tolerated well, gradually increase to a cup or two every 1 to 2 hours. Large amounts of even clear fluids will cause vomiting.

CASTS

In order for your injury to heal, it must be splinted for a period of time in a plaster cast.

Since damage to the nerves and blood vessels can take place at the site of the injury, the doctor will count on you to report any of the following complications:

1. An increase in swelling.
2. Fingers or toes that become swollen, cold, numb, white or blue.
3. Inability to move fingers or toes.
4. Pain that gets worse or persists beyond 48-hours.
5. Cracked or broken casts.
6. A foul odor from the cast.

The cast must be checked by your doctor 24-hours after it was applied.

Dos and don'ts

Dos

1. To prevent swelling, keep the injured part elevated above the level of your heart. This is especially important during the first 24 hours, and to a lesser extent over the next 3 days. A leg cast should be elevated on three pillows. Arm casts for fractures of the hand or forearm should point up, with the hand as the highest point, for the first 12 hours. After that, use a sling for support.
2. Wiggle fingers and toes of the casted arm or leg frequently.
3. It takes 48 hours for a cast to dry completely. Be particularly careful of your cast during this period. If you have a walking cast, don't walk on it at all for the first 48 hours.
4. Keep cast open to air so it will dry.

Dont's

1. Don't get your cast wet.
2. Don't put anything into your cast.
3. Don't rest your cast on hard or sharp surfaces.

CERVICAL SPRAIN

Rest as much as possible until improved. This is best achieved by wearing a cervical collar to hold the neck in slight flexion. Collar should be worn day and night for _____ days. In the presence of severe pain, bedrest for _____ days is necessary.

How to wear your cervical collar. The purpose of the collar is to hold your head and neck still so it should be worn snugly. The collar fastens at the back.

Use of heat on the affected area. Apply moist heat or heating pad to sore neck for ___ minutes every _____ hours until pain is relieved. The collar should be removed to do this.

Medication for relief of pain and muscle spasm. Take prescriptions as directed. *Caution:* Do not drive while taking medicaiton.

Neck position. Neck should be maintained slightly flexed in all daily activities. Avoid positions and movements that hurt.

COLDS

The doctor believes you have a cold. These illnesses are caused by viruses for which there is no cure. Fortunately, these illnesses are self-limited and usually last only 7 to 10 days. Medications offered for this illness will make you more comfortable but will not provide a cure. We do advise the following to aid in recovery and minimize symptoms.

1. Increase fluids to one 8-ounce glass every 2 hours while awake.
2. If your throat feels dry or sore, gargle with salt water: 1 tablespoon of table salt in an 8-ounce glass of warm water.
3. Two to three times a day take a home "steam bath." This may be done by closing the bathroom door and turning on the hot water in the shower so that the room fills with steam. Inhaling this for 5 to 10 minutes will open the air passages, decrease the thickness of secretions, and help restore normal function to the nose, throat, and sinuses.
4. Refrain from smoking and exposures to other persons' smoke.
5. Maintain proper nutrition and adequate rest.
6. Take the medications you have been given as prescribed. If they disagree with you or if new symptoms arise, contact your physician.

USE OF CRUTCHES
Standing

1. Stand with injured foot off ground. Place tips of crutches about 18 inches apart and 6 inches in front of the good foot.
2. Position hands on handgrips with tops of crutches against ribs. Keep elbows slightly bent and close to your body. Try to bear most of your weight on hands, not on underarms!

Walking

1. Do not place tips of crutches too close to feet; it would result in a loss of balance.
2. Push down on handgrips, lift good leg, and swing forward through the crutches, placing weight back on good leg.

Sitting

1. Stand with back of good leg touching front edge of chair.
2. Place both crutch grips in the hand on the side of the injured leg and support yourself.
3. Then lean down and grasp front edge of chair with your free hand and slowly sit down.
4. Reverse procedure to get up.

Going up stairs

1. Put both crutches in your strongest hand, and use the crutches as a single crutch.
2. Put your other hand on the railing.
3. Next, put your weight on both hands, and lift your good leg up to the next step.
4. Then move the crutches to the same step, and move your hand up the railing.
5. Repeat 1 through 4 to go higher.

Going down stairs

1. Put both crutches in your strongest hand, and use the two crutches as a single crutch.
2. Put your other hand on the railing.
3. Move the crutch tips down to the next step, and also move your hand down on the railing.
4. Then lower your injured leg to the level of the next step, but don't put any weight on it.
5. Bring your good leg to the same step, and put your weight on it.
6. Repeat 1 through 5 to go further.

Precautions

1. Never lean on crutches with underarms.
2. Never stand on injured leg without physician's approval.
3. Be careful on wet or waxed floors.
4. Slow down in crowds and confined areas.
5. Never stand with feet in line with crutches. Always maintain a balanced position.
6. Be careful when walking across carpeting. Remove any loose rugs or mats from the floor.
7. Wear sturdy, low-heeled, tie shoes.

HEAD INJURY

We find no evidence of internal head injury at this time and the patient is being sent home. However, it is very important that the patient be observed for 24 hours by some responsible adult. The patient may be allowed to sleep but should be awakened every _____ hours for the next _____ hours to a normal state of alert wakefulness. If the patient cannot be fully aroused or any of the following signs of internal head injury occur, contact your physician immediately. If unable to reach, call the emergency department phone number, or return to the emergency department at once, day or night.

Signs to look for

1. Behavior changes
   a. Confusion.
   b. Irritability.
   c. Difficulty arousing to full alert wakefulness.
   d. Convulsions (fits).
2. Headache: A headache is to be expected. If it lasts more than 1 or 2 days or increases in severity, medical advice should be sought.
3. Nausea and vomiting: This is frequent after head trauma, especially in children. If it lasts for more than 2 hours, medical advice must be sought.

HYPERTENSION AFTERCARE

You had high blood pressure (hypertension) when you were in the emergency department. Uncontrolled high blood pressure over a period of years leads to strokes, heart attacks, and kidney failure. These problems can largely be prevented through modern treatment of high blood pressure. It is important that you have your blood pressure checked again by your private doctor in the next week or so to see if you still have high blood pressure.

Remember, high blood pressure is often present without any symptoms for years before a complication occurs. The only way to know if you have hypertension is to see your doctor.

YOUR BLOOD PRESSURE TODAY: _____
DATE: _____

NOSEBLEEDS

There are a number of ways a nosebleed may be stopped by a physician. Follow the suggestions below for the first 24 hours after any of these treatments. Save this sheet because it contains directions on how to treat nosebleeds at home should this problem ever arise again.

You should

1. Keep your nose and head above the level of your heart. Sit up or stand up. Sleep on your back with your upper body elevated on pillows.

You should not

1. Blow your nose or touch your nose at all.
2. Sneeze or cough.
3. Drink hot liquids or apply hot packs to the face.
4. Take any medication with aspirin in it. Read labels!
5. Drink alcohol.

Home management of nosebleeds

Although bleeding from the nose is an alarming event, it rarely signifies a serious underlying condition, nor is it usually a threat to life. The average adult has within him roughly 10 pints (5 quarts) of blood. The amount lost during any single nosebleed, although it may seem like a great deal, rarely exceeds several fluid ounces.

We recommend the following steps to stop a nosebleed. They are effective in over 90% of cases.

1. Sit up. Do not lie down.
2. Pinch the *lower one half* of the nose between thumb and index finger. These fingers should compress as much of the soft cartilagenous lower half of the nose as possible, not just the "tip" of the nose (see illustration).
3. Keep pinching for *10 minutes* by the clock! Breathe through your mouth. By now the bleeding has probably stopped.
4. After the full 10 minutes, if you are still bleeding, call your doctor or report to the nearest emergency department.

SPRAINS

A sprain is an injury to a ligament or a joint capsule. Ligaments and joint capsules are connective tissues that help hold joints together and in normal position. The usual sprain is a stretching or tearing injury that results in pain and swelling. Sprains are best treated in the following ways:

1. *Immobilization.* Wear the splint or the Ace wrap provided. This rests the injured part and allows it to heal.
2. *Elevation.* Elevate the injured part above the level of your heart, when possible. This is most important for the first 12

hours and is not necessary after 2 days. This reduces swelling.

3. *Cold*. Apply cold packs for _____ minutes _____ times daily for 2 days. This also reduces swelling.

4. *Heat*. After the first 2 days, apply warm packs or warm soaks for _____ minutes _____ times daily for _____ days. This speeds healing.

5. Rest the injured joint as much as possible. Avoid any strenuous use of the joint as much as possible. Avoid any strenuous use of the joint until all pain or tenderness is gone. Check with your doctor before returning to heavy work or sports activity.

WOUND CARE
Wound care instructions

☐ Keep the wound clean and dry for _____ days.

☐ Keep the wound clean and dry until stitches are removed.

☐ Change the dressing if it becomes soiled or wet.

☐ Remove the dressing after 12-24 hours and continue to protect the wound with bandages.

☐ Leave the dressing in place until you see your doctor.

☐ When possible, keep the injured part elevated above the level of the heart for _____ days to help prevent swelling.

☐ Other: _____

CALL YOUR DOCTOR IF ANY OF THE FOLLOWING OCCUR

1. Persistent or increasing pain at the site of the wound.

2. Temperature over 100° F.

3. Swelling or numbness at a point below the wound.

4. Red streaks away from the wound.

5. Drainage of pus from the wound.

Tetanus information

Tetanus infection, commonly called lockjaw, can be acquired through even tiny breaks of the skin. Following the advice of a physician is essential for your safety.

Tetanus immunization instructions

☐ Within the next 24 hours consult your physician to see if you should receive injections to protect you against tetanus.

☐ You have been started on a tetanus immunization series today. Please complete the series with your private doctor. See him 4 to 6 weeks from today for a second injection. A third injection is necessary 6 to 12 months from today. This will complete your tetanus immunization.

☐ You received a tetanus toxoid immunization today that will protect you from tetanus for at least 1 year and probably 5 years. Please record this date for future reference.

Incubation periods*

Disease	Duration of incubation
Asiatic cholera	24 hr. to 5 days
Anthrax	2 to 4 days; may be as long as 7 days
Bacillary dysentery (shigellosis)	1 to 7 days; average of 4 days
Blastomycosis	Unknown
Botulism (food poisoning)	Less than 24 hr.; several days after ingestion of food containing the toxin
Brucellosis (undulant fever)	5 to 30 days
Chickenpox (varicella)	14 to 16 days
Coccidioidomycosis (valley fever)	7 to 21 days
Common cold	1 to 3 days
Diarrhea, viral	3 to 5 days
Diphtheria	2 to 6 days; may be longer
Encephalitis	5 to 15 days; range of 4 to 21 days; varies as to the type
Food infection, *Salmonella*	7 to 72 hr.
Hansen's disease (leprosy, hansenosis)	Short as 5½ mo. or as long as 15 hr.; average about 5 yr.
Hepatitis	
Infectious (epidemic—virus A, catarrhal jaundice)	15 to 50 days
Serum (virus B)	2 to 6 mo.
Herpes simplex (cold sore, fever blister)	2 to 12 days; average of 4 days
Herpes zoster (singles)	4 to 24 days; average of 4 days
Histoplasmosis (Darling's disease)	5 to 18 days; average of 10 days
Infectious mononucleosis (glandular fever)	Children, less than 14 days; adults, 33 to 49 days; average period, 4 to 14 days
Influenza, epidemic	24 to 72 hr.
Malaria	Varies with particular species; 12 to 14 days or as long as 30 days; some strains from 8 to 10 mo.
Measles (rubella, red measles)	9 to 14 days; about 10 days from exposure to onset of fever, and about 14 days to appearance of rash
Meningitis, bacterial	2 to 7 days
Mumps (epidemic parotitis)	14 to 28 days
Paratyphoid fever	1 to 10 days
Pertussis (whooping cough)	5 to 21 days

*From McInnes, M. E.: Essentials of communicable disease, ed. 2, St. Louis, 1975, The C. V. Mosby Co.   *Continued.*

Disease	Duration of incubation
Plague (pasturella pestis)	
Bubonic	2 to 6 days
Pneumonic	2 to 4 days
Pneumococcal pneumonia, bacterial	1 to 3 days
Poliomyelitis (infantile paralysis)	7 to 14 days
Psittacosis (ornithosis, parrot fever)	4 to 15 days but may vary from 5 to 28 days; the most common interval after exposure is 10 days
Rabies (hydrophobia)	Dogs, 3 to 8 wk,; humans, 10 days to 2 yr. with an average of 2 to 6 wk.
Rocky Mountain spotted fever (tick fever)	2 to 12 days; may be as long as 14 days; average of 7 days
Rubella (German measles)	14 to 21 days; usually 18 days after exposure
Scarlet fever (scarlatina) and septic sore throat	24 hr. to 10 days but first clinical signs generally appear between 2 to 5 days
Smallpox (variola)	7 to 16 days; average of 12 days
Tetanus	3 to 21 days; average of 10 days
Tularemia (rabbit fever)	1 to 10 days; average of 3 days
Typhoid fever	10 to 14 days; may be as short as 7 days or as long as 21 days
Typhus fever	10 to 14 days; variation depending on the size of the dose of the infecting organism
Venereal diseases: syphillis, gonorrhea	10 to 90 days; average of 3 to 4 wk.; short as 2 to 10 days or as long as 21 days; average of 3 to 5 days
Viral pneumonia (atypical pneumonia)	Varies widely, depending on specific virus; may be from a few days to a week or longer
Yellow fever	3 to 6 days

Major drug categories*

Every effort has been made to ensure that drug dosage schedules are accurate and in accord with standards accepted at the time of publication. Check the product information sheet included in the package of each drug to be certain that changes have not been made in the recommended dosage or in the contraindications for administration.

GENERAL GUIDELINES FOR DRUG ADMINISTRATION

1. When possible, evaluate the patient's previous history of drug responses, including adverse side effects, allergies, and idiosyncrasies, before giving drug. Document any pertinent findings.
2. Determine the patient's usual drug therapy routine or any use of nonprescription agents, including alcohol. Validate exact name, dose, and administration schedule of drugs when possible. Note recent alcohol intake by time and amount of ingestion as well as by type of beverage.
3. Validate all drug orders. Repeat all verbal orders. List (a) *name* of drug, (b) *dosage,* (c) *route* of administration, and (d) *rate* of delivery.
4. Do not give any medication for which you do not know *usual* actions, *uses* or *indications, contraindications, incompatibilities, adverse reactions, available preparations, dosage range, precautions in administration, route of delivery,* and *rate of administration.*
5. Document the delivery of all drugs, including the following:
   Name
   Dosage
   Route and site
   Rate of delivery
   Time of administration
   Response if noted
6. Request explanation or clarification for any "unusual" order that violates general protocols for your unit.

---

*Modified from Barber, J. M.: Handbook of emergency pharmacology, St. Louis, 1978, The C. V. Mosby Co.

Albumin (Albuspan, Albuminar-5, Albumisol, Albutein, Buminate, Pro-Bumin, Proserum-25)

Major actions
Expands blood volume.
Reduces edema.

Primary emergency uses
Shock.
Burns.
Cerebral edema.

Notes on administration
Contraindicated in cardiac failure.
Adverse reactions include the following:

Circulatory failure	Hypotension
Dyspnea	Pulmonary edema

Preparation and dosage
Consult product literature for dosage guidelines and clinical consideratons for usage.
Draw blood for type and crossmatch (T & C) before administration.

Aminophylline (Aminodur, Lixaminol, Rectalad-Aminophylline, theophylline ethylenediamine, others)

Major actions
Bronchodilator.
Smooth muscle relaxant.
Increases coronary blood flow.
Enhances effectiveness of mercurial diuretics (inhibits tubular reabsorption of electrolytes).

Primary emergency uses
Bronchospasm associated with asthma or pulmonary edema.
Stimulates respiration, increases heart rate, and decreases venous pressure in acute congestive heart failure. Used with digitalizing preparation.

Notes on administration
Can cause cardiac arrest if administered too rapidly (see below).
Anticipate seizures, hypotension, nausea, vomiting, and cardiac dysrhythmias (premature ventricular contractions [PVCs] and tachycardia) as adverse reactions.
Incompatible with codeine, hydroxyzine pamoate (Vistaril), phenytoin (Dilantin), meperidine (Demerol), morphine, promethazine hydrochloride (Phenergan), and prochlorperazine (Compazine).
Note: Give with extreme caution in cases of severe hypoxia.

Preparation and dosage
Dosage is calculated and adjusted to maintain plasma level in therapeutic range.
Adult: 250 to 500 mg in 20 to 30 ml D/5/W (controlled volume) IV over 30 minutes.
Pediatric: Calculated according to age and weight. See product literature.

Atropine sulfate

Major actions

Anticholinergic.
Parasympathetic blocking agent.

Primary emergency uses

Sinus bradycardia, especially with hypotension or ventricular ectopy.
Asystole.
High degree AV block and slow ventricular rates.
Antidote for pilocarpine.
Ureteral and biliary colic.

Notes on administration

Administer with extreme caution to patients with glaucoma.
Incompatible with epinephrine, heparin, metaraminol, warfarin, sodium bicarbonate, most barbiturates, and several antibiotics, including ampicillin sodium, chlortetracycline hydrochloride, methicillin, and novobiocin.
Adverse reactions include coma, hypertension, respiratory failure, atrial dysrhythmia, AV dissociation, tachydysrhythmias, ventricular fibrillation, postural hypotension, fever, and visual disturbances.
May increase the size of a myocardial infarction.
Increases intraocular pressure.
Do not add to IV solution flask.

Preparation and dosage

Adult: 0.5 to 1.0 mg IV over 2 minutes. Repeat every 5 minutes until pulse is above 60.
• Maximum dose is total of 2 mg.
Pediatric: 0.01 to 0.03 mg/kg IV push over 2 minutes.

Bretylium tosylate (Bretylol)

Major actions

Antidysrhythmic; chemical defibrillator. Suppresses ventricular dysrhythmias, including fibrillation.
Dampens effects of sympathetic nerve stimulation in heart and helps to restore normal electrical homogeneity of the conduction system.
Produces positive inotropic effect on myocardium.

Primary emergency uses

Refractory ventricular fibrillation.*
Life-threatening dysrhythmias, for example, ventricular tachycardia.

Notes on administration

Must be used only in settings in which patient can be constantly monitored.
Relatively contraindicated if dysrhythmic episode occurs as a result of digitalis toxicity.
Avoid use with patients with fixed cardiac output (such as severe aortic stenosis or pulmonary hypertension).
Drop in BP may occur after administration; keep patient supine during administration (dopamine or norepinephrine may be used to counteract hypotension).
Correct coexistent volume depletion.
Side effects may include transient hypertension, increase in PVCs, and other dysrhythmic activity.
Suppresses ventricular fibrillation in minutes following IV dose; suppresses ventricular tachycardia and other ventricular dysrhythmias more slowly (that is, 20 minutes to 2 hours after parenteral administration).
Do not initiate digitalis therapy concurrently with bretylium administration.

---

*Used when traditional first-line therapy (other drugs and electrical defibrillation) have not been effective.

Preparation and dosage

Adult: *Immediate life-threatening ventricular dysrhythmias:* 5 mg/kg by rapid IV push. If fibrillation persists, dosage may be increased to 10 mg/kg and repeated at intervals of 15 to 30 minutes until a total dose of not more than 30 mg/kg has been given.

Other ventricular dysrhythmias

• Dilute 1 amp (10 ml = 500 mg) to a minimum of 50 ml with D/5/W or normal saline (N/S). Administer 5 to 10 mg/kg by IV infusion over time period greater than 8 minutes. (More rapid infusion may cause nausea and vomiting.) Dose may be repeated in 1 to 2 hours if dysrhythmia persists.

• IM injection (5 to 10 mg/kg) may be given undiluted. (May be repeated in 1 to 2 hours if dysrhythmias persists.) Vary sites of injection.

• For maintenance therapy intermittent bolus infusion or constant infusion may be employed. *Intermittent infusion:* 5 to 10 mg/kg over time period greater than 8 minutes, every 6 hours. *Constant infusion:* 1 to 2 mg/minute diluted as described above.

Pediatric: Not established.

Calcium chloride

Major actions

Increases myocardial contractility, prolongs systole, and enhances ventricular automaticity.

Primary emergency uses

Cardiac resuscitation
1. Converts fine ventricular fibrillation to coarse ventricular fibrillation.
2. Enhances cardiac output when there is an electrical complex, but no detectable perfusion.

Certain allergic reactions.
Antidote for magnesium sulfate.
Drug of choice in asystole.

Notes on administration

Contraindicated for digitalized patient.
Precipitates in the presence of sodium bicarbonate. Flush line before and after administration.
Expect drop in BP after administration.
Can induce bradycardia and cardiac arrest.

Preparation and dosage

Adult: 5 to 10 ml of 10% solution, IV bolus over 5 to 10 minutes. May be given intracardiac (IC). Dose may be repeated in 5 to 10 minutes if necessary.

Pediatric: 1 to 2 ml of a 1% solution, IV bolus over 5 to 10 minutes. May be given intracardiac. Dose may be repeated in 5 to 10 minutes if necessary.

Note: Calcium chloride is three times more potent than calcium gluconate. Do not interchange these preparations.

Clonidine (Catapres)

Major actions

Effects changes in CNS mechanisms (probably alpha receptors) to lower blood pressure.
May also act on cardiovascular centers in medulla.

Primary emergency uses

Antihypertensive.
Relieves migraine pain.

Notes on administration

Onset of action is rapid within 30 to 60 minutes after oral dose.
Initially may cause rise in BP.
Monitor for rebound rise in BP after sudden withdrawal.
Side effects include drowsiness, constipation, and dry mouth.
Tricyclic antidepressants interfere with antihypertensive effects.

Preparation and dosage

Adult: 0.1 mg (tablet) twice daily initially. (Increments of 0.1 to 0.2 mg/day may be tried until desired response is obtained.) Daily therapeutic doses range from 0.2 to 0.8 mg given in divided doses.
Pediatric: Not established.

Dexamethasone (Decadron, Dezone, Haxadrol Phosphate)

Major actions

Antiinflammatory agent.
Synthetic adrenocortical steroid.

Primary emergency uses

Cerebral edema.
Thyroid crisis.

Notes on administration

Contraindicated in states of myasthenia gravis, thromboembolic tendencies, pregnancy, renal insufficiency, diabetes mellitus, and acute psychosis.
Action inhibited by phenytoin.
Incompatible with phenytoin, prochlorperazine edisylate, and *any drug* in syringe or solution.
Sensitive to extremes in temperatures. Protect from heat and freezing.
Anticipate adverse reactions, including anaphylaxis, hypertension, thromboembolism, hyperglycemia, and peptic ulcer perforation and hemorrhage.
Expect central nervous system excitement after drug is circulated.

Preparation and dosage

Dosage varies widely with indications for emergency use. Check rationale for treatment and calculate all doses accordingly.

Dextran 40 (Gentran 40, Rheomacrodex)

Major actions

Plasma-volume expander; pulls three or four times its volume into circulation.
Increases cardiac output.
Improves microcirculation.
Increases urine output.

Primary emergency uses

Hemorrhage.
Burns.
Trauma.

Notes on administration

Contraindicated in renal shutdown, pregnancy and lactation, blood dyscrasias, pulmonary edema, and congestive heart failure.
Incompatible with aqueous solution of phytonadione, whole blood, ascorbic acid, promethazine, and chlortetracycline hydrochloride.
Correct dehydration before administering.
Monitor pulse, BP, CVP, and intake and output at 5- to 15-minute intervals.
Flush line with normal saline before and after any blood administration in conjunction with dextran 40.
May crystalize at low temperatures.
Adverse reactions include hypotension, anaphylaxis, dehydration, fever, platelet adhesion, and decreased blood coagulation.

Note: Benadryl and Adrenalin are useful in treating severe adverse reactions.

Preparation and dosage

Adult: 500 ml; infused at 20 to 40 ml/minute.
 • Baseline: Draw blood for T & C before administration.
Pediatric: 500 ml; infused at 20 ml/minute.
 • Baseline: Draw blood for T & C before administration.

Dextrose (50%)

Major actions

Osmotic diuretic.
Reverses hypoglycemia.

Primary emergency uses

Cerebral and meningeal edema.
Hypoglycemic shock or other hypoglycemic states.
Shock.
Diuresis.
Hyperkalemia.
Unconsciousness, unknown illness.

Notes on administration

Contraindicated in intracranial hemorrhage, delirium tremens, dehydration, and intraspinal or intracranial hemorrhage.
May elevate insulin requirements.
Incompatible with sodium bicarbonate, warfarin, whole blood, cyanocobalamin, kanamycin sulfate.
Adverse reactions include thrombosis, hypokalemia, and hyperosmolar syndrome.
Will slough tissue if IV is infiltrated. Check IV patency *before* administration.
Administer thiamine before D/50/W in known chronic alcoholics.
Draw serum glocuse *before* administration.

Preparation and dosage

Adult: D/50/W solution: 50 ml IV bolus.
Pediatric: D/50/W solution: 1 ml/kg IV bolus.

Diazepam (Valium)

Major action

Nervous system depressant (central, peripheral, and autonomic).

Primary emergency uses

Psychoneurotic conditions.
Acute alcoholism withdrawal.
Muscle spasms.
Status epilepticus.
Before cardioversion.

Notes on administration

Incompatible with any other drug in syringe or solution.
Contraindicated in pregnancy, acute alcohol intoxication, and glaucoma.
Give with extreme caution to children under 12 years of age. Some authorities deem it contraindicated for these patients.
Do not use in the presence of an allergic reaction.
Prepare to deal with adverse reactions, including apnea and cardiac arrest.
Can cause respiratory depression.

Preparation and dosage

Adult: 2 to 10 mg IV titrated over period of 3 to 4 minutes. Do not add to IV solution. Consider size of patient and nature of problem before giving 10 mg IV in single dose.
Pediatric: 0.25 mg/kg IV over period of 3 to 4 minutes. Do not add to IV solution.

Note: The half-life of diazepam is short (7 minutes). Monitor patient closely for such reactions as repeated seizures after this time period and be prepared to administer additional dose.

Diazoxide (Hyperstat IV)

Major actions

Arterial vasodilator, accelerates heart rate and enhances cardiac output.
Creates state of hyperglycemia.

Primary emergency uses

Hypertensive crises.
Hypoglycemia that is unresponsive to other agents.

Notes on administration

Must be given by rapid IV push to achieve effect.
Must be administered concurrently with potent diuretic.
Potentiates the action of warfarin (Coumadin).
Contraindicated in the presence of dissecting aortic aneurysm, congestive heart failure, and pheochromocytoma. Give with caution to known diabetics because of its hyperglycemic action.
Watch for the following adverse reactions: angina, dysrhythmias, cellulitis at the infusion site, headache, seizures, coma, sodium and water retention, and hypotension.

Note: Keep patient flat during administration and for 30 minutes after administration. Monitor BP closely. The usual response to diazoxide is BP falling rapidly in 1 to 5 minutes and gradually rising over 10- to 30-minute period after administration. IF BP continues to fall after this initial period, suspect a cause other than the effect of the drug for the hypotension.

Preparation and dosage

Adult: 300 mg rapid (10 to 20 seconds) IV push. Large antecubital vein is preferred site for administration.
Pediatric: 5 to 10 mg/kg rapid (10 to 20 seconds) IV push. Large antecubital vein is preferred site for administration. Use with extreme caution.

Digoxin (Davoxin, Lanoxin)

Major actions

Increases strength of myocardial contraction and enhances cardiac output.

Alters electrical behavior of myocardium by increasing block at AV node.

Increases sensitivity of carotid sinus bodies.

Primary emergency uses

Congestive heart failure.

Atrial fibrillation or flutter.

Cardiogenic shock.

Paroxysmal tachycardia.

Shock not responsive to fluid therapy.

Notes on administration

Incompatible with calcium.

Use with caution if patient has taken phenytoin (Dilantin), reserpine (Serpasil), or epinephrine (Adrenalin).

Contraindicated in potassium depletion, second degree AV block, and hypersensitive carotid sinus without artificial pacemaker.

Note: Monitor ECG to evaluate reponse to the drug.

Preparation and dosage

Digitalizing and maintenance dosages for adult and pediatric patients are calculated and administered on a highly individual basis. Consult product literature.

Diphenhydramine hydrochloride (Benadryl)

Major actions

Antihistaminic.

Anticholinergic.

Antiemetic.

Primary emergency uses

Allergic reactions.

Anaphylaxis.

Antidote for phenothiazine-induced parkinsonism.

Severe nausea and vomiting.

Notes on administration

Contraindicated in states of asthma, pregnancy, hypertension, and glaucoma.

Potentiates atropine and other anticholinergics, alcohol, and CNS depressants.

Incompatible with barbiturates, phenytoin, dexamethasone, methylprednisolone, amphotericin B, furosemide, and cephalothin.

Adverse reactions may include hypotension, palpitations, anaphylaxis, atrial tachycardia, seizures, visual disturbances, vomiting and hemolytic anemia.

Inhibits the actions of anticoagulants and some steroids.

Preparation and dosage

Adult: 10 to 50 mg (rarely 100 mg) IV over 1 to 4 minutes.
 • Maximum daily dose is 400 mg.
 • Usually used with epinephrine.

Pediatric: 2 mg/kg IV over 1 to 4 minutes initially in emergency situations or 5 mg/kg/24 hours or 150 mg/M^2/24 hours (divided into 4 doses).
 • Maximum daily dose is 300 mg.

Disopyramide phosphate (Norpace)

Major action
Antidysrhythmic.

Primary emergency uses
Unifocal and multiform PVCs.
Ventricular tachycardia unresponsive to cardioversion or other drugs.

Notes on administration
Peak blood levels are obtained within 39 minutes to 3 hours.
Half-life is prolonged in patients with renal insufficiency or liver disease.
Contraindicated with cardiogenic shock and in individuals with preexisting second or third degree AV block if no pacemaker is present.
Interacts with warfarin.
Side effects include nausea, vomiting, and urinary retention.
Postadministration hypotension can occur in patients with poorly compensated cardiac disease.
Administer after appropriate ECG assessment—not recommended for prehospital care.
Available in Canada in IV form.

Preparation and dosage
Adult: 300 mg oral loading dose followed by 150 mg every 6 hours. Maintenance range is 400-800 mg/day in 4 divided doses.
Pediatric: Not established.

Note: Available only as 100- and 160-mg capsules.

Dopamine hydrochloride (Intropin)

Major actions
Decreases peripheral resistance and increases cardiac output.
Maintains mesenteric and renal perfusion.

Primary emergency uses
Shock sydrome resulting from myocardial infarction, trauma, endotoxic septicemia, renal failure, and congestive heart failure.

Notes on administration
Do not add to any alkaline solution.
Hypovolemia must be corrected before administration.
Monitor blood pressure, pulse, and urinary output.
Anticipate nausea, vomiting, tachycardia, dyspnea, precordial pain, and headache as side effects.
Short-acting agent.
Contraindicated in pheochromocytoma and tachydysrhythmias.
Extravasation may cause necrosis.
Administer into large vein.
Observe frequently for signs of extravasation or flow impediment.
Reverse any local peripheral ischemia with phentolamine (Regitine).

Note: Use microdrip set; titrate for effect. Half-life of less than 2 minutes. Effects dissipate within 10 minutes of discontinuation.

Preparation and dosage
Adult: See dosage chart on p. 722.
Pediatric: Not established.

Note: For extravasation use phentolamine (Regitine) 5 to 10 mg in 10 to 15 ml of N/S and inject liberally throughout infiltrated area with small-gauge needle and hypodermic syringe.

Intropin®
(dopamine HCl)
Dosage Chart

The chart at the right is intended for quick reference. It is based on the concentration of **1600 mcg dopamine HCl/ml** obtained when *FOUR* 5 ml ampuls (200 mg dopamine HCl/ampul) of Intropin are added to 500 ml of a compatible IV solution or *TWO* 5 ml ampuls are added to 250 ml of a compatible IV solution.

Because fluid management is often a concern in shock patients, a different and higher concentration might be necessary for long-term therapy in order to restrict fluid intake while maintaining the therapeutic dose of the drug. An *Intropin Flow Rate Converter* is available for calculating dosage and flow rate for other concentrations. **Always titrate to patient response** since individual dosage requirements may differ widely.

FOR A CONCENTRATION OF 1600 mcg DOPAMINE HCl/ml (4-5 ml AMPULS INTROPIN/500 ml OR 2-5 ml AMPULS INTROPIN/250 ml)

Body Wt lbs	77	88	99	110	121	132	143	154	165	176	187	198	209	220	231	242
kgs	35	40	45	50	55	60	65	70	75	80	85	90	95	100	105	110
5	3.8	3.4	2.9	2.6	2.4	2.2	2.0	1.9	1.8	1.6	1.55	1.5	1.4	1.3	1.25	1.2
10	7.6	6.7	5.9	5.3	4.9	4.5	4.1	3.8	3.6	3.3	3.1	3.0	2.8	2.7	2.5	2.4
15	11	10	8.9	8.0	7.3	6.6	6.1	5.7	5.3	5.0	4.7	4.4	4.2	4.0	3.8	3.6
20	15	13	12	11	9.7	8.9	8.2	7.6	7.1	6.7	6.3	5.9	5.6	5.3	5.1	4.9
25	19	17	15	13	12	11	10	9.5	8.9	8.4	7.8	7.4	7.0	6.6	6.3	6.0
30	23	20	18	16	15	13	12	11	11	10	9.4	8.9	8.4	8.0	7.6	7.3
35	27	23	21	19	17	16	14	13	12	12	11	10	9.8	9.3	8.9	8.5
40	31	27	24	21	19	18	16	15	14	13	13	12	11	11	10	9.7
45	34	30	27	24	22	20	18	17	16	15	14	13	13	12	11	11
50	38	33	30	27	24	22	21	19	18	17	16	15	14	13	13	12
55	42	37	33	29	27	24	23	21	20	18	17	16	15	15	14	13
60	46	40	36	32	29	27	25	23	21	20	19	18	17	16	15	15
70	53	47	42	37	34	31	29	27	25	23	22	21	20	19	18	17
80	61	53	47	43	39	36	33	31	28	27	25	24	23	21	20	19
90	69	60	53	48	44	40	37	34	32	30	28	27	25	24	23	22
100	76	67	59	53	49	45	41	38	36	33	31	30	28	27	25	24

FLOW RATE IN DROPS* PER MINUTE

DOSAGE = mcg DOPAMINE HCl/kg/min

*Based on a microdrip calibration of 60 drops equal to 1.0 milliliter.   Note: All dosages of 10 mcg/kg/min and above have been rounded off to the nearest mcg/kg/min.

Intropin®
(dopamine HCl)
Dosage Phenomena

The Effects of Intropin at Three Dose Ranges:	2-5 mcg/kg/min	5-20 mcg/kg/min	over 20 mcg/kg/min
Cardiac Output	no change	increase	increase
Stroke Volume	no change	increase	increase
Heart Rate	no change	there is an initial increase followed by a decrease toward normal rates as infusion continues	
Myocardial Contractility	no change	increase	increase
Potential for Excessive Myocardial Oxygen Demands	low* coronary blood flow increased	low* coronary blood flow increased	data unavailable
Potential for Tachyarrhythmias	low*	low*	moderate
Total Systemic Vascular Resistance	slight decrease to no change	no change to slight increase	increase
Renal Blood Flow	increase	increase	decrease
Urine Output	increase	increase	decrease

*Low but needs monitoring.

See reverse for full prescribing information

Courtesy Arnar-Stone Laboratories, Inc., McGraw Park, Ill.

Edrophonium chloride (Tensilon)

Major actions

Anticholinesterase.
Antagonist for skeletal muscle relaxants.
Increases parasympathetic stimulation to the heart.

Primary emergency uses

Paroxysmal atrial tachycardia (PAT).
Myasthenia crisis.
Antagonist to tubocurarine, curare, and other similar agents.

Notes on administration

Has rapid onset of action (30 to 60 seconds) and short duration of action (approximately 10 minutes).
Use with caution for patients with asthma or hypotension.
Prolongs muscle relaxant effect of succinylcholine (Anectine).
Contraindicated in pregnancy.
Incompatible in syringe or solution with other drugs.
Serious side effects include cardiac arrest, seizures, laryngospasm, bronchial spasm, respiratory arrest, and vomiting.

Note: Atropine must be at hand for antidote to reverse serious side effects: 0.5 to 1 mg (IV bolus) may be repeated every 3 to 5 minutes as necessary. Administer *only* where all resuscitation equipment is at hand and a physician is present.

Preparation and dosage

Adult: 2 to 10 mg IV push over 2 to 4 minutes *or* may be given by continuous drip in selected situations.
Pediatric: 0.05 mg/kg up to 5 mg IV push over 2 to 4 minutes or may be given by continuous drip in selected situations.

Epinephrine (Adrenalin)

Major actions

Sympathomimetic agent.
Vasoconstrictor.
Cardiac stimulant (inotropic and chronotropic).
Dilates smooth muscle, for example, bronchial tree.
Relaxes bronchial tree.

Primary emergency uses

Cardiac resuscitation; stimulates asystolic heart to contract and converts fine ventricular fibrillation to coarse fibrillation.
Anaphylaxis.
Allergies including bronchial asthma.
Stokes-Adams syndrome.
Histamine antidote.

Notes on administration

Contraindicated in hypertension, hyperthyroidism, glaucoma, and for digitalized patients.
Incompatible with alkaline solutions; flush IV line after administering sodium bicarbonate.
May induce hypertensive crisis if given with monoamine oxidase (MAO) inhibitor drugs.
Relatively ineffective in acidotic patient. Correct acidosis before administration.
Protect drug from light and heat.
Adverse effects include hypertension, pulmonary edema, tachydysrhythmias, and ventricular fibrillation (especially after repeated doses).
Toxic hypertensive reactions should be treated with phentolamine (Regitine).
Neostigmine (Prostigmin) may be useful for other toxic responses.
Do not give epinephrine in oil solution intravenously!

Preparation and dosage

Adult: *Cardiac arrest:* 5 to 10 ml of 1 : 10,000 IV or IC. (May be administered directly into trachea via endotracheal tube if other route cannot be established.) Repeat every 5 minutes during arrest. *Asthma:* 0.3 to 0.5 ml of 1 : 1000 subcutaneously.
Pediatric: *Cardiac arrest:* 0.1 mg/kg of 1 : 10,000 IV or IC. (May be administered directly into trachea via endotracheal tube if other route cannot be established.) Repeat every 5 minutes during arrest. *Asthma:* 0.1 to 0.5 ml of 1 : 1000 subcutaneously calculated to weight (0.01 ml/kg of 1 : 1000 to a maximum of 0.5 ml).

Furosemide (Lasix)

Major actions

Rapid-acting loop diuretic.
Blocks reabsorption of sodium and potassium; produces venous pooling.
May be used in head trauma if other drugs are unavailable.

Primary emergency uses

Acute pulmonary edema/congestive heart failure.
May be used to stimulate urinary output in shock states after volume deficit is corrected.

Notes on administration

Acts within 5 to 10 minutes with maximum effect in 30 minutes.
Potentiates other antihypertensive drugs.
Watch for circulatory collapse associated with rapid diuresis and hypovolemia.
Monitor urinary output; Foley catheter may be indicated.
Contraindicated in pregnancy or with history of sulfonamide sensitivity.
Prolonged use can lead to hypokalemia; observe patient for electrolyte imbalances.
Incompatible with corticosteroids and with any other drug (in syringe or IV solution).

Preparation and dosage

Adult: 20 to 80 mg IV push over 1 to 4 minutes.
Pediatric: 1 mg/kg/dose IV bolus over 1 to 4 minutes.

Note: To stimulate urinary output in shock states after volume deficit has been corrected, 5 to 10 mg may be initially given IV followed by a doubled dose every 15 minutes until satisfactory output is obtained (50 to 100 ml/hour) or until single dose of 500 to 1000 mg has been reached.

Glucagon hydrochloride

Major actions

Enhances inotropic action of digitalis, but not chronotropic action.
Decreases AV conduction time and augments contractility.
Increases myocardial oxygen consumption and coronary blood flow.
Accelerates conversion of glycogen to glucose in liver.

Primary emergency uses

Congestive heart failure.
Myocardial depression.
Reversal of beta-adrenergic blockers.
Not drug of choice for profound hypoglycemia that requires aggressive therapy. Mainly reserved for outpatient basis for self-administration subcutaneously.

Notes on administration

Incompatible with any other drug in IV or syringe.
Unpleasant side effect is nausea and vomiting; protect patient from aspiration. Other side effects include anaphylaxis, hyperglycemia, and hypotension.
Correct existing hypvolemia before IV administration.
May produce microaggregation.
Contraindicated in pheochromocytoma.
Use with caution in conjunction with MAO inhibitors.
Enhances anticoagulant effects of warfarin.
Acute overdose may be treated with insulin.

Preparation and dosage

Adult: *Hypoglycemia:* 5 to 10 mg IV, IM, or subcutaneously. May be repeated in 20 minutes if necessary. Dextrose 50% should be used as first line with glucagon as supplement. *Other uses:* Dissolve in D/5/W. Infuse at rate of 2.5 to 15 mg/hour.
Pediatric: 50 μg/kg every 4 hours, up to 1 mg.

Heparin sodium (Heprinar, Liquaemin, Panheprin)

Major action

Anticoagulant.

Primary emergency uses

Preparation of blood gas syringes.
Autotransfusion.
Disseminating intravascular coagulation (DIC).
Prevention of cerebral thrombosis in evolving stroke.
Atrial fibrillation with embolization.

Notes on administration

Give cautiously to patients with diseases carrying an increased risk of hemorrhage, such as blood dyscrasia, gastrointestinal ulceration, hypertension, and pregnancy.

Avoid concurrent use of salicylates.

Use with extreme caution in patients with allergies to animal tissue derivatives; prepare to manage anaphylaxis.

Avoid concurrent administration of acid citrate dextrose-converted blood (collected in heparin sodium), since anticoagulant activity persists, despite conversion, under certain circumstances.

When giving subcutaneously, neither aspirate before injection nor massage site after injection.

Preparation and dosage

Blood gas syringe: 0.5 ml is sufficient for preparing blood gas syringe. Discard excess after coating barrel and needle.

Autotransfusion: Highly individualized based on manufacturer's guidelines for autotransfuser equipment.

DIC: *Adult:* 5000 to 10,000 units by rapid IV injection followed by a constant infusion of 500 to 1500 units/hour; titrate to maintain thrombin or clotting time two and a half to three times normal or partial thromboplastin time of 70 to 80 seconds. *Pediatric:* Not established.

Others: IV or subcutaneous dosages highly individualized based on coagulation studies.

Note: Have protamine sulfate (1%) at hand as antidote. Never accept orders for heparin specified only by volume (ml), since several strengths (units per ml) are available with widely varying potencies.

Caution: Protamine given IV too rapidly can cause severe hypotension. Normal dose of protamine is 1 mg/1000 units heparin. If 30 minutes or more have elapsed since heparin was given, the dosage of protamine is 0.5 mg/1000 units heparin.

Hydralazine (Apresoline)

Major actions

Direct relaxation of vascular smooth muscle.
Increases cardiac rate and output.
Accelerates renal blood flow.

Primary emergency uses

Hypertensive crisis.
Toxemia of pregnancy.

Notes on administration

Onset of action is at least 5 to 10 minutes.

Contraindicated in rheumatic or coronary heart disease.

Incompatible with phenobarbital sodium.

Tachycardia, atrial flutter, ileus, and toxic psychosis are among recognized side effects.

Do not add to IV solution flask. (Apresoline drips are not used.)

Monitor BP every 5 minutes during administration.

Preparation and dosage

Adult: 10 to 40 mg IV bolus given over 1 to 4 minutes. May be repeated if necessary with increased dose.

Pediatric: 1.7 to 3.5 mg/kg/24 hours IM or IV in 4 to 6 divided doses.

Ipecac (syrup)

Major action
Acts on brain stem and locally on gastric mucosa to produce vomiting.

Primary emergency use
Emetic.

Notes on administration
Contraindicated in patient with depressed level of consciousness or decreased gag reflex.

Should not be used to induce vomiting after ingestion of caustic substances.

Acts within 15 to 20 minutes for most adults and children.

Do not use fluid extract of ipecac (extremely toxic) in place of syrup of ipecac.

Produces myocardial irritability if absorbed systemically in large amounts.

Ambulate patient if possible. Protect the airway from aspiration during vomiting.

Should be given in conjunction with several glasses of water.

Assess airway after administration.

Preparation and dosage
Adult: 1 ounce (30 ml) orally with 1 or 2 glasses of water. May be repeated in 20 to 30 minutes if necessary. Lavage if second dose is ineffective.

Pediatric: 10 to 15 ml orally with 1 or 2 glasses of water. May be repeated in 20 to 30 minutes if necessary. Lavage if second dose is ineffective.

Isoproterenol hydrochloride (Isuprel)

Major actions
Cardiac stimulant (chronotropic and inotropic).
Increases coronary and renal blood flow.
Improves A V conduction.
Bronchial smooth muscle relaxant.
Increases systolic blood pressure.

Primary emergency uses
Sinus bradycardia, unresponsive to atropine.
A V block, unresponsive to atropine.
Septic shock.
Bronchospasm.
Asystole.
Cardiogenic shock, postinfarction.
Idioventricular rhythms.

Notes on administration
Contraindicated in states of hypokalemia, hypovolemia, hyperthyroidism, coronary insufficiency, diabetes, or tachycardia from digitalis intoxication or any other cause.

Should be used cautiously if at all in patients receiving MAO inhibitors and propranolol (Inderal).

Action is of short duration. Must be administered by way of continuous drip and titrated for effect for dependable results.

Adverse reactions include palpitations, anginal pain, headache, ventricular tachycardia, and cardiac arrest.

Observe for PVCs, ventricular fibrillation, and evidence of pulmonary edema. CVP and BP should be monitored closely.

Preparation and dosage
Preparation and dosage rates vary widely for each indication. Consult product literature.

Adult (for cardiac problems): 1 to 2 mg in 500 ml D/5/W titrated for effect. May be given IC (0.02 mg) if IV line is unavailable.

Pediatric (for cardiac problems): 1 mg in 500 ml D/5/W titrated for effect.

Levarterenol bitartrate (Levophed, norepinephrine)

Major actions

Increases force of myocardial contraction.
Sympathomimetic.
Dilates coronary arteries.
Peripheral arteriolar vasoconstriction.
Reduces splanchnic and renal blood flow.

Primary emergency uses

Hypotension.
Blood and drug reactions.
Hemorrhage (rare).

Notes on administration

Administer through plastic catheter in large vein.
Contraindicated in mesenteric thrombosis and patients taking MAO inhibitors.
Nothing should be added to infusion.
Incompatible with amobarbital sodium (Amytal), phenytoin (Dilantin), heparin sodium (Heprinar, Liquaemin, Panheprin), warfarin (Coumadin), whole blood, sodium bicarbonate, metaraminol bitartrate (Aramine, Pressonex), oxytocin (Pitocin, Syntocinon), Phenobarbital sodium, (Eskabarb, Luminal Sodium), and sulfisoxazole (Gantrisin).
Watch for adverse reactions, including bradycardia, chest pain, ischemia, and necrosis caused by extravasation.
Observe for hypotension after discontinuation because of decrease in plasma volume.
Do not use in endotoxic shock or renal shutdown.

Preparation and dosage

Adult: Dilute 4 to 8 mg in 500 mg D/5/W. Use micropdrip. Titrate for effect. Do not allow BP to rise above 110 systolic. Use Regitine* 15 to 30 mg injected with fine needle in blanched area of extravasation.
Pediatric: 2 to 4 mg in 500 ml D/5/W infused at 0.2 to 1 μg/kg/minute. Use microdrip. Titrate for effect. Do not allow BP to rise above 110 systolic.

---

*Prevents excessive vasoconstriction and local necrosis in the event of extravasation.

Lidocaine (Xylocaine) 2%

Major actions

Reduces myocardial excitability; elevates fibrillatory threshold.
Local anesthetic (discussion of use as an anesthetic will not be discussed below).

Primary emergency uses

Supraventricular rhythms with aberrant conduction. Ventricular dysrhythmias, especially PVCs and tachycardia.
Useful in managing acute myocardial dysrhythmias after 1 hour from onset of symptoms if heart rate is between 60 and 100 beats per minute.
Prophylactically in patients who appear to be experiencing acute myocardial infarction.

Notes on administration

Use bolus and drip together or another bolus. Effect of bolus without drip or another bolus dissipates in 10 to 15 minutes. A drip alone does not become effective for 20 to 30 minutes.
Seizures may occur as side effect. Have Valium and Luminal Sodium at hand.
Use with caution in presence of reduced cardiac output or liver disease.
Contraindicated in instances of heart block, bradycardia, congestive heart failure, or chronic obstructive lung disease.
Ineffective in refractory ventricular fibrillation.
Incompatible with procaine amide and quinidine.
Patients may be refractory to lidocaine during the first hour after myocardial infarction.

Preparation and dosage

Adult: 50 to 100 mg IV bolus followed by IV infusion at 1 to 4 mg/minute. (Dilute 2 gm in 500 ml D/5/W.) *Bolus only* (especially recommended in prehospital care: 75 mg IV bolus *initially* followed by additional 50 mg bolus in 5 minutes, then 50 mg bolus every 10 minutes up to 275 to 325 mg.
Pediatric: *IV bolus:* 0.5 mg/kg given over 3 minutes. *Drip:* 0.02 to 0.03 mg/kg/minute (100 mg in 500 ml D/5/W).

Note: Use microdrip set: titrate for effect. Rapid bolus injection may result in hypotension, severe bradycardia or tachycardia, and seizures.

Mannitol (Osmitrol)

Major action
Osmotic diuretic.

Primary emergency uses
Increased intracranial pressure.
Drug overdose. (Check references for specific drugs.)
Generalized edema or ascites.

Notes on administration
Contraindicated in states of pregnancy, anuria or severe renal impairment, congestive heart failure, fluid and electrolyte depletion, and dehydration.
Incompatible with any drug in syringe or solution and with whole blood.
Rare adverse reactions include seizures, dehydration, hypertension or hypotension (rapid volume depletion—rare occurrence in adults but not so rare in children), pulmonary edema, tachycardia, visual disturbances, chest pain, chills, thrombophlebitis, and urinary retention.

Preparation and dosage
Adult: 50 to 200 mg of 20% solution over 20 to 60 minutes. (1.5 to 4.5 mg/kg may also be given by slow IV bolus.)
• Use blood filter for administration.
Pediatric: 2 to 3 gm/kg of 20% solution over 20 to 60 minutes. May also be given by slow IV bolus.

Metaraminol bitartrate (Aramine, Pressonex)

Major actions
Peripheral arteriolar vasoconstrictor.
Increases cardiac contractility.

Primary emergency uses
Rapid correction of hypotension.
Terminate supraventricular tachycardia.

Notes on administration
Incompatible with heparin solution (Heprinar, Liquaemin, Panheprin), phenytoin (Dilantin), hydrocortisone succinate (Solu-Cortef), norepinephrine (Levophed), penicillin G potassium (Orapen, Penalev, Penasoid, Pentids), sulfisoxazole (Gantrisin), warfarin sodium (Coumadin), sodium bicarbonate, and Ringer's lactate injection.
Watch for adverse reactions, including dysrhythmias, hypertension, and cardiac arrest.

Preparation and dosage
Adult: 15 to 100 mg in 500 ml D/5/W titrated for effect. (Unusual circumstances may warrant 150 to 500 mg in 500 ml D/5/W.) A bolus of 0.5 to 5.0 mg IV push *followed by* an infusion of 15 to 100 mg in 500 ml D/5/W (titrated for effect) is an alternate regimen.
Pediatric: 0.3 to 2 mg/kg in 500 ml D/5/W titrated for effect. Use microdrip.

Methyldopate hydrochloride (Aldomet, methyldopa)

Major actions
Decreases sympathetic activity.
Lowers renal vascular resistance.

Primary emergency use
Hypertensive or pheochromocytoma crisis.

Notes on administration
Should be given concurrently with diuretics.
Monitor urinary output.
May cause death if administered with MAO inhibitors or CNS depressants.
Potentiates levarterenol and other antihypertensives.
Contraindicated in pregnancy and for patients with depression or liver dysfunction.
Incompatible with tetracycline, amphotericin B, and sulfadiazine sodium in same solution.
Side effects include dizziness, fever, postural hypotension, and unusual mental phenomena including nightmares and depression.
Effects may be reversed by metaraminol.

Preparation and dosage
Adult: 250 to 500 mg every 6 hours. Dilute in 100 to 200 ml of D/5/W and administer by infusion over 30 to 60 minutes.
Pediatric: 20 to 40 mg/kg/24 hours in 4 divided IV doses at 6-hour intervals. Dilute in 100 to 200 ml of D/5/W and administer each dose over 30 to 60 minutes.

Methylergonovine maleate (Methergine)

Major actions
Contracts uterus.
Constricts uterine vessels.

Primary emergency uses
Routine, after placenta delivery.
Postpartum atony and hemorrhage.

Notes on administration
May be ineffective if patient is hypocalcemic.
May create hypertension or bradycardia if used with regional anesthetics or vasopressors.
Contraindicated in toxemia.
Do not mix with any other drug.
Monitor BP before administration.
Side effects include chest pain, dilated pupils, diaphoresis, dyspnea, nausea, vomiting.

Preparation and dosage
Keep refrigerated. Use within 60 days if stored at room temperature.
Adult: 0.2 mg IM. (May be repeated in 2 to 4 hours.) IV administration is reserved for extremely urgent situations. See product literature.
Pediatric: Not established.

Methylprednisolone sodium succinate (Solu-Medrol)

Major actions

Antiinflammatory agent.
Adrenocortical steroid.

Primary emergency uses

Allergies.
Cerebral edema.
Septic shock.
Infections with toxicity.
Shock states unresponsive to conventional therapy.
Bronchial asthma unresponsive to conventional therapy.
Esophageal burns.
Croup.

Notes on administration

Incompatible with anticonvulsants, some antihistamines, barbiturates, digitoxin (Crystodigin), propranolol (Inderal), meperidine (Demerol), and promethazine (Phenergan).
Contraindicated in systemic fungal infections with long-term use of steroids.
Watch for adverse reactions including anaphylaxis, hypertension, increased intracranial pressure, seizures, and thromboembolism.
Increases requirements for insulin or oral hypoglycemic agents in diabetes.

Note: Dosage varies widely with rationale for use.

Preparation and dosage

Dosage varies widely with indications for emergency use. Check rationale for treatment and calculate all doses accordingly.

Morphine sulfate

Major actions

Narcotic analgesic; alters perception of pain; elevates pain threshold.
Increases venous capacitance.

Primary emergency uses

Relieves pain from coronary occlusion.
Acute pulmonary edema secondary to cardiac failure.
Relieves pain from biliary or renal colic.
Severely burned patients who do not have associated trauma.

Notes on administration

Use with extreme caution for patients with chronic obstructive lung disease.
Contraindicated for patients with asthma, head injuries, increased intracranial pressure, and chronic cor pulmonale.
Correct volume depletion or hypotension before administration.
Expect maximum respiratory depression in 7 to 10 minutes after IV administration.
Analgesic effect is immediate and peaks at 20 minutes.
Incompatible in syringe with aminophylline, phenytoin (Dilantin), meperidine (Demerol), phenobarbital (Eskabarb, Luminal Sodium), heparin, sodium bicarbonate, and sulfisoxazole (Gantrisin).

Preparation and dosage

Adult: 2 to 15 mg IV, given over 3 to 5 minutes. Titrate for effect.
Pediatric: 0.1 to 0.2 mg/kg IV dose, given over 3 to 5 minutes.

Note: Side effects, especially respiratory depression, can be reversed with naloxone (Narcan) (0.4 to 0.8 mg IV or IM every 2 to 5 minutes as needed) after a delay of 4 to 5 minutes. Treat resultant hypotension with shock position.

Naloxone (Narcan)

Major actions

Narcotic antagonist.
Useful in reversing respiratory depression induced by depressant drugs.

Primary emergency uses

Antidote for narcotics and dextropropoxyphene (Darvon), pentazocine lactate (Talwin), and diphenoxylate (Lomotil).
Differentiates coma that is induced by narcotics or dextropropoxyphene and pentazocine from other causes.

Notes on administration

Elevates partial thromboplastin time.
Will precipitate narcotic withdrawal in drug-abusing patient. Be prepared to deal with a combative patient after administration.

Preparation and dosage

Adult: 0.4 to 0.8 mg or more (given by IV, IM, subcutaneous, or sublingual injection). May repeat two or three times at intervals of 2 to 3 minutes.
Pediatric: 0.01 mg/kg dose given by IV, IM, subcutaneous, or sublingual injection. May repeat two or three times at intervals of 2 to 3 minutes.

Note: May be used in place of morphine sulfate. May be used in conjunction with morphine sulfate *but not simultaneously.* Trial of nitroglycerin first after initiation of IV is recommended.

Nitroglycerin (glyceryl trinitrate)

Major actions

Vasodilator; pools venous blood, thus decreasing myocardial workload and oxygen requirements.
Relaxes smooth muscle.
Redistributes coronary blood flow; preferential dilatation of conducting vessels.
Pools venous blood.

Primary emergency uses

Relieves pain from angina pectoris and acute myocardial infarction.
Minimizes infarct size by reducing preload.
Relieves pain from biliary or renal colic.
Pulmonary edema.

Notes on administration

Effective in 1 or 2 minutes after administration.
Headache and flushing of the face and neck are expected transient side effects.
Drug may lose potency after prolonged storage.
Store in brown glass bottle only. Protect from air, light, and heat. Procure fresh supply every 4 to 6 months.

Preparation and dosage

Adult: Gr 1/150 sublingually (0.4 mg). May repeat one time after 5 minutes if BP continues to be in acceptable range. *In pulmonary edema with normotension or hypertension: Mild:* 0.8 mg (gr $\frac{1}{150}$ × 2 tablets) sublingually. *Moderate:* 1.2 mg (gr $\frac{1}{150}$ × 3 tablets) sublingually. *Severe:* 1.6 mg (gr $\frac{1}{150}$ × 4 tablets) sublingually.
Pediatric: Dosage not established.

Note: Patient should be sitting or supine during and immediately after administration. Treat resultant hypotension with shock position.

Oxygen

(See also Chapters 8 and 17.)

Major actions

Decreases ventilatory and myocardial effort to maintain alveolar and arterial oxygen tensions, respectively.

Increases alveolar oxygen tensions.

Primary emergency uses

Shock states.

Head injuries.

Cardiac or pulmonary complaints.

Poisonings or toxic states resulting in respiratory depression, acidosis, or decreased levels of conciousness.

Sickle cell anemia crisis.

Agitation and confusion that may be the result of cerebral hypoxia.

Cardiac or pulmonary arrest.

Multiple trauma.

Notes on administration

Humidify oxygen if possible, since it has a rapid drying effect on nasal and pulmonary mucosa. This is a crucial consideration when an artificial airway is in use.

Do not attempt to supply humidity when using a bag-mask device for assisting breathing, since water can be aspirated into the tubing and valve mechanisms of the bag, thus interfering with gas delivery.

Oxygen, even 100% concentration, has no adverse effects for brief periods in emergency situations. Do not withhold oxygen during initial transpor-tation or resuscitation while waiting for arterial blood gas analyses on the ruling out of chronic obstructive pulmonary states. The detrimental and often irreversible effects of hypoxia and hypoxemia develop quickly. Most adverse effects of excessive oxygen delivery (such as oxygen toxicity) develop slowly, usually after 24 hours of therapy. When in doubt, employ concentrations less than 50% for supportive management of the cardiopulmonary mechanisms while awaiting results of arterial blood gas analyses and other clinical validation.

Ensure airway efficiency by proper positioning, suctioning, and employment of an adjunctive device if necessary.

Never deliver less than 5 liters by mask, since expired air can accumulate in the device and be rebreathed, thus increasing carbon dioxide inhalation and resulting in a concurrent decline in oxygen delivery.

Low-flow oxygen delivery (less than 35%) should be reserved for patients with regular, consistent ventilations of normal volume and a rate less than 25 per minute.

High-flow oxygen delivery (greater than 60%) is usually reserved for patients with primary cardiopulmonary disease or those who cannot maintain a consistent ventilatory pattern.

Never discontinue oxygen at the same time that mechanical ventilatory support is discontinued. When oxygen therapy is no longer indicated, administration should be gradually reduced while carefully monitoring ventilatory indices and cardiac activity.

Oxytocin (Pitocin, Syntocinon)

Major action
Contracts uterine muscles; constricts uterine blood vessels.

Primary emergency use
Controls postpartum hemorrhage.

Notes on administration
Adverse reactions include anaphylaxis, cardiac dysrhythmias, subarachnoid hemorrhage, hypotension, tachycardia, and water intoxication.

Preparation and dosage
Adult: 10 to 20 units in 1000 ml D/5/W or D/5/½NS infused at 0.5 to 1 ml/minute.
Pediatric: Not established.

Pentazocine lactate (Talwin)

Major action
Depresses central nervous system.

Primary emergency uses
Analgesia and sedation.

Notes on administration
Contributes to respiratory depression and intracranial pressure. May precipitate narcotic withdrawal symptoms.
Naloxone (Narcan) is specific antidote.
Avoid concurrent use with alcohol, tranquilizers, antihistamines, and general anesthetic agents.

Preparation and dosage.
Adult: 30 to 60 mg every 3 to 4 hours; IV bolus over 2 minutes. Can also be given IM.
Pediatric: Not established.

Phenobarbital sodium (Eskabarb, Luminal Sodium)

Major actions
Anticonvulsant.
Sedative, hypnotic.

Primary emergency use
Status epilepticus.

Notes on administration
Contraindicated with respiratory depression.
Incompatible with any drug in any solution.
Incompatible with Compazine, Keflin, insulin, morphine, Thorazine, codeine, Dramamine, Benadryl, Dilantin, Solu-Cortef, Vistaril, Levophed, and Demerol.
Avoid mixing; flush line before delivery.
Adverse reactions include asthma, bronchospasm, hypotension, respiratory depression, pulmonary edema, and coma.
May stimulate CNS in children.

Preparation and dosage
Adult: 30 to 130 mg IV bolus over period of 5 to 10 minutes until seizure is controlled.
- Support respirations, especially if Valium (or any drug that can produce CNS depression, such as morphine or pentazocine) has been administered previously.

Pediatric: 3 to 5 mg/kg/dose IV bolus over 5 minutes until seizure is controlled.
- Support respirations, especially if Valium has been administered previously.

Phenylephrine (Isophrin, Neo-Synephrine)

Major actions

Sympathomimetic.
Increases stroke volume.

Primary emergency uses

PAT.
Reversal of hypotensive crisis, especially drug induced.
Antidote for hypotension produced by chlorpromazine (Thorazine).

Notes on administration

Administer cautiously to patients who are elderly or who have known myocardial disease.
Potentiated by other sympathomimetics, tricyclic antidepressants, and MAO inhibitors.
Contraindicated in states of hypertension or ventricular tachycardia.
Incompatible with alkaline solutions.
Side effects include bradycardia, ventricular extrasystoles, ventricular tachycardia, and hypertensive crisis.
Phentolamine (Regitine) is agent of choice for reversing severe hypertensive response.
Monitor BP at least every 2 to 3 minutes.

Preparation and dosage

Adult: *IV bolus:* dilute 1 mg with 9 ml of IV solution (0.1 mg/ml); 0.1 to 0.5 mg over 20 to 30 seconds to treat PAT. Rate is over 1 to 2 minutes for all other uses. *Drip:* dilute 10 mg in 250 ml of D/5/W or N/S. Use microdrip. Titrate for effect.
Pediatric: 0.1 to 0.5 μg/kg/minute IV over 1 to 2 minutes.

Phenytoin (Dilantin, diphenylhydantoin)

Major actions

Anticonvulsant.
Stabilizes seizure threshold and depresses seizure activity.
Decreases sinus node pacemaker activity, speeds conduction time, shortens refractory period and reduces myocardial contractility.

Primary emergency uses

Status epilepticus. (Drug of choice is Valium).
Neurological trauma with seizures.
Ventricular premature contractions.
PAT with block.
Junctional or ventricular tachycardia.

Notes on administration

Contraindicated in bradycardia, complete heart block, and second degree heart block.
Use only when completely dissolved and clear.
Ensure vein patency before administration. Extravasation can cause sloughing.
Incompatible with any drug in syringe or solution.
Inhibits corticosteroids.
Action inhibited by alcohol, antihistamines, and barbiturates.
Potentiates antihypertensives, CNS depressants, diuretics, and muscle relaxants.
Do not administer in same solution with aminophylline, insulin, meperidine, disulfiram, digitalis, metaraminol, diphenhydramine, and levarterenol bitartrate.
Adverse reactions include heart block, bradycardia, hypotension, respiratory arrest, ventricular fibrillation, cardiac arrest, and phlebitis resulting from local irritation.

Preparation and dosage

Adult: *Anticonvulsant:* 150 to 250 mg over 5 minutes, IV bolus. *Antidysrhythmic:* 100 mg to maximum of 300 mg/24 hours.
  • Heart block or bradycardia may be reversed with atropine.
Pediatric: 1 to 2 mg/kg IV over 5 minutes to maximum of 5 to 7 mg/kg/day.

Note: Monitor ECG during administration. Half-life is 24 hours.

Physostigmine salicylate (Antilirium, Eserine)

Major action

Inhibits cholinesterase.

Primary emergency uses

Reverses atropine-like drugs.

Indicated for anticholinergic findings with hypertension, hallucinations, seizures, coma, and dysrhythmias.

Notes on administration

Too rapid administration may induce seizures.

Should not be used in asthma, diabetes, cardiovascular disease, gangrenous states, or obstructions of the intestinal or urinary tract.

Preparation and dosage

Adult: 0.5 to 2 mg IV (over 2 minutes) or IM. May be repeated if life-threatening circumstances prevail (1 to 4 doses). Have atropine ready at one half the dose of the physostigmine. Monitor ECG.

Pediatric: 0.5 mg IV over 2 minutes. May be repeated at 5-minute intervals.

Potassium chloride

Major actions

Depresses ectopic impulse generation.

Affects (enhances and depresses) conduction velocity of myocardium.

Primary emergency use

Hypokalemia resulting from diuretic therapy, diabetic ketoacidosis, digitalis toxicity, and other causes.

Notes on administration

Contraindicated in second degree AV block, oliguria, dehydration, acidosis, shock with hemolytic reactions, and kidney failure.

Incompatible with amphotericin B and protein hydrolysate.

Adverse reactions include bradycardia, AV block, ventricular fibrillation, ventricular asystole, cardiac arrest, respiratory distress, and voluntary muscle paralysis.

Ensure continuous cardiac monitoring and obtain periodic serum electrolyte levels during administration.

Potentiated by spironolactone.

Preparation and dosage

Adult: Dilute 20 to 40 mEq in 1000 ml. Deliver at rate of 10 mEq/hour or less.

Pediatric: Daily pediatric dose should not exceed 3 mEq/kg of body weight.

Note: Hyperkalemia ECG manifestations: narrowed, peaked T wave; shortened QT interval; widened QRS; lengthened PR interval; P wave may diminish or disappear; ST segment may shift.

Procainamide (Pronestyl)

Major actions

Slows and depresses conduction across excitable tissue.
Reduces myocardial contractility; slows heart.
Prolongs refractory period.
Decreases membrane permeability.

Primary emergency uses

Supraventricular and ventricular dysrhythmias, PAT, atrial fibrillation, PVCs, and others.
Useful in managing dysrhythmias after myocardial infarction that are refractory to lidocaine (such as first hour).

Notes on administration

Contraindicated for patients with heart block or myasthenia gravis.
Use with caution for digitalis-related ventricular dysrhythmias.
Incompatible with phenytoin (Dilantin).
Rapid administration results in a negative inotropic effect or heart block with resultant hypotension.
Be prepared for adverse reactions, including ventricular tachycardia, ventricular fibrillation, and asystole.

Preparation and dosage

Adult: *IV bolus:* 100 mg given slowly over 2 minutes. Dose may be repeated every 5 minutes up to 1 gm maximum. *Drip:* 1 gm in 500 ml D/5/W given at a rate of 1 to 3 ml/minute.
Pediatric: *IV bolus:* 2 mg/kg/dose given over 2 to 4 minutes. *Drip:* 10 to 100 mg in 500 ml D/5/W.

Note: Use microdrip set; titrate for effect. Bolus rate of administration should never exceed 50 mg/minute.

Propranolol (Inderal)

Major actions

Beta-adrenergic blocker; decreases heart rate and myocardial contractility.
Reduces myocardial oxygen requirements.
Prolongs AV junction conduction.
Suppresses atrial and ventricular ectopic foci.
Increases airway resistance.

Primary emergency uses

Severe angina attacks.
Tachydysrhythmias associated with digitalis toxicity or thyrotoxicosis.
Acute myocardial infarction after first hour with heart rate above 100 and normal or elevated BP.
Acute anxiety attacks.
Atrial extrasystoles unresponsive to other drugs.

Notes on administration

Use with digitalizing drugs if patient has not been digitalized.
Contraindicated in asthma, sinus bradycardia, or heart block beyond first degree.
Prepare to treat bronchoconstriction and severe asthmatic attack.
May precipitate congestive heart failure (reduction in contractility).
Tends to exaggerate digitalis-induced bradycardia, which may be reversed with atropine (0.5 [never less] to 1 mg).
Monitor ECG and BP during administration.
Observe for hypotension and AV block, AV dissociation, and cardiac arrest.
Can induce hypoglycemia. Use with caution in insulin-dependent diabetics.
Onset of action is rapid (1 to 3 minutes). Peaks in 10 to 15 minutes.
Incompatible with any other antihypertensive agent and with any other drug (in syringe).

Preparation and dosage

Dosage varies widely with indications for emergency use. Check rationale for treatment and calculate all doses accordingly.

Note: Have pacemaker equipment at hand. Half-life is 2 to 3 hours.

Quinidine gluconate (injection)

Major actions

Prolongs atrial and ventricular refractory period.
Decreases ectopic impulse generation.
Depresses myocardial contractility.
Vagal-blocking agent.

Primary emergency uses

Atrial fibrillation or flutter.
Paroxysmal atrial and ventricular tachycardia.
Premature systoles.

Notes on administration

Contraindicated in conduction pathology, myasthenia gravis, myocardial damage, digitalis intoxication.
Keep patient supine during administration.
Monitor patient's ECG and BP.
Potentiated by thiazides, neuromuscular blocking agents, anticholinergics, muscle relaxants, and anticoagulants.
Use cautiously with procaine amide, propranolol, and digitalis.
May increase prothrombin time.
Adverse reactions include hypotension, tachycardia, visual disturbances, idioventricular rhythms and ventricular fibrillation, AV block, asystole, quinidine syncope (ventricular tachydysrhythmias with loss of consciousness).
Sodium bicarbonate, procaine amide, lidocaine, isoproterenol, levarterenol bitartrate, and metaraminol are useful in treating adverse conduction disturbances and vascular collapse.

Preparation and dosage

Adult: 800 mg (10 ml) in 40 ml D/5/W. Administer 1 ml of infusion over 1-minute period.
Pediatric: 30 mg/kg/24 hours given in 5 divided doses diluted 5:1 with D/5/W. Administer 1 ml over 1-minute period.

Note: Discontinue drug when normal sinus rhythm returns or if P waves disappear.

Sodium bicarbonate

Major actions

Alkalizing agent; buffering agent in blood.
Elevates pH promptly.

Primary emergency uses

Cardiac arrest.
Acidosis of severe shock.
Status asthmaticus.
Salicylate intoxication.

Notes on administration

Contraindicated in edema, hypertension, impaired renal function, and respiratory alkalosis.
Incompatible with calcium chloride, Ringer's lactate injection, dextrose solutions, levarterenol, and morphine.
Adverse reactions include alkalosis, hyperexcitability, tetany, congestive heart failure (CHF) precipitated by sodium excess, hypernatremia, and hyperosmolality.

Preparation and dosage

Adult: In cardiac arrest 1 to 2 amps IV bolus stat, then 1 amp every 10 minutes while patient is pulseless (1 amp = 44.8 mEq $NaHCO_3$) or calculate according to arterial blood gas values.
Pediatric: In cardiac arrest 1 mEq/kg IV every 5 to 10 minutes.

Note: Excessive $NaHCO_3$ can displace the oxyhemoglobin dissociation curve and can decrease the oxygen released at the tissue level.

Sodium nitroprusside (Nipride)

Major actions

Direct dilation of arterioles and veins.
Improves left ventricular function.
Increases cardiac output.

Primary emergency uses

Pulmonary edema with hypertensive response.
Chronic refractory heart failure and acute myocardial infarction.
Hypertensive emergencies including dissecting aneurysms.
Minimizes bleeding during surgical procedures.

Notes on administration

Use only fresh solution. Discard in 4 hours.
Solution is sensitive to light. Cover IV flask with aluminum foil or other opaque material.
Administer concurrently with diuretic.
Do not mix with any other drug.
Anticipate nausea, vomiting, headache, sweating, restlessness, and substernal pain.
Guard against infiltration.
Never leave patient unmonitored, even for 1 minute!
For prolonged usage of greater than 8 mcg/kg/minute or renal dysfunction there may be an accumulation of thiocyanate. Watch for excessive thiocyanate toxicities: tinnitus, blurred vision, or delirium.

Preparation and dosage

Adult: 50 mg in 250 ml D/5/W infused at rate of 0.5 to 10 μg/kg/minute. Average dose is 3 μg/kg/minute.
Pediatric: Same as adult.

Note: Use microdrip set; titrate for effect. BP will fall drastically within 2 minutes but will rise in 1 to 10 minutes to pretreatment level upon discontinuation. Monitor BP, pulse, and flow rate on a minute-to-minute basis.

Trimethaphan camsylate (Arfonad)

Major actions

Vasodilator.
Blocks sympathetic reflexes.
Ganglionic blocking.
Liberates histamine.
Lowers BP by vasodilation and a drop in cardiac output.

Primary emergency uses

Hypertensive crises.
Cardiogenic shock.
Pulmonary edema caused by hypertension.

Notes on administration

Short-acting potent drug. Must be administered in presence of physician.
Drug must be prepared just before use, and unused portion refrigerated.
Patient should remain flat during receipt of drug. Continuous monitoring of BP and ECG is mandatory. Concurrent oxygen administration may be required.
Potentiated by other antihypertensives, diuretics, alcohol, and anesthetic agents.
Contraindicated for patients with anemia, hypovolemia, pregnancy, shock, respiratory insufficiency, and those who have had MAO inhibitor drugs within past 21 days.
Incompatible with any other drug in syringe, solution, or IV tubing.
Side effects include visual disturbances, depressed respirations, tachycardia, urinary retention, and obstipation.
Overdose may be managed by vasopressors such as phenylephrine or levarterenol.
Keep head of bed elevated during administration to assist in controlling BP.

Preparation and dosage

Adult: Dilute 500 mg in 500 ml of D/5/W (1 ml = 1 mg). Administer 2 to 15 mg/minute. Titrate for effect. Monitor BP continuously.
Pediatric: Not established.

Sample performance review*

Your performance will be reviewed with you in all of the categories below. Please complete the form evaluation yourself before your appraisal interview. All staff will be reviewed using the same format in the first four categories. Remaining section(s) are specific to job classifications.

PART I

	1 Always	2 Usually	3 Infrequently
Professional conduct			
Work habits			
1. Shows willingness to help colleagues	☐	☐	☐
2. Completes all assigned duties	☐	☐	☐
3. Is punctual	☐	☐	☐
4. Is well organized in work	☐	☐	☐
5. Anticipates patient care needs (set-ups, undressing patients, and so on)	☐	☐	☐
6. Looks for things to do during slow times	☐	☐	☐
7. Follows through on problems (takes responsibility for resolution and/or reporting)	☐	☐	☐
8. Meets schedule commitments	☐	☐	☐

COMMENTS: _____

	1 Always	2 Usually	3 Infrequently
Perspective			
1. Is receptive to needs of client groups	☐	☐	☐
2. Understands need for change	☐	☐	☐
3. Takes appropriate measures to correct problems	☐	☐	☐
4. Solicits feedback concerning performance	☐	☐	☐
5. Has positive, cheerful attitude toward work	☐	☐	☐
6. Uses good judgment and common sense in problem solving	☐	☐	☐

COMMENTS: _____

*Courtesy Department of Emergency Medicine, Brotman Medical Center, Culver City, California. *Continued.*

PART I—cont'd

	1 Always	2 Usually	3 Infrequently
Professional conduct—cont'd			
Appearance			
1. Wears appropriate uniform	☐	☐	☐
2. Uniform clean and pressed	☐	☐	☐
3. Shoes clean and in good repair	☐	☐	☐
4. Wears name tag	☐	☐	☐
5. Hair neat and well groomed	☐	☐	☐

COMMENTS: _____

	1 Always	2 Usually	3 Infrequently
Involvement			
1. Contributes suggestions	☐	☐	☐
2. Takes responsibility for problem solving (finds answers if unknown, follows through, reports appropriately)	☐	☐	☐
3. Attends educational conferences and staff meetings	☐	☐	☐
4. Takes responsibility for awareness and understanding of policy/ procedures and change(s)	☐	☐	☐

COMMENTS: _____

	1 Always	2 Usually	3 Infrequently
Record keeping			
1. Completes all necessary forms and logs	☐	☐	☐
2. All documentation is thorough and accurate	☐	☐	☐

COMMENTS: _____

	1 Always	2 Usually	3 Infrequently
Adaptability			
1. Accepts change easily	☐	☐	☐
2. Is able to set priorities	☐	☐	☐
3. Is able to set priorities during census increase	☐	☐	☐
4. Accepts constructive suggestion with ease	☐	☐	☐

COMMENTS: _____

	1 Always	2 Usually	3 Infrequently
Interpersonal relationship			
Co-workers			
1. Gets along well with co-workers	☐	☐	☐
2. Resolves interpersonal conflicts on own	☐	☐	☐
3. Is supportive of co-workers	☐	☐	☐
4. Carries fair share of work load	☐	☐	☐

COMMENTS: _____

PART I—cont'd

	1 Always	2 Usually	3 Infrequently
Interpersonal relationship—cont'd			
Patients/families			
1. Is sensitive to patients' and families' feelings	☐	☐	☐
2. Keeps patients and families informed	☐	☐	☐
COMMENTS:			

	1 Always	2 Usually	3 Infrequently
Leadership ability			
1. Uses good judgement and perspective in problem-solving	☐	☐	☐
2. Is a role model in attitude and perspective	☐	☐	☐
3. Is responsible in work commitments	☐	☐	☐
4. Is supportive of department goals/objectives	☐	☐	☐
5. Communicates clearly without alienating or attacking co-workers	☐	☐	☐
6. Solicits feedback concerning performance	☐	☐	☐
7. Has thorough understanding of department policies, procedures, and duties	☐	☐	☐
8. Motivates others successfully	☐	☐	☐
9. Provides input regarding department problems (personnel and systems)	☐	☐	☐
10. Anticipates patient care needs	☐	☐	☐
COMMENTS:			

PART II

	1 Superior	2 Above average	3 Satis-factory	4 Needs im-provement
RNs				
Knowledge				
1. Drugs	☐	☐	☐	☐
2. Dysrhythmias	☐	☐	☐	☐
3. Laboratory values	☐	☐	☐	☐
4. Anatomy and physiology	☐	☐	☐	☐
5. Medical/legal considerations	☐	☐	☐	☐
6. Pathophysiology of disease entities	☐	☐	☐	☐
COMMENTS:				
Assessment				
1. History taking	☐	☐	☐	☐
2. Physical assessment	☐	☐	☐	☐
a. Cardiovascular	☐	☐	☐	☐
b. Respiratory	☐	☐	☐	☐
c. Musculoskeletal	☐	☐	☐	☐
d. ENT	☐	☐	☐	☐
e. Skin	☐	☐	☐	☐
f. GYN/GU	☐	☐	☐	☐

Continued.

PART II—cont'd

	1 Superior	2 Above average	3 Satis- factory	4 Needs im- provement
RNs—cont'd				
Assessment — cont'd				
g. GI	☐	☐	☐	☐
h. OB	☐	☐	☐	☐
i. Neurological	☐	☐	☐	☐
j. Psychological/social	☐	☐	☐	☐
3. Integration of input with appropriate decision making	☐	☐	☐	☐

COMMENTS: _____

---

	1 Superior	2 Above average	3 Satis- factory	4 Needs im- provement
Intervention				
1. Priority setting	☐	☐	☐	☐
a. Patient specific	☐	☐	☐	☐
b. Multiple patients	☐	☐	☐	☐
c. Departmental	☐	☐	☐	☐
2. Procedural skills	☐	☐	☐	☐
a. IV/venipuncture	☐	☐	☐	☐
b. CVPs	☐	☐	☐	☐
c. Pacing/cardiac	☐	☐	☐	☐
d. Sternotomy	☐	☐	☐	☐
e. Chest tubes	☐	☐	☐	☐
f. Peritoneal lavage	☐	☐	☐	☐
g. Arterial lines	☐	☐	☐	☐
h. Intracranial pressure monitoring	☐	☐	☐	☐
i Splinting	☐	☐	☐	☐
j. Cardioversion/defibrillation	☐	☐	☐	☐
k. Childbirth	☐	☐	☐	☐
l. MAST	☐	☐	☐	☐
3. Patient teaching	☐	☐	☐	☐
4. Crisis intervention				
a. Counseling	☐	☐	☐	☐
b. Referrals	☐	☐	☐	☐

COMMENTS: _____

Certifications
- ☐ BCLS provider
- ☐ BCLS instructor
- ☐ ACLS provider
- ☐ ACLS instructor
- ☐ CEN
- ☐ MICN
- ☐ CCRN

PART II—cont'd

	1 Superior	2 Above Average	3 Satis- factory	4 Needs im- provement
Emergency medical technicians (EMTs)				
Knowledge				
1. Knowledge of the signs and symptoms of patient illness/ severity of illness	☐	☐	☐	☐
2. Knowledge of the principles of emergency procedures	☐	☐	☐	☐
3. Knowledge of uses of emergency equipment, supplies, and instruments	☐	☐	☐	☐
4. Knowledge of restocking and supply system	☐	☐	☐	☐

COMMENTS: _____

Skills				
1. Procedures for all EMTs	☐	☐	☐	☐
a. Suture set-up and dressings	☐	☐	☐	☐
b. Chest tube set-up	☐	☐	☐	☐
c. MAST	☐	☐	☐	☐
d. Lavage set-up	☐	☐	☐	☐
e. Patient discharge teaching	☐	☐	☐	
2. EMT II procedures				
a. Splinting	☐	☐	☐	☐
b. Gait training	☐	☐	☐	☐
c. Foley catheter	☐	☐	☐	☐
d. Tetanus	☐	☐	☐	☐
e. NG tubes/Ewald tubes	☐	☐	☐	☐

COMMENTS: _____

Patient representatives				
Knowledge				
1. Principles of patient triage and screening	☐	☐	☐	☐
2. Logistics of patient care (flow of patients through the ED)	☐	☐	☐	☐
3. Referral system	☐	☐	☐	☐
4. Admitting, discharge, and transfer procedures	☐	☐	☐	☐
5. Paper work processing	☐	☐	☐	☐
6. Communications systems (intercom, beepers, HEAR, telephones)	☐	☐	☐	☐
7. Knowledge of patient and family needs	☐	☐	☐	☐
8. Medicolegal aspects of emergency care	☐	☐	☐	☐
9. Prehospital care system	☐	☐	☐	☐

COMMENTS: _____

Continued.

PART II—cont'd

	1 Superior	2 Above average	3 Satis- factory	4 Needs im- provement
Patient representative—cont'd				
Skills				
1. Scribing	☐	☐	☐	☐
2. Crisis intervention	☐	☐	☐	☐
3. Registration: speed, accuracy, thoroughness	☐	☐	☐	☐
4. Triage and screening	☐	☐	☐	☐
5. Interaction with patients and families	☐	☐	☐	☐
6. Telephone interactions	☐	☐	☐	☐
7. Communication with colleagues	☐	☐	☐	☐

COMMENTS: _____

	1 Superior	2 Above average	3 Satis- factory	4 Needs im- provement
Controllers				
1. Delegation (with tact)	☐	☐	☐	☐
2. Perspective of entire department	☐	☐	☐	☐
3. Anticipation	☐	☐	☐	☐
4. Patient charges (if applicable)	☐	☐	☐	☐

COMMENTS: _____

Index

A

ABCs, 132; *see also* Airway; Breathing; Circulation
  in assessment, 105-106
  in pediatric cardiopulmonary resuscitation, 192
Abdomen
  "cold," 400
  emergencies of, 399-418
    acute abdomen as, 399-406
      assessment of pain in, 399-402
      baseline data for, 402-405
      diseases producing, 400
      pain in, radiation of, 400
      trauma-related, 399
    bowel obstruction as, 411-415
      bowel sounds in, 411
      cecal volvulus as, 413
      ingested foreign bodies as, 412-415
      management of, 411-412
      sigmoid volvulus as, 413
      x-ray and clinical evidence of, 412
    gastrointestinal bleeding as, 408-411
      acute, 408-409
      insertion of nasogastric tube for, 409-410
      lower, 409
      Sengstaken-Blakemore tube for, 410-411
    inflammatory conditions as, 406-408
      abscesses as, 407
      appendicitis as, 407-408
      pancreatitis as, 406
      ulcerative colitis as, 406-407
    trauma as, 415-418
      blunt, 415-418
      penetrating, 415
  examination of, 129-130, 402
  "hot," 400
  "silent-peritonitis," 407
  "warm," 400
Abdominal pain in children, 513
Abdominal thrust maneuver, 136
Abortion, 474-475
  incomplete, 491
Abrasion, 229, 422, 616
Abruptio placentae, 489-490, 492

Abscess, 230
  abdominal, 407
  Bartholin gland, 481
  dental, 347
  ovarian, 479-480
Abusive, angry patient, 532-533
Accidents of children, 500-502
Acetaminophen
  and appendicitis, 408
  and fever in children, 511
  overdose of, 626-627
Acetazolamide, 322, 335
  and salicylate poisoning, 625
Acetylcysteine, 627
Acetylsalicylic acid; *see* Aspirin
Achilles tendon, ruptured, 424
Achromycin; *see* Tetracycline
Acid, 388
Acid burns, 615
Acid-base balance in shock, 253
Acidosis, 388
Acromioclavicular dislocation, 448
Acute abdomen, 399-406
Acute organic brain syndrome, 548-549
Addison's disease, 560-561
Administration; *see* Management, emergency
    department
Administrative structure and change, 59-62
  creativity in, 60-61
  defining needs in, 59-60
  matching process in, 61
  organizational chart for, 59
Adrenal crisis, 560-561
Adrenalin; *see* Epinephrine
Adrenergic agents in cardiogenic shock, 251
Adult burn chart, 601
Adult respiratory disease syndrome, 381-382
Advanced life support, 132-195
  airway management in, 142-150
    endotracheal intubation and, 146-148
    esophageal obturator airway in, 143-146
    nasopharyngeal airway in, 143, 144
    oropharyngeal airway in, 142-143

Advanced life support—cont'd
　airway management in—cont'd
　　surgery in, 148-150
　　　cricothyrotomy as, 149
　　　tracheostomy as, 149-150
　　　transtracheal catheter ventilation as, 148-149
　　ambulance equipment for, 15
　　basic life support and, 132-137
　　breathing in, 150-156
　　cardiopulmonary arrest in, 137-142
　　　arrest phase in, 141-142
　　　flow sheet for, 184
　　　prearrest phase in, 137-141
　　circulation in, 156-193
　　　cardioversion in, 187-188
　　　carotid sinus massage in, 189
　　　defibrillation in, 186-187
　　　drugs and, 182-183, 185
　　　dysrhythmias and, 157-181; see also Dysrhythmias
　　　electromechanical dissociation in, 190
　　　open chest massage in, 188-189
　　　pacemakers in, 190-192
　　　for infants and children, 192-193
　　　and near drowning, 382
Adventitious sounds, 114-116
Advertising in recruiting, 64
"AEIOU TIPS" for assessing seizure disorders, 304
Aftercare instructions, 223-227, 706-710
　for back strain, 223
　for bland diet, 706-707
　for casts, 224-226, 458, 707
　for cervical sprain, 707
　for clear liquid diet, 707
　for colds, 707-708
　for crutches, 708
　for fever, 224-225
　for head injury, 223, 708-709
　for nosebleeds, 709
　for overdose, 223
　for sprains, 709-710
　for sutured lacerations, 223-224
　and tetanus information, 710
　for upper respiratory infection, 226
　for vomiting, 226-227
　for wounds, 710
Age of patient as assessment barrier, 102-103
Air embolism, 589
Air splints, 457
Airway
　assessment of, in multiple trauma, 263-264
　burns and, 606
　establishment of, 132-133
　　head tilt maneuver in, 132
　　jaw thrust maneuver in, 132, 133
　management of, in advanced life support, 142-150
　obstruction of, 134-136, 338
　　in children, 506-509
　　　bronchiolitis as, 509
　　　croup as, 508
　　　epiglottitis as, 507-508

Airway—cont'd
　obstruction of—cont'd
　　in children—cont'd
　　　foreign bodies as, 509
　　　intrathoracic, 508-509
　　　laryngeal, 508
　　　nasopharyngeal, 507
　　　oropharyngeal, 507
　　　upper, 506-507
　　cross-finger technique in, 134
　　Heimlich maneuver in, 135, 136
　　in petroleum distillate ingestion, 621
　　poisoning and, 617
　　in shock management, 252-253
Akathisia, 625
Albumin, 714
　salt-poor, 359
　　and adult respiratory disease syndrome, 381-382
Albuminar-5; see Albumin
Albumisol; see Albumin
Albuspan; see Albumin
Albutein; see Albumin
Alcohol abuse, compared with brain injuries, 551
Alcohol levels in blood, 201
Alcohol withdrawal, 553
Alcohol-related emergencies, 539-542, 550-554
Alcoholic hallucinosis, 541-542
Aldomet; see Methyldopa
Alkalosis, 388
Allen's sign, 384, 386
　test for, 384
Allografts, 613
Alternatives, in problem solving, 33
Alveoalgia, 347
Ambulance, 14-15
　equipment for, 15
Aminodur; see Aminophylline
Aminophylline, 714
　and advanced life support, pediatric dosage for, 193
　and asthma, 379, 509
　and chronic obstructive pulmonary disease, 380
　and dyspnea, 378
　and pulmonary edema, 371
　and status asthmaticus, 379
Ammonia levels in blood, 201
Amobarbital
　abuse of, 543
　and alcohol abuse, 552
Ampicillin, 508
Amputations, traumatic, 456
Amylase, serum, 127
Amytal; see Amobarbital
Analeptic drugs and alcohol abuse, 552
Analgesia, 372, 374
　and crush injuries, 422
　and impaling injuries, 423
　and severe strains, 424
Anaphylaxis, 251-252
　emergency management of, 252
　and insect stings, 574

Anaphylaxis—cont'd
  and iron poisoning, 621
  signs and symptoms of, 252
  and snakebite, 571-572
Ancillary services in disaster, 675
Anesthesia, dental, 347
Aneurism, aortic, and chest pain, 376-377
Angina pectoris, 365-366
  and chest pain, 376-377
  differential diagnosis of, 366
Angiocatheter, 207
Angiography, cerebral, 283
Angry patient, 532-533
Ankle
  dislocation of, 455
  fracture of, 443-445
Antabuse; *see* Disulfiram
Antibiotics; *see also* specific drug
  and abdominal trauma, 415
  and abortion, 476
  and acid burns, 615
  and Bartholin gland abscess, 481
  and bowel obstruction, 411
  and bronchitis, 379
  and burns, 613
  and epiglottitis, 508
  and hypovolemic shock, 247
  and near drowning, 382
  and ovarian abscess, 479
  and pancreatitis, 406
  and pericarditis, 372
  and pneumonia, 375
  and septic abortion, 476
  and septic shock, 244
  and snakebite, 571
  and urinary tract infection, 470
  and vomiting and diarrhea, 510
Anticoagulants and adult respiratory disease syndrome, 382
Antidotes, 619
  for chemical burns of eye, 327
Antihistamines and laryngeal obstruction, 508
Antihypertensives
  and aortic dissection, 373
  and dialysis-related emergencies, 471
Antilirium; *see* Physostigmine
Antipyretics
  and delirium tremens, 554
  and fever, 511
  and thyrotoxic storm, 562
  and vomiting and diarrhea, 510
Antishock trousers, medical, 247-249, 264, 357, 363
  and abdominal trauma, 415
  and burns, 604
  and gastrointestinal bleeding, 408
  and pediatric shock, 503
  and pelvic fracture, 438
Antitoxin for botulism, 628
Antivenin therapy and snakebite, 571-572

Anxiety, 25
  as psychiatric emergency, 523-526
  panic reaction in, 525-526
AOBS; *see* Acute organic brain syndrome
Aorta, dissection of, 372-373
Apgar score, 485
Apnea, posthyperventilation, 285
Apomorphine and poisoning, 619
Appearance of patient
  as assessment barrier, 102
  in neurological assessment, 279
Appendicitis, 407-408
  perforation in, 407
  radiation of pain in, 400, 401
Apresoline; *see* Hydralazine
Aramine; *see* Metaraminol
Arfonad; *see* Trimethaphan
Arm, fracture of, 430-434
Arm board use, 208
Arrest, cardiopulmonary; *see* Cardiopulmonary arrest
Artane; *see* Trihexyphenidyl
Arterial blood gases, 127-128
  measurement of, 384-388
  reference chart for, 387
Artery
  brachial, 384
  femoral, 384, 385
  radial, 384, 385, 386
  selection of, for blood sample, 384-385
Arthropods, stings and bites of, 572-577
ASA; *see* Aspirin
Ascorbic acid and disulfiram reaction, 554
Aspirin
  and appendicitis, 408
  and fever in children, 511
Assessment
  of abdomen, 402
  of chest, 362
  documentation of, 103-105
    problem-oriented medical record in, 103-105
    SOAP process in, 104-105
  general survey in, 129
  head-to-toe examination in, 129-131
  history as, 106-108
  of multiple trauma; *see* Trauma, multiple, assessment of
  neurological, 272-277
    initial, 272
    of motor tone and posture, 275-276
    of ocular movements, 274
    of pupillary signs, 272-274
    of reflex activity, 276-277
  patient, 96-131
    barriers to, 97-103
      institutional, 98-100
      patient-related, 100-103
      professional, 97-98
  of patients in crisis, 27
    guidelines for, 28-29
  of peripheral nerve injuries, 425

Assessment—cont'd
  of poison ingestion, 618
  primary, 105-106
  primary survey in, 128-129
    ABCs in, 128
  setting priorities for, 105
  of vaginal bleeding, 475-476
  of vital signs, 129
Asthma, 379, 508-509
Asystole, 181
Ataxic breathing, 285, 286
Atrial fibrillation, 165
Atrial flutter, 164
Atropine, 335, 715
  and advanced life support, 185
    pediatric dosage for, 193
  and asystole, 181
  and belladonna abuse, 544
  and cardiogenic shock, 251
  and first degree AV block, 170
  and idioventricular rhythm, 180
  and jimsonweed toxicity, 624
  and mushroom poisoning, 628
  and nodal rhythm, 166
  and premature ventricular contractions, 176
  and rapid AV dissociation, 175
  and second degree AV block, 172
  and sinus bradycardia, 159
  and third degree AV block, 173-174
  toxicity of, 274
  and ventricular fibrillation, 179
Attitude of patient as assessment barrier, 102
Auscultation, 114-118, 129, 130
Autotransfusion
  and hemothorax, 357
  and hypovolemic shock, 249-250
AV block, 170-174
  first degree, 170
  second degree
    Mobitz type I, 171
    Mobitz type II, 172
  third degree
    complete, 174
    Stokes-Adams syndrome, 173
Avulsion, 229
Avulsion fracture, 427
Axis, plotting of, with electrocardiogram, 394-397

B

Back
  examination of, 130-131
  strain of, aftercare for, 223
Bag-valve-mask device, 146, 148, 151, 152-154
Ballance's sign, 402
Barbiturates; *see also* specific drugs
  abuse of, 543-544
  and heat stroke, 587
  and salicylate poisoning, 625
Barriers
  goal, 55-57

Barriers—cont'd
  to patient assessment, 97-103
  people versus system, 56-57
Bartholin gland abscess, 481
Base, 388
Base hospital, 15-16
  radio communication with, 11-13
Basic life support, 132-137; *see also* Advanced life support
  airway in, 132-133
  breathing in, 133-136
  circulation in, 136-137
Battered child syndrome, 41-42
Battle's sign, 296
Baxter formula, 608, 609
"Because" technique, 56-57
Beck's triad, 360, 372
Bee stings, 572-573, 574
Belladonna abuse, 544
Bellevue bridge, 470
Benadryl; *see* Diphenhydramine
Bends, 589-590
Benztropine, 625
  and phenothiazines, 547
Bigeminy, ventricular, 177
Biocommunications radio, 12
Biomedical communications system, 16-17
  elements of, 16
  equipment for, 16-17
  jargon, standard, in, 17
  rules for, 17
  techniques for, 17
Biopsy, endometrial, 474
Biot respirations, 285, 286
Bites
  arthropod, 572-577
  dog and cat, 235
  human, 234-235
Bladder, trauma to, 463, 465
Bladder tap, suprapubic, in children, 511-512
Bland diet, 706-707
Bleeding; *see also* Hemorrhage
  in children, 511-512
    hematuria as, 511-512
    rectal, 511
  dysfunctional uterine, 491
  gastrointestinal, 408-411
  vaginal, 473-476
    assessment of, 475-476
    endometrial biopsy for, 474
    caused by fibroid tumors, 473-474
    postpartum, 475
    with pregnancy and abortion, 474-475
Blepharitis, marginal, 33
Blood
  alcohol levels in
    analysis of, 43-44
    and symptoms, 552
  and blood components
    and hemophilia, 513
    and near drowning, 382

Blood—cont'd
  and blood components—cont'd
    and pulmonary contusion, 359
    for blood gas measurement, 384-388
      aftercare for, 388
      equipment for, 384-385
      interpretation of values for, 387, 388
      selection of site for
        brachial artery as, 384
        femoral artery as, 385
        radial artery as, 384
      specimen for, 385-386
        care of, 386-388
  dyscrasias of, in children, 513-514
  and gastrointestinal bleeding, 408
  normal values for, 693-699
  sampling of, 196-202
    femoral vein punctures in, 200-201
    pediatric, 200
    sequence of, 201
    syringe technique for, 199-200
    vacuum tube system for, 196-199
      procedure for, 197-199
      site selection for, 196-197
  and snakebite, 570
  tubes for drawing, 126
Blood chemistry, 693-699
Blood count
  complete, 127
  white, and differential, 124
Blood gases, arterial, 127-128
  in pulmonary edema, 371
  reference chart for, 387
  sampling of, 203
Blood glucose, 127
Blood pressure in patient assessment, 121-122
Blood urea nitrogen, 127
Blow-out fracture, 322
Body restraint, 497
Bone, 419
Botulism, 627-628
  infant, 628
Boxer's fracture, 435
Boyle's law, 588
Brachial artery, 384
Bradycardia
  in myocardial infarction, 141
  sinus, 159
Brain injuries, 296-302
  compared with alcohol abuse, 551
  concussion as, 296-297
  contusion as, 297-298
  dural lacerations as, 298
  hemorrhage and hematoma as, 298-301
  summary of, 301
Brainstorming session, 59
BRAT diet, 510
Breach of contract, 36
Breath sounds, 120-121

Breathing, 133-136
  airway obstruction in, 134-136
  assessment of, in multiple trauma, 264
  ataxic, 285, 286
  cluster, 285
  devices for management of, in advanced life support, 150-156
    bag-valve-mask as, 151, 152-155
    face mask as, 151, 152
    nasal cannula as, 150-151
    oxygen reservoir mask as, 151, 152, 153
    oxygen-powered, 151, 155-156
    pocket mask as, 151, 152, 154
    Venturi mask as, 151, 152, 153
  mouth-to-mouth, 133, 134
    on infant, 134, 135
  mouth-to-nose, 133-134
  mouth-to-stoma, 134
Bretylium, 715-716
  and premature ventricular contractions, 176
  and ventricular fibrillation, 179
Bretylol; see Bretylium
Bridge, Bellevue, 470
Bromide toxicity, 544-545
Bronchiolitis, 509
Bronchitis, 379
Bronchodilators, 379, 381
  and bronchiolitis, 509
  and burns, 606
  and laryngeal obstruction, 508
  and pulmonary embolism, 374
Bronchus, rupture of, 363
Bronkosol; see Isoetherine
Brown-Sequard syndrome, 311-315
Brudinski's sign in meningeal irritation, 294
Buccolingual crisis, 547, 625
Buminate; see Albumin
Bupivacaine, 230
Burns, 599-616
  airway and, 606
  charts of,
    adult, 601
    pediatric, 602
  chemical, 615
  classification of, 599-602, 603
  electrical, 613-615
  emergency management of, 605-613
  of eye; see Eye, burns of
  fluids and, 608
  hydrofluoric acid, 615
  major, 602
  minor, 613
  nasogastric intubation and, 608
  noxious gases in, 607
  pain relief and, 608-609
  pathophysiology of, 599
  prehospital care of, 602-605
  severity of, 602
  shock and, 606-608
  sunburn as, 616

Burns—cont'd
tar, 615
tetanus prophylaxis for, 613
wound care and, 609-613
Burrow's solution and snakebite, 571
Butterfly infusion device, 204-207
Butyrophenone reactions, 625-626

C

Calcium
in hypovolemic shock, 247
and salicylate poisoning, 625
Calcium chloride, 716
and advanced life support, pediatric dosage for, 193
and idioventricular rhythm, 180
and ventricular fibrillation, 179
Calcium gluconate
and advanced life support, 185
and asystole, 181
Calculi
ureteral, radiation of pain in, 401
urinary tract, 468-469
Caloric stimulation test, 274
Candida albicans, 482
Cane, 459
Cannula, nasal, 150-151
Carbachol, 335
Carbamycholine; *see* Carbachol
Carbocaine; *see* Mepivacaine
Carcholin; *see* Carbachol
Cardiac arrest flow sheet, 184; *see also* Circulation
Cardiac cycle, 116
Cardiac enzymes, 127
Cardiac injuries, 360-362
contusions as, 360
penetrating, 360
tamponade as, 360-362
pericardiocentesis for, 361-362
Cardiac tamponade, 360-362
Cardiopulmonary arrest; *see also* Myocardial infarction
drug therapy for, 182-183
flow sheet and, 184
phases of, 137-142
Cardiopulmonary resuscitation; *see also* Advanced life
support
body position for, 137
of infants and children, 192-193
Cardiovascular phenomena in dialysis patients, 471
Cardiovascular system, effect of septic shock on, 242
Cardioversion, 187-188
Career seekers, 63
Carotid sinus massage, 189
Carpal fractures, 435-437
Cartilage, 419
Casts
aftercare for, 224-226, 458, 707
plaster, 457-459
Casualty collection point, 650
Casualty distribution log, 659
Catapres; *see* Clonidine

Catheter over needle device, 205
Catheters
insertion of internal jugular, 208-209
and needles, 204-208
Cavernous sinus thrombosis, 330
CCP; *see* Casualty collection point
Cecal volvulus, 413
Cellulitis, orbital, 330
Center for Communicable Diseases, 628
Central retinal artery occlusion, 330
Cephalosporin, 476
Cephalothin, 233
Cerebellum, 270
Cerebral angiography, 283
Cerebral edema; *see* Edema, cerebral
Cerebrospinal fluid, normal laboratory values for, 704
Cerebrovascular accident, 287
Cerebrum, 270
Cervical collar, 307, 309
Cervical spine films, 283
Cervical sprain, aftercare of, 707
Chain of evidence, 45
Chalazion, 325-329, 332
Change, 61-62
Charting
example of, 107-108
problem-oriented, examples of, 104
Chemical burns, 615
Chest
anatomical reference lines of, 350-351
anatomy and physiology of, 349-350
assessment of, in multiple trauma, 264
examination of, 129
flail, 352, 353-354
injuries to
of diaphragm, 360
of lung, 359
of parenchyma, 359
of tracheobronchial tree, 357
open massage of, 188-189, 268-269
pain in, 365-378
of aortic origin, 372-373
of cardiac origin, 365-372
acute pericarditis as, 372
angina pectoris as, 365-366
cardiac tamponade as, 372
congestive heart failure as, 371
myocardial infarction as, 366-367
pulmonary edema as; *see* Edema, pulmonary
in children, 512-513
differential diagnosis of, 376
hyperventilation syndrome and, 375-378
of pulmonary origin, 373-375
pleurisy as, 374
pneumonia as, 374-375
pulmonary embolus as, 373-374
spontaneous pneumothorax as, 374
sucking wound of, 356
trauma to, 349-364
assessment and intervention for, 362

Chest—cont'd
  trauma to—cont'd
    flail chest as, 352, 353-354
    hemothorax as, 356-357
    pneumothorax as, 354-356
      simple, 354-355
      tension, 355-356
    rib fractures as, 352
    sternal fracture as, 352
    sucking chest wound as, 356
    tubes and drainage for, 357-359
Chest tube, 354, 355, 357, 359, 363, 374, 375
  and chest drainage, 357-359
Cheyne-Stokes respirations, 285, 286
Chief complaint
  evaluation of, 92-93
  and history, 106-107
Childbirth, 483-485
Children; *see also* Pediatric emergencies
  accidents of, 500-502
    risks and age levels of, 500-501
  anatomical variations and, 502
  blood sampling in, 200
  chest compression in, 137
  communicating with, 494-499
    and history and examination, 494-499
    techniques of, 494
  estimated weights of, 499
  genital trauma in, 482-483
  mouth-to-mouth breathing on, 134, 135
  procedural restraints for, 495, 496-498
  shock in, 502-505
  triage of, 499-500
Chloramphenicol, 335
Chlordiazepoxide
  abuse of, 543
  and alcohol abuse, 552
  and delirium tremens, 553, 554
  in psychiatric emergencies, 538-539
Chloromycetin; *see* Chloramphenicol
Chlorpheniramine, 554
Chlorpromazine
  and fever, 511
  and heat stroke, 586-587
  and psychosis, 538
Chlor-Trimeton; *see* Chlorpheniramine
"Chocolate cyst," 480
Cholecystitis
  and chest pain, 376
  radiation of pain in, 400, 401
Choroid, injury to, 325
Chronic illness in exacerbation, 514
Chronic obstructive lung disease, 380
Cimino-Brescia fistula, 471
Circulation, 136-137
  in advanced life support, 156-189
    cardiac dysrhythmias in; *see* Dysrhythmias, cardiac
    cardioversion in, 187-188
    carotid sinus massage in, 189
    defibrillation in, 186-187

Circulation—cont'd
  in advanced life support—cont'd
    drugs used in, 183, 185
      dosages for, 193
    electrical mechanical dissociation in, 190
    in infants and children, 192-193
    open chest massage in, 188-189
  assessment of, in multiple trauma, 264
  cardiac massage in, 136
  chest compression in, 136-137
Clavicle, fracture of, 428, 429
Clindamycin, 476
Clinical skill, 83
Clonidine, 717
Clostridium botulinum, 627, 628
Clostridium tetani, 233
Clotting time, Lee White, 128
Cloxacillin and shunt infections, 471
Cluster breathing, 285
Coagulation studies, 128
Cocaine, 545
Codeine, 542, 546
Cogentin; *see* Benztropine
Cold, aftercare for, 226, 707, 708
Colitis, ulcerative, 406-407
Collar, cervical, 307, 308
Colles fracture, 435
Color changes in skin, 124
Coma, barbiturate-induced, 290
Coma Scale, Glasgow, 278, 280
Comatose patient
  management of, 556
  rostral-caudal dysfunction signs in, 273
Combustion, toxic products of, 381
Command post in disaster, 663
Comminuted fracture, 425, 426
Commitment in setting goals, 53
Common sense in setting goals, 53
Communicable Diseases, Center for, 628
Communicable diseases, incubation periods for, 711-712
Communication, 516-518
  with children and adolescents, 517
  in crisis, 21-34
  in disaster, 653
  with the elderly, 517-518
  by leaders, 82-83
  in management, 68-69
  nonverbal, in crisis intervention, 27-30
  radio, 11-13
  verbal, in crisis intervention, 30
Communications center, 6
Community planning for disaster, 647-651
Community standard, 36
Compazine; *see* Prochlorperazine
Complaints, staff involvement in, 70
Complete blood count, 127
Compound fracture, 425
Compression of chest, 136-137
Compression fracture, 425, 426
Compressors, chest, 156

Compromise in setting goals, 53
Computerized axial tomography, 283
Concussion, 296-297
  postconcussion syndrome in, 297
Confrontation skills, 81
Confusion as coping mechanism, 25
Congenital falciform folds, 186
Congestive heart failure, 371
Conjunctiva
  foreign bodies in, 322-323
  lacerations of, 324
Conjunctivitis, acute, 330, 332
Consciousness, level of, in patient assessment, 122-123
"Conspiracy of silence," 37
Constructive criticism, 69
Contact lenses
  problems with, 325
  removal of, 325, 326
Contour of chest, 120
Contractions
  premature atrial, 161
  premature nodal, 168
  premature ventricular, 176-177
Contracture, Volkmann's ischemic, 433
Contrecoup, in contusions, 297, 298
Contusion, 229, 297-298, 422
  cardiac, 360
Conversions and equivalencies, 705
Cooperation in teamwork, 87-88
  conflict recognition as, 87
  conflict resolution as, 87-88
  empathy as, 87
Coping mechanisms, 25
  in crisis, 27
    confronting crisis as, 32
    identifying feelings as, 32-33
    promoting problem solving as, 33
Cord, prolapsed, 488
Cornea
  abrasions of, 324, 332
  fluorescein staining of, 324
  foreign body in, 323
  lacerations of, 324
  ulcers of, 324-325
Coroner's office, 46-47
Corticosteroids; *see* Steroids
Cortisone in anaphylaxis, 252
Cortisporin; *see* Polymyxin B with neomycin
Cortril; *see* Terramycin/oxytetracycline/hydrocortisone
Couplet, 177
CPK, 367
CPR; *see* Cardiopulmonary resuscitation
Cranial nerves
  involved in facial trauma, 341
  testing of, 283
Cranial surgery, techniques of, 299
Cravats, 307, 309
Creatinine, serum, 127
Creativity
  in administrative structure and change, 60-61

Creativity—cont'd
  in project management, 58-59
"Crib death," 514-515
Cricothyrotomy, 149
  and burns, 606
Crime, reporting to police, 40-42
Crisis
  confronting of, 32
  and crisis intervention, 26-33, 520-521
    assessment in, 27
    balancing factors in, 26-27
      coping mechanisms as, 27
      perception as, 26
      situational supports as, 26-27
    focus of, 27
    techniques of, 27
      coping mechanisms as, 32-33
      perception as, 31-32
      situational support as, 27-33
  definition of, 520
  factors that produce, 23-25
    coping mechanisms as, 25
    precipitating event as, 23-24
    threat to securities as, 24-25
  impact of, 28-29
  phases of reaction to, 22-23
    impact as, 22
    posttraumatic phase as, 23
    recoil as, 22-23
Crisis-prone people, 25-26
Critical care teams in disaster, 672-674
Criticism, constructive, 69
Croup, 508
Crush injuries, 422-423
Crutches, 708
  fitting of, 459
Culdocentesis, 405, 406
Cullen's sign, 402
Cultures
  blood, 201-202
  throat and sputum, 203
Cutdown, venous, 209-211, 212
Cyclogyl; *see* Cyclopentolate
Cyclopentolate, 335
Cyst
  "chocolate," 480
  dermoid, 479
  ovarian, 478-479
    ruptured, 491

D

Dacryocystitis, 331
Dactylitis and sickle cell crisis, 513
Darvon, 546
Data base, 103
Davoxin; *see* Digoxin
D & C after abortion, 476
DCC; *see* Disaster coordinating center
Death in emergency department, 46-47
Death rattle, 115

Decadron; *see* Dexamethasone
Decision making
  by leaders, 83
  in staff selection, 66
Decompression sickness, 589
Deferoxamine and iron poisoning, 621
Defibrillation, 186-187
Degenerative disk disease and chest pain, 376-377
Dehydration, 564
  in cerebral edema, 289-290
Delayed (Class III) patient, 90, 95
Delirium, 544
Delirium tremens, 541, 553-554
Delivery of baby, 484-485
Dental emergencies, 345-347
  abscess as, 347
  avulsed teeth as, 346-347
  chipped teeth as, 346
  dry socket as, 347
  neuralgias as, 345-346
  pain as, 346
  periodontal, 347
  postoperative bleeding as, 347
  toothaches as, 346
Depression, 533-534
Depression fracture, 427
Dermatomes, 307, 310-311
Detachment, retinal, 333
Dexamethasone, 309, 336, 717
  and asthma, 509
  and heat stroke, 587
  and idioventricular rhythm, 180
Dextran
  and hypovolemia, 266
  and pregnancy, 417
  low molecular weight, and lightning injuries, 577
Dextran 40, 718
Dextrose 5%
  in half normal saline, and cerebral edema, 289
  in normal saline
    and adrenal crisis, 561
    and hypovolemia, 265
    and mushroom poisoning, 628
    and thyrotoxic crisis, 562
  in Ringer's lactate
    and ectopic pregnancy, 478
    and obstetrical emergencies, 489
    and placenta previa, 489
    and shock, 291
    and spinal cord injuries, 307
  in water
    and alcohol abuse, 552
    and anaphylaxis, 252
    and aortic dissection, 373
    and asthma, 379
    and bowel obstruction, 411
    and cardiac tamponade, 372
    and carotid sinus massage, 189
    and chronic obstructive pulmonary disease, 380
    and delirium tremens, 553

Dextrose 5%—cont'd
  in water—cont'd
    and dyspnea, 378
    and hypertension, 306
    and iron poisoning, 620
    and ketoacidosis, 557
    and pancreatitis, 406
    and paroxysmal atrial tachycardia, 163
    and poisoning, 617
    and pulmonary edema, 368-369
    and pulmonary embolism, 374
    and smoke inhalation, 380
    and spinal cord injuries, 310
    and spontaneous pneumothorax, 374
    and status asthmaticus, 379
    and status epilepticus, 303
    and unconscious patient, 281
Dextrose 10% in water and half-normal saline, 353
Dextrose 50%, 718
  in water
    and hypoglycemia, 560
    and newborn resuscitation, 485
    and seizures, 305
    and unconscious patient, 281
Dezone; *see* Dexamethasone
DFP; *see* Isoflurophate
Diabetes, 554-560
Dialysis and alcohol abuse, 553
Dialysis-related emergencies, 471
Diamox; *see* Acetazolamide
Diaphragm, injuries to, 360
Diarrhea in children, 510
Diazepam, 719
  and alcohol abuse, 552
  in cardioversion, 188
  and delirium tremens, 554
  and drug withdrawal, 543
  and eclampsia, 491
  and hallucinogens, 544
  and heat stroke, 587
  and panic reaction, 526
  and phencyclidine abuse, 546
  and psychiatric emergencies, 538-539
  and salicylate poisoning, 625
  and seizures, 303-304
  and status epilepticus, 303-304
Diazoxide, 719
  and hypertensive crisis, 305, 306
DIC; *see* Disseminated intravascular coagulation
Diencephalon, 270
Diet
  bland, 706-707
  clear liquid, 707
Digitalis
  and atrial fibrillation, 165
  and atrial flutter, 164
  and congestive heart failure, 371
  and hypovolemic shock, 247
  and premature atrial contractions, 161
  and pulmonary edema, 371

Digitalis—cont'd
  and shock, 253
  and sinus tachycardia, 158
  toxicity of, 622
Digoxin, 720
  and cardiac injuries, 360
  and paroxysmal atrial tachycardia, 163
Dihydromorphinone, 546
Dilantin; *see* Phenytoin
Dilaudid; *see* Dihydromorphinone
Diphenhydramine, 720
  and cardiogenic shock, 252
  and disulfiram reaction, 554
  and phenothiazines, 547, 625
  and renal trauma, 463
Diphenylhydantoin; *see* Phenytoin
Disaster; *see also* Triage
  assignment sheet for, 664
  casualty distribution log for, 659
  emergency department plan for, 660-676
    ancillary services in, 675
    command post in, 663
    critical care teams in, 672-674
    personnel in, 663-665
    phases of, 660
    supplies in, 674-675
    training and drills in, 675-676
    triage area in, 665-672
  emergency report for, 661
  field operations in, 651-660
    communications in, 653
    prewarning and evacuation as, 652-653
    transport in, 658-660
    triage in, 653-658
      activity flow in, 657
      civilian, 653-654
      immediate and delayed cases in, 655-656
      military, 653, 654
      rating systems for, 655
  hazards after, 678
  levels of, 647-650
  mass casualty incident as, 643-646
  multiple casualty incident as, 643
  multiple patient incident as, 642-643
  natural, 676-678
  nuclear, 676-678
  obtaining safe drinking water after, 677-678
  planning for, 646-651
    community, 647-651
      federal, 647
      local, 640-651
      state, 647-650
    family, 646-647
  staff assignment in, 665
  staff call roster for, 664
  staff duty cards in, 665, 666-668
  staff identification in, 665
Disaster action card for triage officer, 670
Disaster coordinating center, 651, 661, 662
Disaster nursing, 641-679

Disaster support area, 650
Disaster tag, 671
Disaster triage tag, 658
Disclaimer clauses, 36
Discomfort as coping mechanism, 25
Diseases versus symptoms, 56
Disk
  degenerative, and chest pain, 376-377
  ruptured, 315-316
Dislocation, 446-456
  acromioclavicular, 448
  of ankle, 455
  of elbow, 448-451
  of finger, 451, 452
  of foot, 455
  of hand, 451
  of hip, 451-452, 453
  of knee, 452-455
  of leg, 452-456
  metatarsophalangeal, 455-456
  of patella, 455
  of shoulder, 448
  of toe, 455-456
  of wrist, 451
Disopyramide, 721
Dissecting aortic aneurysm and chest pain, 376-377
Disseminating intravascular coagulation, 259, 490
  and heat stroke, 585, 587-588
Dissociation
  electrical mechanical, 190
  isorhythmic, 175
  rapid AV, 175
Dista; *see* Sulfisoxazole
Disulfiram
  and alcohol abuse, 551
  reaction to, 554
Diuretics; *see also* specific drug
  and adult respiratory disease syndrome, 381
  and cardiac injuries, 360
  and congestive heart failure, 371
  digitalis toxicity and, 623
  and hypovolemic shock, 247
  and intracranial pressure increase, 289
  osmotic, 289
  and pulmonary contusion, 359
  and pulmonary edema, 369-371
Diving emergencies, 588-598
  air embolism and, 589
  decompression sickness and, 589-590
  decompression tables and, 591-596
  depth of dive and gas volume in, 588-589
  hyperpnea exhaustion syndrome and, 590
  nitrogen narcosis and, 589
  safety rules and, 590
Doll's eye maneuver, 274, 275
Donnagel, 544
Donnatal, 544
Dopamine, 721-722
  and advanced life support, 185
    pediatric dosage for, 193

Dopamine—cont'd
  for hypotension, 266
  and hypovolemic shock, 247
  and poisoning, 617
  and septic shock, 244
Doptone, 489
Doriden; *see* Glutethimide
Doryl; *see* Carbachol
Drainage, chest, 357-359
Drills for disaster, 675-676
Drop-ins in recruiting, 64
Drowning, near, 382-384
  dry, 382
  salt water and fresh water aspiration in, 383
  secondary, 382
  wet, 382
Drugs
  abuse of, 542-548; *see also* Alcohol-related emergencies;
      Poisonings and toxicology
  in advanced life support, 185
  antihypertensive, 306
  in cardiac arrest, 182-183
  categories of, 713-738
  in hypertensive crisis, 305
  ophthalmological, 335-337
  overdoses of, 40-41, 542-548
  pediatric dosages of, for cardiopulmonary resuscitation,
      538-539
  used in psychiatric emergencies, 538-539
Dry socket, 347
DSA; *see* Disaster support area
DTs; *see* Delirium tremens
Dura, lacerations of, 298
Dysfunction, rostral-caudal, 272, 273
Dysfunctional uterine bleeding, 491
Dyskinesias, 625
Dyspnea, 378
Dysrhythmias, cardiac, 157-181
  algorithm for drug therapy for, 182-183
  management of, 140
  originating in atria, 161-165
    atrial fibrillation as, 165
    atrial flutter as, 164
    paroxysmal atrial tachycardia as, 163
    premature atrial contractions as, 161
    wandering atrial pacemaker as, 162
  originating in AV node, 166-175
    first degree AV block as, 170
    nodal (junctional) rhythm as, 166-167
    nodal (junctional) tachycardia as, 169
    premature nodal contractions as, 168
    rapid AV dissociation, 175
    second degree AV block as, 171, 172
    third degree AV block as, 173, 174
  originating in sinus node, 157-160
    bradycardia as, 159
    sinus dysrhythmia as, 160
    sinus tachycardia as, 158
  originating in ventricles, 176-181
    asystole as, 181

Dysrhythmias—cont'd
  originating in ventricles—cont'd
    idioventricular rhythm as, 180
    premature ventricular contractions as, 176-177
    ventricular fibrillation as, 179
    ventricular tachycardia as, 178
  sinus, 160
Dystonia, 625
Dystonic reactions to phenothiazines, 547-548

E

EACA; *see* Epsilon aminocaproic acid, 259
Ear
  emergencies of, 340
    acute otitis media as, 340
    otitis externa as, 340
    vertigo as, 340
  foreign bodies in, 337
Ecchymosis and snakebite, 570
ECG; *see* Electrocardiogram
Echoencephalography, 283, 291
Echothiophate, 335
Eclampsia, 490-491, 492
Ectopic pregnancy, 477-478, 491, 492
Ectropion, 331
Edema, 564
  cerebral
    CT scan of, 290
    management of, 289-290
      airway and oxygenation as, 289
      dehydration and fluid therapy as, 289-290
      intracranial shifts as, 290
  of eyelid, 331
  heat, 580-581
  pulmonary
    high altitude, 371
    intervention for, 367-371
      aminophylline as, 371
      arterial blood gas analysis as, 371
      digitalis as, 371
      diuretics as, 369-371
      high Fowler position as, 368
      IV line as, 368-369
      morphine sulfate as, 369
      oxygen as, 368
      phlebotomy as, 371
      rotating tourniquets as, 369, 370
  and snakebite, 570
Edrophonium chloride, 723
  and paroxysmal atrial tachycardia, 163
Ego strength, 80
Eight-ball hemorrhage, 322
EKG; *see* Electrocardiogram
Elbow
  dislocation of, 448-451
  fracture of, 433
Elecath, 191
Electrical injuries, 613-615
Electrocardiogram
  dysrhythmias and, 157-181

Electrocardiogram—cont'd
  heat stroke and, 585-586
  hyperkalemia and, 563
  hypocalcemia and, 563
  hypokalemia and, 563
  hypothermia, 579-580
  infarct on, 392, 393, 394
  injury on, 392
  ischemia on, 392
  monitoring of, 388-394
    on four-lead system, 388, 389
    on three-lead system, 390
    on 12-lead system, 390, 391
  normal, 392
  plotting simple axis with, 394-397
    equipment for, 394
    procedure for, 394-397
Electrocardiogram strip recorder, 389
Electroencephalography, 283
Electrolyte and fluid disturbances, 562-565
Electrolytes, serum, 127
Embolism, air, 589
Embolus, pulmonary, 373-374
Emergency department
  disaster plan for; see Disaster, emergency department
    plan for
  explaining procedures of, 31-32
  hospital, 6-8
  physical facilities in, 9
Emergency Department Nurses' Association, 3, 4
Emergency facilities, classification of, 7
Emergency medical service
  communications center and, 6
  history of, 4-5
  manpower for, 5-6
  systems approach to, 8
Emergency Medical Services Systems Act, 5
Emergency medical technicians, 5, 15
Emergency medicine residency training, 6
Emergency nurse practitioner, 4
Emergency nursing, 3-10
Emergency operations center, 651
Emergency services
  Joint Commission on Accreditation of Hospitals require-
    ments for, 683-691
  parent education about, 515
Emergency situation report for hospitals, 661
Emergent (Class I) patient, 90, 94-95
Emesis, specimen of, 202
Emetics and laxatives, administration of, 45-46
EMT; see Emergency medical technicians
Endotracheal intubation, 146-148
Entenox; see Nitrous oxide
Enthusiasm of leaders, 82
Entropion, 331
Envenomation, 568-569
  grading of, 570
Environment as assessment barrier, 99-100
Enzymes, cardiac, 127
EOC; see Emergency operations center

Ephedrine, 335
Epididymitis, 470
Epilepsy, 303
Epinephrine, 335, 723
  and advanced life support, 185
    pediatric dosage for, 193
  and anaphylaxis, 252
  and asthma, 379, 509
  and asystole, 181
  and burns, 606
  and laryngeal obstruction in children, 508
  and myocardial infarction, 141-142
  racemic, and croup, 508
  and septic shock, 244
  and status asthmaticus, 279
  and ventricular fibrillation, 179
  and wound management, 230
Epistaxis, 337-338, 339
Epitrate; see Epinephrine
Epsilon aminocaproic acid, 259
Equilibrium, maintaining; see Crisis and crisis
    intervention
Equivalencies and conversions, 705
Ergotamine tartrate, 305
  with caffeine, 305
Erythromycin, 335
Escharotomy and burns, 610
Escherichia coli, 234, 240
Eserine; see Physostigmine
Eskabarb; see Phenobarbital
Esophageal obturator airway, 143-146
Esophagus, rupture of, 363
Ethacrynic acid, 369-371
Ethanol intoxication; see Alcohol-related emergencies
Evacuation in disaster, 652-653
Evidence, helping police gather, 43-45
Examination, physical, 108-118
  in assessment of multiple trauma, 267
  of eye, 110-111
  of reflexes, 111
  techniques of, 111-118
    auscultation as, 114-118
      of heart sounds, 116-118
      of lung sounds, 114-116
    inspections as, 112
    palpation as, 112
    percussion as, 112-114
  tools for, 109-111
    ophthalmoscope as, 109-111
    otoscope as, 109-110
    reflex hammer as, 111
    stethoscope as, 109
Exhaustion, heat, 581-582
Exophthalmos, 331
Expectancy theory, 67-68
Expectations as motivation, 69
Expectorants, 379
Express understanding, 46
Extrasystoles, 161
Extremities, examinations of, 130

Eye, 318-337
  anatomy of, 318-319
  burns of, 325-328
    caused by liquids and solids, 327
    chemical, 325-327
      antidotes for, 327
    radiation, 327-328
      infrared, 327-328
      ultraviolet, 327
    thermal, 327
  examination of, 109-111, 319-321
  injuries to, 324-325
    conjunctival lacerations as, 324
    corneal abrasions as, 324
    corneal lacerations as, 324
    corneal ulcers as, 324-325
    iris injury as, 325
    lens injury as, 325
    optic nerve avulsion as, 325
    retina and choroid injury as, 325
  irrigation of, 328, 329
    continuous, using Morgan therapeutic lens, 328, 329
  medical problems of, 328-332
    acute conjunctivitis as, 330
    acute iritis as, 330
    blepharitis as, 328
    cavernous sinus thrombosis as, 330
    central retinal artery occlusion as, 330
    chalazion as, 328-329
    hordeolum as, 328
    uveitis as, 330
  medications for, 335-337
    drops as, instilling of, 336
    ointment as, instilling of, 336-337
  trauma to, 321-324
    blow-out fracture as, 322
    blunt, 322
    eyelid injuries as, 321-322
    foreign bodies as, 322-323
      to conjunctiva, 322-323
      to cornea, 323
      intraocular, 323-324
    orbital rim injuries as, 322
Eyelid
  edema of, 331
  everting of, 323
  injuries of, 321-322

F

Face mask, 151, 152
Failure, pump, 250-251
Family interference as assessment barrier, 101
Family support in crisis intervention, 30
Fasciotomy
  and frostbite, 579
  and snakebite, 571
Fear as coping mechanism, 25
Federal Disaster Relief Act, 647
Federal planning for disaster, 647, 649
Feedback as motivation, 69

Feeling, identification of, 32-33
Felonies, 44
Femoral artery, 384, 385
Femur, fracture of, 439-442
  Hare traction splint for, 439-441
Fetal emergencies, 488
Fever
  aftercare for, 224-225
  in children, 510-511
  in meningeal irritation, 294
  in septic shock, 242
  of unknown origin, 511
Fibrillation
  atrial, 165
  ventricular, 179
Fibula, fracture of, 443, 444
Field operations in disaster; *see* Disaster, field operations in
Figure eight support, 428, 429
Finger
  dislocation of, 451, 452
  fracture of, 436, 437
Fingertip, injuries to, 233, 423
"Fire-fighting" syndrome, 52
Fistula, Cimino-Brescia, 471
Flaccidity in neurological assessment, 276
Flagyl; *see* Metronidazole
Flail chest, 352, 353-354
Float nurse staffing as assessment barrier, 98-99
Floor burns, 616
Floropryl; *see* Isoflurophate
Flow sheet for cardiac arrest, 184
Fluid and electrolyte disturbances, 562-565
Fluid therapy
  in cerebral edema, 289-290
  in fever in children, 511
  intravenous, 203-208
    devices for, 204
    needles and catheters for, 204-208
      angiocatheter as, 207
      butterfly, 204-207
      intracatheter as, 207-208
  in pediatric shock, 504-505
    calculation of, 505
  in vomiting and diarrhea, 510
Fluorescein staining, 324
Flush method for taking blood pressure, 122
Flutter, atrial, 164
Flutter valve, 509
Folic acid, 259
Food poisoning, 627-631
Food toxins, 629-631
Foot
  dislocation of, 455
  fracture of, 445-446
  prolapsed, 488
Forearm fracture, 433-434
Foreign bodies
  in eye, 322-324
  in genitourinary tract, 466
  intraocular, 323-324

Foreign bodies—cont'd
  intrathoracic, 509
  of nose and ear canals, 337
  of throat, 337
Forensic specimen, 203
Fracture(s), 424-448
  of ankle, 443-445
  of arm, 430-434
  assessment of, 427
    in multiple trauma, 266
  avulsion, 427
  blow-out, 322
  boxer's, 435
  carpal and metacarpal, 435-437
  clavicular, 428, 429
  closed, 425
  Colles, 435
  comminuted, 425, 426
  compound, 425
  compression, 425, 426
  depression, 427
  of elbow, 433
  facial, 342-345
  of femur, 439-442
    Hare traction splint for, 439-441
  of fibula, 443, 444
  of foot, 445-446
  of forearm, 433-434
  greenstick, 425-427
  healing of, 446
  of heel, 445-446
  of hip, 438-439
  of humerus, 430-433
  impacted, 425, 426
  intervention for, 427-428
  of knee, 442
  LeFort, 344, 345
  of leg, 439-445
  mandibular, 344
  maxillary, 344
  oblique, 425
  open, 425
  of os calcis, 445
  of patella, 442-443
  of pelvis, 437-438
  of penis, 467
  of phalange, 436, 437, 446, 447
  of radius, 433-434
  of rib, 352, 464
  of scapula, 430, 431
  of shoulder, 428-430
  simple, 425
  signs and symptoms of, 424-425
  skull, 294-296
    basilar, 296
  spiral, 425, 426
  sternal, 352
  tarsal and metatarsal, 445, 446
  of tibia, 443, 444
  of toe, 446, 447

Fracture(s)—cont'd
  transverse, 425
  of ulna, 433-434
  of upper arm, 430-433
Friction burns, 616
Frostbite, 578-579
FUO; *see* Fever of unknown origin
Furosemide, 724
  and advanced life support, 185
  and hypertensive crisis, 305
  in hypovolemic shock, 247
  and pulmonary edema, 369-371
  and septic shock, 244

G

Gait training, 459-461
Gantrisin; *see* Sulfisoxazole
Garamycin; *see* Gentamicin
Gas inhalation, 607
Gastric fluid, normal laboratory values for, 704
Gastric ulcer, acute, radiation of pain in, 400
Gastroenteritis, radiation of pain in, 400
Gastrointestinal tract
  bleeding and, 408-411
  disturbances of, and chest pain, 376-377
  emergencies of, 399-418; *see also* Abdomen
  obstruction of, 411-415
  perforation of, 414, 415
Gaze, tonic, 274
Genital herpes, 482
Genitourinary emergencies, 463-472
  acute urinary retention as, 467-468
  dialysis-related, 471
  epididymitis as, 470
  foreign bodies as, 466
  gross hematuria as, 469
  infections as, 469-470
  orchitis as, 470-471
  penis fracture as, 467
  testicular torsion as, 467
  trauma as, 463-465
    of bladder and urethra, 463, 465
    renal, 463, 464
  urinary tract calculi as, 468-469
  zipper injuries as, 466
Gentamicin, 335, 476
Gentran 40; *see* Dextran 40
Gila monsters, 572
Gingivitis, 347
Glasgow Coma Scale, 278, 280
"Glass-blower's cataracts," 328
Glaucoma, 333-336
  acute, 334
  congenital, 334
  measurement of, with tonometer, 334-336
  open-angle, 334
Glucagon, 724
Glucose
  and alcohol abuse, 552
  and delirium tremens, 553

Glucose—cont'd
  and thyrotoxic storm, 562
Glutethimide
  abuse of, 543
  overdose of, 274
Glyceryl trinitrate; *see* Nitroglycerine
Goals
  barriers to, 55-57
  communication of, 69
  and objectives, setting of, 52-55
  staff involvement in, 71
"Good samaritan" act, 40
Gram-negative organisms, 234
Gram-positive organisms, 234, 240
Grand mal seizures, 303
Grease gun injuries, 423
Great vessel injuries, 362-363
Greenstick fracture, 425-427
Grey Turner's sign, 402
Gross hematuria, 469
Guanethidine and thyrotoxic crisis, 562
Guanidine and botulism, 628
Gunshot wounds, 233, 423
Gynecological emergencies, 473-483; *see also* Bleeding,
      vaginal; Obstetrical emergencies
  differential diagnosis of, 491
  pain in, 480-482
    Bartholin gland abscess and, 481
    pelvic inflammatory disease and, 480-481
    vaginal infections and, 482
  shock as, 476-480
    caused by ectopic pregnancy, 477-478
    caused by ovarian abscess, 479-480
    caused by ovarian cyst, 478-479
  trauma as, 482-483
    sexual, 483
Gynergen; *see* Ergotamine tartrate

H

Habitual abortion, 474
Half-normal saline
  and ketoacidosis, 555-557
  and petroleum distillate ingestion, 622
Hallucinogens, abuse of, 544
Hallucinosis, bromide, 544-545
Haloperidol
  and alcohol-related emergencies, 540
  and delirium tremens, 553
  and paranoia, 538
  and phencyclidine abuse, 546
  and phenothiazines, 547
  reactions to, 625-626
Hammer, reflex, 111
Hand, dislocation of, 451
Hare traction splint, 439-441, 457
Haxodrol; *see* Dexamethasone
Hazards after disaster, 678
Head, examination of, 129
Head injury, 287-296
  aftercare for, 223, 708-709

Head injury—cont'd
  assessment of, 287-289
  cerebral edema in, 289-290
  intracranial monitoring in, 290-291, 292
  pathophysiology of, 284
    cardiovascular factors in, 286-287
    metabolic factors in, 284
    respiratory factors in, 285-286
  scalp lacerations as, 294
  seizures after, 293
  shock accompanying, 291-293
Headache in meningeal irritation, 293
Head-to-toe examination, 129-131
HEAR network, 643, 645, 653
Heart; *see also* Circulation
  contusions and penetrating injuries of, 360
Heart attack; *see* Myocardial infarction
Heart sounds, auscultation of, 116-118
  cardiac cycle in, 116
  evaluation of, 118
  murmurs as, 117-118
  pericardial friction rubs as, 118
Heat syndromes, 580-588
  clinical presentation of, 584-586
  etiology of, 582-583
  heat edema as, 580-581
  heat exhaustion as, 581-582
  heat stroke as, 582-588
  heat syncope as, 581
  pathophysiology of, 583-584
  therapy for, 586-588
Heel, fracture of, 445-446
Heimlich maneuver, 135, 136
Helplessness as coping mechanism, 25
Hematoma, 422
  in brain injury, 298-301
    extradural and epidural, 298-299
    subdural, 299-301
      acute, 300
      chronic, 300-301
  in IV infusions, 211
  and penis fracture, 467
  of vulva, 491
Hematuria
  in children, 511-512
  gross, 469
Hemodynamic monitoring; *see* Monitoring, hemodynamic
Hemodynamics of hypovolemic shock, 244
Hemophilia, 513
Hemophilus, 330
Hemophilus influenzae, 507
Hemorrhage; *see also* Bleeding
  and burns, 604
  in abruptio placentae, 489
  in brain injury, 298-301
    brainstem contusion and, 298
    cerebral, 298
    intracerebral, 298
    subarachnoid, 298
  eight-ball, 322

Hemorrhage—cont'd
  in placenta previa, 488-489
  retrobulbar, 322
Hemothorax, 356-357
Henry's law, 589
Heparin, 725
  and disseminating intravascular coagulation, 259
  and heat stroke, 587
Heprinar; *see* Heparin
Hernia, hiatus, and chest pain, 376-377
Herniated nucleus pulposus, 315-316
Herniation, cingulate and tentorial, 290
Herpesvirus hominis, 482
HHNC; *see* Hyperosmolar hyperglycemic nonketotic
        coma
Hiatus hernia and chest pain, 376-377
Hip
  dislocation of, 451-452, 453
  fracture of, 438-439
History
  in assessment of multiple trauma, 267
  elements of, 107
  pediatric, 494-499
  taking of, 106-108
    in crisis intervention, 31
Homatrocel; *see* Homatropine
Homatropine, 355
Home care instruction sheets, 221-222; *see also* Aftercare
        instructions
Homeostasis, 21-22
Homosexual panic, 537
Hordeolum, 328, 332
Hospital emergency department, 6-8
Humerus, fracture of, 430-433
Hydralazine, 725
  as antihypertensive, 306
  and hypertensive crisis, 305
Hydrocarbon ingestion, 621-622
Hydrofluoric acid burns, 615
Hydrogen peroxide and friction burns, 616
Hydron burn dressings, 611-612
Hydroxyamphetamine, 335
Hydroxyzine pamoate, 552
Hymenoptera, 572-573
Hyoscine; *see* Scopolamine
Hyperkalemia, 563, 564
  and heat stroke, 588
Hypernatremia, 565
Hyperosmolar hyperglycemic nonketotic coma, 558-560
  pathophysiology of, 558
Hyperpnea exhaustion syndrome, 590
Hyperpyrexia, 511
Hyperstat; *see* Diazoxide
Hyperstat IV: *see* Diazoxide
Hypertension, aftercare of, 709
Hypertensive emergencies, 305-306
  antihypertensive drugs for, 306
  drug selection in, 305
  management of, 306
  signs and symptoms of, 305

Hyperventilation, 285-286
  and chest pain, 375, 376-377
  and panic reaction, 526
Hyperventilation syndrome, 375-378
Hyphema, 322
Hypocalcemia, 563, 565
Hypofibrinogenemia, 490
Hypoglycemia, 560
Hypokalemia, 563, 564
  and digitalis toxicity, 623
Hypomagnesemia, 565
Hypomania, 531
Hyponatremia, 565
Hypotension, 238
  causes of, 240
  and heat stroke, 584-585
  and poisoning, 617
Hypothalamus, 270
Hypothermia, 579-580
Hypovolemia; *see also* Shock, hypovolemic
  assessment of, in multiple trauma, 264-266
  therapy for, 265-266
Hypoxia, mechanism of, 239

I

Idoxuridine, 336
Ilotycin; *see* Erythromycin
Imbalance in volume as assessment barrier, 99
Impact as reaction to crisis, 22
Impacted fracture, 425, 426
Impaled object, 422, 423
Impaling injuries, 423
Implied consent, 40
  laws for, 43, 44-45
In loco parentis, 39
Incomplete abortion, 474
Incubation periods, 711-712
Incubator, transfer, 486
Inderal; *see* Propranolol
Inevitable abortion, 474
Infants; *see also* Children
  botulism and, 628
  delivery of, 484-485
  mouth-to-mouth breathing on, 134, 135
Infarction, myocardial; *see* Myocardial infarction
Infections
  food, 627
  of genitourinary tract, 469-470
  upper respiratory tract, aftercare for, 226
  vaginal, 481-482
    herpes progenitalis as, 482
    monilial vaginitis as, 482
    trichomonal, 481-482
Infiltration in IV infusion, 211
Inflammatory disease, pelvic, 480-481
Infrared radiation burn of eye, 327-328
Infusion, intravenous; *see* Intravenous infusion
Infusion site, 201
Ingestion, caustic, 337
Initiative by leaders, 83

Injuries; *see also* Trauma
  crush, 422-423
  on electrocardiogram, 392
  fingertip, 233, 423
  head; *see* Head injury
  impaling, 423
  to knee, 423
  peripheral nerve, 424, 425
  soft tissue; *see* Soft tissue injuries
  wringer, 422-423
  zipper, 466
Inotropic agents, 247
  and cardiogenic shock, 251
  and hypovolemic shock, 247
Insects, stings and bites of, 572-577
Inspection, 112
Inspiratory/expiratory ratio, 120-121
Insulin, 557-558, 559
  and alcohol abuse, 552
Interference, family, as assessment barrier, 101
Interpersonal skills, 80-81
Intervention; *see* Assessment, patient; Crisis, and crisis
    intervention
Interview, psychiatric, 518-520
Interviewing
  staff involvement in, 71
  in staff selection, 64-66
  responsibilities of interviewer in, 65-66
    techniques of, 64-65
      one-to-one method as, 65
      one-to-one series method as, 65
      one-to-two method as, 65
Intoxication; *see also* Alcohol-related emergencies
  bromide, 544
  food, 627
Intracatheter, 207-208
Intracranial shifts, 290
Intravenous infusion, 203-213
  arm board use in, 206-207, 208
  disruption of, 211
  hematoma in, 211
  infiltration of, 211
  needles and catheters for, 204-208
  sites for, 208-211
    internal jugular vein as, 208-209, 210
    subclavian vein as, 208
    venesection as, 209-211, 212
  termination of, 213
Intropin; *see* Dopamine
Intubation, endotracheal, 146-148
Ipecac, 726
  and poisoning, 619, 621-622, 624
Iris, injury to, 325
Iritis, acute, 330, 332
Iron poisoning, 620-621
Irrigation of eye, 328, 329
Irritation, meningeal, 293-294
Ischemia on electrocardiogram, 392
Isoetherine, 509
Isoflurophate, 335

Isophrin; *see* Phenylephrine
Isoproterenol, 726
  and advanced life support, 185
    pediatric dosage for, 193
  and asystole, 181
  and cardiogenic shock, 251
  and first degree AV block, 170
  and heat stroke, 586
  and hypovolemic shock, 247
  and idioventricular rhythm, 180
  and near drowning, 382
  and nodal rhythm, 166
  and rapid AV dissociation, 175
  and second degree AV block, 172
  and septic shock, 244
  and sinus bradycardia, 159
  and status asthmaticus, 378
  and third degree AV block, 173, 174
  and ventricular fibrillation, 179
Isopto Atropine; *see* Atropine
Isopto Carbachol; *see* Carbachol
Isopto Carpine; *see* Pilocarpine
Isopto Homatropine; *see* Homatropine
Isuprel; *see* Isoproterenol

J

Jacksonian seizures, 303
Jargon in biomedical communication, 17
Job seekers, 63
Joint Commission on Accreditation of Hospitals require-
    ments for emergency services, 683-691
Jimsonweed, 623-624
Junctional rhythm, 166-167

K

Kaopectate and drug withdrawal, 543
Kayexalate, 172
Keflin; *see* Cephalothin
Kehr's sign, 477
Keratitis, 329
Keratoconjunctivitis, 329-330
Kernig's sign in meningeal irritation, 294
Ketoacidosis, 554-558
  insulin therapy for, 557
  pathophysiology of, 555
Kidney, trauma to, 463, 464
Klebsiella, 234
Klebsiella pneumoniae, 240
Knee
  dislocation of, 452-455
  fracture of, 442
  injuries to, 423
Korsakoff syndrome, 539, 541, 542

L

Labor, stages of, 484
Laboratory analysis in assessment, 126-128
  blood tests in, 126-127
    tubes for, 126
  urinalysis in, 127

Laboratory evaluation of multiple trauma, 267
Laboratory values, normal, 692-704
  for cerebrospinal fluid, 704
  for gastric fluid, 704
  for urine, 700-703
  for whole blood, serum, and plasma, 693-699
Laceration, 229-230, 422
  dural, 298
  facial, 342
  of parenchyma, 359
  scalp, 294
  sutured, aftercare for, 223-224
  of vagina, 491
Language as assessment barrier, 100-101
Lanoxin; *see* Digoxin
Laryngotracheobronchitis, 508
Lasix; *see* Furosemide
Lavage
  and hypothermia, 580
  iced saline gastric, 409
  and poisoning, 619-620, 622, 623
    mushroom, 628
  peritoneal, 402-405
Laxatives and emetics, administration of, 45-46
LDH, 367
Leadership
  as effect on motivation, 72-73
  "natural," 79-80
  styles of, 83-84
Lee White clotting time, 128
LeFort fractures, 344, 345
Leg
  dislocation of, 452-456
  fracture of, 439-445
Legal considerations
  in emergency department, 35-50
  in gynecological emergencies, 492
Leiomyomata uteri, 473-474
Lens
  contact, removal of, 325, 326
  injury to, 325
Lesions
  of shoulder and ribs, and chest pain, 376-377
  of spinal cord, 314
Levarterenol, 727
  and advanced life support, 185
  and cardiogenic shock, 252
Levine Scale, 117-118
Levophed; *see* Levarterenol
Liability, 36-40
  civil, 37-38
Librium; *see* Chlordiazepoxide
Lidocaine, 727
  and advanced life support, 185
    pediatric dosage for, 193
  in myocardial infarction, 140-141
  and premature ventricular contraction, 140-141,
    176
  and seizures, 304
  and testicular torsion, 467

Lidocaine—cont'd
  and uremic seizures, 304
  and urinary retention, 468
  and ventricular tachycardia, 178
  and wound management, 230
  and zipper injuries, 466
Lido-Pen, 141
Life Care Pump, 504
Ligament, 419
Lightning injuries, 577-578
Limb trauma, 419-462; *see also* Dislocation; Fracture; Soft
    tissue injuries
  crutch and cane fitting for, 459
  gait training in, 459-461
  and injuries to peripheral nerves, 424, 425
  pediatric, 456
  and plaster casts, 457-459
  splinting in, 457
  traumatic amputations as, 456
Liquaemin; *see* Heparin
Liquid diet, clear, 707
Lithium carbonate, 531
Lixaminol; *see* Aminophylline
Lofstrand crutches, 459
Longboards, 457, 458
Long-leg splint, 439-441
LSD, 544
Luminal; *see* Phenobarbital
Lung disease, chronic obstructive, 380
Lung injuries, 359
Lung sounds, auscultation of, 114-116
  adventitious, 114-116
    pleural friction rub as, 115
    rales as, 114-115
    rhonchi as, 115
  bronchial, 114
  bronchovesicular, 114
  vesicular, 114

M

Mafenide and burns, 610-611
Magnesium and botulism, 628
Magnesium sulfate and delirium tremens, 553
Mallory-Weiss syndrome, 408
Management, emergency department, 51-89
  by crisis, 52
  of people, 62-88
    leadership in, 79-85
      qualities for, 79-81
      recruiting for, 81-82
      responsibilities of, 82-83
      skills for, 84-85
      styles of, 83-84
    motivation in, 66-73
      communication as, 68-69
      expectations as, 69
      feedback as, 69
      goals as, 69
      leadership as effect on, 72-73
      recognition as, 69

Management, emergency department—cont'd
  of people—cont'd
    motivation in—cont'd
      staff involvement as, 69-72
      theories of, 66-68
    performance review systems in, 74-79
      sample of, 739-744
    personnel conflicts in, 85-88
    scheduling in, 73-74
    staff member selection in, 62-66
      decisions in, 66
      defining needs in, 63
      interviewing in, 64-66
      recruiting in, 63-64
    teamwork in, 85-88
      atmosphere of, 85-87
      cooperation in, 87-88
    problem solving in, 55-57
      "because" technique in, 56-57
      people barriers versus system barriers in, 56-57
      symptoms versus diseases in, 56
    project management in, 57-59
  of system, 51-62
    setting goals and objectives in, 52-55
      annual, 52-53
      status survey in, 53-55
      strategic, 52-53
      tactical, 55
      task outline in, 55
Manic psychosis, 531
Manipulative patient, 537
Mannitol, 728
  and cardiogenic shock, 251
  and electrical injuries, 615
  and eye trauma, 322
  and heat stroke, 587
Marcaine; *see* Bupivacaine
Marijuana, 545
Masks, for oxygen, 151-154
Maslow's hierarchy of needs, 66-67
Massage
  carotid sinus, 189
  open chest, 188-189, 268-269
MAST: *see* Antishock trousers, medical
MAST program; *see* Military Assistance to Safety and
        Traffic program
Maxillofacial trauma, 340-345
  ABC assessment of, 340-341
  fractures as, 342-345
    nasal, 343
    mandibular, 344
    maxillary, 344
      LeFort, 345
    of zygomatic arch, 343-344
  lacerations as, 342
Measurement and monitoring, 384-397
Measurements and temperature conversions, 705
Medical antishock trousers; *see* Antishock trousers,
    medical
Medications; *see* Drugs

Medulla oblongata, 270-271
Meninges, irritation of, 293-294
Meperidine, 546
  abuse of, 542
  and burns, 608
  and pulmonary embolism, 374
  and sickle cell crisis, 514
  and ulcerative colitis, 406
  and urinary calculi, 469
Mepivacaine, 230
Meprobamate, 543
Mescaline, 544
Metabolic emergencies, 555-566
  adrenal crisis as, 560-561
  alcohol-related, 550-554
  diabetes-related, 554-560
  fluid and electrolyte disturbances as, 562-565
  thyroid crisis as, 561-562
Metabolism in head injury, 284
Metacarpal fractures, 435-437
Metaraminol, 728
  and advanced life support, 185
  and anaphylaxis, 252
  and cardiogenic shock, 251
  and hypovolemic shock, 247
  and paroxysmal atrial tachycardia, 163
Metatarsal, fracture of, 445, 446
Metatarsophalangeal dislocation, 455-456
Methadone, 543
Methergine; *see* Methylergonovine maleate
Methimazole, 562
Methyldopa, 729
  and hypertensive crisis, 305, 306
Methylergonovine maleate, 729
Methylprednisolone, 730
  and renal trauma, 463
  and spinal cord injuries, 309
Methyprylon, 543
Metimyd; *see* Prednisolone
Metronidazole
  and alcohol abuse, 551
  and vaginal infections, 482
MIC; *see* Mobile intensive care
MICN; *see* Mobile intensive care nurse
Microcirculation, 237-238
MICU: *see* Mobile intensive care unit
Midbrain, 270
Migraine, 305
Military Assistance to Safety and Traffic program, 6
Miltown; *see* Meprobamate
Misdemeanors, 44
Mnemonics
  ABCs as, 132
  AEIOU TIPS as, 304
  BRAT diet as, 510
  PQRST as, 92, 107, 126, 138
  SOAP as, 104-105
  TABS for resuscitation of newborn as, 485
  TIDES as, 344
Mobile intensive care, 13; *see also* Prehospital care

Mobile intensive care nurse, 13
  role of, 17-19
    definition of, 17
    qualifications for certification of, 18-19
    responsibilities of, 17-18
Mobile intensive care paramedic, 14, 15
Mobile intensive care unit, 14-15
  equipment for, 15
Mobitz AV blocks, 171, 172
Monitoring
  cardiac, 138, 139
  hemodynamic, 250-251, 254-259
    invasive, 254-259
      arterial pressure as, 254-256
      central venous pressure as, 256-257
      intraarterial lines in, 258-259
      pulmonary artery wedge pressure as, 257-258
  intracranial, 290-291, 292
Morgan therapeutic lens, 328
Morphine, 545, 730
  and burns, 605
  and cardiogenic shock, 251
  and drug abuse, 543
  and hypertensive crisis, 305
  and myocardial infarction, 140
  and pulmonary edema, 369
  and urinary calculi, 469
Motivation-hygiene theory, 68
Motor tone and posture in neurological assessment, 275-276
Mouth-to-mouth breathing, 133, 134, 135
Mucomyst; see Acetylcysteine
Multigravida, 483
Multipara, 483-484
Multipurpose staging area in disaster, 650
Multivitamins and alcohol abuse, 552
Mummy restraint, 496
Murine, 336
Murmurs, heart, 117-118
Murphy's sign, 402
Muscle cramps and heat exhaustion, 581-582
Mushroom poisoning, 628, 631, 638
Mycostatin; see Nystatin
Mydriacyl; see Tropicamide
Mydriaticum; see Tropicamide
Myocardial infarction, 132, 137-142, 366, 367
  anterior wall, 393
  arrest phase of, 141-142
  and chest pain, 376-377
  on electrocardiogram, 392, 393, 394
  inferior wall, 393
  lateral wall, 393
  posterior wall, 394
  prearrest phase of, 137-141
    cardiac monitoring during, 138
    dysrhythmias in, 140-141
    PQRST in, 138
Myxedema coma, 561

N
N Ach theory, 67
Naloxone, 731
  and advanced life support, pediatric dosage for, 193
  and heroin overdose, 546
  and ketoacidosis, 557
  and myocardial infarction, 140
  and poisoning, 617, 619
  and pulmonary edema, 369
  and respiratory distress, 140
Narcan; see Naloxone
Nasal cannula, 150-151
Nasogastric tube, 360, 381, 399, 406, 408, 411, 479
  insertion of, 409-410
  and near drowning, 382
Nasopharyngeal airway, 143, 144
National Center for Poison Information, 638
National Highway Safety Act, 5
Neck trauma, 338-340
Needle over catheter device, 205
Needles and catheters, 204-208
Needs, defining of
  in administrative structure, 59-60
  in staff member selection, 63
Negligence, 37
Neisseria, 234
Neisseria gonococcus, 330, 480
Nembutal; see Pentobarbital
Neonatal resuscitation tips, 192-193
Neonatal seizures, 303
Neo-Cortef; see Neomycin and hydrocortisone
Neo-Delta-Cortef; see Neomycin with methylprednisolone
Neo-Medrol; see Neomycin with methylprednisolone
Neomycin
  and hydrocortisone, 336
  with methylprednisolone, 336
Neo-Polycin; see Polymixin B with neomycin
Neosporin; see Polymixin B
Neostigmine; see Physostigmine
Neo-Synephrine; see Phenylephrine
Nerves
  cranial
    involved in facial trauma, 341
    testing of, 283
  peripheral, injuries to, 424, 425
Nervous system, central, 270-272
Neuralgia
  glossopharyngeal, 346
  trigeminal, 345-346
Neurological dysfunction, patterns of respiration in, 285
Neurological emergencies, 270-317
  assessment of, 272-277
  brain injuries as, 296-302
  cerebrovascular accident as, 287
  checklist for, 302
  head injuries as, 287-296
  hypertensive, 305-306
  migraine as, 305
  seizures as, 303-305
  spinal cord injuries as, 306-316

Neurological emergencies—cont'd
  syncope as, 306
  unconsciousness as, 277
Newborn
  evaluation of, 485
  resuscitation of, 485
  transfer of
    form for, 487
    incubator for, 486
Nipride; *see* Sodium nitroprusside
Nitrogen narcosis, 589
Nitroglycerine, 731
  for angina pectoris, 366
  and myocardial infarction, 138
Nitroprusside, 251
Nitrous oxide, 140
Nodal rhythm, 166-167
Noludar; *see* Methyprylon
Nonverbal communication, 27-30
Norepinephrine; *see* Levarterenol
Normal saline
  and adrenal crisis, 561
  and amputated part, 456
  and asthma, 509
  and bronchiolitis, 509
  and burns of eye, 325-327
  and delirium tremens, 553
  and eyelid injuries, 321
  and flail chest, 352
  and gastrointestinal bleeding, 409
  and heat stroke, 586
  and hypovolemia, 264, 265
  and ketoacidosis, 555-557
  and poisoning, 617
  and snakebite, 569, 572
  and tension pneumothorax, 355-356
Norpace; *see* Disopyramide
Nose
  emergencies of, 337-340
    epistaxis as, 337-338, 339
    foreign bodies as, 337
  fracture of, 343
Nosebleed, 337-338, 339
  aftercare of, 709
Nuclear disaster, 676-678
  safe drinking water after, 677-678
Nulligravida, 483
Nullipara, 483
Numbness as coping mechanism, 25
Nurse contact, multiple, as assessment barrier, 98
Nystatin
  and burns, 613
  and monilial vaginitis, 482
Nytol, 544

O

Oblique fracture, 425
Obstetrical emergencies, 483-493
  delivery as, 484-485
  and fetal, 488

Obstetrical emergencies—cont'd
  maternal complications as, 488-491
    abruptio placentae as, 489-490
    disseminated intravascular coagulation as, 490
    placenta previa as, 488-489
    preeclampsia and eclampsia as, 490-491
  resuscitation of newborn as, 485-488
  stress factors in, 491-493
Ocular movements in neurological assessment, 274
Oculogyric crisis, 547, 625
Ocusol, 336
Ophthalmological medications, 335-337
Ophthalmoscope, 109-111, 320-321
Ophtheine; *see* Procaracaine
Opiates, 546-547
Opisthotonic crisis, 547, 625
Opisthotonus in meningeal irritation, 294
Optic nerve, avulsion of, 325
Optimyd; *see* Prednisolone
Orbital cellulitis, 330
Orbital rim injuries, 322
Orchitis, 470-471
Organizational chart, 59
Organizational skill, 83
Orientation, staff involvement in, 71
Oropharyngeal airway, 142-143
  and children, 507
Os calcis, fracture of, 445-446
Osmitrol; *see* Mannitol
Otitis
  externa, 340
  media, acute, 340
Otoscope, 109-110
Outdoor emergencies, 567-598
  arthropod bites and stings as, 572-577
  diving emergencies as, 588-598
  frostbite as, 578-579
  heat syndromes as, 580-588
  hypothermia as, 579-580
  lightning injuries as, 577-578
  snakebite as, 567-572
Ovarian abscess, 479-480
Ovarian cyst, 478-479
Overdose
  aftercare for, 223
  drug, 40-41, 542-548
Oxacillin and shunt infections, 471
Oxazepam, 539
Oxycodone, abuse of, 542
Oxygen, 732
  and adult respiratory disease syndrome, 381
  and advanced life support, 150-156
  and air embolism, 589
  and amputations, 456
  and aortic dissection, 373
  and asthma, 509
  and asystole, 181
  and bronchiolitis, 509
  and burns, 604, 606
  and cardiac contusions, 360

Oxygen—cont'd
  and cardiac tamponade, 361
  and cardiovascular accident, 287
  and carotid sinus massage, 189
  and cerebral edema, 289
  and chest pain in children, 512
  and chronic obstructive lung disease, 380
  and congestive heart failure, 371
  and croup, 508
  and decompression sickness, 590
  and disulfiram reaction, 554
  and dyspnea, 378
  and ectopic pregnancy, 478
  and epiglottitis, 508
  and esophageal rupture, 363
  and fetal emergencies, 488
  and first degree AV block, 170
  and flail chest, 352
  and gastrointestinal bleeding, 408-409
  and great vessel injuries, 363
  and head injury, 286
  and heat stroke, 586
  and high-altitude pulmonary edema, 371
  and hypovolemic shock, 246
  and intrathoracic foreign bodies, 509
  and lightning injuries, 577
  and maxillofacial trauma, 341
  and multiple trauma, 264
  and newborn resuscitation, 192-193, 485
  and oropharyngeal obstruction in children, 507
  and paroxysmal atrial tachycardia, 163
  and pediatric shock, 503
  and pelvic fracture, 438
  and pericarditis, 372
  and petroleum distillate ingestion, 621
  and pleurisy, 374
  and pneumonia, 375
  and poisoning, 617
  and premature atrial contractions, 161
  and premature ventricular contractions, 176
  and pulmonary contusion, 359
  and pulmonary edema, 368
  and pulmonary embolism, 374
  and ruptured bronchus, 363
  and salicylate poisoning, 625
  and second degree AV block, 172
  and septic shock, 243
  and shock, 243, 246, 252
  and sickle cell crisis, 514
  and simple pneumothorax, 355
  and sinus bradycardia, 159
  and smoke inhalation, 380
  and spinal cord injuries, 307
  and spontaneous pneumothorax, 374
  and status asthmaticus, 379
  and status epilepticus, 303
  and sucking chest wound, 356
  and tension pneumothorax, 355
  and tracheobronchial tree injuries, 359
  and unconscious patient, 281

Oxygen—cont'd
  and vaginal bleeding, 476
  and ventricular fibrillation, 179
  and ventricular tachycardia, 178
Oxygen reservoir mask, 151, 152, 153
Oxygenation in management of head injury, 289
Oxytocic drugs and pregnancy, 417
Oxytocin, 733
  and abortion, 476
  and postpartum bleeding, 476

P

PAC; *see* Premature atrial contraction
Pacemakers, 190-192
Pain, 537
  abdominal, in children, 513
  assessment of, in abdominal emergencies, 399-
    402
  and burns, 608-609
  chest; *see* Chest, pain in
  and eclampsia, 490
  and ectopic pregnancy, 477
  evaluation of, 125-126
    PQRST mnemonic in, 126
  and eye trauma, 321
  and myocardial infarction, 138-140
  radiation of, in abdominal emergencies, 400, 401
  and urinary tract calculi, 468
Paint gun injuries, 233, 423
Palpation, 112, 129, 130
Pancreatitis, acute, 406
Panheprin; *see* Heparin
Panic, homosexual, 537-538
Panic reaction, 525-526
Papoose board, 498
Paraldehyde and seizures, 304
Paranoia, 529
Paratonia, 275
Paredrine; *see* Hydroxyamphetamine
Parenchyma, lacerations of, 359
Parkinsonism, 625
Paroxysmal atrial tachycardia, 163
Pasteurella multocida, 235
PAT; *see* Paroxysmal atrial tachycardia
Patella
  dislocation of, 455
  fracture of, 442-443
Patient education for parents, 515
Patient teaching in emergency department, 214-227
  home care instruction sheets for, 221-222
  process of, 215-221
    assessment of learner as, 216-217
    documentation of, 221
    establishment of goals as, 218-219
    evaluation of, 221
    facilities and time for, 220-221
    identification of learning needs as, 216
  rationale for, 215
  responsibility of nurses in, 214
PAWP; *see* Pulmonary artery wedge pressure

PCP; *see* Phencyclidine
PCWP; *see* Pulmonary capillary wedge pressure
Pediatric burn chart, 600
Pediatric emergencies; *see also* Children
  abdominal pain as, 513
  bleeding as, 511-512
  blood dyscrasias as, 513-514
  chest pain as, 512-513
  diarrhea as, 510
  fever as, 510-511
  respiratory distress as, 505-510
  shock as, 502-505
  suddent infant death syndrome as, 514-515
  vomiting as, 510
Pediatric limb trauma, 456
Pediatric vital signs, 503
Pelvic inflammatory disease, 480-481, 491
Pelvis, fracture of, 437-438
Penicillin
  and burns, 613
  and sexual trauma, 483
Penis
  fracture of, 467
  injury to, 466
Pentazocine, 542, 733
Pentobarbital, 543
People skill, 83
Perception
  in crisis intervention, 31-32
  of events as balancing factor, 26
Percussion, 112-114, 129, 130, 131
Performance review, 74-79
  formal, 74-76
    objectives of, 75-76
  formats of, 78-79
  informal, 76
  responsibilities in, 76
    of reviewer, 78
    of staff member, 76-78
  sample of, 739-744
Pericardial friction rub, 118
Pericardiocentesis, 361-362
Pericarditis, 372
  and chest pain, 376-377
Pericoronitis, 347
Periodontal emergencies, 347
Peritoneal lavage, 402-405
  and hypothermia, 580
Personality in staff selection, 63
Personnel problems, staff involvement in, 71
Petit mal seizures, 303
Petroleum distillate ingestion, 621-622
pH, 388
Phalange, fracture of, 436, 446, 447
Phenazopyridine, 470
Phencyclidine, 545-546
Phenobarbital, 733
  abuse of, 543
  and seizures, 304
  and status epilepticus, 304

Phenothiazines, 547-548
  and heat stroke, 586-587
  and mushroom poisoning, 628
  reactions of, 625-626
Phentolamine and hypertensive crisis, 305
Phenylephrine, 734
  and hypertensive crisis, 335
Phenytoin, 734
  and delirium tremens, 554
  and premature ventricular contraction, 176
  and seizures, 293, 304
  and status epilepticus, 304
Phlebotomy for pulmonary edema, 371
Phospholine; *see* Echothiophate
Physostigmine, 735
  and belladonna abuse, 544
  and hypertensive emergencies, 335
  and jimsonweed toxicity, 623-624
Physostol; *see* Physostigmine
PID; *see* Pelvic inflammatory disease
Pilocar; *see* Pilocarpine
Pilocarpine, 335
Pitocin; *see* Oxytocin
Placebos, 537
Placenta accreta, 475
Placenta previa, 488-489, 492
Plants, poisonous, 632-637
Plasma
  and burns, 608, 609
  and near drowning, 382
  and pulmonary contusion, 359
Plaster casts, 457-459
Platelet count, 128
Pleur-evac, 358
Pleural friction rub, 115
Pleurisy, 374
PNC; *see* Premature nodal contractions
Pneumonia, 374-375
Pneumothorax
  and chest pain, 376-377
  simple, 354-355
  spontaneous, 374
  tension, 355-356
Pocket mask, 151, 152, 154
Poisindex system, 638
Poison control center, 9
Poison control systems, 638-639
Poison Information, National Center for, 638
Poisoning, mushroom, 628, 631, 638
Poisonous house plants, 632-637
Poisons and toxicology, 617-640; *see also* Drugs, abuse of
  acetaminophen and, 626-627
  airway in, 617
  antidotes and, 619
  assessment in, 618
  butyrophenones in, 625-626
  cardiovascular status in, 617
  digitalis in, 622-623
  food poisoning in, 627
  iron, 620-621

Poisons and toxicology—cont'd
  jimsonweed in, 623-624
  lavage in, 619
  petroleum distillate in, 621-622
  phenothiazines in, 625-626
  plants in, 632-637
  prevention of, 638-639
  salicylates in, 624-625
  seizures in, 617-619
  vomiting in, 619
Polyhydramnios, 488
Polymyxin B
  with neomycin, 335
  and tar burns, 615
POMR; *see* Problem-oriented medical record
Pontocaine; *see* Tetracaine
Positive end expiratory pressure, 252
Postconcussion syndrome, 297
Postpartum bleeding, 475
Posttraumatic phase as reaction to crisis, 23
Postural vital signs, 121, 255
Posturing, decorticate and decerebrate, 275-276
Potassium and burns, 608, 609
Potassium chloride, 735
  and ketoacidosis, 557
Potassium iodide, supersaturated solution of, 562
PQRST device, 92, 107, 126, 138
  case example of, 107-108
Prednisolone, 336
  with sulfacetamide, 336
Preeclampsia, 490-491, 492
Prefrin, 336
Pregnancy
  blunt abdominal trauma in, 416-418
  ectopic, 477-478, 491, 492
Prehospital care, 11-20
  assessment considerations in, 19-20
  components of, 14-17
    base hospital as, 15-16
    biomedical communications systems as, 16-17
    mobile intensive care paramedic as, 15
    mobile intensive care unit as, 14-15
  history of, 13-14
  innovations in, 14
  patient evaluation in, 19-20
  radio communication in, 11-13
Prejudgment as assessment barrier, 101-102
Premature atrial contractions, 161
Premature nodal contractions, 168
Premature ventricular contractions, 176-177
Preservation of amputated part, 456
Pressonex; *see* Metaraminol
Pressure
  arterial, 254-256
    pressure veil method to measure, 266
  central venous, 256-259
Pressure sore, 458-459
Pressure veil method to measure arterial pressure, 266
Prewarning in disaster, 652-653
Primigravida, 483

Primipara, 483
Prinzmetal angina, 366
Problem solving, 33, 55-57
  by leaders, 82
Problem-oriented medical record, 103-105
Pro-Bumin; *see* Albumin
Procainamide, 736
  and advanced life support, 185
  and atrial flutter, 164
  and myocardial infarction, 141
  and premature atrial contractions, 161
  and premature nodal contractions, 168
  and premature ventricular contractions, 176
  and ventricular fibrillation, 179
Procaine and wounds, 230
Procaracaine, 335
Prochlorperazine, 543
Project management, 57-59
  creativity in, 58-59
Prolapsed cord, 488, 492
Prolapsed foot, 488
Promethazine and sickle cell crisis, 514
Pronestyl; *see* Procainamide
Propranolol, 736
  and advanced life support, 185
  and atrial flutter, 164
  and hypertensive crisis, 305
  and paroxysmal atrial tachycardia, 163
  and premature ventricular contractions, 176
  and thyrotoxic crisis, 562
Propylthiouracil and thyrotoxic crisis, 562
Proserum-25; *see* Albumin
Prostaglandins and abortion, 476
Protamine in disseminating intravascular coagulation, 259
Proteus, 234, 240
Prothrombin time, 128
Pseudomonas, 234, 240, 324, 330
Pseudomonas aeruginosa, 325
Psychiatric emergencies, 516-549
  abusive angry patient as, 532-533
  alcohol-related, 539-542
  anxiety as, 523-526
  crisis intervention in, 520-521
  depression as, 533-534
  drug-related, 542-548
  homosexual panic as, 537-538
  manipulative patient as, 537
  panic reactions as, 525-526
  psychosis as, 528-531
  psychosomatic illness as, 536-537
  rape victims as, 521-523
  suicide as, 534-536
  violence as, 531-532
Psychiatric medications, 538-539
Psychiatric patients, commitment of, 42-43
Psychomotor seizures, 303
Psychosis, 528-531
  manic, 531
Pterygium, 332
Pulmonary artery wedge pressure, 259

Pulmonary capillary wedge pressure, 257
Pulmonary edema; *see* Edema, pulmonary
Pulmonary embolus, 373-374
  and chest pain, 376-377
Pulmonary system, effect of septic shock on, 242
Pulse
  paradoxical, 372
  in patient assessment, 119-120
Pump failure, 250-251
Puncture, femoral vein, 200-201
  site of, 200
Puncture wound, 230, 422
  of snakebite, 570
Pupillary signs in neurological assessment, 272-277
Pus, specimens of, 202
P.V. Carbachol; *see* Carbachol
P.V. Carpine Liquifilm; *see* Pilocarpine
PVB; *see* Premature ventricular contractions
PVC: *see* Premature ventricular contractions
Pyribenzamine and disulfiram reaction, 554
Pyridium; *see* Phenazopyridine

Q

Quinidine, 737
  and atrial flutter, 164
  and paroxysmal atrial tachycardia, 163
  and premature atrial contractions, 161
  and premature nodal contractions, 168

R

Rabies, 235
Radial artery
  location of, 385
  puncture of, 386
  as site for blood gas drawing, 384
Radiation burns of eye, 327-328
Radio
  biocommunications, 12
  field, 11
Radio communication, 11-13
  rules for, 17
  standard jargon in, 17
Radiological evaluation of multiple trauma, 267
Radius, fracture of, 433-434
Rales, 114-115
Rape, 483
  physical evidence in, 47-48
Recognition as motivation, 69
Recoil as reaction to crisis, 22-23
Recruiting
  for leaders, 81-82
  staff involvement in, 71
  in staff selection, 63-64
Rectal bleeding in children, 511
Rectalad-Aminophylline; *see* Aminophylline
References, checking, in interviewing, 66
Referrals in recruiting, 64
Reflex hammer, 111
Reflexes
  oculocephalic, 274, 275

Reflexes—cont'd
  oculovestibular, 274
  positions for testing, 277
  tendon, testing of, 277
Regionalization, 8
Reimplantation, 456
Renal system
  effect of septic shock on, 242
  trauma to, 463, 464
Res ipsa loquitur, 37
Reserpine, 306
  and hypertensive crisis, 305
  and thyrotoxic crisis, 562
Resolution of conflict, 87-88
Respirations
  apneustic, 285
  Biot, 285, 286
  Cheyne-Stokes, 285, 286
  in head injury, 285-286
    patterns of, 285
  in patient assessment, 120-121
Respiratory disease syndrome, adult, 381-382
Respiratory disorders, 378-384
  adult respiratory disease syndrome as, 381-382
  asthma as, 379
  bronchitis as, 379
  chronic obstructive lung disease as, 380
  dyspnea as, 378
  near drowning as, 382-384
  smoke inhalation as, 380-381
  status asthmaticus as, 379
Respondeat superior, 37, 38, 39
Restraints, procedural, for children, 495, 496-497
Retention, acute urinary, 467-468
Reticular formations, 271
Retina
  detachment of, 333
  injury to, 325
Retinitis, focal, 328
Review, performance, 74-79, 739-744; *see also* Performance review systems
Rheomacrodex; *see* Dextran 40
RhoGAM, 476
Rhonchi, 115
Rhythm
  idioventricular, 180
  nodal, 166-167
Rib, fractures of, 352, 464
Rigidity
  decorticate and decerebrate, 275-276
  nuchal, in meningeal irritation, 293-294
Ringer's lactate
  and amputated part, 456
  and appendicitis, 408
  and asthma, 509
  and bowel obstruction, 411
  and bronchiolitis, 509
  and burns, 604, 605, 609
  and electrical injuries, 615
  and flail chest, 352

Ringer's lactate—cont'd
and gastrointestinal bleeding, 409
and heat stroke, 586
and hypovolemia, 264, 265
and shock, 246, 253, 291
pediatric, 503, 505
and tension pneumothorax, 355-356
Role modeling, 82
Rum fits, 553
Rupture
of Achilles tendon, 424
of bronchus, 363
of disk, 315-316
of esophagus, 363
of ovarian cyst, 491
of spleen, 415-416, 417
of urethra, 465

S

Salicylate poisoning, 624-625
Salpingectomy, 478
Sampling
arterial blood gas, 203
blood, sequence for, 201
icing, 201
Sandbags, 307, 309
Scapular fracture, 430, 431
Scheduling, 73-74
staff involvement in, 71
Schiøtz tonometer, 334-336
Schizophrenia, 530-531
transitory, 544-545
Sclerema neonatorum, 502
"Scoop and run," 264
Scopolamine, 335
and belladonna abuse, 544
overdose of, 274
toxicity of, 274
Scorpions, 573, 574
Screen, toxic, 127
SCUBA, 588, 590
Secobarbital, abuse of, 543
Seconal; see Secobarbital, abuse of
Seizures, 303-305
"AEIOU TIPS" for assessing, 304
classification of, 303
epilepsy as, 303
grand mal, 303
after head injury, 293
jacksonian, 303
neonatal, 303
petit mal, 303
and poisoning, 617-619
psychomotor, 303
status epilepticus as, 303
emergency management of, 303-305
Self-assessment, 81
Self-confidence, 80
Semantics, 55-56
in teamwork, 86-87

Sengstaken-Blakemore tube, anchoring of, 410-411
Septic abortion, 474-475
Serax; see Oxazepam
Serratia marcescens, 240
Serum
human or equine, 235
normal values for, 693-699
Serum amylase, 127
Serum creatinine, 127
Serum drug level, 127
Serum salicylate level, 624
Sexual trauma, 483
SGOT, 367
SGPT, 367
Shifts, intracranial, 290
Shock, management of, 237-260
anaphylactic; see Anaphylaxis
cardiogenic, 250-251
cause of, 250
hemodynamic monitoring in, 250-251
arteriovenous oxygen saturation difference in, 251
cardiac output in, 251
left heart function in, 250-251
oxygen saturation in, 251
right heart function in, 250
signs and symptoms of, 251
treatment for, 251
in children, 502-505
complications of, 259-260
disseminating intravascular coagulation as, 259
shock lung as, 259-260
definition of, 237
degree of severity of, 245-246
and head injury, 291-293
and hemorrhage, 238
hypovolemic, 244-250
cause of, 244
emergency management of, 244-250
antishock trousers in, 247-249
autotransfusion in, 249-250
drug therapy in, 247
hemodynamics of, 244
pathophysiology of, 237-238
at cellular level, 237
hypotensive events as, 238
microcirculation in, 237-238
therapy for, 252-259
acid-base balance in, 253
airway and ventilation in, 252-253
digitalization in, 253
drug therapy in, 253-254
fluids in, 253
hemodynamic monitoring in, 254-259
shock position for, 254
septic, 240-244
assessment of, 243
cause of, 240-241

Shock, management of—cont'd
  septic—cont'd
    effect of
      on cardiovascular system, 242
      on pulmonary system, 242
      on renal system, 242
    fever in, 242
    pathology of, 241-242
    pathophysiology of, 241
    predisposition to, 241
    signs and symptoms of, 242-243
    treatment of, 243-244
  types of, 238
Shock lung, 259-260
Shortboards, 457, 458
Shoulder
  dislocation of, 448, 449
  fracture of, 428-430
Shunt clotting and infections, 471
Sickle cell disease, 513-514
SIDS; *see* Sudden infant death syndrome
Sigmoid volvulus, 413
Signs
  Allen's, 384, 386
  Ballance's, 402
  Brudinski's, 294
  Cullen's, 402
  Grey Turner's, 402
  Kehr's, 477
  Kernig's, 294
  Murphy's, 402
  Thompson's, 424
Silvadene; *see* Silver sulfadiazine
Silver sulfadiazine, 610
Sinus bradycardia, 159
Sinus dysrhythmia, 160
Sinus tachycardia, 158
Situational support as crisis intervention technique, 26-27
Skeleton, 420-421
Skills in management, 83
Skin
  color changes in, 124
  moisture of, 125
  temperature of, 125
  vital signs of, 123-125
Skull films, 283
Skull fractures; *see* Fracture, skull
Sling and swath, 429-430
Smoke inhalation, 380-381
  of toxic products of combustion, 381
Snakebite, 567-572
  antivenin therapy and, 571-572
  emergency care for, 569-571
  first aid for, 569
  wound care and follow-up for, 571
Snellen visual acuity chart, 320
SOAP process, 104-105
Socket, dry, 347
Sodium bicarbonate, 737
  and advanced life support, 185

Sodium bicarbonate—cont'd
  and advanced life support—cont'd
    pediatric dosage for, 193
  and asthma, 379
  and asystole, 181
  and decompression sickness, 590
  and electrical injuries, 615
  and idioventricular rhythm, 180
  and iron poisoning, 620
  and ketoacidosis, 557
  and myocardial infarction, 141-142
  and ventricular fibrillation, 179
Sodium iodide and thyrotoxic crisis, 562
Sodium nitroprusside, 738
  and hypertensive crisis, 305, 306
Sodium sulfate and botulism, 628
Soft tissue injuries, 422-424
  crush injuries as, 422-423
  fingertip injuries as, 233, 423
  gunshot wounds as, 423
  impaling injuries as, 423
  knee injuries as, 423
  ruptured Achilles tendon as, 424
  sprains as, 424
  strains as, 423-424
  wringer injuries as, 422-423
Solu-Medrol; *see* Methylprednisolone
Sominex, 544
Sore, pressure, 458-459
Sounds
  breath, 120-121
  beart, 116-118
  lung, 114-116
Specimens
  emesis, 202
  forensic, 203
  laboratory, 196-203
  percutaneous fluid, 202
  pus, 202
  sputum, 203
  stool, 202-203
  urine, 202
Spiders, 573, 575
Spinal cord
  injuries to, 306-316
    airway management of, 309
    immobilization of, 307, 309
    level of, 311-315
    management of, 315
    motor and sensory examination of, 310-311
    neurogenic shock in, 307
    radiological studies of, 311
    ruptured disk as, 315-316
    steroid therapy for, 309-310
    types of, 311-315
    whiplash injury as, 316
  lesions of, 314
Spine, cervical, assessment of in multiple trauma, 264
Spiral fracture, 425, 426

Spleen, ruptured, 415-416, 417
  radiation of pain in, 401
Splints, 457
  Hare traction, 439-441, 457
  long-leg, 439-441
  traction, 457
  types of, 457
"Split" in heart sounds, 117
Sprains, 424
  aftercare of, 709-710
  cervical, aftercare of, 707
Sputum specimen, 203
Squeeze, 590
SSKI; *see* Potassium iodide, supersaturated solution of
Staff
  attitudes of, as assessment barrier, 101
  call-in of, in disaster, 663-665
  float nurse, as assessment barrier, 98-99
  involvement of, 69-72
  lack of, as assessment barrier, 99
  selection of, and personnel conflicts, 86
  as support in crisis, 27-30
Staff call roster for disaster, 664
Standstill, ventricular, 181
Staphylococcus aureus, 234, 328
State planning for disaster, 647-650
Status asthmaticus, 379
Status epilepticus, 303-305
Status survey, emergency department, 53-55
Sternum, fracture of, 352
Steroids; *see also* specific drug
  and adult respiratory disease syndrome, 382
  and burns, 606
  and heat stroke, 587
  and hypovolemic shock, 247
  and laryngeal obstruction, 508
  and near drowning, 382
  and pulmonary contusion, 359
  and septic shock, 244
  and smoke inhalation, 381
  and spinal cord injuries, 309
  and status asthmaticus, 379
  and sunburn, 616
Stethoscope, 109
Stimulation, painful, 123
Stokes-Adams syndrome, 173
Stool specimen, 202-203
Stoxil; *see* Idoxuridine
Strabismus, 332
Strains, 423-424
Street burns, 616
Streptococcus, 234
Stress, 23-24
  as factor in obstetrical and gynecological emergencies, 491-493
Strip recorder, 389
Stroke, 287
  heat, 582-588
Subpoena duces tecum, 47
Subpoenas, 48-49

Sucking chest wound, 356
Sudden infant death syndrome, 514-515
Suicide, 534-536
Sulamyd; *see* Sulfacetamide
Sulfacetamide, 335
Sulfamylon; *see* Mafenide and burns
Sulfisoxazole, 335
Sunburn, 616
Supplies, emergency department, for disaster, 674-675
Support, figure eight, 428-429
Support/perspective of leaders, 82
Surgery, cranial, 299
Survey
  general, 128
    in assessment, 106
  primary, 128-129
    in assessment, 105-106
Susphrine; *see* Epinephrine
Suture
  absorbable, 230
  buried, 232
  continuous, 232
  horizontal mattress, 231
    half-buried, 231
  nonabsorbable, 230
  removal of, 230
  simple interrupted, 231
  subcuticular, 232
  vertical mattress, 231
Swimmer's ear, 340
Symptoms versus diseases, 56
Syncope, 306
  heat, 581
Syndromes
  acute organic brain, 548-549
  Brown-Sequard, 311, 314
  central, 272
  heat; *see* Heat syndromes
  hyperpnea exhaustion, 590
  Korsakoff, 539, 541, 542
  lateral, 272
  Mallory-Weiss, 408
  postconcussion, 297
  sudden infant death, 514-515
  third space, 564
  Wernicke, 539, 541, 542
Synocinon; *see* Oxytocin
Syringe technique, 199-200

T

TABS for resuscitation of newborn, 485
Tachycardia
  junctional, 169
  nodal, 169
  paroxysmal atrial, 163
  sinus, 158
  ventricular, 178
Tamponade, cardiac, 360-362, 372
  paradoxical pulse in, 372
Tapazole; *see* Methimazole

Taping procedures for IV devices, 206-207
Tar burns, 615
Tarsal, fracture of, 445, 446
Task outline, 55, 58
Team, management of, 83-84
Teamwork, 85-88
  groundwork of, 86
  roles in, 86
  semantics in, 86-87
Teeth
  avulsed, 346-347
  chipped or broken, 346
Temperature conversions, 705
Temperature in patient assessment, 119
Tendon, 419
  Achilles, ruptured, 424
Tensilon; see Edrophonium chloride
Terra-Cortril; see Terramycin/oxytetracycline/hydrocorti-
    sone
Terramycin/oxytetracycline/hydrocortisone, 336
Testicular torsion, 467
Tetanus, 233
  information on, 710
  prophylaxis for, 233-234
    and burns, 606, 613
    and frostbite, 578
    immunization series for, 233-234
    for injuries, 234
    and lightning injuries, 578
    in multiple trauma, 268
    and snakebite, 571
Tetracaine, 335
  and wounds, 230
Tetracycline, 335
Tetrahydrocannabinol, 544
Tham; see Tromethamine
THC; see Tetrahydrocannabinol
Theophylline ethylenediamine; see Aminophylline
Therapy, intravenous fluid; see Fluid therapy, intravenous
Thiamine
  and alcohol abuse, 552-553
  and delirium tremens, 553
Thiotic acid and mushroom poisoning, 628
Third space syndrome, 564
Thomas splint, 439
Thompson's sign, 424
Thoracotomy, open, 188-189
Thorazine; see Chlorpromazine
Threatened abortion, 474
Throat emergencies, 337-340
  airway obstruction as, 338
  caustic ingestion as, 337
  foreign bodies as, 337
  neck trauma as, 338-340
Throat and sputum specimen, 203
Thyroid crises, 561-562
Thyroid storm, 561-562
Thyrotoxic crisis, 561-562
Tibia, fracture of, 443, 444
Tic douloureux, 345-346

Ticks, 573-574
TIDES mnemonic, 344
Tilt test, 121
Tissue, soft, injuries of; see soft tissue injuries
Todd's paralysis, 304
Toe
  dislocation of, 455-456
  fracture of, 446, 447
Tonic gaze, 274
Tonometer, Schiøtz, 334-336
Toothache, 346
Torsion, testicular, 467
Tort, 36-37
Torticollic crisis, 547, 625
Tortipelvic crisis, 547, 625
Tourniquets, rotating, for pulmonary edema, 369, 370
Toxic conditions, 529
Toxic reactions, 539-548
  alcohol-related, 539-542
  drug-related, 542-548
Toxic screen, 127
Toxins, food, 629-631
Tracheobronchial tree injuries, 359
Tracheostomy, 149-150
Tracheotomy, needle, 149
Traction, cervical, with tongs, 315
Training for disaster, 675-676
Transfer incubator, 486
Transport in disaster, 658-660
Transverse fracture, 425
Trauma
  abdominal, 415-418
  of bladder and urethra, 463, 465
  to genital organs, 482-483
  multiple, assessment of
    in emergency department, 266-268
      history as, 267
      intervention in, 267-268
      physical examination as, 267
      radiological and laboratory evaluation as, 267
    in prehospital setting, 263-266
      of airway, 263-264
      algorithm for, 269
      of breathing, 264
      of cervical spine, 264
      of chest, 264
      of circulation, 264
      of fractures, 266
      of hypovolemia, 264-266
  renal, 463, 464
  sexual, 483
Traction splints, 457
Triage, 90-95; see also Disaster
  activity flow in, 657
  administrative needs in, 91, 92
  casualty distribution log for, 659
  of children, 499-500
  civilian, 653-654
  considerations in, 91-92
  definition of, 90

Triage—cont'd
evaluation of chief complaint in, 92-93
PQRST technique for, 92
SOAP technique for, 92-93
examples of, 93-95
classifications of, 94-95
field, in disaster, 653-658
function of, 665-669
location of, 665-669
mass casualty, 656
medical needs in, 91, 92
military, 653, 654
paperwork in, 670-671
personnel required for, 669-670
problem-oriented medical records in, 92-93
rating systems for, 655
simple, 655-656
spatial needs in, 91, 92
supplies for, 671-672
temporal needs in, 91, 92
Triage nurse, 90-92
qualifications and requirements of, 91
Triage officer, 669
disaster action card for, 670
Triage tag, 658, 671
Trichomonas vaginalis, 482
Trigeminy, ventricular, 177
Trihexyphenidyl, 625
and phenothiazines, 547
Trimethaphan, 306, 738
and hypertensive crisis, 305
Tromethamine, 625
Tropicamide, 335
Trumpet tube, 143
Tubes
chest, 357-359
for drawing blood, 126
nasogastric, insertion of, 409-410
Sengstaken-Blakemore, 410-411
trumpet, 143

U

Ulcer
acute gastric, radiation of pain in, 400
duodenal, radiation of pain in, 401
Ulna, fracture of, 433-434
Ultraviolet radiation burns of eye, 327
Unconscious patient, 277-283
causes of brain dysfunction in, 278
initial approach to, 278-281
management of, 281-283
cranial nerve testing in, 283
diagnostic tests in, 283
Urea, 322
Ureter, trauma to, 465
Ureteral calculus, radiation of pain in, 401
Urethra
rupture of, 465
trauma to, 463, 465
Urgency as coping mechanism, 25

Urgent (Class II) patient, 90, 95
Urinalysis in assessment, 127
Urinary retention, acute, 467-468
Urinary tap, suprapubic, in children, 511-512
Urinary tract calculi, 468-469
Urine
normal laboratory values for, 700-703
specimen of, 202
Uterus, fibroid tumors of, 473-474
Uveitis, 330

V

V tach; *see* Ventricular tachycardia
Vaccine, duck embryo, 235
Vacuum tube system, 196-199
Vagina, laceration of, 491
Vaginal bleeding; *see* Bleeding, vaginal
Valium; *see* Diazepam
Vaponefrin; *see* Epinephrine, racemic, and
croup
Vasodilators, 251
and cardiogenic shock, 251
and septic shock, 244
Venesection, 209-211, 212
Venipuncture, sites for, 196
Venom, snake, 567-568
Ventilation
in shock management, 252-253
transtracheal catheter, 148-149
Ventricular bigeminy, 177
Ventricular fibrillation, 179
Ventricular tachycardia, 178
Ventricular trigeminy, 177
Venturi mask, 151, 152, 153
Verbal communication, 30
Vertigo, 340
Vessel, great, injuries to, 362-363
Vial-of-Life, 108
Vidarabine, 336
Violence as psychiatric emergency, 531-532
Vira-A; *see* Vidarabine
Visine, 336
Vistaril; *see* Hydroxyzine pamoate
Visual acuity examination, 319-320
Vital signs, assessment of, 118-125, 129
blood pressure as, 121-122
level of consciousness as, 122-123
orthostatic, 121
pediatric, 503
postural, 255
pulse as, 119-120
respirations as, 120-121
of skin, 123-125
color changes in, 124
temperature as, 119
Vitamins
B, 562
B complex, 553
B$_{12}$, 259
C, 562

Vitamins—cont'd
  K
    and disseminating intravascular coagulation, 259
    and salicylate poisoning, 625
Volkmann's ischemic contracture, 433
Volume, tidal, estimation of, 120
Volume imbalance as assessment barrier, 99
Volvulus, 413
Vomiting
  aftercare for, 226-227
  in children, 510
  and poisoning, 619
VPB; *see* Premature ventricular contractions
Vulva, hematoma of, 491

W

Wandering atrial pacemaker, 162
Water, purifying, 677
Weight equivalencies, 705
Weights, table of estimated, 499
Well child in emergency department, 514
Wenckebach phenomenon, 171
Wernicke syndrome, 539, 541, 542
Whiplash injury, 316
White blood count and differential, 128
Willful neglect, 41, 42
Wounds; *see also* Soft tissue injuries
  abrasion as, 229
  abscess as, 230
  aftercare of, 710
  avulsion, 229
  burn, care of, 609-613

Wounds—cont'd
  contusion as, 229
  gunshot, 233, 423
  healing of, 228
  laceration as, 229-230
  management of, 228-233
    anesthesia for, 230
    general, 228-229
    infection in, 229
    penetrating, 230-233
      gunshot wounds as, 233, 423
      high-pressure grease/paint gun injuries as, 233, 423
  puncture, 230, 422
  snakebite, care of, 571
  suturing in, 230, 232-232
Wringer injuries, 422-423
Wrist
  dislocation of, 451
  fracture of, 434-435

X

Xenografts, 613
Xylocaine; *see* Lidocaine

Y

Y-board, 496

Z

Zinc levels in blood, 201
Zipper injuries, 466
Zygomatic fracture, 343-344